Bioequivalence and Statistics in Clinical Pharmacology

Second Edition

Chapman & Hall/CRC Biostatistics Series

Published Titles

Adaptive Design Methods in Clinical Trials, Second Edition
Shein-Chung Chow and Mark Chang

Adaptive Designs for Sequential Treatment Allocation
Alessandro Baldi Antognini and Alessandra Giovagnoli

Adaptive Design Theory and Implementation Using SAS and R, Second Edition
Mark Chang

Advanced Bayesian Methods for Medical Test Accuracy
Lyle D. Broemeling

Applied Biclustering Methods for Big and High-Dimensional Data Using R
Adetayo Kasim, Ziv Shkedy, Sebastian Kaiser, Sepp Hochreiter, and Willem Talloen

Applied Meta-Analysis with R
Ding-Geng (Din) Chen and Karl E. Peace

Basic Statistics and Pharmaceutical Statistical Applications, Second Edition
James E. De Muth

Bayesian Adaptive Methods for Clinical Trials
Scott M. Berry, Bradley P. Carlin, J. Jack Lee, and Peter Muller

Bayesian Analysis Made Simple: An Excel GUI for WinBUGS
Phil Woodward

Bayesian Designs for Phase I–II Clinical Trials
Ying Yuan, Hoang Q. Nguyen, and Peter F. Thall

Bayesian Methods for Measures of Agreement
Lyle D. Broemeling

Bayesian Methods for Repeated Measures
Lyle D. Broemeling

Bayesian Methods in Epidemiology
Lyle D. Broemeling

Bayesian Methods in Health Economics
Gianluca Baio

Bayesian Missing Data Problems: EM, Data Augmentation and Noniterative Computation
Ming T. Tan, Guo-Liang Tian, and Kai Wang Ng

Bayesian Modeling in Bioinformatics
Dipak K. Dey, Samiran Ghosh, and Bani K. Mallick

Benefit-Risk Assessment in Pharmaceutical Research and Development
Andreas Sashegyi, James Felli, and Rebecca Noel

Published Titles

Benefit-Risk Assessment Methods in Medical Product Development: Bridging Qualitative and Quantitative Assessments
Qi Jiang and Weili He

Bioequivalence and Statistics in Clinical Pharmacology, Second Edition
Scott Patterson and Byron Jones

Biosimilars: Design and Analysis of Follow-on Biologics
Shein-Chung Chow

Biostatistics: A Computing Approach
Stewart J. Anderson

Cancer Clinical Trials: Current and Controversial Issues in Design and Analysis
Stephen L. George, Xiaofei Wang, and Herbert Pang

Causal Analysis in Biomedicine and Epidemiology: Based on Minimal Sufficient Causation
Mikel Aickin

Clinical and Statistical Considerations in Personalized Medicine
Claudio Carini, Sandeep Menon, and Mark Chang

Clinical Trial Data Analysis using R
Ding-Geng (Din) Chen and Karl E. Peace

Clinical Trial Methodology
Karl E. Peace and Ding-Geng (Din) Chen

Computational Methods in Biomedical Research
Ravindra Khattree and Dayanand N. Naik

Computational Pharmacokinetics
Anders Källén

Confidence Intervals for Proportions and Related Measures of Effect Size
Robert G. Newcombe

Controversial Statistical Issues in Clinical Trials
Shein-Chung Chow

Data Analysis with Competing Risks and Intermediate States
Ronald B. Geskus

Data and Safety Monitoring Committees in Clinical Trials
Jay Herson

Design and Analysis of Animal Studies in Pharmaceutical Development
Shein-Chung Chow and Jen-pei Liu

Design and Analysis of Bioavailability and Bioequivalence Studies, Third Edition
Shein-Chung Chow and Jen-pei Liu

Design and Analysis of Bridging Studies
Jen-pei Liu, Shein-Chung Chow, and Chin-Fu Hsiao

Design & Analysis of Clinical Trials for Economic Evaluation & Reimbursement: An Applied Approach Using SAS & STATA
Iftekhar Khan

Design and Analysis of Clinical Trials for Predictive Medicine
Shigeyuki Matsui, Marc Buyse, and Richard Simon

Design and Analysis of Clinical Trials with Time-to-Event Endpoints
Karl E. Peace

Design and Analysis of Non-Inferiority Trials
Mark D. Rothmann, Brian L. Wiens, and Ivan S. F. Chan

Difference Equations with Public Health Applications
Lemuel A. Moyé and Asha Seth Kapadia

DNA Methylation Microarrays: Experimental Design and Statistical Analysis
Sun-Chong Wang and Arturas Petronis

DNA Microarrays and Related Genomics Techniques: Design, Analysis, and Interpretation of Experiments
David B. Allison, Grier P. Page, T. Mark Beasley, and Jode W. Edwards

Dose Finding by the Continual Reassessment Method
Ying Kuen Cheung

Dynamical Biostatistical Models
Daniel Commenges and Hélène Jacqmin-Gadda

Elementary Bayesian Biostatistics
Lemuel A. Moyé

Empirical Likelihood Method in Survival Analysis
Mai Zhou

Published Titles

Essentials of a Successful Biostatistical Collaboration
Arul Earnest

Exposure–Response Modeling: Methods and Practical Implementation
Jixian Wang

Frailty Models in Survival Analysis
Andreas Wienke

Fundamental Concepts for New Clinical Trialists
Scott Evans and Naitee Ting

Generalized Linear Models: A Bayesian Perspective
Dipak K. Dey, Sujit K. Ghosh, and Bani K. Mallick

Handbook of Regression and Modeling: Applications for the Clinical and Pharmaceutical Industries
Daryl S. Paulson

Inference Principles for Biostatisticians
Ian C. Marschner

Interval-Censored Time-to-Event Data: Methods and Applications
Ding-Geng (Din) Chen, Jianguo Sun, and Karl E. Peace

Introductory Adaptive Trial Designs: A Practical Guide with R
Mark Chang

Joint Models for Longitudinal and Time-to-Event Data: With Applications in R
Dimitris Rizopoulos

Measures of Interobserver Agreement and Reliability, Second Edition
Mohamed M. Shoukri

Medical Biostatistics, Third Edition
A. Indrayan

Meta-Analysis in Medicine and Health Policy
Dalene Stangl and Donald A. Berry

Mixed Effects Models for the Population Approach: Models, Tasks, Methods and Tools
Marc Lavielle

Modeling to Inform Infectious Disease Control
Niels G. Becker

Modern Adaptive Randomized Clinical Trials: Statistical and Practical Aspects
Oleksandr Sverdlov

Monte Carlo Simulation for the Pharmaceutical Industry: Concepts, Algorithms, and Case Studies
Mark Chang

Multiregional Clinical Trials for Simultaneous Global New Drug Development
Joshua Chen and Hui Quan

Multiple Testing Problems in Pharmaceutical Statistics
Alex Dmitrienko, Ajit C. Tamhane, and Frank Bretz

Noninferiority Testing in Clinical Trials: Issues and Challenges
Tie-Hua Ng

Optimal Design for Nonlinear Response Models
Valerii V. Fedorov and Sergei L. Leonov

Patient-Reported Outcomes: Measurement, Implementation and Interpretation
Joseph C. Cappelleri, Kelly H. Zou, Andrew G. Bushmakin, Jose Ma. J. Alvir, Demissie Alemayehu, and Tara Symonds

Quantitative Evaluation of Safety in Drug Development: Design, Analysis and Reporting
Qi Jiang and H. Amy Xia

Quantitative Methods for Traditional Chinese Medicine Development
Shein-Chung Chow

Randomized Clinical Trials of Nonpharmacological Treatments
Isabelle Boutron, Philippe Ravaud, and David Moher

Randomized Phase II Cancer Clinical Trials
Sin-Ho Jung

Sample Size Calculations for Clustered and Longitudinal Outcomes in Clinical Research
Chul Ahn, Moonseong Heo, and Song Zhang

Published Titles

Sample Size Calculations in Clinical Research, Second Edition
Shein-Chung Chow, Jun Shao, and Hansheng Wang

Statistical Analysis of Human Growth and Development
Yin Bun Cheung

Statistical Design and Analysis of Clinical Trials: Principles and Methods
Weichung Joe Shih and Joseph Aisner

Statistical Design and Analysis of Stability Studies
Shein-Chung Chow

Statistical Evaluation of Diagnostic Performance: Topics in ROC Analysis
Kelly H. Zou, Aiyi Liu, Andriy Bandos, Lucila Ohno-Machado, and Howard Rockette

Statistical Methods for Clinical Trials
Mark X. Norleans

Statistical Methods for Drug Safety
Robert D. Gibbons and Anup K. Amatya

Statistical Methods for Healthcare Performance Monitoring
Alex Bottle and Paul Aylin

Statistical Methods for Immunogenicity Assessment
Harry Yang, Jianchun Zhang, Binbing Yu, and Wei Zhao

Statistical Methods in Drug Combination Studies
Wei Zhao and Harry Yang

Statistical Testing Strategies in the Health Sciences
Albert Vexler, Alan D. Hutson, and Xiwei Chen

Statistics in Drug Research: Methodologies and Recent Developments
Shein-Chung Chow and Jun Shao

Statistics in the Pharmaceutical Industry, Third Edition
Ralph Buncher and Jia-Yeong Tsay

Survival Analysis in Medicine and Genetics
Jialiang Li and Shuangge Ma

Theory of Drug Development
Eric B. Holmgren

Translational Medicine: Strategies and Statistical Methods
Dennis Cosmatos and Shein-Chung Chow

Chapman & Hall/CRC Biostatistics Series

Bioequivalence and Statistics in Clinical Pharmacology

Second Edition

Scott Patterson

Pfizer Vaccines Clinical Research & Development

Collegeville, Pennsylvania

Byron Jones

Novartis Pharma AG

Basel, Switzerland

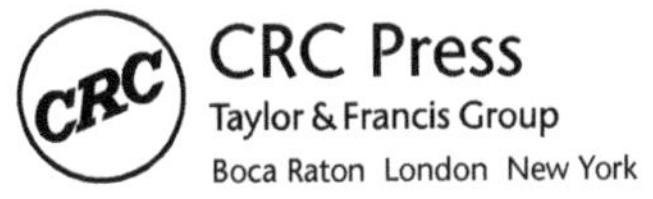

CRC Press is an imprint of the
Taylor & Francis Group, an **informa** business
A CHAPMAN & HALL BOOK

CRC Press
Taylor & Francis Group
6000 Broken Sound Parkway NW, Suite 300
Boca Raton, FL 33487-2742

First issued in paperback 2020

ISBN-13: 978-1-4665-8520-1 (hbk)
ISBN-13: 978-0-367-78244-3 (pbk)

Visit the Taylor & Francis Web site at
http://www.taylorandfrancis.com

and the CRC Press Web site at
http://www.crcpress.com

This book is for

– my dearest Karen, who has given me the most precious gift in life, and our children Daniel, Mary Grace, Michael, Joseph, Robert, Thomas, and Little Bit, who have given us even more. (SDP)

– my wife Hilary, for her love, support and encouragement. (BJ)

Contents

List of Figures xv

List of Tables xvii

Preface to the Second Edition xxiii

I Bioequivalence and Biopharmaceutical Development 1

1 Drug Development and Clinical Pharmacology 3
1.1 Aims of this Book 4
1.2 Biopharmaceutical Development 5
1.3 Clinical Pharmacology 7
1.4 Statistics in Clinical Pharmacology 11
1.5 Structure of Book 14

2 History and Regulation of Bioequivalence 15
2.1 When and How BE Studies Are Performed 16
2.2 Why Are BE Studies Performed? 22
2.3 Deciding When Formulations Are Bioequivalent 22
2.4 Potential Issues with TOST Bioequivalence 25
2.5 Current International Regulation 28
2.6 Some Practical Notes 29

3 Testing for Average Bioequivalence 31
3.1 Background 31
3.2 Linear Model for 2×2 Data 35
3.3 Applying the TOST Procedure 39
3.4 Carry-Over, Sequence, and Interaction Effects 42
3.5 Checking Assumptions Made about the Linear Model 45
3.6 Power and Sample Size for ABE in the 2×2 Design 46
3.7 Example in Which Test and Reference Are Not ABE 49
3.8 Nonparametric Analysis 56

4 BE Studies with More Than Two Periods 63
4.1 Background 64
4.2 Three-Period Designs 64
4.2.1 Examples of Analysis of BE Trials with Three Periods 66
4.3 Within-Subject Variability 71
4.4 Robust Analyses for Three-Period Designs 72
4.5 Four-Period Designs 73
4.5.1 Choice of Design 73
4.5.2 Examples of Data Analysis for Four-Period Designs 74
4.6 Designs with More Than Two Treatments 79

4.7 Adjusting for Multiple Testing . . . 86
4.8 Nonparametric Analyses of Tmax . . . 88
4.8.1 Three Treatments . . . 88
4.8.1.1 Single Stratum . . . 90
4.8.1.2 Multiple Strata . . . 95
4.8.2 Four Treatments . . . 96
4.9 Technical Appendix: Efficiency . . . 97
4.9.1 Theory and Illustration . . . 97
4.9.2 Comparison of Three Alternative Designs for Three Periods . . . 99
4.10 Tables of Data . . . 99

II Special Topics in Bioequivalence **111**

5 Dealing with Special BE Challenges **113**
5.1 Restricted Maximum Likelihood Modelling . . . 114
5.2 Failing BE and the DER Assessment . . . 117
5.3 Simulation . . . 121
5.4 Data-Based Simulation . . . 122
5.5 Carry-Over . . . 124
5.6 Optional Designs . . . 129
5.7 Determining Trial Size . . . 133
5.8 What Outliers Are and How to Handle Their Data . . . 137
5.9 Bayesian BE Assessment . . . 138

6 Adaptive Bioequivalence Trials **141**
6.1 Background . . . 141
6.2 Two-Stage Design for Testing for ABE . . . 142
6.3 TOST Using the Standard Combination Test . . . 144
6.4 Example of Using the Standard Combination Test . . . 145
6.5 Maximum Combination Test . . . 148
6.6 Using the Maximum Combination Test . . . 149
6.7 Conditional Errors and Conditional Power . . . 151
6.8 Algorithm for Sample Size Re-Estimation . . . 152
6.9 Operating Characteristics . . . 155
6.10 Conclusions . . . 167
6.11 Technical Appendix: R code . . . 167
6.11.1 Power and sample size for single-stage design . . . 167
6.11.2 Critical values for standard combination test . . . 169
6.11.3 Simulation of data for first stage and application of TOST at interim . . . 171
6.11.4 Application of TOST at interim . . . 171
6.11.5 Decision at interim and sample size re-estimation . . . 173
6.11.6 Simulation of data for second stage . . . 174
6.11.7 Estimation and TOST for second stage . . . 176
6.11.8 Application of the standard combination test . . . 177
6.11.9 Critical values for maximum combination test . . . 178
6.11.10 Sample size re-estimation using the maximum combination test . . 179
6.11.11 Power of first stage using the maximum combination test . . . 180
6.11.12 Simulation of data for second stage when maximum combination test is used . . . 180

6.11.13 Estimation and TOST for second stage when maximum combination test is used . . . 181
6.11.14 Apply maximum combination test . . . 182
6.11.15 Conditional errors for second stage . . . 183
6.11.16 Power of second stage using conditional errors . . . 184
6.11.17 Conditional power at interim . . . 185
6.11.18 Conditional errors for maximum combination test . . . 185
6.11.19 Sample size for maximum combination test using conditional errors . . . 186

7 Scaled Average Bioequivalence Testing **189**
7.1 Background . . . 190
7.2 Scaled Average Bioequivalence in Europe . . . 193
7.3 Scaled Average Bioequivalence in the USA . . . 198
7.4 Discussion and Cautions . . . 201

III Clinical Pharmacology **203**

8 Clinical Pharmacology Safety Studies **205**
8.1 Background . . . 206
8.2 First-Time-in-Humans . . . 208
8.3 Sub-Chronic Dosing Studies . . . 219
8.4 Food Effect Assessment and Drug-Drug Interactions (DDIs) . . . 229
8.5 Dose Proportionality . . . 238
8.6 Technical Appendix . . . 242

9 QTc **245**
9.1 Background . . . 246
9.2 Modelling of QTc Data . . . 248
9.3 Interpreting QTc Modelling Findings . . . 250
9.4 Design of a Thorough QTc Study in the Future . . . 254

10 Clinical Pharmacology Efficacy Studies **257**
10.1 Background . . . 258
10.2 Sub-Chronic Dosing . . . 261
10.3 Phase IIa and the Proof of Concept . . . 268

11 Population Pharmacokinetics **279**
11.1 Population and Pharmacokinetics . . . 279
11.2 Absolute and Relative Bioavailability . . . 285
11.3 Age and Gender Pharmacokinetic Studies . . . 287
11.4 Ethnicity . . . 291
11.5 Liver Disease . . . 295
11.6 Kidney Disease . . . 298
11.7 Technical Appendix . . . 302

IV Vaccines and Epilogue **305**

12 Vaccine Trials **307**
12.1 Brief Introduction to Vaccine Research and Development 308
12.2 Phase I Vaccine Studies 311
12.3 Proof-of-Concept and Phase II 316
12.4 Lot Consistency 319
12.5 Concomitant Vaccination 327
12.6 Cross-Over Trials in Vaccines 331

13 Epilogue **339**

V Bibliography **341**

Index **431**

List of Figures

1.1 Critical Path in Drug Development 6
1.2 Plasma Concentration (ng/mL) versus Time (h) 8

2.1 Normal Distribution (Mean = 1, SD = 1) 19
2.2 Log-Normal Distribution 21
2.3 Normal Distribution Arising from Log-Transformation for AUC Data of Figure 2.2 21

3.1 Example 3.1: Subject Profiles Plot 33
3.2 Examples of Patterns in a Paired-Agreement Plot 34
3.3 Example 3.1: Paired-Agreement Plots 35
3.4 Example 3.1: Mean Differences versus Totals Plot 38
3.5 Example 3.1: Fitted Normal Densities for $\hat{\mu}_T - \hat{\mu}_R$ 41
3.6 Example 3.1: 90% Confidence Intervals for $\exp(\hat{\mu}_T - \hat{\mu}_R)$ 42
3.7 Groups-by-Periods Plot 43
3.8 Example 3.1: Groups-by-Periods Plot 45
3.9 Example 3.1: Normal Probability Plots 46
3.10 Example 3.2: Subject Profiles Plot 52
3.11 Example 3.2: Paired-Agreement Plots 52
3.12 Example 3.2: Groups-by-Periods Plot 54
3.13 Example 3.2: Mean Differences versus Totals Plot 54
3.14 Example 3.2: Fitted Normal Densities for $\hat{\mu}_T - \hat{\mu}_R$ 55
3.15 Example 3.2: Normal Probability Plots 56
3.16 Example 3.1: Studentized Residuals for Tmax 60

4.1 Example 4.1: Subject Profiles Plot 66
4.2 Example 4.1: Groups-by-Periods Plot 67
4.3 Example 4.1: Subject Contrasts versus Means Plot 69
4.4 Example 4.2: Subject Profiles Plot 69
4.5 Example 4.2: Groups-by-Periods Plot 70
4.6 Example 4.2: Subject Contrasts versus Means Plot 71
4.7 Example 4.3: Subject Profiles Plot 74
4.8 Example 4.3: Groups-by-Periods Plot 75
4.9 Example 4.3: Subject Contrasts versus Means Plot 76
4.10 Example 4.4: Subject Profiles Plot 77
4.11 Example 4.4: Groups-by-Periods Plot 78
4.12 Example 4.4: Subject Contrasts versus Means Plot 79
4.13 Example 4.5: Subject Profiles Plot: Sequences 1 and 2 80
4.14 Example 4.5: Subject Profiles Plot: Sequences 3 and 4 80
4.15 Example 4.5: Subject Profiles Plot: Sequences 5 and 6 81
4.16 Example 4.5: Groups-by-Periods Plot 82
4.17 Example 4.6: Subject Profiles Plot: Sequences 1 and 2 83

4.18 Example 4.6: Subject Profiles Plot: Sequences 3 and 4 84
4.19 Example 4.6: Groups-by-Periods Plot 85
4.20 Example 4.5: Histograms of Bootstrap Distribution of Estimates 96

5.1 A Potentially Bioinequivalent Test and Reference Product: Fitted Normal Densities for $\hat{\mu}_T - \hat{\mu}_R$ 118

6.1 Planning and Analysis of First Stage 153
6.2 Decisions Made at the End of the First Stage 154
6.3 Sample Size Re-Estimation 154
6.4 Analysis at End of Trial 154
6.5 Flow Diagram for the Method of Maurer et al. 156
6.6 Flow Diagram for Method B of Potvin et al. 156
6.7 Simulation-Based Power Estimates for Method B when True Ratio = 0.95 158
6.8 Simulation-Based Power Estimates for Maximum Combination Test ($w = 0.5, w^* = 0.25$) when True Ratio = 0.95 160
6.9 Simulation-Based Type I Error Rate Estimates for Maximum Combination Test ($w = 0.5, w^* = 0.25$) when True Ratio = 0.80 and Futility Rule Applied 163
6.10 Simulation-Based Power Estimates for Maximum Combination Test ($w = 0.5, w^* = 0.25$) when True Ratio = 0.95 and Futility Rule Applied 165

8.1 Estimated logDose versus logAUC Curve with Individual Data Points from Example 8.2.1 213
8.2 Estimated Dose versus AUC Curve (90% CI) with Individual Data Points from Example 8.2.2 216
8.3 Estimated Proportion of DLTs versus logDose from Example 8.2.3 218
8.4 Estimated Concentration versus Time (h) Profile from Phase I Concentration Data in `conc.sas7bdat` 225
8.5 Dose-to-Exposure (AUC or Cmax) Relationship for β from 0.8 to 1.2 . . . 239

9.1 A Typical 12-Lead ECG Interval 246
9.2 Mild and Moderate QTc Prolongation ($n = 41$) in Example 9.1 249

11.1 Estimated AUCs versus Dose from a Simulated Population Pharmacokinetic Study 284
11.2 Boxplot of Estimated Clearance versus Dose from a Simulated Population Pharmacokinetic Study 285

12.1 Model Estimates for Proportion of Events (Fevers) versus Dose in a Phase I Study 315
12.2 Mean ln-Transformed Titer Data by Vaccine Sequence versus Time Matrix Plot for Antibody Types 1–6 for Periods 1 and 2, prior to and 1 Month following Vaccination 333

List of Tables

1.1 Selected Regulatory Authorities . . . 5
1.2 Potential Errors When Interpreting Bioequivalence Data . . . 12

2.1 Schematic Plan of a 2 × 2 Cross-Over Study . . . 17
2.2 Example of a Random Allocation of Sequences to Subject in a 2 × 2 Cross-Over Design . . . 18

3.1 Example 3.1 . . . 32
3.2 Fixed Effects in the Linear Model for the 2 × 2 Design . . . 35
3.3 Fixed Effects: Alternative Parametrization for the 2 × 2 Design . . . 36
3.4 Random Effects in the Linear Model for the 2 × 2 Design . . . 36
3.5 Example 3.1: Groups-by-Periods Means . . . 38
3.6 Example 3.1: TOST Procedure Results . . . 40
3.7 Fixed Effects Model Including Interactions for a 2 × 2 Design . . . 43
3.8 Fixed Effects Model Including Interactions for a 2×2 Design: After Applying Constraints . . . 44
3.9 Fixed Effects Model Including Carry-Over Effects for a 2 × 2 Design . . . 44
3.10 Fixed Effects Model Including Carry-Over Effects for a 2 × 2 Design: After Applying Constraints . . . 44
3.11 Sample Sizes to Achieve Powers of 0.8 or 0.9 for Ratios of 0.9, 0.95, and 1.00 . . . 48
3.12 Power Values Corresponding to the Sample Sizes in Table 3.11 . . . 49
3.13 Example 3.2 . . . 50
3.14 Example 3.2: Groups-by-Periods Means . . . 53
3.15 Example 3.2: TOST Procedure Results . . . 55
3.16 Example 3.2: TOST Procedure Results (all subjects) . . . 56
3.17 Example 3.1: Tmax . . . 58
3.18 Example 3.1: TOST Procedure Results for Tmax . . . 60

4.1 Expectations of $\bar{y}_{ij.}$ for Design 1 . . . 65
4.2 Example 4.1: Group-by-Period Means . . . 67
4.3 Example 4.1: TOST Procedure Results . . . 68
4.4 Example 4.2: Group-by-Period Means . . . 70
4.5 Example 4.2: TOST Procedure Results . . . 70
4.6 Efficiencies of Designs 1 through 7 . . . 74
4.7 Example 4.3: Group-by-Period Means . . . 75
4.8 Example 4.3: TOST Procedure Results . . . 76
4.9 Example 4.4: Group-by-Period Means . . . 77
4.10 Example 4.4: TOST Procedure Results . . . 78
4.11 Example 4.5: Group-by-Period Means . . . 81
4.12 Example 4.5: TOST Procedure Results . . . 82
4.13 Example 4.6: Group-by-Period Means . . . 84

4.14 Example 4.6: TOST Procedure Results 85
4.15 Example 4.5: Tmax, Williams Design for Three Treatments 89
4.16 Example 4.5: Tmax, Williams Design for Three Treatments 89
4.17 Example 4.5: Tmax, Williams Design for Three Treatments 89
4.18 Williams Design for Three Treatments: Stratified for Comparing T and R 90
4.19 Williams Design for Three Treatments: Stratified for Comparing T and S . 90
4.20 Period Differences for Comparing T and R: Stratum I 93
4.21 Period Differences for Comparing T and R: Stratum II 93
4.22 Period Differences for Comparing T and R: Stratum III 94
4.23 Components of the Stratified Test for Comparing T and R 94
4.24 Efficiencies of Three Alternative Designs 99
4.25 Example 4.1: Sequence RTT 99
4.26 Example 4.1: Sequence TRR 101
4.27 Example 4.2: Sequence RTT 102
4.28 Example 4.2: Sequence TRR 103
4.29 Example 4.3: Replicate Design 104
4.30 Example 4.4: Replicate Design 105
4.31 Example 4.4: Replicate Design 105
4.32 Example 4.5: Williams Design for Three Treatments 106
4.33 Example 4.5: Williams Design for Three Treatments 107
4.34 Example 4.5: Williams Design for Three Treatments 108
4.35 Example 4.6: Williams Design for Four Treatments 108
4.36 Example 4.6: Williams Design for Four Treatments 109
4.37 Example 4.6: Williams Design for Four Treatments 109
4.38 Example 4.6: Williams Design for Four Treatments 109
4.39 Example 4.6: Tmax, Williams Design for Four Treatments 110

5.1 REML Results from PROC MIXED for Standard Bioequivalence Designs . 116
5.2 REML Results from PROC MIXED for Chapter 5 Examples of Replicate Designs 117
5.3 Number of Successful BE Trials 123
5.4 Example 5.1: AUC and Cmax Data from a Replicate Cross-Over Study Design with Test and Reference Formulations and Carry-Over (C) 125
5.5 Example 5.1: Adjusted Cmax and AUC Data for Subjects 1 and 10 128
5.6 Example: Variability Estimates for Use in Designing a Bioequivalence Study 136
5.7 Statistics for δ and σ_W^2 Inverse Probabilities Given AUC and Cmax Data Observed in Example 3.1 140

6.1 Schematic Plan of Two-Stage Design 143
6.2 Decisions at the End of the First Stage 143
6.3 Simulated Cmax Data for First Stage of a Two-Stage Design 146
6.4 Simulated Cmax Data for Second Stage of a Two-Stage Design 147
6.5 Simulated Cmax Data for Second Stage of a Two-Stage Design when Using Maximum Combination Test 150
6.6 Summary of Steps in Analysis of a Two-Stage Design, Using the Maximum Combination Test 155
6.7 Simulation-Based Estimates of Power for Method B When True Ratio = 0.95 158
6.8 Simulation-Based Estimates of Power for Algorithm that Uses the Maximum Combination Test 159
6.9 Average Total Sample Sizes for Method B When True Ratio = 0.95 161

6.10 Average Total Sample Sizes for Maximum Combination Test 161
6.11 Difference in Average Total Sample Sizes for the Two Methods When True Ratio = 0.95 161
6.12 Average Total Sample Sizes for Maximum Combination Test 162
6.13 Stopping Rates When the Maximum Combination Test Is Used and the Futility Rule is Applied after the First Stage When True Ratio = 0.80 . . 162
6.14 Average Total Sample Sizes for Maximum Combination Test 162
6.15 Stopping Rates When the Maximum Combination Test Is Used and the Futility Rule Is Applied after the First Stage When True Ratio = 0.95 . . 164
6.16 Average Total Sample Sizes for Maximum Combination Test 164
6.17 Average Total Sample Sizes for Maximum Combination Test 165
6.18 Simulation-Based Estimates of Power for Maximum Combination Test . . 166
6.19 Simulation-Based Estimates of Power for Algorithm That Uses the Maximum Combination Test 166
6.20 Average Total Sample Sizes for Maximum Combination Test 167

7.1 Sample Sizes for the European Scaled Average Bioequivalence Requirements in Three-Period Studies 197
7.2 Sample Sizes for the European Scaled Average Bioequivalence Requirements in Four-Period Studies 197
7.3 Sample Sizes for the Scaled Average Bioequivalence Requirements of the FDA in Three-Period Studies 200
7.4 Sample Sizes for the Scaled Average Bioequivalence Requirements of the FDA in Four-Period Studies 201

8.1 Schematic Plan of a First-Time-in-Humans Cross-Over Study 210
8.2 Example 8.2.1: AUC and Cmax Data from a Cross-Over First-Time-in-Humans Study Design 212
8.3 Parameter Estimates from Example 8.2.1 214
8.4 Example 8.2.2: AUC and Cmax Data from a Cross-Over First-Time-in-Humans Study Design 214
8.5 Parameter Estimates from Example 8.2.2 215
8.6 Example 8.2.3: Dose Limiting Toxicity Data from a First-Time-in-Humans Trial 216
8.7 Schematic Plan of a Sub-Chronic Dosing Cross-Over Study 220
8.8 Example 8.3.1: AUC and Cmax Data from a Sub-Chronic Dosing Cross-Over Study Design 221
8.9 Parameter Estimates from Example 8.3.1 223
8.10 Stationarity of Clearance Assessment from Example 8.3.1 223
8.11 Pharmacokinetic Concentration Data from Subject 47 of `conc.sas7bdat` following a Single Dose of 5 mg 224
8.12 Estimated PK Model Parameters from Phase I Concentration Data in `conc.sas7bdat` 226
8.13 ALT Data from Subject 4 of `liver.sas7bdat` 227
8.14 Estimated ALT Data (based on `liver.sas7bdat`) from the Sub-Chronic Dosing Study Design 228
8.15 Example 8.4.1: AUC and Cmax Data from a 2×2 Food Effect Cross-Over Study Design 231
8.16 Example 8.4.2: AUC and Cmax Data from a 2×2 Drug Interaction Cross-Over Study Design for Metabolic Inhibition 233

8.17 Example 8.4.3: AUC and Cmax Data from a Drug Interaction Cross-Over Study Design for Metabolic Induction 235
8.18 Example 8.5.1: AUC and Cmax Data from a Randomized Dose Proportionality Cross-Over Study 240
8.19 Exposure Estimates from a Preclinical Species 242
8.20 Exposure Estimates for a 50 kg Human from a Preclinical Species 242

9.1 First Subject's Data in Example 9.1 248
9.2 Mean Changes (90% CI) between Regimens Following a Single Dose in Example 9.1 ($n = 41$) 250
9.3 Mean Changes (90% CI) between Test Drug and Positive Control Following a Single Dose in Example 9.1 ($n = 41$) 255

10.1 Example 10.2.1: Pharmacodynamic Biomarker Data from an Exploratory Sub-Chronic Dosing Study 262
10.2 Example 10.2.2: Dose, Pharmacokinetic, and Low Density Lipoprotein Data from a Sub-Chronic Dosing Study 264
10.3 LDL Dose-Response (Ratio Relative to Baseline LDL) with 95% Confidence Intervals in Sub-Chronic Dosing Study Example 10.2.2 267
10.4 Example 10.3.1: Low-Density Lipoprotein Data from a Proof-of-Concept Study 269
10.5 LDL Effect Size (Ratio Relative to Baseline LDL) from a Bayesian Statistical Analysis of a Proof-of-Concept Study Example 10.3.1 ($n = 8$) 270
10.6 Example 10.3.2: QTc Data from One Subject in a Proof-of-Concept Study 271
10.7 Example 10.3.2: Plasma Pharmacokinetic-Pharmacodynamic Data from One Subject in a Proof-of-Concept Study . . 272
10.8 QTc Response on Placebo on Days 1 and 8 in a Proof-of-Concept Study from Modelling of Dose-QTc Data in Example 10.3.2 274

11.1 Estimated AUC Parameters from `conc.sas7bdat` 282
11.2 Selected Sparse Concentration Data from Patient Studies 283
11.3 Estimated Population PK Parameters from Sparse Population Data 283
11.4 Selected Estimates for AUC from Sparse Concentration Data Obtained in Patient Studies 284
11.5 Dose-Normalized (DN) AUC from an Absolute Bioavailability Cross-Over Trial 287
11.6 AUC and Cmax Data from a Pediatric (PED) and Adult (ADT) Bioavailability Trial 288
11.7 AUC and Cmax Data from a Gender Bioavailability Trial 289
11.8 Mean AUC Findings from a Gender Bioavailability Trial 291
11.9 AUC and Cmax Data from a Population Pharmacokinetic Assessment of South Korean and Western Subjects 293
11.10 Estimated Population Parameters from Evaluation of logAUC as a Function of Ethnicity, logDose, and Weight 295
11.11 Pharmacokinetic Data from a Clinical Pharmacology Hepatic Impairment Trial 296
11.12 Estimated Population Parameters from Evaluation of logAUC as a Function of Group 298
11.13 Pharmacokinetic Data from a Clinical Pharmacology Renal Impairment Trial 300

11.14 Estimated Population Parameters from Evaluation of logAUC as a function of Creatinine Clearance 302

12.1 Schematic Plan of a Phase I Study 312
12.2 Number of Fevers Observed in Each Dose Group in a Phase I Study 313
12.3 Findings from a Phase I Study 314
12.4 Strain 1 Pre-vaccination and Post-vaccination Geometric Mean Titres (GMT) from Proof-of-Concept Vaccine Trial 317
12.5 Schematic Plan of a Concomitant Vaccination Study 329
12.6 Data from a Concomitant Influenza Vaccination Study 331
12.7 Schematic Plan of a Balaam Design Cross-Over Study 332
12.8 Example: Traditional Analysis of Differences in Mean ln-Titer between Vaccine Groups and Following Sequences of Dosing from a Cross-Over Vaccine Trial 334
12.9 Example: Traditional Analysis of Period 2-1 ln-Titer Following Sequences of Dosing from a Cross-Over Vaccine Trial 334
12.10 Example: Traditional Analysis of Pre-Vaccination Adjusted Differences in Period 2-1 for ln-Titer between Sequences of Dosing from a Cross-Over Vaccine Trial 335
12.11 Example: Model-Based Cross-Over and Carry-Over Analysis of ln-Titer from a Cross-Over Vaccine Trial 336

Preface to the Second Edition

This book remains concerned with the use of statistics in an area of study known as clinical pharmacology but contains updates and is an enhancement to the first edition. With the increasing size, duration, and cost of drug and biological development, increased attention is being paid to clinical pharmacology research with a corresponding increase in attention to the use of statistics. This second edition covers the relevant topics of the original edition but also addresses several recent developments in the field, namely:

An additional chapter on adaptive bioequivalence studies and sample size re-estimation - Chapter 6.

Scaled Average Bioequivalence - Chapter 7 is now dedicated to this topic.

An additional chapter on Bioequivalence and topics related to Clinical Pharmacology in Vaccines - Chapter 12.

The focus of this second edition remains those areas of statistics which we regard as most important from a practical perspective in day-to-day clinical pharmacology and related work. It is not intended to be comprehensive but to provide a starting point for those engaged in research. In writing this book we have taken from our own experiences of working in the biopharmaceutical industry. To emphasize this, each chapter begins with a brief vignette from Scott's experiences updated from the first edition (when appropriate) for more recent experiences. All the sets of data in the book are taken from real trials unless otherwise indicated.

Following a chapter devoted to biopharmaceutical development and clinical pharmacology, describing the general role of statistics, we start with several chapters wholly devoted to the study of bioequivalence – a topic where successful studies are required for regulatory approval. The aim was that this should be, to a large extent, self-contained and mostly at a level that was accessible to those with some statistical background and experience.

In Part II, following a chapter on special topics, we develop two more specialized aspects of bioequivalence testing involving sample size re-estimation followed by a chapter on scaled average bioequivalence.

The statistical tools developed in Parts I and II are useful for other topics – namely, general safety testing, testing for pro-arrythmic potential, population pharmacokinetics and dose selection. These and other related topics are covered in Part III of the book.

The book concludes in Part IV with a chapter on vaccines.

A suggested course outline may be found on the website accompanying this edition. As with the first edition, data and code used in the examples throughout the book are also available for download at the book's website.

The bibliography (and citations in text) have been updated in this edition to include recent publications on relevant topics. Computing code has been added and enhanced to address the emerging practical needs of statisticians for application to clinical trial simulations and study design, and computing code was updated to address analysis procedure updates in the SAS software used for some analyses. The text from the first edition has been revised, updated, and corrected as appropriate.

For this second edition, we wish to add our thanks to the following individuals for their advice, discussions, and communications on the topics of this edition: Bob Kohberger, James Trammel, Bill Gruber, Laszlo Endrenyi, Mike Kenward, Kevin Chartier, Cyrus Hoseyni, Emilio Emini, Tom Jacobs, Thomas Mathew (and his students at the University of Maryland, Baltimore County), Garry Anderson, Dieter Hauschke, Steven Julious, Karen Patterson, Benjamin Lang, Tobias Bluhmki, Qin Jiang (who very kindly supplied some of the vaccine data), Willi Maurer, Ying Chen, Frank Bretz, Tim Friede, Johanna Mielke, and Detlew Labes.

Some of the plots in Chapters 3 and 4 used Splus code based on examples in [879]. The description of the nonparametric method for estimating confidence intervals for stratified data, given at the end of Chapter 4, was based on notes written by Gunter Heimann. The sample size tables given in Chapter 7 are reproduced from [1249] with the kind permission of Professor Laszlo Endrenyi.

We remain indebted to those who helped with their advice and discussions, over many years, on the topics of this book: Névine Zariffa, Bob Schriver, Kate Howland, Ken Waltham, Lynda Waltham, Frank Rockhold, Mike Tydeman, Darryl Downing, Lynne Collins, Dan Patterson, Vicky Patterson, Matt Huber, Andy Huber, Todd Patterson, John Whitehead, Bob Harris, Bernie Ilson, Stephen Senn, Mike Kenward, John Matthews, Dieter Hauschke, Vern Chinchilli, Frank Harrell, Lloyd Fisher, Dallas Johnson, Laszlo Endrenyi, Val Fedorov, Andy Grieve, Gary Koch, Lutz Harnisch, Vlad Dragalin, Sergei Leonov, Peter Lane, Steven Julious, Ashwini Mathur, Nick Bird, Duane Boyle, Marty Hyneck, John Finkle, Phil Sager, Delyth Jones, Paul Stober, Annabel Mortimer, Lisa Benincosa, Marty Freed, Dave Tenero, Dawn Webber, Mick Ireson, Jeff Barrett, Klaus Hinkelmann, Carl Peck, Lewis Sheiner, Nick Holford, Terry Hyslop, Walter Hauck, Marilyn Agin, Rich Anziano, Tracy Burgess, Christy Chuang-Stein, Alex Dmitrienko, Georg Ferber, Margarida Geraldes, Kalyan Ghosh, Ron Menton, Rob Muirhead, Jaya Natarajan, Walt Offen, Jay Saoud, Brian Smith, and Ram Suresh; and to those who helped us to find relevant data: Venkat Sethuraman, Ruwei Zhi, Tim Montague, Alka Preston, Willi Maurer, Ying Chen, Frank Bretz, Tim Friede, and Steven Kathman.

We are also grateful to our employers, Pfizer® and Novartis®, and our former employers, GlaxoSmithKline® and Wyeth®, for their support and permission to publish.

This edition has been typeset using the pdfLaTeX system, and we are grateful to the staff at Chapman & Hall/CRC Press for their help with this and in particular to Shashi Kumar, Jessica Vakili, Rachel Holt, Sarah Gelson, Sarfraz Khan, Alexander Edwards, and Rob Calver for all their assistance.

We take full responsibility for any errors or omissions in the text.

Karen J. Simon and Robin Starkes to the list of folks from Chapman & Hall / CRC Press acknowledged.

Computer software used in the text

GenStat: Lawes Agricultural Trust. Supplied by VSN International, Wilkinson House, Jordan Hill Road, Oxford, UK.

R: R Core Team (2015). R: A language and environment for statistical computing. R Foundation for Statistical Computing, Vienna, Austria. URL https://www.R-project.org/

SAS: SAS Institute Inc., SAS Campus Drive, Cary, North Carolina 27513, USA.

Splus: Insightful Corporation, 1700 Westlake Avenue N, Suite 500, Seattle, Washington 98109, USA.

StatXact: Cytel Software Corporation, 675 Massachusetts Avenue, Cambridge, Massachusetts 02139, USA.

WinBUGS: MRC Biostatistics Unit, Institute of Public Health, University Forvie Site, Robinson Way, Cambridge CB2 2SR, UK.

Part I

Bioequivalence and Biopharmaceutical Development

1

Drug Development and Clinical Pharmacology

Introducing Drug Development

It was anti-climactic when I left the company where I had worked for many years. I drove away, seeing the sign and the building where I had worked in the rear-view mirror. It was January in Pennsylvania, and the solid gray sky and freezing temperature reminded me of when work there had started....

Fourteen years earlier, it was the depths of winter, and I drove up to Philadelphia to begin working in the clinical pharmacology unit for SmithKline Beecham Pharmaceuticals Research and Development as a brand new biostatistician, only four days out of school. The unit is gone now, and the name of the company has changed. The folks working in clinical pharmacology still do the same thing though — studies to bring new drug products to market and to optimise the use of drugs which are already there.

It was pretty confusing when I walked into our offices. Fresh from school, I thought the toughest part of my day was finding a parking space in West Philadelphia, but little did I know that much more fun was soon to come. Clinicians were wandering around doing clinical things, and scientists and nurses were rushing around with findings, lab samples, and dosing schedules. In the midst of all this, subjects were showing up for their studies, and getting their physical exams and being dosed.

We (the clinical pharmacology statistics group) consisted of three people then (my boss, another statistician, and me). My boss had been there for two years, and the other statistician had joined a month or two before. We were located right alongside the clinical staff, the subjects in the trials, and the laboratory personnel. It was nice to start out as a new statistician co-located with the people whom I'd work with on studies as it gave me a very practical understanding of the implications of what 'really happens' in the clinic, and we hope to convey that experience in this book.

I also caught the worst case influenza that I had ever had (prior to having children — I have had worse since) when one of the subjects vomited while I was passing by the clinic on the way to my office, so after a couple years, you will prefer an office in another building.

My boss showed me my desk and my (desktop) computer. She then sent me a dataset analyzed by a statistician at a contract research organization (the dataset is reproduced in Chapter 3). These contract research organizations are businesses hired by drug companies to do research and/or analyses for them (i.e., on contract).

It was a collection of times in a cross-over study (see Chapters 2 and 3). She asked that I verify their findings from a nonparametric analysis (because nobody else could, the thought was the contract research organization had done it wrong).

This brought several issues to mind: To what do these times correspond? What is this for? What treatments were these subjects on? Where is the rest of the study data and the protocol? What is a cross-over study (we had studied those in school, but not like this)? What is a nonparametric analysis, and which one did they use? When is lunch?

Statistically speaking, I probably should have asked the last question first. That is the first thing you need to sort out in drug development. If I had it to do over again, I would have taken a longer break before starting work too.

More important, however, is asking how such data fit into drug development, what are we trying to do with them, and what depends on the outcome? By the end of this book, you will be able to analyze these data, design studies to generate such data, and know the ins and outs of where, when, and how such data impact drug development.

...Fourteen years later, it was good to reminisce, but I was not sorry to leave my former company. I am not sure of the cause-and-effect relationship (or even sure if there is one), but over the course of years, it is clear that companies can begin to take their employees for granted and that, vice versa, employees can begin to become cynical about their company. When a company begins taking one for granted or one notes a cynical personal attitude appearing with regard to working there, it is time to make a change. One should write a book, take up a worthy cause, change jobs — in brief, do something! One should never, ever just sit marking time.

1.1 Aims of this Book

The main purpose of this book is to provide statisticians and other personnel in clinical pharmacology and drug development, teachers, and students with the methods needed to design, analyze, and interpret bioequivalence trials; when, how, and why these studies are performed as part of drug development; and to motivate the proposed methods using real-world examples. The topic is a vast one and encompasses ethics, recruitment, administration, clinical operations, and regulatory issues. Some of these aspects will have a statistical component, but it must be borne in mind throughout this book that the statistical features of the design and analysis constitute only one aspect of the role of clinical pharmacology.

Once the foundations of clinical pharmacology drug development, regulatory applications, and the design and analysis of bioequivalence trials are established, we will move to related topics in clinical pharmacology involving the use of cross-over designs. These include (but are not limited to) safety studies in Phase I, dose-response trials, drug interaction trials, food-effect and combination trials, QTc and other pharmacodynamic equivalence trials, dose-proportionality trials, and vaccine trials.

We have tried to maintain a practical perspective and to avoid those topics that are of largely academic interest. Throughout the book we have included examples of SAS code [1073] so that the analyses we describe can be immediately implemented using the SAS statistical analysis system. In particular, we have made extensive use of the `proc mixed` procedure in SAS [795].

In each chapter, we will begin with the practical utility, objectives, and real-world examples of the topic under discussion. This will be followed by statistical theory and applications to support development of the area under study. Technical theory and code (where extensive) will be included in technical appendices to each chapter. Each topic will include worked examples to illustrate applications of the statistical techniques and their interpretation, and to serve as problems for those situations where this book serves as the basis for course work.

1.2 Biopharmaceutical Development

Biopharmaceutical development is the process of changing someone's mind. To clarify, industrialized nations today have (pretty much uniformly) created governmental "watchdog" bureaucracies to regulate the use of biopharmaceutical products (drugs, biologics, and vaccines) in human beings. These groups were created in response to historical events in a variety of settings where such products, which were unsafe, ineffective, or poorly made, were used in human populations. Such regulatory agencies are meant to protect public health by ensuring that marketed products are safe, benefit the patients taking them, and are manufactured to standards of high quality (so when one takes one pill, for example, it is the same as the next, and the next, etc.).

The regulatory agencies one will frequently hear about when working in biopharmaceutical development are listed in Table 1.1.

TABLE 1.1
Selected Regulatory Authorities

Nation	Agency
Australia	Therapeutic Goods Administration (TGA)
Canada	Therapeutic Products Directorate (TPD)
China	State Food and Drug Administration (SFDA)
European Union	European Agency for the Evaluation of Medical Products (EMEA)
Japan	Ministry of Health and Welfare (MHW)
United States of America	Food and Drug Administration (FDA)

These regulatory agencies are, in general, gigantic in size and the scope of their activities. They employ hundreds if not thousands of people worldwide — clinicians, physicians, nurses, epidemiologists, statisticians, and a variety of other personnel. Regulatory agencies are charged with specific roles to protect the public health. Under the assumptions that all drugs, biologics, and vaccines are unsafe, or will not benefit the patients taking them, or cannot be manufactured to high quality standards, these people are charged with finding the few biopharmaceutical products that are safe, will benefit patients, and are manufactured to high quality.

What is usually not mentioned in the charters and laws establishing these agencies are that they are also to do this as quickly as possible (people who are sick do not like to wait) without sacrificing safety on a shoestring budget. It is a challenging job.

We will typically refer to biopharmaceutical products as "drugs" for simplicity. Technically, drugs are small-molecule chemical products that have been shown to be of some benefit to public health, can be safely administered, and can be manufactured to high quality. Large-molecule products (e.g., insulin) known as "biologics" are being developed and marketed on a more routine basis. Vaccines have a long history of use in this context for the prevention of disease [918]. For simplicity, we will refer to drug development for the remainder of this chapter. However, these concepts apply to vaccines.

The job of any sponsor (or drug company) is to show regulators that benefit, safety, and quality are present and to get their drug to patients needing it as soon as possible thereafter. In essence, drug companies are charged with changing the regulators' minds (i.e., proving them wrong). They must show that their product is safe, effective, and made to high-quality standards.

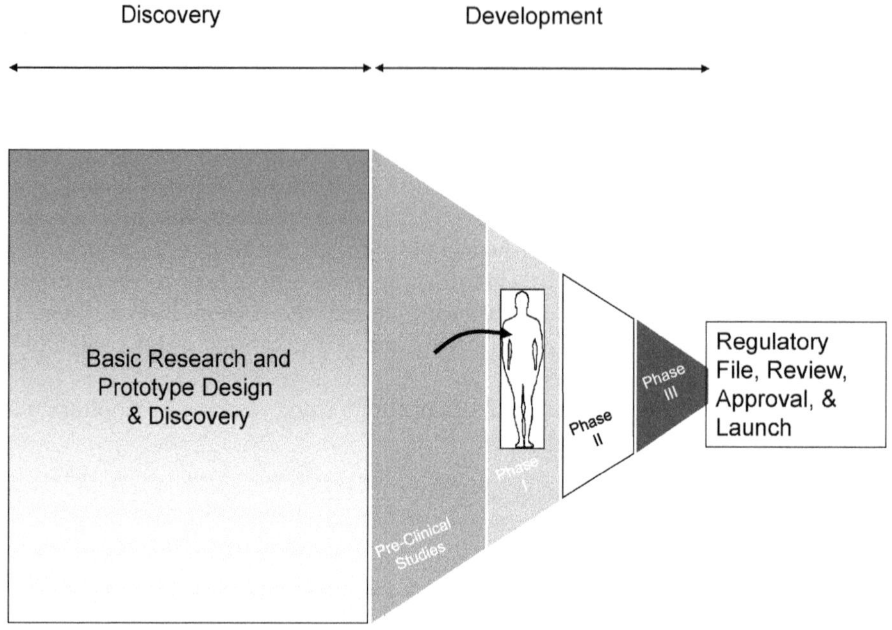

FIGURE 1.1
Critical Path in Drug Development

Sponsors (e.g., drug companies) develop drugs on what has been termed the critical path [377]; see Figure 1.1.

A drug is generally discovered in the context of basic science — in that it causes a biological response in vitro (in a lab setting) which is thought to have the potential to provide benefit. Following an extensive battery of in vitro, animal, and manufacturing testing, and following regulatory review, it is administered to humans (a first-time-in-humans study) in a clinic. Clinical pharmacology work begins then, and extensive human and animal testing follows to evaluate safety and medical utility in parallel with scale-up of manufacturing to provide large amounts of drug substance. If all this is successful, a data package is filed with the regulatory agency where a sponsor wishes to market the product.

Generally, from the time a drug enters the clinic to the time it is approved by regulators and ready to market, 10.4 years on average elapse [261]. The cost is also substantial, with estimates ranging from 0.8 to 1.7 billion dollars being spent in research and development to bring **one** new product to market [377]. Of the drugs which clear the various hurdles to human testing, only one in ten will be approved for the marketplace, failing for reasons of lack of efficacy (benefit), unacceptable safety profile, poor manufacturing, or lack of economic benefit.

What is done over this 10-plus years and a billion dollars? In a nutshell, a drug is developed by finding a dose or set of doses which produce the desired beneficial response (like lowering blood pressure: a surrogate marker or predictor of cardiac benefit) without producing an undesirable response (e.g., nausea, vomiting). One also has to be able to make the product (manufacture it) to a standard of high quality, and in a consistent manner [1355].

1.3 Clinical Pharmacology

Clinical pharmacology is the study of drugs in humans [30]. It blends the science of laboratory assessment of chemicals with the clinical and medicinal art of their application. Many textbooks are devoted to the proper study of clinical pharmacology, and we shall dwell only on those aspects which will be important for the subsequent chapters of this book.

First, some concepts. The study of pharmacokinetics (PK) is defined as "movements of drugs within biological systems, as affected by uptake, distribution, binding, elimination and biotransformation; particularly the rates of such movements [1186]". In layman's terms, PK is what the body does to a drug (as opposed to what a drug does to the body, which we'll cover later).

When a tablet of a drug is taken orally, in general, it reaches the stomach and begins to disintegrate and is absorbed (A). When dissolved into solution in the stomach acid, the drug is passed on to the small intestine [1058]. In the small intestine, many things can happen. Some of the drug will pass right on through and be eliminated (E) from the body. Some will be metabolized (M) into a different substance right in the intestine, and some drug will be picked up by the body and distributed (D) into the body through the portal circulation. This last bit of drug substance passes through the liver first, where it is often metabolized (M). The remainder passes through the liver and reaches the bloodstream where it is circulated throughout the body. Pharmacokinetics is thus the study of ADME [30].

This process, however, is difficult to measure. Modern technology provides many options (e.g., one might tag a molecule using a radio-label and follow the progress of the molecule using X-ray imaging and similar techniques); however, the most common means is to measure how much drug substance is put into the body (i.e., dose) and how much drug reaches the systemic circulation by blood sampling. Figure 1.2 provides a typical plasma concentration profile (vertical axis) versus time (horizontal axis) for a dose of drug administered orally to an individual at 0 hours.

As the drug is absorbed and distributed, the plasma concentration rises and reaches a maximum (called the Cmax or maximum concentration). Plasma levels then decline until the body completely eliminates the drug. The overall exposure to the drug is measured by computing the area under the plasma concentration curve (AUC). AUC is derived in general by computing the area for each triangle or quadrangle as appropriate to each time point and then adding them up.

This is known as the trapezoidal rule [30] and, following the principles given in Chapter 8 of [30], AUC is derived for each triangle or quadrangle by taking the sum of the expression

$$AUC_{i-1}^{i} = \frac{1}{2}[C_{t_i} + C_{t_{i-1}}](t_i - t_{i-1})$$

where $i = 1, 2, 3, ...$ and t_i is the time at which concentration C_{t_i} is observed. Specifically, this type of approach to summarization of data is called a noncompartmental analysis. No rate or elimination assumptions are made about how the drug enters into and exits the bloodstream. Concentrations are just summarized using various measures of the observed data. In practice, this sort of calculation and others that are described have been automated into a number of commercial software packages used in practice. We therefore do not dwell further upon noncompartmental analysis topics here.

The points on the concentration versus time curve are derived based upon measurement by an assay. These assays have performance limits including the limit of detection (LOD, the point below which the assay cannot detect a concentration), the lower limit of quantification (LLOQ, the point below which the concentration may not reliably be quantified), and the

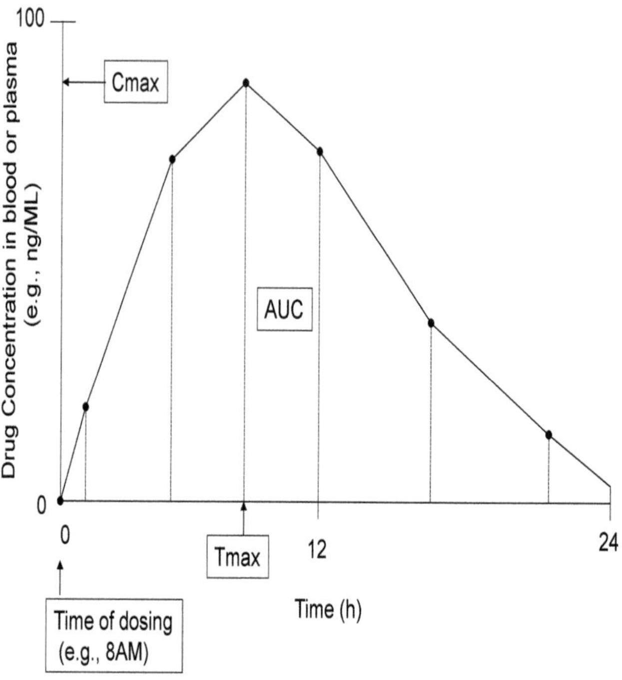

FIGURE 1.2
Plasma Concentration (ng/mL) versus Time (h)

upper limit of quantification (ULOQ, the point above which the concentration may not reliably be quantified). In the context of AUC(0-t), the t is the last time point at which a concentration above or equal to the LLOQ is observed.

To conclude, some summary measures [1058] for the plasma concentration versus time curve are derived as

- AUC(0-t) (i.e., Area under the curve from time zero to t where t is the time of last quantifiable concentration),
- Cmax (maximum concentration),
- Tmax (time of maximum concentration),
- $T_{\frac{1}{2}}$ (half-life of drug substance), and

$$AUC(0-\infty) = AUC(0-t) + \frac{C_t}{\lambda} \tag{1.1}$$

where C_t is the last quantifiable concentration at time t and λ is -2.303 times the slope of the terminal phase of the $\log_e$-concentration time curve. See [1192] for other summary measures. More details of techniques used in the derivation of the AUC may be found in [1376]. We could also fit a model to summarize a plasma concentration curve and will develop the methods used for doing so in a later chapter.

The endpoint $AUC(0-\infty)$ is less frequently used in regulatory applications, as there is error associated with the extrapolation after the last quantified time point, and there is no scientifically valid way to verify the extrapolation, as the assay is not quantified below the LLOQ. Therefore AUC(0-t) is used as the standard endpoint, in general.

Turning back now to what is happening with the drug itself, once a drug is ingested, the substance (or active metabolite) passes through the blood and hopefully reaches a site of action, thereupon provoking what is termed a pharmacodynamic (PD) response in the body. This response is measured by looking at a biomarker or a surrogate marker.

Biomarkers are "a characteristic that is objectively measured and evaluated as an indicator of normal biological processes, pathogenic processes, or pharmacologic responses to a therapeutic intervention" [82]. In contrast, a surrogate marker is "a biomarker that is intended to substitute for a clinical endpoint. A surrogate endpoint is expected to predict clinical benefit (or harm or lack of benefit or harm) based on epidemiologic, therapeutic, pathophysiologic, or scientific evidence" [82]. Alternative definitions exist, for example, "a laboratory measurement or physical sign that is used in therapeutic trials as a substitute for a clinically meaningful endpoint that is a direct measure of how a patient feels, functions, or survives and is expected to predict the effect of therapy", [1219].

For example, blood pressure [1219] can be considered as a surrogate marker for clinical benefit, as numerous clinical studies have shown that lowering blood pressure improves patient survival (i.e., decreases the rate of mortality seen in patients with high blood pressure). HDL (high density lipoprotein) cholesterol is a biomarker. Increasing HDL was thought to have therapeutic cardiac benefit [1181], but findings from clinical studies have not borne it out as a valid surrogate marker.

Large numbers of biomarkers are used in early-phase clinical development to characterize the pharmacodynamic and clinical effects of drug treatment. The purpose of clinical development at this early stage is to provide a safe and potentially effective range of doses to be fully evaluated for safety and efficacy to regulatory standards in later-phase trials (Phases II and III). Generally, biomarkers are qualitatively evaluated for their predictive value in supporting later-phase development. However, recent developments highlight the need to apply quantitative tools to biomarker data to enhance their utility in support of company decisions regarding the prediction of subsequent surrogate marker and clinical outcome measures [757].

Surrogate markers have been used to support successful regulatory applications in drug development [1219]. Criteria for demonstrating that an endpoint is a surrogate marker for clinical outcome are not well established [82, 757, 1219]; however, some qualitative principles have been repeatedly discussed. These principles are "Biological Plausibility, Success in Clinical Trials, Risk-Benefit, and Public Health Considerations" [1219].

It should be noted, however, that, at the same time as a drug is giving a "good" PD response, the drug (or a metabolic by-product) may attach itself to a different site of action, thereby provoking unwanted side effects. The study of pharmacodynamics, is in layman's terms, "what the drug does to the body."

In combination, dose, PK, and PD relationships contain the necessary and sufficient information we need to begin convincing people that use of a drug is worthwhile and to learn about the behavior of a drug product. This is sometimes also referred to as the dose-exposure-response (DER) relationship [372, 621, 1139].

How do we go about developing drugs under this approach to clinical pharmacology? Early-stage development should focus on learning about the compound, understanding its safety and efficacy in patients by means of varying dose and measuring PK and PD. Once sufficient confidence is reached that the compound does what is beneficial and is safe enough to dose, sponsors begin conducting large confirmatory trials. These are trials designed to convince regulatory authorities that the drug is safe to use in the marketplace and will be of public benefit. A more comprehensive review may be found in [1142].

Let us revisit our earlier discussion of drug development (Figure 1.1) in light of what we now know about clinical pharmacology and to break down the critical path of clinical drug development in more detail. Prior to the first-in-human study in clinic, in vitro and animal preclinical experimentation should establish a range of safe doses for study in humans. Doses are then selected for introduction into clinical studies in humans [1027].

Clinical development of a drug product, with the exception of only the most toxic products targeted for the treatment of cancer, then initiates with the study of the drug product in normal healthy male volunteers in what is known as Phase I. These studies are typically small, well controlled, data intensive, dose escalating, and placebo controlled (we will get into this in a later chapter).

In this stage of human drug development, the primary objective of a clinical study is to determine a safe range of doses and dosing regimens (e.g., once-a-day or twice-a-day) for later dosing in studies involving patients with the disease state under study. Dose and dosing regimen are examined with respect to their impact on the pharmacokinetics of the drug product. Additionally, should biomarker or surrogate markers be present to characterize the activity of the drug in normal healthy volunteers, these data are characterized relative to dose and PK.

By the end of Phase I, dose-finding studies in normal healthy volunteers or patient studies (e.g., for oncology compounds) should provide a range of safe (and potentially efficacious) doses for further study in patients, an initial description of pharmacokinetic exposure levels and/or biomarker/surrogate marker levels at each dose to facilitate choice of dose, dose titration, dosing intervals for Phase II studies, and the development of initial models for use in pharmacokinetic-pharmacodynamic modelling for both desirable and undesirable effects.

Subsequent Phase II clinical studies in patients establish the minimum starting and maximum effective dose as well as the maximum tolerated dose in patients with the disease state using pharmacodynamic endpoints or surrogate markers of therapeutic response. Dose titration and the length of time needed to see an effect (desirable or undesirable) are also established. In these studies, models relating dose to PK and to PD are developed to understand the mechanism of the drug's action and to search for relevant covariates (e.g., age or gender) to control later Phase II or Phase III confirmatory trial designs [621].

Dose-finding studies in Phase II in the target population should establish the therapeutic window by identifying a minimum effective starting dose (the lowest dose yielding a desirable effect), a maximum effective dose (the dose beyond which further escalation lacks further desirable benefit), and a maximum tolerated dose (the dose beyond which there is an unacceptable increase in undesirable effects) in the target population. In addition, these studies should identify the time interval needed to see an effect (desirable and/or undesirable) and reasonable, response-guided, titration steps along with the time intervals at which to dose titrate, to develop updated pharmacokinetic-pharmacodynamic models for both desirable and undesirable effects in the population of interest, and to identify potential covariates to be studied for dose adjustment in Phase III (e.g., age, gender).

Once a dose or set of efficacious doses are chosen from Phase II trials and the characteristics of Figure 1.2 are mapped out, confirmatory Phase III trials are performed to support regulatory acceptance. These trials, in large numbers of patients with the disease under study, should characterize the risk relative to benefit in clinical use of the compound. These studies in Phase III should be used to establish the risk:benefit ratio and pharmacokinetic-pharmacodynamic relationship (if any) for doses chosen to be in the therapeutic window established in Phase II.

Additional clinical pharmacology studies will also be conducted in Phase III to determine how to dose the drug in patients with particular health problems (like kidney disease) and for patients taking a variety of concomitant medications. Additionally, clinical pharmacology studies will be done to confirm that new formulations of drug product are equivalent to those used in clinical development when scale-up of the manufacturing process for mass production occurs. These are bioequivalence studies and will be the subject of Chapters 2–7.

1.4 Statistics in Clinical Pharmacology

What is a statistic? It is numerical information about a given object or event. This information is derived from a sample (a study or trial) of a population (as it would often be impossible to collect information from an entire large population that is too numerous for exhaustive measurement). On its own, a statistic is just a number. However, decisions are made based on statistics, and that is where statistical sciences come into play.

James Bernoulli described nine "general rules dictated by common sense" [499] (see Chapter 15 on Bernoulli's Ars Conjectandi, 1713) for making decisions based on statistics, and most statisticians follow these (in principle):

1. One must not use conjecture (i.e., use statistics) in cases where complete certainty is obtainable.
2. One must search for all possible arguments or evidence concerning the case (i.e., show due diligence).
3. One must take into account both arguments for and against the case.
4. For a judgment about general events, general arguments are sufficient; for individual events, however, special and individual arguments have to be taken into account.
5. In case of uncertainty, action should be suspended until more information is at hand; however, if circumstances permit no delay, the action that is most suitable, safe, wise, and probable should be chosen.
6. That which can be useful on some occasion and harmful on no occasion is to be preferred to that which is useful and harmful on no occasion.
7. The value of human actions must not be judged by their outcome.
8. In our judgments we must be wary of attributing more weight to a thing than its due and of considering something that is more probable than another to be absolutely certain.
9. Absolute certainty occurs only when the probability nearly equals the whole certainty (i.e., when the probability of some event is equal to one, such that we know it will occur).

Statisticians are applied mathematicians. In drug development, these people are responsible for quantifying the uncertainty inherent in the scientific and regulatory process of developing new drug products. The focus of our discussion will be on the techniques statisticians apply to the design and analysis of clinical pharmacology trials, but statisticians are involved in a variety of other topics associated with drug development (see [434] for more details).

As any statistic is derived from a sample, there is **always** uncertainty involved in its use. There is always a chance that the sample and the statistic derived from it got something "wrong" relative to the truth of the situation. Statisticians and the art of statistics are therefore employed in drug development to ensure that the probability of a "wrong answer" is quantified and understood so that the implications can be considered.

Consider the main topic of this book, bioequivalence. At certain times in drug development, drug companies must show that a new formulation of drug (i.e., a new capsule or tablet) is equivalent to an old formulation. It is assumed (i.e., the hypothesis) that the formulations are not equivalent, and a study must be performed to generate data to show that they are.

Obviously it is completely impossible to assess every new tablet and compare each one to each and every old tablet to ensure high quality is present. It would take forever and be too time consuming to even contemplate, and even if we could devise a test to ensure that each and every tablet is exactly the same as each and every old one, we are more interested in whether the two formulations will give us the same results when patients take them anyway. So it may not matter if they are not exactly the same.

Therefore, a clinical study is used to do the job. Data are generated in the study, and statistics are derived to compare the results of the new formulation to the old formulation. When the data come in, we use them to decide whether we have sufficient evidence to throw out our hypothesis (that the formulations are not equivalent) and that we have sufficient data to conclude they are.

We approach this topic like a regulator would — i.e., assume that they are not equivalent until data shows that they are. The two formulations may in fact (i.e., in truth) be equivalent, but until we have conclusive data to show that, it is best to err on the side of caution.

When the data come in, they will give us information to conclude whether the drugs are equivalent or not. We can make two errors in this situation (see Table 1.2). We can conclude from the data that they are equivalent, when in fact they are not (a Type 1 error), or we could conclude that the formulations are not equivalent when in fact they are (a Type 2 error). Bernoulli's second and third principles are applied in this manner, and we will get into the application of the other Bernoulli principles in this setting later in the book.

Statisticians use tools to design and analyze studies to ensure that the probabilities of a Type 1 or 2 error are controlled and held at a quantified rate of occurrence. These tools are randomization, replication, blocking, blinding, and modelling, and their definition and specific application will be discussed in great detail in later chapters. Application of these tools enables those using the statistics (i.e., the drug companies and regulators) to know the implications of their decision on whether the two formulations are equivalent or not and to make a reasoned decision on whether to provide the new formulation to the patients who need it.

TABLE 1.2
Potential Errors When Interpreting Bioequivalence Data

		The Truth	
		Formulations are NOT equivalent	Formulations ARE equivalent
Statistics from study show that	Formulations are NOT equivalent	Right answer!	Wrong answer (Type 2 error)
or that	Formulations ARE equivalent	Wrong answer (Type 1 error)	Right answer!

A few words here on blinding and randomization are necessary, as these design factors are too often taken for granted in clinical trials, ignoring their purpose and importance.

Blinding [588] of a clinical trial is defined as disguising of the treatment given to a study's subject to ensure that subsequent observations (either by the subject, study staff, and laboratory measurements) are not biased by knowledge of the treatment assignment. The level of the blind may be Open label (subjects and study staff know the treatment administered), Single blind (subjects do not know the treatment), Double blind (Subjects and study staff do not know the treatment), and sometimes "Triple" blind (subjects, study staff, and sponsor staff such as those in the laboratory or assessing safety data do not know the treatment assignment). This is done to ensure that the study's results are not biased by knowledge of the treatment given to a particular subject and is common practice (where possible and practical) in modern clinical trials.

Randomization is another step taken to ensure unbiased results. Subjects are randomly assigned to treatment groups to eliminate sources of bias due to treatment allocation (also, unknown sources of bias). Its application is typically viewed as a common sense requirement — one would not play cards (for money and items of significance) without shuffling the deck. By randomising (in clinical trials), one ensures that the effects of treatment are not biased by other factors (e.g., subjective investigator judgment, subject disease status) and unknown things which could occur during a study (a mishap at the lab, for example). Beyond this, however, there are statistical reasons why randomisation must be done [737, 738, 1043, 1337]. In brief, randomization is required to ensure that the probabilities of a Type 1 error and a Type 2 error are controlled as expected. Use of randomization ensures that these probabilities can be reliably estimated, and ensures that those using products which were approved based upon clinical trials are reasonably well protected from false findings.

Not much is 100% certain, and studies like those described above are no exception. It is not unusual for studies to give misleading (i.e., Type 1 or 2 error) results when one considers that thousands of clinical trials are performed worldwide each year. Even as small an error rate as 5% can result in five Type 1 errors when a hundred studies are run. Clinical trials are only a sample of the truth, and it is unusual for Bernoulli's ninth principle to ever have application in biopharmaceutical development. In the context of uncertainty being present, use of blinding and randomization ensures that clinical trials have quantified value in protection of human populations and in the company's intrinsic interests in approval and use of a pharmaceutical product, satisfying Bernoulli's seventh principle.

This sort of approach is used often in clinical pharmacology when looking at data from which one wants to make a regulatory claim of some sort — i.e., to convince a regulator that there is sufficient basis to grant approval to market for reasons of quality, safety, or efficacy.

In other, more experimental studies, an inductive approach is used, and dose is varied in different patient and volunteer populations to estimate the PK and PD properties of the drug to evaluate its potential safety and efficacy attributes. The focus here is on unbiased and precise estimation, and less on Type 1 and 2 errors and their impact on decision making.

To quantify this, we will call Θ the set of PK and PD properties we wish to estimate. Before we conduct clinical trials to characterize Θ, we will have only a rough idea (from previous experiments) or, at worst, no idea, about what Θ is. Once the study or set of studies is complete, statistics will be used to quantify Θ based on the data and give the clinical pharmacologists an understanding of how the various factors involved in Θ behave.

The statistical tools of randomization, replication, blocking, blinding, and modelling are also used in this situation, but for a different purpose. Here they are applied to ensure that the statistics give a clear idea about what Θ is (i.e., is not confounded or biased by other factors) and to meet the desired level of precision in understanding the behavior of Θ. These sorts of studies are conducted to enhance the drug company's and regulators' knowledge of the compound's properties in preparation for confirmatory trials. They do not (except in unusual circumstances) constitute sufficient evidence to permit regulators to grant market access. In part, this is due to blinding and randomization not being as rigorously applied as would be required to precisely control Type 1 and 2 errors.

1.5 Structure of Book

Now that drug development, clinical pharmacology, and the role of statistics have been discussed, we turn to bioequivalence. We will begin with the history of bioequivalence and an in-depth discussion of current regulatory requirements. This will be followed by a lengthy chapter on the design and analysis of bioequivalence trials using 2×2 cross-over designs. Alternative designs for demonstrating bioequivalence will then be discussed and followed by discussion devoted to special challenges encountered in bioequivalence studies. Following this we will cover studies where the sample size is re-estimated and potentially adjusted to ensure a conclusive finding. There follows a discussion of more recent proposals on alternative means of assessing bioequivalence.

In subsequent chapters, we consider statistical approaches to the design and analysis of clinical pharmacology experiments to study safety, QTc prolongation, efficacy, population pharmacokinetics, and vaccines.

Readers not interested in in-depth discussions of statistical theory and applications will find Chapters 1 and 2 most useful for their research on bioequivalence and statistics in clinical pharmacology.

Where permitted, data and code for examples used in text may be found on the website accompanying the book. Users should note that a read-me file on the website is available to assist in identification of which set of data and code pertains to each example.

2

History and Regulation of Bioequivalence

Introducing Bioequivalence

It was a rainy day, and I was looking forward to another day at the Clinical Pharmacology Unit. We called it "The Unit" for some reason. I think it was a sign of the times in the 1990s. We worked at "The Unit"; people from FDA worked at "The Center"; people with the CIA probably worked for "The Agency." It is good that times have changed.

It had been about a year and a half since I started working in statistics in clinical pharmacology, and I was starting to feel like I knew what was going on when working with the teams which were making the potential drugs and designing and performing the clinical pharmacology trials. By this time, I had worked on a couple of submissions to regulatory agencies (under supervision), had been through a regulatory audit by the FDA (they come in occasionally to check all the paperwork — as long as you follow your standard operating procedures and document what you have, this is no problem and nothing to worry about), and had figured out when lunch was.

I felt like I had it made until a ClinPharm physician and a scientist came into my office that morning while I was drinking my coffee. We will call them "Lenny" and "Denny", and they both looked like they were having a bad day. They were characters. Both of them talked a lot and at great velocity most of the time, but today they were pretty quiet. They had both been at work since 6 a.m. (clinical staff usually come in early — I think it gives them more time to make mischief) and both looked like they would rather be out in the Pennsylvania thunderstorm that was now cutting loose.

Over the monsoon, Denny filled me in on what the problem was. Lenny just nodded and groaned occasionally and looked like he wanted to go home and go back to bed. I figured he brought it on himself coming to work at 6 a.m.

In brief, one of our drugs was in the late stages of drug development. The confirmatory trials were close to finishing, and the scale-up of manufacturing to make sufficient drug to supply the marketplace had been completed about three months ago. Everything looked pretty good — the drug was safe and well tolerated in addition to being efficacious, and we expected the Regulators to approve it once we submitted it in about six to eight months.

The company had spent a lot of money to buy this product (we had bought it from whomever had invented it) and to develop it (estimates were in the range of what was discussed in Chapter 1) in addition to spending about five years in clinical development. It was a tremendous effort.

The problem was that the new formulation we wanted to mass produce and prepare to market clearly did not demonstrate bioequivalence to the formulation being used in the confirmatory clinical trials. It was close, but the bioequivalence study did not fully meet the regulatory standard. Lenny groaned here, but I just kept drinking my coffee. I was still too new to know how bad this was. We had a quality issue in the manufacture of the drug.

This essentially meant that, even if the regulators at the FDA approved the product for safety and efficacy, the company would not be able to market it. We could not (at that time) confirm that the new formula was of a sufficiently high quality to deliver the same safety and efficacy results when used in the marketplace as achieved in the confirmatory clinical trials. When Denny explained that, suddenly my coffee did not taste as good (it was always pretty bad, actually — it was free, though).

After reminding myself that I knew when lunch was supposed to be and had gotten more sleep the night before than Lenny and Denny combined (both positive factors in my view in this situation), I got a crash course in the history of bioequivalence. We then started working through the issue of how to get the quality assessment for this drug product back on track.

2.1 When and How BE Studies Are Performed

Biopharmaceutical statistics traditionally has focused on differentiating between products (or placebo) to provide new and enhanced treatments for the public's benefit [1104]. However, this is generally expensive and time consuming (see Chapter 1) and over time steps have been taken to reduce costs and to increase supply of pharmaceutical products while maintaining the potential for innovation. One such example pertains to bioequivalence.

To call something equivalent implies a context or set of criteria for the determination of equivalence. There are several stakeholders who have a say in choosing such criteria:

- Regulatory and public health considerations: The approach used must protect public health in that the risk of a false positive (Type 1 error — see Chapter 1 for more details) market access must be controlled at a predetermined rate.
- Statistical considerations: The approach should be quantifiable, accurate, precise, well understood, and should be transparent in interpretation.
- Sponsor considerations: Using a well-designed, controlled, and reasonably sized study (or set of studies), the sponsor should be able to show the criteria have been met with a quantified chance of success (Type 2 error — see Chapter 1 for more details).

Bioequivalence (BE) studies are performed to demonstrate that different formulations or regimens of drug product are similar to each other in terms of their therapeutic benefit (efficacy) and nontherapeutic side-effects (safety). They play a key and pivotal role in the drug development process by ensuring that, when a patient switches to a new formulation in the marketplace, safety and efficacy will be maintained. Primarily, these studies are used in the study of solid oral dosage forms (i.e., drugs administered as a tablet or capsule when ingested), and this chapter will be confined to discussion of this type of drug product.

When the new and old formulations use exactly the same substance (i.e., are pharmaceutically equivalent [59]), why do these studies need to be done? It is a known fact that rate and extent of bioavailability (i.e., how much drug gets into the bloodstream and is available at the site of action after one takes a dose — see Chapter 1) can be affected by very small changes in formulation. Factors like the constituent content of the formula, small changes to the lining of the formula, and by compaction into tablet (versus administration as a capsule), for example, may result in big changes in bioavailability. See [762] and [37] for examples.

Many changes are made to the formulation while Phases I and II of drug development are ongoing in clinic prior to it being approved for market access. Prior to submission to regulatory agencies and while the trials are ongoing, drug companies commonly check that these changes in formulation do not drastically change bioavailability by what are known as relative bioavailability studies. These studies are primarily used by pharmaceutical sponsors of new drug entities to ensure that the formulation to be used in Phase II or in later confirmatory trials is sufficiently similar to that used in Phase I drug development and are not performed to the high requirements of true bioequivalence trials. When one wants access to the marketplace for a new formulation, a higher standard is to be met.

The bioequivalence study is used to demonstrate that the formulation used in Phase III confirmatory clinical trials is sufficiently similar to the final commercial formulation to be marketed following approval.

Bioequivalence studies are primarily used by pharmaceutical sponsors of new drug entities who have conducted pivotal confirmatory trials with a specific formulation of a drug therapy but need market access for a more commercially suitable formulation (i.e., that can be mass produced). BE studies can be viewed as providing necessary and sufficient reassurance to regulators that the formulation to be marketed is the same as that used in the clinical confirmatory trials without the need to repeat the development program or to perform a therapeutic equivalence study in patients with clinical endpoints [609]. Obviously, it is impossible to repeat a drug development program with a new formulation when it is expected to last over 10 years and cost approximately a billion dollars. Such an effort is not sustainable even with modern industrial power.

Bioequivalence studies must also be performed following substantial postmarketing formulation alteration. They are also used by what is termed the "generic" pharmaceutical industry to gain market access for formulations of established drug therapies when the patent of the original sponsor's formulation expires. When the original sponsors themselves perform a formulation change (for instance, change the site of manufacture) following approval, they often also must do a bioequivalence study to convince regulators that the new formula is safe and effective to market.

Multiple companies may produce and market similar formulations to the original marketed product following patent expiration, provided they can demonstrate bioequivalence to the original product. *Generic substitution* has thus provided a means of supplying the market with inexpensive, efficacious, and safe drug products without the need to repeat an entire clinical and clinical pharmacology development package following patent expiration.

We have now addressed when these studies are done, and we now turn to how the studies are performed. Bioequivalence studies are conducted to meet documented, legislated regulatory standards, and cross-over study designs [652], [1113] are typically used to study bioequivalence. The design and application of such studies will be discussed at length in Chapter 3 but are summarized briefly here.

Bioequivalence studies are usually conducted in male and female healthy volunteer subjects. Each individual subject is administered two formulations (T=Test or R=Reference) in one of two sequences of treatments (e.g., RT and TR); see Table 2.1. R is the "standard" and T is the "new" formulation.

Each administration is separated by a washout period appropriate to the drug under study; see Table 2.2. This washout period consists of five half-lives between administrations. Half-life is determined by looking at the elimination (after Cmax) part of the PK

TABLE 2.1
Schematic Plan of a 2×2 Cross-Over Study

Sequence Group	Period			Number of Subjects
	1	Washout	2	
1(RT)	R	—	T	$n/2$
2(TR)	T	—	R	$n/2$
R=Reference, T=Test n =total number of subjects				

TABLE 2.2
Example of a Random Allocation of Sequences to Subject in a 2×2 Cross-Over Design

Subject	Sequence	Period 1	Washout period of 5 half-lives	Period 2
1	TR	T	—	R
2	RT	R	—	T
3	RT	R	—	T
.	.	.	...	.
.	.	.	...	.
.	.	.	...	.
n	TR	T	—	R

concentration versus time curve (see Figure 1.2) and is simply the length of time it takes the body to eliminate one-half of the amount of whatever drug is in the body at any given time. In general, if five half-lives go by, little to no drug should be left in the systemic circulation.

Such a design is termed a 2×2 cross-over [652] and is a type of design typically applied in bioequivalence trials. Of the potential list of designs (alternatives are discussed in Chapter 5) for application in bioequivalence trials, by far the most common is the 2×2 cross-over design (with sequences RT, TR). A potential complication for this design is that the effect of a formulation given in the first period may last into the second period, i.e., the washout period is inadequate. In the presence of such carry-over effects, the interpretation of the statistics from such trials are known to be complicated [1114, 1115]. When an adequate washout period is included, carry-over effects are generally considered to be negligible ([237, 1115, 1388, 1389]). Let's go through the 2×2 BE design in a bit more detail.

The dose of drug substance in each formulation is pharmaceutically equivalent, and typically the formulations are not blinded (i.e., not disguised to the patient or investigator). It obviously would be difficult for a subject or clinician to bias or influence a subject's PK levels by knowing what treatment the subject received (one presumably cannot change one's PK by just thinking about it). Clinical staff do confirm that each subject has taken their pill(s) as randomly assigned, and those subjects who subsequently throw up their pill are excluded from analysis (for example, see [373]).

Random allocation of subject to sequence is done here to ensure that time-related effects (i.e., period to period differences in blood sampling timings or laboratory handling of the samples, for example) can be accounted for in the analysis and are not confounded with the estimate for the difference between formulations. This is an example of the practice of randomization and is one of the tools used to ensure bias does not creep into the study. Blood samples will be collected at predetermined, regular intervals prior to and following each dose of formulation [373] to generate the concentration versus time curves described in Chapter 1.

Each subject serves as their own control (i.e., we can compare T to R on each subject). This is referred to as blocking and ensures that a precise measurement of the difference in formulations can be made. We will develop the model used for doing this in Chapter 3.

Replication (i.e., the number of patients assigned to each sequence) is chosen to ensure that the regulatory standards for demonstrating bioequivalence can be met. This topic will be discussed further in Chapters 3 and 5.

To demonstrate equivalence in plasma concentration profiles, *rate* and *extent* of bioavailability of the drug substance in plasma must be sufficiently similar so as to meet the regulatory standard for showing that exposure of the body to the drug substance is the same between formulations [59]. For this purpose, Cmax (rate) and AUC (extent) are typically used as summary measures for the plasma concentration curves and are required to be demonstrated as equivalent under preset decision rules to achieve regulatory approval. As discussed in Chapter 1, AUC(0-t) is generally used, and we neglect the (0-t) in the following without loss of generality. The other pharmacokinetic endpoints discussed in Chapter 1 provide supporting information but do not directly impact approvability of the new formulation.

AUC and Cmax are looked at in this situation as surrogate markers [82] for clinical efficacy and safety. For example, if Cmax increases too much with the new formulation, this could lead to unwanted side effects. On the other hand, if it decreases too much, the drug may not be effective in treating the illness. Similar arguments apply to AUC. Hence the quality of manufacturing assessment focuses on ensuring these do not change "too much" in the new formulation. The definition of "too much" is quite involved and will be the subject of the next section.

Looking more closely at the endpoints we are concerned with, the pharmacokinetic endpoints AUC and Cmax are generally assumed to be what is referred to as log-normally distributed. A distribution is a mathematical description of the state of nature from which individual observations (like AUC and Cmax collected in our BE studies) arise. What follows is a nontechnical description of distribution theory relating to bioequivalence. Those interested in the specifics of distributional theory in this setting should review [229].

An example of a normal distribution is plotted in Figure 2.1. The density of the distribution is on the vertical axis and the corresponding AUC values are on the horizontal

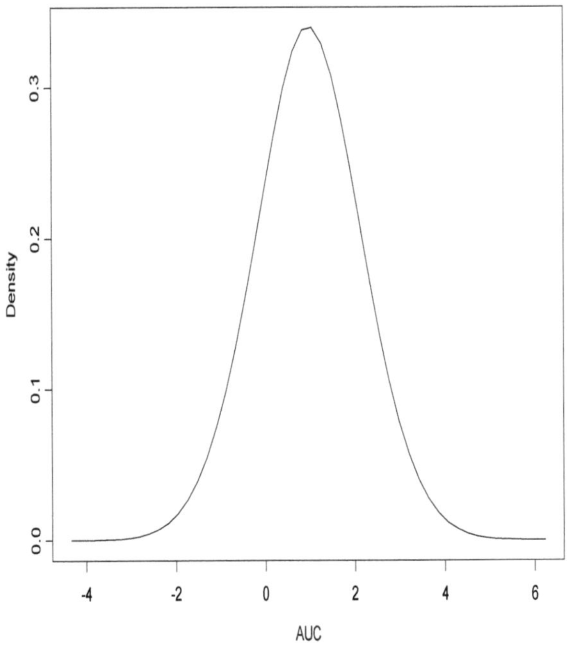

FIGURE 2.1
Normal Distribution (Mean = 1, SD = 1)

axis. For a given interval on the horizontal axis, the area under the curve is the probability of observing the AUC values in that interval. The larger the area of the density, the more likely are we to observe the values in the given interval. The frequency of occurrence of a lot of data in nature is well described by such a distribution. The bulk of the distribution is centered around a parameter known as the mean (μ, the measure of centrality) and is spread out to a certain extent described by the standard deviation (σ, a measure of spread). Half of the distribution falls above μ, and half falls below. Obviously, we do not know a priori what the values of μ and σ are, so we collect data and estimate them using statistics.

The role of a statistician is to use randomization, replication, blocking, and blinding [561] in study design and proper application of models to ensure that the statistics for the parameters we are interested in are accurate and precise.

A great variety of statistical tools have been developed over the last 100 to 200 years [499, 500] to precisely model the behavior of such normally distributed data. However, it is not uncommon for actual data not to behave themselves! AUC and Cmax data are two such examples.

Let us look at Figure 2.1 again to determine why we cannot use it directly here. Note that negative AUC or Cmax values are allowed to occur! Obviously, it doesn't make sense to use this distribution directly to describe AUC or Cmax data. One cannot physiologically have a negative blood concentration level, nor therefore a negative AUC. This situation is just not possible. The lowest they can go is 0.

Statisticians (e.g., [104]) have devised a variety of ways to mathematically "transform" non-normal data such that they can be modelled using the plethora of powerful tools involving the normal distribution which are available [732].

Westlake [1323] determined that AUC and Cmax data were consistent with a log-normal distribution (see [660, 730, 873] for more details). This essentially means that the data are skewed such that AUC and Cmax observations must always be greater than or equal to 0. See Figure 2.2.

Mathematically, this is useful and quite convenient. If AUC and Cmax are log-normal in distribution, by taking the natural logarithm of AUC and Cmax (i.e., by taking a mathematical *transformation*), the resulting log-transformed AUC and Cmax are normally distributed. Hence the name — if one takes the log of a log-normal variable like AUC or Cmax, the resulting log-variable is normal in distribution.

To clarify, we take AUC as described in Figure 2.2 and recognize that the distribution is skewed and log-normally distributed. We then take the natural logarithm of the AUC values, and we get the distribution of **log**AUC plotted in Figure 2.3. Note that, in Figure 2.3, the horizontal axis denotes the natural logarithm of AUC (which is denoted mathematically as ln- or log_e-transformed AUC), which we refer to as logAUC (not AUC as in Figures 2.1 and 2.2). It is permissible for logAUC or logCmax data to have a negative value, as we can always transform their value (by exponentiating) back to their original distribution where the data are always greater than or equal to 0.

To be specific, if AUC is log-normally distributed with mean $\exp(\mu + (1/2)\sigma^2)$ and variance $\exp(2\mu + \sigma^2)(\exp(\sigma^2) - 1)$, then logAUC is normally distributed with mean μ and variance σ^2 [228, 229]. This will become important later in the book as we begin modelling AUC and Cmax data.

There have been debates centered around whether AUC and Cmax are the best endpoints to use for the assessment of bioequivalence. Some findings indicate that AUC and Cmax are not always sufficient to completely demonstrate bioequivalence [729, 1031, 1192]; however, international regulatory authorities have depended on these endpoints since the early 1990s. Pharmacodynamic data or safety data may be required for some drug products (for an example, see [845]). Those interested in looking further into metrics for bioequivalence will find [338] and [302] informative.

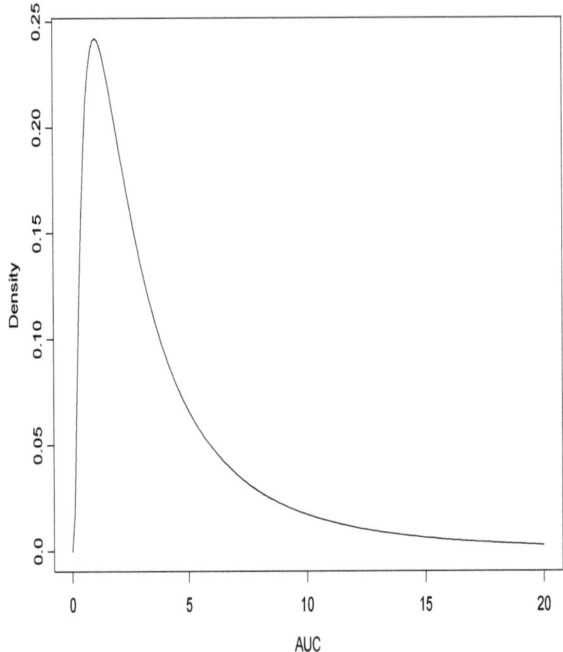

FIGURE 2.2
Log-Normal Distribution

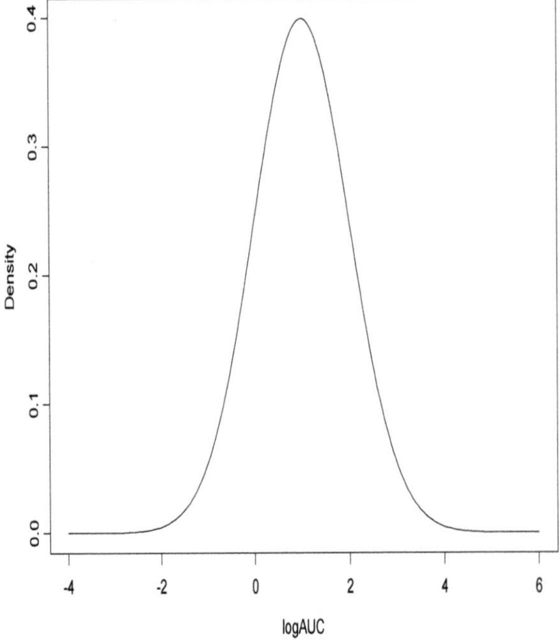

FIGURE 2.3
Normal Distribution Arising from Log-Transformation for AUC Data of Figure 2.2

Recall that AUC is held by international regulators [148, 300, 555] to be a standard measure for extent of bioavailability. Cmax as a measure of rate of bioavailability has been found to be confounded with extent of bioavailability in studies [43] and is known to not characterize the rate of bioavailability particularly well in some situations [148].

Cmax is obviously dependent on the a priori choice of blood sampling scheme. It is known to be generally more variable than AUC and is sometimes problematic in the assessment of bioequivalence [127, 1254]. Regardless of this, however, Cmax has been held to be more reliable in the eyes of regulators than several alternatives [91].

Other measures of rate of absorption have been proposed in the literature, such as Direct Curve Metrics [840] and Cmax/AUC [325], and indirect metrics [1038]. However, simulation-based assessment of alternatives has demonstrated such measures to be less desirable than the use of Cmax to date [1250, 1251]. Recent work in alternative measures of absorption rate such as Partial AUCs [330] is ongoing in response to workshop and regulatory considerations [958, 1131] but these measures have yet to be accepted as useful in bioequivalence assessment [40].

Cmax thus seems to be held as the least undesirable measure available at present for rate of bioavailability [300].

Why did something this complex ever come about? We'll go into that now.

2.2 Why Are BE Studies Performed?

In the late 1960s and 1970s, advances in chemical engineering increased the capability to create inexpensive copies of patented drug products (since termed generics). Following patent expiration, such new formulations could potentially be marketed [1202].

This was desirable from a governmental perspective for public health. Such a practice would be expected to increase the supply of the products in demand in the marketplace, and thereby reduce prices for consumers. This offered substantive benefit to public health (lower costs).

However, when some pharmaceutically equivalent copies of drug products were produced, reports of therapeutic failure received a great deal of public attention in the United States. These failures included lack of desired effect (Amitriptyline, Carbamazepine, Glibenclamide, Oxytetracycline) and undesirable side effects like intoxication (Carbamazepine, Digoxin, Phenytoin). Development of a set of regulated standards for market access was necessary [1034],[25]. The FDA was authorized under the 1984 Drug Price Competition and Patent Term Restoration Act to create an approval process for generic drug products.

The years following revealed increasing trends in market access for generic products [1202]. For approval to market, the FDA decided to require a bioequivalence study for market access with prespecified decision rules for acceptability based on the data collected. Such studies were also required for extension of patent protection for innovators seeking to maintain market exclusivity [608].

2.3 Deciding When Formulations Are Bioequivalent

The FDA initially proposed Decision Rules (sometimes referred to as uniformity requirements) to assess bioequivalence such as the 80/20 and 75/75 rule. The 75/75 rule was defined

such that 75% of subjects' individual ratios of Test to Reference, AUC or Cmax, values must be greater than or equal to the value of 0.75 for bioequivalence to be demonstrated.

While the 75/75 rule would protect against a lack of efficacy associated with decreased plasma concentrations, it obviously would not protect against undesirable side-effects potentially brought about by increased concentrations from a new formulation. Additionally, Haynes [549] established, using simulation studies, that the proposed 75/75 uniformity requirement was highly dependent on the magnitude of within-subject variation. Finally, individual ratios are confounded with period effects. As these effects are known to frequently appear as significant in cross-over studies in normal healthy volunteers [1089], due, for example, to changes in assay procedures between periods, use of the 75/75 rule criteria for bioequivalence assessment was quickly observed to be inappropriate for a large variety of drug products and was dismissed from regulatory practice.

Another idea proposed for testing bioequivalence was to simply test to see whether the formulations were different, and if the test did not demonstrate a significant difference of 20%, then one would accept bioequivalence. This was the 80/20 rule. Let μ_T (μ_R) denote the mean value of logAUC or logCmax, for T (R). Under these criteria, the study first must **not** have rejected the hypothesis H_0 that

$$H_0: \quad \mu_T = \mu_R \tag{2.1}$$

versus

$$H_1: \quad \mu_T \neq \mu_R. \tag{2.2}$$

The estimator, $\hat{\mu}_T - \hat{\mu}_R$, of $\mu_T - \mu_R$, has certain statistical properties (described in the next chapter). These may be used to derive a test statistic and p-value to assess the above null hypothesis H_0.

A p-value is a statistic measuring how convincing is the evidence in the data in favor of H_0. Traditionally, if its value is less than 0.05, the hypothesis H_0 is rejected in favor of its alternative H_1.

Additionally, the study must have had a sufficient number of subjects to rule out the occurrence of a Type 2 error at the rate of 20% when planned to detect a clinically important difference. The use of such a procedure (known as post hoc power calculation, where power equals 1 minus the probability of a Type 2 error) is inappropriate in this context for a variety of reasons [566]. However, the clinically relevant difference was determined to be $\ln 1.25 = 0.2231$ on the log_e scale (a 20% difference on the natural scale). See [40] for details on how this value was chosen by the FDA.

Criticisms of the 80/20 approach to bioequivalence are obvious. Absence of evidence of a significant difference does not imply evidence of absence (for more discussion see [647]). The goal of a bioequivalence study is to generate data to confirm that a difference is **not** present, not to confirm there is one. One could presumably demonstrate BE under the 80/20 rule by running a poorly conducted trial!

The statistical community had been aware, for some time, of better methods to test the hypothesis of equivalence of two treatments relative to a preset, clinically relevant goalpost. Cox [227] related Fieller's theorem [405] for the ratio of two normally distributed means to the conditional distributions used to obtain similar regions based on traditional Neyman–Pearson theory (for the testing of hypotheses; see also [808]). Alteration of the traditional hypothesis tested in clinical trials (Equations (2.1) and (2.2)) to a framework appropriate for equivalence testing was introduced in [290]. In this paper, Dunnett and Gent [290] compared two binomial samples relative to a prespecified goalpost Δ to assess equivalence of the responses to treatment. Westlake ([1321–1323]; for summary of work performed in the 1970s see [1324]) applied similar concepts to the analysis of bioequivalence trials.

In brief, when a bioequivalence study is conducted, the confidence interval for the difference in $\mu_T - \mu_R$ is derived using a model appropriate to the data and the study design. If the confidence interval falls within prespecified goalposts, the formulations are declared bioequivalent. Implementation of the approaches proposed by Westlake [1321–1323] to the question of bioequivalence was initially assessed by Schuirmann [1087] at the FDA and the approaches were subsequently adopted as the regulatory standard of choice.

This procedure was designated the "two one-sided testing procedure" (known as the "TOST").

To clarify, one hypotheses that the AUC and Cmax data in the new formulation are "too low" (H_{01}) relative to the reference formulation or also that they are "too high" (H_{02}). If both hypotheses are rejected by the data in favor of their alternatives (H_{11}, H_{12}), then the new formulation is deemed to be bioequivalent to the reference formulation.

To be specific, under this approach to inference, the usual null hypothesis was reformulated to correspond to the structure of testing the question of bioequivalence:

$$H_{01}: \quad \mu_T - \mu_R \leq -\Delta \tag{2.3}$$

versus the alternative

$$H_{11}: \quad \mu_T - \mu_R > -\Delta$$

and

$$H_{02}: \quad \mu_T - \mu_R \geq \Delta \tag{2.4}$$

versus the alternative

$$H_{12}: \quad \mu_T - \mu_R < \Delta$$

Inference was based on the use of the central t-distribution using a model in a randomized, two-period cross-over design. Summaries of the implementation of such a TOST procedure may be found in [951] and [1190].

The goalpost Δ was again chosen to be equal to $\ln 1.25 = 0.2231$ (corresponding to a 20% range on the natural scale). Schuirmann subsequently refined his work in a publication in 1987 [1088]. For each of the hypotheses H_{01} and H_{02} it was determined that the FDA wanted no more than a 5% chance of a Type 1 error. Recall that this means that the FDA wanted no more than a 5% chance that a study would demonstrate bioequivalence when in truth the formulations were not bioequivalent. Examples of the application of the TOST procedure are given in Chapter 3.

Operationally, the TOST corresponds to showing that a 90% confidence interval for $\mu_T - \mu_R$ is contained in the interval $-\ln 1.25$ to $\ln 1.25$.

Blackwelder [84] and Anderson and Hauck [21] published similar work. These ideas were further developed in [525] and [1045], and general approaches to the question of statistical inference were subsequently summarized under the framework of fiducial probability and inference in [945]. Practical considerations in the design and Type 2 error properties and sample size of such studies were further developed in [1089].

The two one-sided testing procedure was easy to implement for nearly any cross-over study design and had the benefit of being easily interpretable in practice. As described in the last section, its regulatory and public health, statistical, and sponsor considerations were well understood.

The confidence interval provides a plausible range of values within which the true difference in formulation means can be expected to fall [526]. Note that often the results are exponentiated to the natural scale following analysis. On the natural scale, the interval 0.80–1.25 is used to assess whether the formulations are bioequivalent for AUC and Cmax.

The ranges of plausible values as expressed by the confidence intervals were used to assess the degree of equivalence or comparability. Type 1 error was termed "consumer" or "regulator" risk — i.e., the risk to the regulator and consumer in making an incorrect decision, i.e., allowing market access when the application in fact should not be approved. Although often the subject of debate, the choice of $\Delta = \ln 1.25$ gave regulators an easy standard under which to assess the results of such studies.

Randomization to sequence and definition of a washout period sufficient to negate potential residual (i.e., carry-over) effects from the previous period were established as desirable properties in bioequivalence study design. The times at which blood samples were taken was noted as being very important for proper consideration and definition of Cmax, and period effects were noted as being a "recurrent phenomenon" in cross-over designs (due to changes in sample storage, environmental conditions, or assay bias between periods). The use of prospectively designed, randomized cross-over designs was established as the norm for bioequivalence assessment.

Regulatory agencies have little direct interest in the Type 2 error properties of bioequivalence studies under the TOST procedure (this is typically referred to as "sponsor's risk" in this context). The regulator's primary concern is with the significance level at which bioequivalence can be concluded and with ensuring that the design of such studies ensures an unbiased comparison of formulations. Under Schuirmann's TOST procedure, the confidence level (α) was set at 5% per test for an overall study-wise Type 1 error rate of up to 5% [352].

The FDA recommended this in the 1992 guidance [352] and thus specified that subjects must be randomized to sequence. A general linear model (see Chapter 3) would be fitted to the log_e-transformed AUC and Cmax for demonstration of bioequivalence in a two-period cross-over design. Between- and within-subject variances were assumed to be homogeneous across formulations, and AUC and Cmax data were assumed to be log-normally distributed. In practical terms, under the 1992 FDA Guidance, equivalence was demonstrated if the 90% confidence interval (calculated using a linear model appropriate to the study design) for $\exp(\mu_T - \mu_R)$ was contained in the interval 0.80–1.25. Different models should be applied if the study design differs from a two-period cross-over design to construct the confidence intervals for $\mu_T - \mu_R$.

The FDA encouraged those conducting bioequivalence studies to conduct single-dose studies at the maximal dose to be marketed in healthy normal subjects and to ensure an adequate washout period between study periods. AUC and Cmax were designated as the primary endpoints of interest to assess extent and rate of absorption, respectively, in the 1992 FDA Guidance.

2.4 Potential Issues with TOST Bioequivalence

This *average bioequivalence* approach (so-called because it pertains to the equivalence of the means of the test and reference formulations) has safeguarded public health since its adoption [40]. However, it was not without issues.

For narrow therapeutic index drugs (for which a slight change in dose or exposure can cause a large alteration in response to treatment), bioequivalence is regarded as particularly problematic under the average bioequivalence approach [58]. Such drugs, e.g., digoxin and warfarin [216], generally exhibit low within-subject variability (i.e., within-subject coefficients of variation less than 10%). Under the average bioequivalence approach, it is possible [985] to demonstrate bioequivalence of means even in the presence of small but statistically significant changes in means — i.e., as the limits of the confidence interval for the ratio of formulation means fall within 0.80 to 1.25, bioequivalence is demonstrated; however, some confidence intervals will not contain the value 1 and thus are slightly (but significantly) different while still being bioequivalent. Such small changes in mean test to reference rate and extent of exposure are potentially clinically meaningful in a small proportion of patients [40], and some have advocated [25] special equivalence definitions for narrow therapeutic index products whereby such drugs would be held to a stricter regulatory standard (e.g., equivalence limits corresponding to a 10% range on the log_e scale, 0.90 to 1.11).

When issues with average bioequivalence are found for a particular product (e.g., [646]), FDA typically issues a special biopharmaceutical guidance on demonstrating bioequivalence for that particular product to safeguard patients. For example, reports of therapeutic failure for the product Clozapine, an antipsychotic, were published [343]. Clozapine was granted market access following "non-standard" bioequivalence studies mandated by FDA under biowaivers applied for by the manufacturers due to the fact that normal healthy volunteers may not be safely exposed to any dose but the lowest of Clozapine. Reports of therapeutic failure followed in the United States where uncontrolled switching in-clinic was allowed, resulting in significant costs, as this condition requires hospitalization. FDA subsequently required the manufacturers of the generic formulations to perform a better bioequivalence study to maintain market access and developed drug-specific guidance on the topic of Clozapine bioequivalence. Examples of such drug-specific guidance include Potassium-Chloride [350], Metaproterenol and Albuterol [351], Cholestyramine [353], Phenytoin [354], Clozapine [357], and Topical Dermatologics [355].

High-variability products (with within-subject standard deviations in excess of 0.30 [87]), require sample sizes in excess of 30 subjects in order to have less than a 10% to 20% chance of a Type 2 error. Some have argued [874, 875] that small changes in rate and extent of exposure for such products are not clinically meaningful and have advocated allowance of a less strict regulatory standard — e.g., equivalence limits corresponding to a 30% equivalence range on the log_e scale, i.e., 0.70 to 1.43 on the natural scale. As an alternative, equivalence limits could be widened based upon the within-subject variability observed in the study [90, 874, 875, 1079] allowing such drug products easier market access. We will discuss such approaches further in Chapter 7.

The concept of switchability of formulations *for the individual patient* is not addressed by the average bioequivalence criterion [615]. Population means are compared, and variation between individual subjects (or patients) is factored out of the variation used to assess the distance between population means, as described above. Peace [977], Anderson and Hauck [22], Hauck and Anderson [528], and Welleck [1311] introduced the concept of *individual* bioequivalence. Under this approach, the question, asked is "Can I safely and effectively switch my patient from their current formulation to another?"

Average bioequivalence is a special case of what in [528] is termed *population* bioequivalence. This type of bioequivalence addresses the question, "Can I safely and effectively start my patient on the currently approved formulation or another?" Differences in variation between formulations should also be considered when determining whether a formulation will be equally effective and safe when administering the commercial formulation of a new drug product relative to that used in clinical trials in Phase III. It is not clear in this context whether comparison of within-subject variances or total variances (so termed as the sum of between- and within-subject variance for a given formulation) is the appropriate variance for comparison between formulations, and arguments [487, 529] have been offered for both in this context.

Techniques for comparing within-subject variances in a two-period cross-over (under the assumption that between-subject variances across formulations are homogeneous) had been developed in [991] and [891]. Alternatively, the total variances between formulations (between- plus within-subject variance) can be compared using a similar procedure.

Most techniques for assessment of the equality of variances assume that variance components are independent [36, 121], a condition not met in the correlated data encountered in cross-over trials. Bristol [113, 114] developed practical maximum likelihood techniques for comparing within-subject variances in this context based on techniques discussed in [832]. Cornell [223] derived nonparametric tests of dispersion for the two-period cross-over design. Chow and Liu [196] described similar procedures, and [1293] and [494, 495] described similar procedures in publications. These techniques reduce to different transformations to assess unequal marginal scales in a bivariate normal population [692], and such comparisons were also addressed in work in [78], [297], [857], and [48]. More recent work is published in [751].

Comparisons of total- or within-subject variance between formulations can be accomplished using such procedures; however, it is known [1388, 1389] that variance components are ill-characterized in cross-over studies of the size usually performed. Increasing sample size [1389] can improve the precision of estimated variance components; however, it is unusual for such studies to be performed except in the case of highly variable drug products [1388].

Moreover, while such procedures are theoretically and statistically viable, they are highly dependent [1271] on the choice of estimation procedure. Estimates for between-subject variance can be negative under a method-of-moments based procedure or maximum-likelihood procedure [114]. Such estimates may be positively biased [334] when using a restricted-maximum-likelihood based estimation procedure as would be expected in a procedure constrained in the likelihood to only permit estimates greater than or equal to zero for between-subject variances and correlation constrained to lie in the range [-1, 1] (see references [241, 652, 961, 1271]).

We will not discuss the comparison of variances further in this book, as such techniques are not applied in the regulatory assessment of bioequivalence. Those interested in further information on the topic should read information on this topic in [196] and the publications noted above.

Consideration of these individual and population bioequivalence ideas (and sundry others) led the FDA to form a bioequivalence working group in the mid-1990s. This body (composed of FDA representatives from clinical, scientific, and statistical disciplines) was tasked with determining whether a public health risk under the average bioequivalence approach could exist [870] and if so to determine a method or methods to evaluate bioequivalence in a manner to protect the public health. A description of the ideas under discussion may be found in [19, 20, 23, 165–167, 483, 529, 957] but will not be discussed further here.

After considering the public comments on the preliminary draft 1997 guidance [358], the FDA reissued two draft guidances on the topic of bioequivalence in August 1999 ([362, 363] replacing the draft guidance issued in 1997). These two guidances described when to perform a relative bioavailability, population, or individual bioequivalence study [362] for drug products in solution, suspensions, aerosols and for topical administration and for the more usual immediate-release and modified-release orally administered drug products. General guidance for study design (discussed earlier in this chapter) was provided.

The FDA acknowledged in the new draft guidance [362] that narrow therapeutic index drugs should be held to a stricter equivalence criterion than the usual 20% range required in the existing FDA guidance [352]. For these drug products, a 10% range on the log_e scale (corresponding to an equivalence range of 0.90–1.11 on the natural scale) was required. However, this requirement was removed in the final revised FDA guidance [373].

The second draft guidance from the FDA [363] described in more detail the study design, model, and approach to statistical inference for average, population, and individual bioequivalence relative to the 1997 draft guidance, but departed from the original approach only in minor respects. Requirements for power and sample size were described in more detail in this draft guidance relative to the original 1997 draft guidance; however, the main departure was in the model used for statistical inference.

The FDA followed up in 2000 [366] with the introduction of the "Biopharmaceutical Classification System." Orally administered drug products are categorized based upon in vitro testing into classes I, II, III, or IV. Class I compounds, known as highly soluble and permeable in that they are quick to dissolve when ingested and are absorbed directly into the body quickly, are exempt from the requirements of demonstrating bioequivalence in a clinical study and only must demonstrate that in vitro dissolution profiles for the formulations under study are equivalent. The choice of reference product is of importance in this setting [1180]. Under the BCS guidance, only Class II, III, and IV drugs are required to demonstrate in vivo bioequivalence before being granted market access. A study of the impact of this approach is given in [221].

The FDA guidance [367] finalized in October 2000 indicated that the agency would adopt the 2000 guidances [366, 367] as final. However, following additional discussion at the 2001 Pharmaceutical Sciences Advisory Committee, the FDA provided revised final guidance [373] which removed the potential for using population and individual bioequivalence for market access. It is possible that in the future the use of these criteria will be reinvestigated if the FDA determines that there is a need for such based upon observations of the marketplace.

2.5 Current International Regulation

To summarise, the debate on how to do bioequivalence trials culminated in 1987 [1088] when Schuirmann's two one-sided testing method for a regulatory set goalpost of $\ln 1.25$ was introduced using the pharmacokinetic measures of AUC and Cmax as surrogate markers for efficacy and safety by the FDA.

In general, the AUC and Cmax refer to the parent compound being administered (not any metabolites produced in the body). However, under unusual circumstances, it may be important to measure metabolite AUC and Cmax also for the assessment of average bioequivalence. See [629] and [631] for more details.

The design of choice was determined to be a randomized, 2×2, two-period cross-over in normal healthy volunteers to isolate and quantify any differences in formulation, and regulatory risk was set at 5% per test. The design and analysis of cross-over studies had been extensively developed by this time [652, 1113], and statistical considerations in power and sample size were described in [260].

For long half-life drugs (where the wash-out period would be so long that a cross-over design is not feasible), a parallel group design where subjects are randomized to receive one or the other formulation may be applied.

This approach was formalized in the 1992 FDA Guidance [352] and applied to both pre- and post-marketing approvals for changes in formulation. Average bioequivalence quickly became an international standard, with most nations utilizing the FDA's 1992 guidance or slight modifications to the approach.

This procedure was adopted as the standard method by European [308] and Canadian [140, 141] regulatory authorities subsequent to finalization of the US FDA guidance in 1992 [148, 1193].

Japan [634], China [183], and Australia [33] also follow this procedure (with minor changes in study design or decision rules) for the assessment of bioequivalence.

To date, the vast majority of products which have utilized this approach have not been observed to have marketplace failures in terms of their safety and efficacy profiles (see [40] for more details). Average bioequivalence testing of $\delta = \mu_T - \mu_R$ has thus been established de facto as a surrogate marker for public safety based primarily upon observation, consistency of knowledge, and replication of findings of the application of the FDA guidance [352] and less upon quantified, scientific assessment of biological plausibility and strength of association.

Average bioequivalence did, however, have the potential for issues in implementation with regard to the regulatory, statistical, and sponsor considerations discussed earlier in this chapter. One potential difficulty was regulatory in nature. The approach was concerned with testing only the formulation means and did not contain any explicit criteria pertaining to individual subjects, and it was felt that the inclusion of criteria relating to variation might address such points. Another potential area of difficulty involved both regulatory and sponsor considerations. The regulatory limits of 20% were also questioned, as they might be too large for low variability products with a narrow therapeutic index, and the 20% acceptance limits created a practical difficulty for sponsors due to the large sample sizes needed to ensure a high probability of success for high variability products.

The FDA addressed the issue presented by low variability drugs by tightening the range in some instances, and it was known alternative designs [1271] and mixed modelling approaches [689] could be used to demonstrate average bioequivalence to address sponsors' considerations for highly variable drug products.

The FDA opened the discussion on the resolution of the theoretical "individual subjects switchability" issue with the publication of the 1997 preliminary draft guidance [358] and significant international debate followed. This debate resolved in 2003 [373] with a decision to continue using average bioequivalence.

Average bioequivalence in practice has been "harmonized" to assess the difference in means between formulations in a relatively standard fashion throughout most of the world today [245].

Recently, the FDA and EMEA both proposed that specific study designs and/or testing procedures be used in certain cases for what is termed highly variable drugs [243, 440]. These "scaled average bioequivalence" approaches (SABE) are not the same mathematically and statistically, and those adopting the approach should plan to consult with the local regulatory authority to ensure acceptability prior to performing the clinical trial. These approaches will be discussed further in Chapter 7.

Readers interested in more information on the USA FDA's perspective will find the review article [1393] of interest. This review article also covers perspectives on unusual products such as inhaled and complex (i.e., combination) drug products.

2.6 Some Practical Notes

In most cases, multiple AUC endpoints are derived in bioequivalence datasets. In general, if half-life ($T_{\frac{1}{2}}$, see Chapter 1) can be estimated, it will be used to calculate AUC(0-∞) as described in Equation (1.1). However, if insufficient concentration data are captured during elimination of the drug, half-life may not be subject to estimation, and therefore AUC(0-t) will be used in statistical evaluation. Recall that, in this context, t denotes the last quantifiable concentration during the period in which samples are captured.

The t in AUC(0-t) may differ across periods for any given subject. In datasets where marked differences between the last quantifiable time t are present between periods and half-life cannot be estimated, it may be preferable to consider an endpoint like AUC(0-t'). Here, t' denotes the last quantifiable concentration time in common across periods for a given subject.

The decision about which AUC endpoint is primary and which will provide supportive information should be made prior to analysis to prevent the introduction of bias into interpretation of the data [1113]. It is unusual for AUC(0-t') to be used, as most BE studies are designed to ensure sufficient samples are taken during elimination to ensure half-life can be estimated. FDA guidance [373] recommends that both AUC(0-t) and AUC(0-∞) be provided in submissions.

In cases where multiple "peaks" in blood concentration are observed, it is common practice for the first [373] to be chosen as Cmax, with the corresponding time relative to dose being Tmax. The value of Tmax is highly dependent on the choice of sampling times. Its use in bioequivalence studies is that of an endpoint providing supportive information. Some nations [140, 141] require that Tmax be analyzed as if it were normally distributed.

3

Testing for Average Bioequivalence

Introduction

There is nothing like a little pressure to brighten up one's day, and this one was no exception. I had arrived as usual at the clinical pharmacology unit and was at work preparing a study design proposal when my boss walked into my office.

She had run up the stairs. My office by this time (about two years after I had hired on) was one floor up and well away from my clinical colleagues, who tended to be a bit noisy and nosy. The first was no problem (get some earplugs), but the second is irritating for a working statistician. They were always stopping by for just a "peek" at the data, but they were full of questions. Answer one and at least a dozen more pop out. After about two years, one figures out that a little distance is not a bad thing (and no peeking).

After she got her breath back, she told me that one of my colleagues from Pharmacokinetics had a bioequivalence dataset that needed to be looked at Stat (an expression the clinicians used all the time). I'm guessing that Stat in clinician-speak means "run the tests as soon as humanly possible." I guess they like to think that we sit around twiddling our thumbs unless they shout Stat repeatedly.

There is one certainty in drug development and statistics that one can depend on: the data are always late. There are always reasons that someone wanted to know the findings yesterday. Sometimes it is even a good reason!

Like the subject of statistics itself, after you get used to it, it does not bother you too much.

In any event, it was 10:30, and the results were needed by lunchtime. After making sure she meant a late lunch (she did not), I hastily pulled the code you will see later in this chapter, grabbed the data, and went to work.

We ***did*** *have a late lunch that day, by the way. Analysis of bioequivalence data is not as simple as pressing a button.*

3.1 Background

In the previous chapter we briefly introduced the 2×2 cross-over trial and the TOST (two one-sided testing) procedure. In this chapter we will describe in some detail how data obtained from a 2×2 trial can be used to test for Average Bioequivalence (ABE). To illustrate the analyses, we will use the data given in Table 3.1.

It can be seen that data were collected on 32 subjects; 17 received the formulations in the order RT and 15 in the order TR. The original design of the trial planned for an equal number of subjects in each group. However, it is usual for such studies to over-enroll to ensure that an adequate number complete the trial (without having to go to the trouble of replacing dropouts). In this case, some of the subjects did not turn up to participate in the trial. We will discuss other such practical issues of the planning of trials in a subsequent chapter.

Before we proceed to test for ABE, we will explore the data graphically. The main reason for using a cross-over design is to make comparisons between the two formulations "within" each subject and as a result to eliminate any between-subject variability. Figure 3.1 is a

TABLE 3.1: Example 3.1

	Sequence RT			
	AUC Period		Cmax Period	
Subject	1	2	1	2
1	2849	2230	499	436
4	2790	2864	733	416
5	2112	1744	344	48
8	1736	1882	342	437
9	1356	1175	357	240
11	1775	1585	442	286
16	2997	2237	425	332
17	1973	1778	423	407
19	1454	1297	256	348
21	2469	2023	392	480
24	1584	1855	316	373
25	4004	2449	465	625
28	1944	1593	502	326
29	1175	1147	248	221
31	1696	1801	390	350
34	1737	1655	425	319
36	2040	2199	464	384
	Sequence TR			
Subject	1	2	1	2
2	2025	2000	438	361
3	2090	1826	535	558
6	2006	1881	443	681
7	2202	1935	446	481
10	1838	1602	310	340
12	1898	2504	323	331
15	1129	1036	308	243
18	2014	1938	552	427
20	1900	1730	355	401
22	1763	1472	213	177
23	1678	1336	487	412
26	2271	2389	422	731
27	1986	1857	560	461
30	2519	1941	537	400
35	1560	1629	463	372
R=Reference, T=Test				

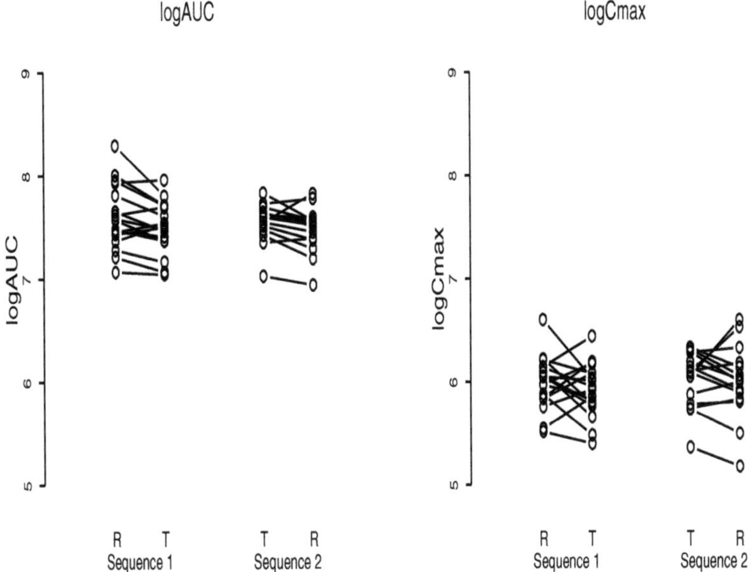

FIGURE 3.1
Example 3.1: Subject Profiles Plot

subject-profiles plot ([652], Ch. 2) and displays the between-subject variability and the difference in response between the two formulations within each subject. The left panel displays the logAUC values and the right panel the logCmax values.

As explained in the previous chapter, the analysis is done on the natural log-transformed data; hence, most of the figures in this chapter will use that scale of measurement. The subject-profiles plot is constructed for each sequence by first plotting on the vertical axis, for each subject, the Period 1 and Period 2 responses against the values 1 and 2, respectively, and then joining the two responses with a line. In our plot we have replaced the axis labels for Period 1 and Period 2 with the corresponding treatment labels, so that the treatment ordering within each sequence is evident. The distance between the periods (i.e., between the R and T labels) on the horizontal axis is a matter of taste.

The expected large variation over the subjects is very evident from the vertical spread of the points in the plot. If the two formulations were identical and there were no variation in the two responses from a subject, then the plot would consist of parallel lines in a "ladder-like" pattern. If, in addition, there were no period effect, the lines would be horizontal: if there were a period effect, all the lines would either slope upward or all the lines would slope downward. In Figure 3.1, within a sequence, some lines go up as the formulation changes within a subject and other lines go down. It is not possible at this preliminary stage of analysis to determine whether the within-patient variability is just random noise or due to a true difference between the two formulations or between the two periods.

Another useful plot is the paired-agreement plot (see [491]). Here the test response is plotted against the reference response for each subject. Figure 3.2 shows, for simulated sets of data, the patterns that might be seen in such a plot. These patterns correspond to (i) no difference between the two responses on a subject (Identity), (ii) a period difference in the absence of a formulation difference (Period difference), (iii) a formulation difference in the absence of a period difference (Formulation difference), and finally (iv) when there is

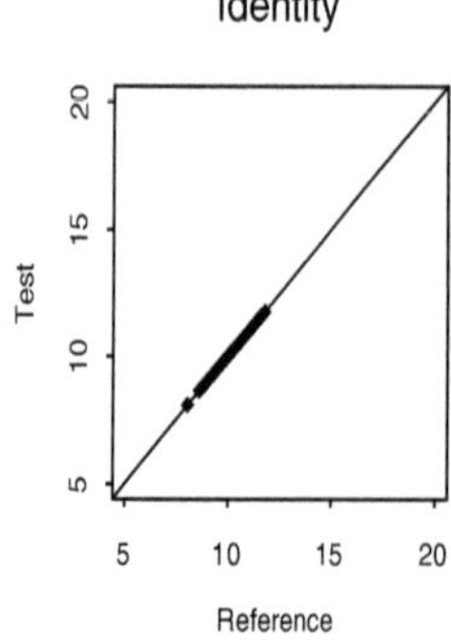

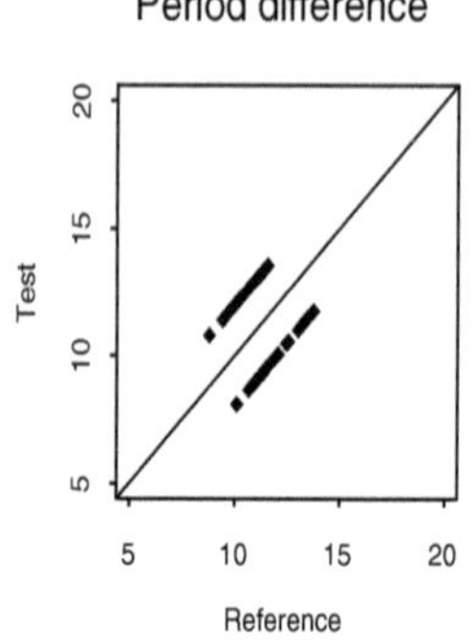

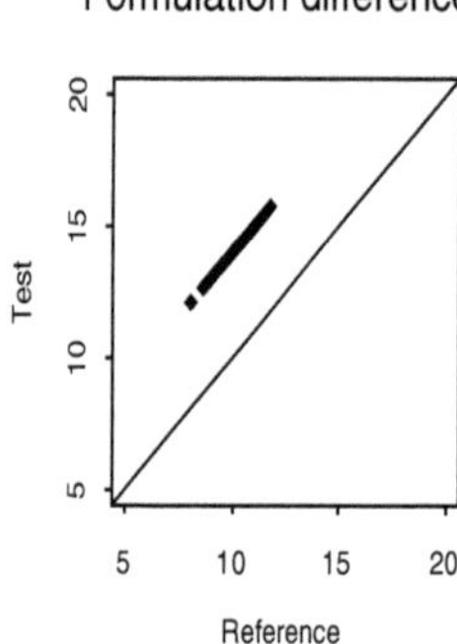

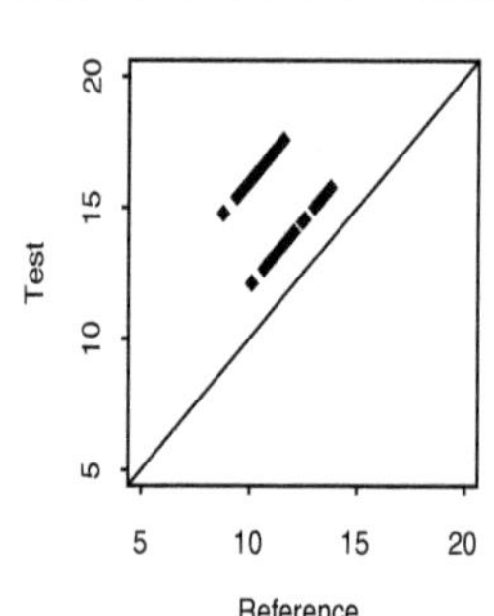

FIGURE 3.2
Examples of Patterns in a Paired-Agreement Plot

both a period difference and a formulation difference. To emphasize the underlying pattern in each plot, we have removed the within-subject variability.

For Example 3.1, the paired-agreement plots for logAUC and logCmax are shown in Figure 3.3. The patterns in the plots suggest there is a period difference but no formulation difference. In addition, we can see larger within-subject variation in the logCmax values.

In order to make a proper determination of any differences in response between formulations, we need to specify a statistical linear model that will allow for any systematic effects that we believe are present in the data a priori. These systematic (fixed) effects are identified during the design phase of the trial and in our case are the sequence, formulation, and period effects. In the previous chapter, reference was briefly made to so-called carry-over effects. If the effect of the formulation given in the first period is still present at the start of the second period, then we refer to that effect as the (first-order) carry-over effect of that formulation. If a long enough washout period is used to separate the two active periods (5 half-lives is recommended) then there should not be any pharmacological carry-over from the first period to the second.

Models will now be developed to generate summary statistics which account for these factors, characterize the distribution of the difference in formulation means, and to allow us to better assess the noise in the data. The essential feature of the TOST procedure is the calculation of a 90% confidence interval for $\mu_T - \mu_R$, the mean difference between the formulations on the log scale. To calculate this confidence interval, we need an estimate of

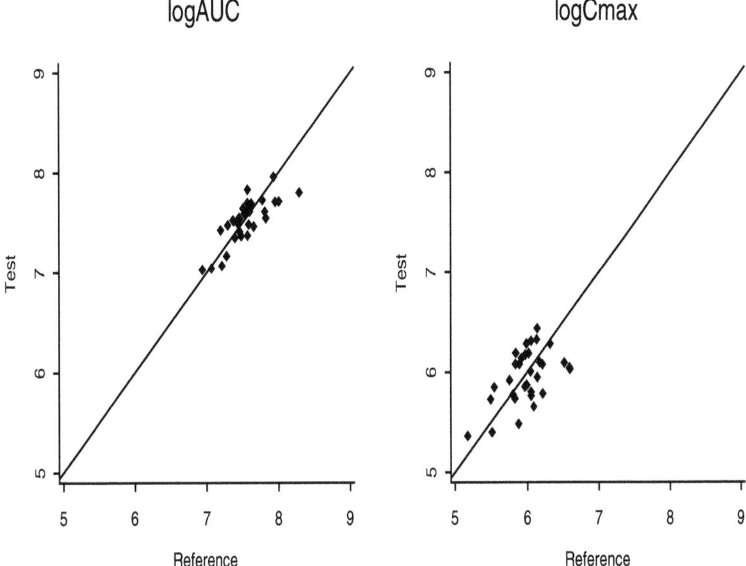

FIGURE 3.3
Example 3.1: Paired-Agreement Plots

$\mu_T - \mu_R$, and this can be done by specifying a statistical (linear) model for the logAUC and logCmax values observed on the subjects.

3.2 Linear Model for 2×2 Data

In order to define the linear model, let y_{ijk} denote the response (i.e., logAUC or logCmax) in period j on subject k in sequence group i, where $i = 1, 2$, $j = 1, 2$, $k = 1, 2, \ldots, n_i$, and n_i is the number of subjects in group i. The total number of subjects in the trial is $n = n_1 + n_2$. The systematic effects we anticipate are due to the periods and formulations. As the subjects are allocated randomly to the two groups, there should be no sequence effect (i.e., a significant difference in mean response between the two sequence groups). However, it is traditional to include such an effect and we will do so here. The notation we will use is that μ denotes the overall mean response, τ_R and τ_T are the formulation effects, π_1 and π_2 are the period effects, and γ_1 and γ_2 are the sequence effects. The fixed effects model (i.e., the systematic effects) for each of the four group-by-period response combinations is displayed in Table 3.2.

TABLE 3.2
Fixed Effects in the Linear Model for the 2×2 Design

Group	Period 1	Period 2
1(RT)	$\mu + \tau_R + \pi_1 + \gamma_1$	$\mu + \tau_T + \pi_2 + \gamma_1$
2(TR)	$\mu + \tau_T + \pi_1 + \gamma_2$	$\mu + \tau_R + \pi_2 + \gamma_2$

TABLE 3.3
Fixed Effects: Alternative Parametrization for the 2×2 Design

Group	Period 1	Period 2
1(RT)	$\mu_R + \pi_1 + \gamma_1$	$\mu_T + \pi_2 + \gamma_1$
2(TR)	$\mu_T + \pi_1 + \gamma_2$	$\mu_R + \pi_2 + \gamma_2$

As we will explain later, the difference in carry-over effects, if any, between the formulations is aliased with (i.e., completely mixed up with) any difference between the sequence effects, so including sequence effects in our model does have some potential benefits, which we will explore later. As regards the parameters themselves, they are all defined with reference to an overall mean response parameter μ. The result of moving from R to T, for example, is to cause an increase or a decrease in response relative to the overall mean. Consequently, as it is only the size of the increase or decrease that needs to be accounted for, two different formulation parameters, τ_R and τ_T, are not needed. To remove this redundancy, a constraint is typically applied such as $\tau_R + \tau_T = 0$. The result of this is that we can refer to $\mu_R = \mu + \tau_R$ and $\mu_T = \mu + \tau_T$ as the means for formulations R and T, respectively. This alternative parametrization is displayed in Table 3.3. For exactly the same reasons, a constraint is also placed on the period and sequence parameters, e.g., $\pi_1 + \pi_2 = 0$ and $\gamma_1 + \gamma_2 = 0$. The choice of constraint is not unique and we could have chosen $\tau_R = 0$ and $\pi_1 = 0$, for example. What is important to remember is that, although the choice of constraint is arbitrary, the difference $\mu_T - \mu_R$ is uniquely identified.

Coming now to the "random-effects" part of our model, we need to allow for the variation between patients that was so evident in Figures 3.1 and 3.3 and for any "residual" random variation that is unexplained by the rest of the terms in the model. This is done by introducing two random variables: $\xi_{k(i)}$, to allow for variation between subjects, and ε_{ijk}, to allow for unexplained variation between the two responses on the same subject. The random effects are displayed in Table 3.4 for a typical subject k in Group 1(RT) and for a typical subject k' in Group 2(TR). Dropping the distinction between k and k', we assume that $\xi_{k(i)}$ and ε_{ijk} are independent random variables such that $\mathrm{E}(\xi_{k(i)}) = 0$, $\mathrm{Var}(\xi_{k(i)}) = \sigma_B^2$, $\mathrm{E}(\varepsilon_{ijk}) = 0$, and $\mathrm{Var}(\varepsilon_{ijk}) = \sigma_W^2$, where σ_B^2 is the between-subject variance and σ_W^2 is the within-subject variance. E denotes the expected value (i.e., population mean) for a given parameter, and Var denotes its variance. We also assume that the $\xi_{k(i)}$ are independent among themselves and that the ε_{ijk} are independent among themselves.

The complete model for y_{ijk} is then

$$y_{ijk} = \mu_{d[i,j]} + \pi_j + \gamma_i + \xi_{k(i)} + \varepsilon_{ijk}, \tag{3.1}$$

where $d[i,j] = R$ or T and identifies the formulation in period j of sequence i.

We note that the variance of a response on subject k in group i in period j is

$$\sigma^2 = \mathrm{Var}(y_{ijk}) = \mathrm{Var}(\xi_{k(i)} + \varepsilon_{ijk}) = \sigma_B^2 + \sigma_W^2. \tag{3.2}$$

TABLE 3.4
Random Effects in the Linear Model for the 2×2 Design

Group	Period 1	Period 2
1(RT)	$\xi_{k(1)} + \varepsilon_{11k}$	$\xi_{k(1)} + \varepsilon_{12k}$
2(TR)	$\xi_{k'(2)} + \varepsilon_{21k'}$	$\xi_{k'(2)} + \varepsilon_{22k'}$

The covariance between two responses on the same subject is

$$\text{Cov}(y_{i1k}, y_{i2k}) = \text{Cov}(\xi_{k(i)} + \varepsilon_{i1k}, \xi_{k(i)} + \varepsilon_{i2k}) =$$
$$\text{Cov}(\xi_{k(i)}, \xi_{k(i)}) = \text{Var}(\xi_{k(i)}) = \sigma_B^2.$$

Hence, the correlation between two responses on the same subject is

$$\rho = \text{Corr}(y_{i1k}, y_{i2k}) = \frac{\sigma_B^2}{\sigma_B^2 + \sigma_W^2}. \tag{3.3}$$

Returning now to the estimation of $\mu_T - \mu_R$, let $\bar{y}_{ij.} = \frac{1}{n_{ij}} \sum_{k=1}^{n_{ij}} y_{ijk}$ denote the mean response of the subjects in period j in sequence group i.

$$\text{For Group 1: E}(\bar{y}_{11.} - \bar{y}_{12.}) = \pi_1 - \pi_2 + \mu_R - \mu_T.$$

$$\text{For Group 2: E}(\bar{y}_{21.} - \bar{y}_{22.}) = \pi_1 - \pi_2 + \mu_T - \mu_R.$$

Hence,

$$\text{E}\left\{\frac{1}{2}\left[(\bar{y}_{21.} - \bar{y}_{22.}) - (\bar{y}_{11.} - \bar{y}_{12.})\right]\right\} = \mu_T - \mu_R. \tag{3.4}$$

This expression in (3.4) is a key fundamental finding in working with cross-over designs and should be emphasized. By taking the difference across periods within sequence, and then combining the data across sequences, the result is an unbiased expression for the finding that is of key interest, the difference between formulations.

That is,

$$\hat{\mu}_T - \hat{\mu}_R = \frac{1}{2}(\bar{y}_{21.} - \bar{y}_{22.} - \bar{y}_{11.} + \bar{y}_{12.}) \tag{3.5}$$

and

$$\text{Var}(\hat{\mu}_T - \hat{\mu}_R) = \frac{1}{4}\left[\frac{\sigma_W^2}{n_1} + \frac{\sigma_W^2}{n_1} + \frac{\sigma_W^2}{n_2} + \frac{\sigma_W^2}{n_2}\right] = \frac{\sigma_W^2}{2}\left[\frac{1}{n_1} + \frac{1}{n_2}\right]. \tag{3.6}$$

If $n_1 = n_2 = n/2$, then

$$\text{Var}(\hat{\mu}_T - \hat{\mu}_R) = \frac{\sigma_W^2}{2}\left[\frac{2}{n} + \frac{2}{n}\right] = \frac{2\sigma_W^2}{n}. \tag{3.7}$$

If $\hat{\sigma}_W^2$ is an estimate of σ_W^2 on $n-2$ degrees of freedom (d.f.) and $t_{0.95}(n-2)$ is the upper 95% percentile of the t–distribution on $n-2$ d.f., the 90% confidence interval for $\mu_T - \mu_R$ is

$$\hat{\mu}_T - \hat{\mu}_R \pm t_{0.95}(n-2)\sqrt{\frac{\hat{\sigma}_W^2}{2}\left[\frac{1}{n_1} + \frac{1}{n_2}\right]}. \tag{3.8}$$

The groups-by-periods means for Example 3.1 are given in Table 3.5.

Finally, we display a plot that is directly linked to the linear model and displays information on both the formulation difference within subjects and their variability. In this "Mean Differences versus Totals" plot we plot for each subject k in Group i, the mean difference $d_{ik} = (y_{i1k} - y_{i2k})/2$ against the total $t_{ik} = y_{i1k} + y_{i2k}$ (see [652] and [491]). The resulting plot is given in Figure 3.4, where open symbols are used for the subjects in Group 1. The two large diamonds on each plot indicate the position of the centroids $[(\bar{t}_{1.}, \bar{d}_{1.}), (\bar{t}_{2.}, \bar{d}_{2.})]$. The vertical difference between the centroids within a plot is the value of $\hat{\mu}_T - \hat{\mu}_R$. We can

TABLE 3.5
Example 3.1: Groups-by-Periods Means (sample size in parentheses)

	logAUC		
Group	Period 1	Period 2	Mean
1(RT)	$\bar{y}_{11.} = 7.60(17)$	$\bar{y}_{12.} = 7.50(17)$	$\bar{y}_{1..} = 7.55$
2(TR)	$\bar{y}_{21.} = 7.55(15)$	$\bar{y}_{22.} = 7.48(15)$	$\bar{y}_{2..} = 7.51$
Mean	$\bar{y}_{.1.} = 7.58$	$\bar{y}_{.2.} = 7.49$	$\bar{y}_{...} = 7.53$
	logCmax		
1(RT)	$\bar{y}_{11.} = 5.99(17)$	$\bar{y}_{12.} = 5.91(17)$	$\bar{y}_{1..} = 5.95$
2(TR)	$\bar{y}_{21.} = 6.02(15)$	$\bar{y}_{22.} = 5.99(15)$	$\bar{y}_{2..} = 6.01$
Mean	$\bar{y}_{.1.} = 6.01$	$\bar{y}_{.2.} = 5.95$	$\bar{y}_{...} = 5.98$

see that, for both logAUC and logCmax, the centroids are close together, suggesting that T and R might be ABE. The solid and dashed lines in each plot give the positions of the convex hulls, one for each group. The convex hull connects the "outermost" points in a group, and is a useful way of displaying the variation in the d_{ik} and t_{ik}. There is an impression that variability is higher in Group 1 for both logAUC and logCmax. The usefulness of plotting the subject totals is that the difference $\bar{t}_{1.} - \bar{t}_{2.}$ is an estimate of the difference in the carry-effects of T and R (see [652], Chapter 2). For BE trials with an adequate washout period, this difference should be zero. Testing for a difference in carry-over effects in the RT/TR design is problematic, and we do not recommend it. We say more on carry-over effects in Section 3.4.

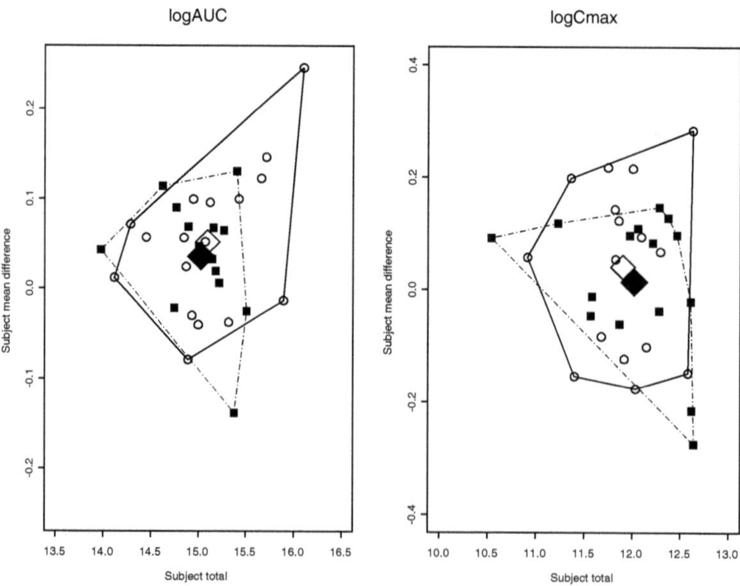

FIGURE 3.4
Example 3.1: Mean Differences versus Totals Plot

3.3 Applying the TOST Procedure

The SAS code to fit Model (3.1) and calculate the 90% confidence interval is given in the following boxes. An edited version of the output produced is given in the boxes immediately following the SAS code. The results of applying the TOST procedure are given in Table 3.6.

The ABE limits are (-0.2231, 0.2231) on the log scale and $(0.8, 1.25)$ on the original scale. Clearly the confidence intervals for both AUC and Cmax are well with the ABE limits and so T and R can be declared equivalent based on the ABE criterion.

A graphical representation of the results is given in Figure 3.5, where the density of the normal distribution based on the fitted mean and standard error for each of logAUC and logCmax are plotted along with the ABE limits. Both densities are well within the limits, indicating that T and R are average bioequivalent. It is also apparent that the density for logCmax is wider than that for logAUC, indicating that Cmax is a more variable metric than AUC in this particular trial.

We note that the estimated correlation between the two responses on the same subject can be estimated from the SAS output. For logAUC $\hat{\sigma}_B^2 = 0.052$ and appears under the output heading of Covariance Parameter Estimates in the row labelled SUBJECT(SEQUENCE). For logAUC, $\hat{\sigma}_W^2 = 0.011$ and appears in the row labelled Residual. The estimated correlation coefficient for logAUC is then $\hat{\rho}_{\text{logAUC}} = 0.052/(0.052 + 0.011) = 0.83$. For logCmax the corresponding value is $\hat{\rho}_{\text{logCmax}} = 0.045/(0.045 + 0.038) = 0.54$. There is a higher level of total variability for logCmax as compared to logAUC, as was already concluded from Figures 3.3 and 3.4.

ABE Example 3.1 — SAS `proc mixed` *Code:*

```
data ABEexample1;
input subject sequence$
formulation$ period AUC CMAX;
logauc=log(AUC);
logcmax=log(CMAX);
datalines;
 1 RT R 1 2849 499
 1 RT T 2 2230 436
 . . . .   .   .
 . . . .   .   .
 . . . .   .   .
35 TR R 2 1629 372
35 TR T 1 1560 463
;
run;

proc mixed data=ABEexample1;
class sequence subject period
formulation;
model logauc=sequence period
formulation/ddfm=kenwardroger;
random subject(sequence);
lsmeans formulation/pdiff cl alpha=0.1;
estimate 'ABE for logAUC' formulation -1 1;
run;
```

ABE Example 3.1 — SAS `proc mixed` *Code, continued:*

```
proc mixed data=ABEexample1;
class sequence subject period formulation;
model logcmax=sequence period formulation/
ddfm=kenwardroger;
random subject(sequence);
lsmeans formulation/pdiff cl alpha=0.1;
estimate 'ABE for logCmax' formulation -1 1;
run;
```

ABE Example 3.1 — Edited SAS Output:

```
Log AUC
Covariance Parameter Estimates
Cov Parm                  Estimate
SUBJECT(SEQUENCE)          0.0516
Residual                   0.0110
                    Standard
Effect  Estimate Error   DF
T-R     -0.0166   0.0263  30
Alpha  Lower    Upper
0.1    -0.0612  0.0280
```

ABE Example 3.1 — Edited SAS Output:

```
Log Cmax
Covariance Parameter Estimates
Estimate SUBJECT(SEQUENCE) 0.04528
Residual                   0.03835
                    Standard
Effect  Estimate Error   DF
T-R     -0.0269  0.0490  30
Alpha  Lower    Upper
0.1    -0.1102  0.0563
```

TABLE 3.6
Example 3.1: TOST Procedure Results

Endpoint	$\hat{\mu}_T - \hat{\mu}_R$	90% Confidence Interval
AUC	-0.0166	(-0.0612, 0.0280)
Cmax	-0.0269	(-0.1102, 0.0563)
Endpoint	$\exp(\hat{\mu}_T - \hat{\mu}_R)$	90% Confidence Interval
AUC	0.98	(0.94, 1.03)
Cmax	0.97	(0.90, 1.06)

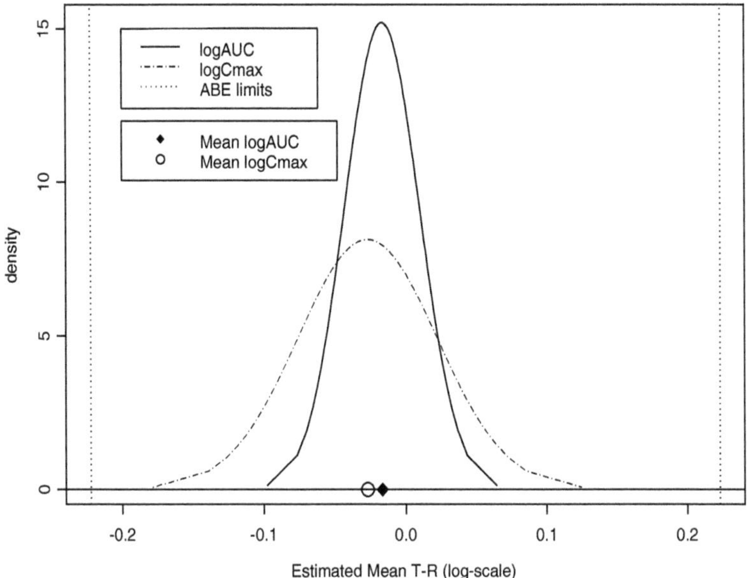

FIGURE 3.5
Example 3.1: Fitted Normal Densities for $\hat{\mu}_T - \hat{\mu}_R$

As a final summary we display the confidence intervals on the natural scale alongside a plot of the ratios T:R for each of AUC and Cmax in Figure 3.6. We note that, for Cmax especially, there are many subjects that have ratios outside the ABE limits of (0.8, 1.25). This example highlights that fact that, to be equivalent on the ABE criterion, it is only necessary to show that the means of T and R do not differ to a significant extent.

Before leaving this section, we demonstrate that the confidence interval testing approach we have used is equivalent to the alternative version of the TOST procedure that requires the testing of two one-sided hypotheses:

$$H_{01}: \quad \mu_T - \mu_R \leq -\Delta \tag{3.9}$$

versus the alternative

$$H_{11}: \quad \mu_T - \mu_R > -\Delta$$

and

$$H_{02}: \quad \mu_T - \mu_R \geq \Delta \tag{3.10}$$

versus the alternative

$$H_{12}: \quad \mu_T - \mu_R < \Delta.$$

Here, it will be recalled, $\Delta = \ln(1.25) = 0.2231$.

We first consider logAUC. The value of the t-statistic for testing (3.9) is $t_{01} = (-0.0166 + \Delta)/0.0263 = 7.86$ on 30 d.f. and the value for testing (3.10) is $t_{02} = (-0.0166 - \Delta)/0.0263 = -9.12$ on 30 d.f. Clearly both of these null hypotheses would be rejected at the 5% level on a one-sided test. For logCmax, the story is similar, with a value of 4.00 for testing (3.9) and a value of -5.10 for testing (3.10), both on 30 d.f.

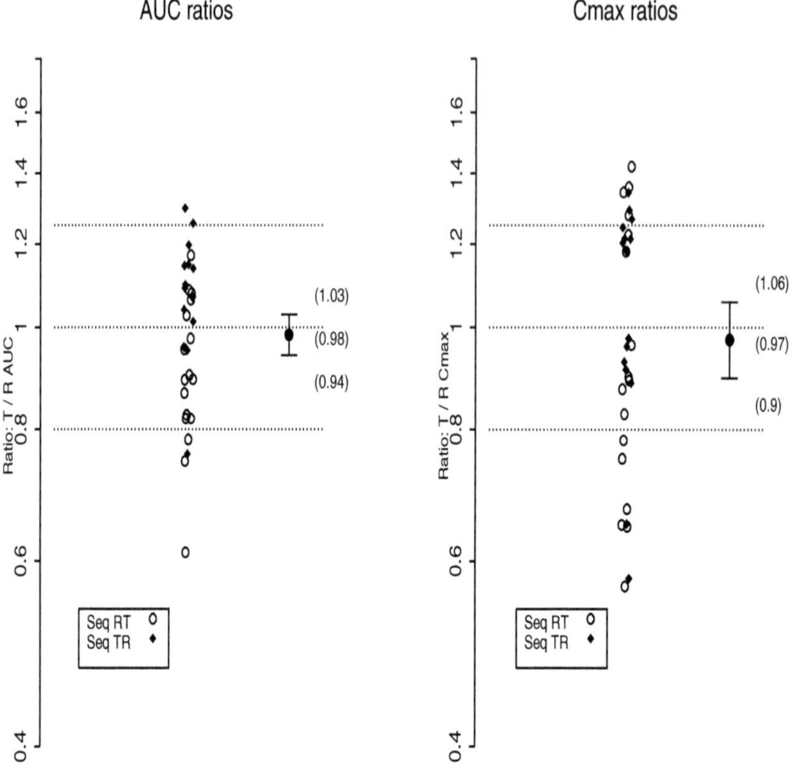

FIGURE 3.6
Example 3.1: 90% Confidence Intervals for $\exp(\hat{\mu}_T - \hat{\mu}_R)$

3.4 Carry-Over, Sequence, and Interaction Effects

We now return to consider the other potential effects that might be present in our data, namely, carry-over and formulation-by-period interaction. The nature of the carry-over effects was described in the Introduction, so we do not repeat that here. The interaction effect, however, is something we have not yet considered. Our current Model (3.1) assumes that the difference between μ_T and μ_R is the same in Period 2 as it is in Period 1. This is the situation when there is no formulation-by-period interaction. The presence of such an interaction implies that the size of the formulation difference in Period 1 is not the same as its size in Period 2. Figure 3.7 contains four examples of a groups-by-periods plot ([652], Ch. 2) which displays the four group-by-period means $\bar{y}_{11.}, \bar{y}_{12.}, \bar{y}_{21.}$, and $\bar{y}_{22.}$. They are given in two versions and each for the cases of no-interaction and interaction. Let us look first at the Version 1 plots. If we assume for the moment that there is no random variation, i.e., the plotted points refer to the true mean values, then the upper left-hand plot is a case where there is no interaction and as a consequence the lines cross at a point midway between Period 1 and Period 2. The lower left-hand plot is a case where there is interaction, and the lines cross at a position that is not midway between the two period labels. Deciding quickly if the crossing point is midway or not may not be easy and so Version 2 offers an alternative. Here the points are in the same positions, but an alternative way of connecting them has been used. If the lines are parallel, then there is no interaction. Readers can decide which

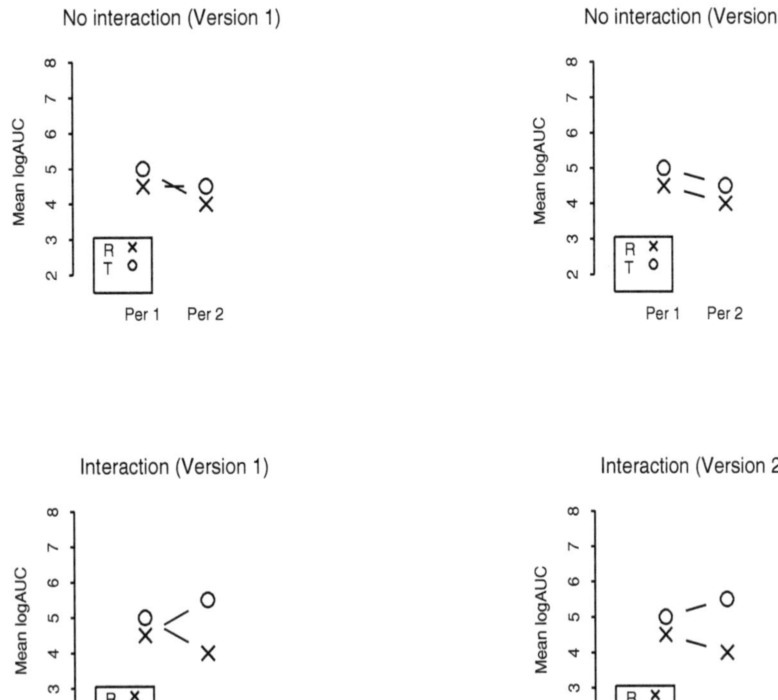

FIGURE 3.7
Groups-by-Periods Plot

version, if any, they find useful. In all the upper plots a period effect is evident that gives a lower response in Period 2. In the presence of random variation, we will not see parallel lines even in the absence of any interaction: a statistical test of significance will be required to determine if there is any evidence of an interaction.

If this is the case, then the fixed effects part of our model, as displayed in Table 3.2, needs to be enlarged to that given in Table 3.7, where there are four new (interaction) parameters $(\tau\pi)_{d[i,j],j}, i = 1, 2, j = 1, 2$ and where $d[i, j] = R$ or T. (Note that we have omitted the sequence parameters for reasons which will be explained shortly.) The inclusion of these parameters implies that a response observed in Group i, Period j under formulation R or T is not just the sum of the individual effects of formulation $d[i, j]$ and period j. However,

TABLE 3.7
Fixed Effects Model Including Interactions for a 2 × 2 Design

Group	Period 1	Period 2
1(RT)	$\mu_R + \pi_1 + (\tau\pi)_{R1}$	$\mu_T + \pi_2 + (\tau\pi)_{T2}$
2(TR)	$\mu_T + \pi_1 + (\tau\pi)_{T1}$	$\mu_R + \pi_2 + (\tau\pi)_{R2}$

TABLE 3.8
Fixed Effects Model Including Interactions for a 2 × 2 Design: After Applying Constraints

Group	Period 1	Period 2
1(RT)	$\mu_R - \pi + (\tau\pi)$	$\mu_T + \pi + (\tau\pi)$
2(TR)	$\mu_T - \pi - (\tau\pi)$	$\mu_R + \pi - (\tau\pi)$

TABLE 3.9
Fixed Effects Model Including Carry-Over Effects for a 2 × 2 Design

Group	Period 1	Period 2
1(RT)	$\mu_R + \pi_1$	$\mu_T + \pi_2 + \lambda_R$
2(TR)	$\mu_T + \pi_1$	$\mu_R + \pi_2 + \lambda_T$

as already mentioned in Section 3.2, our linear model is over-parameterized and we need to apply constraints to remove the redundancy. The constraints on the formulation and period parameters have already been described. For the interaction parameters, we assume $(\tau\pi)_{R1} = (\tau\pi) = -(\tau\pi)_{R2} = -(\tau\pi)_{T1} = (\tau\pi)_{T2}$. The model containing the interaction parameters is displayed in Table 3.8. From this table it is also clear that the sequence parameter for Sequence $1(-\gamma)$ and the interaction parameter $(\tau\pi)$ are interchangeable in Group 1 and (γ) and $-(\tau\pi)$ are interchangeable in Group 2. Hence, the statistical test for a group difference is identical to the test for a nonzero formulation-by-period interaction. In this situation we say that the sequence and interaction effects are aliased. The same can be said about the carry-over difference. To see this we need to apply a different constraint to the four interaction parameters (recall the choice of constraint is arbitrary). Table 3.9 displays the model with carry-over effects. There is no carry-over effect in Period 1 and $\lambda_R(\lambda_T)$ denotes the carry-over effect of formulation $R(T)$. If we apply the constraint $\lambda_R = -\lambda = -\lambda_T$, then the model is as displayed in Table 3.10. If we return to Table 3.7 and apply the constraints $(\tau\pi)_{R1} = (\tau\pi)_{T1} = 0$, $(\tau\pi)_{R2} = -\lambda$, and $(\tau\pi)_{T2} = \lambda$, we will reproduce Table 3.10. In other words, the carry-over effects and the interaction effects are aliased.

We may now be tempted to test for a nonzero formulation-by-period interaction (or carry-over difference or group difference). However, such a test is pointless and has undesirable side effects. The reasons why this is the case were first given by [427] and subsequently described and discussed thoroughly by Senn (see [1103], [1104], [1114], [1115]), for example) and [652]. We therefore do not consider or recommend such testing for trials that use the RT/TR design.

TABLE 3.10
Fixed Effects Model Including Carry-Over Effects for a 2 × 2 Design: After Applying Constraints

Group	Period 1	Period 2
1(RT)	$\mu - \tau - \pi$	$\mu + \tau + \pi - \lambda$
2(TR)	$\mu + \tau - \pi$	$\mu - \tau + \pi + \lambda$

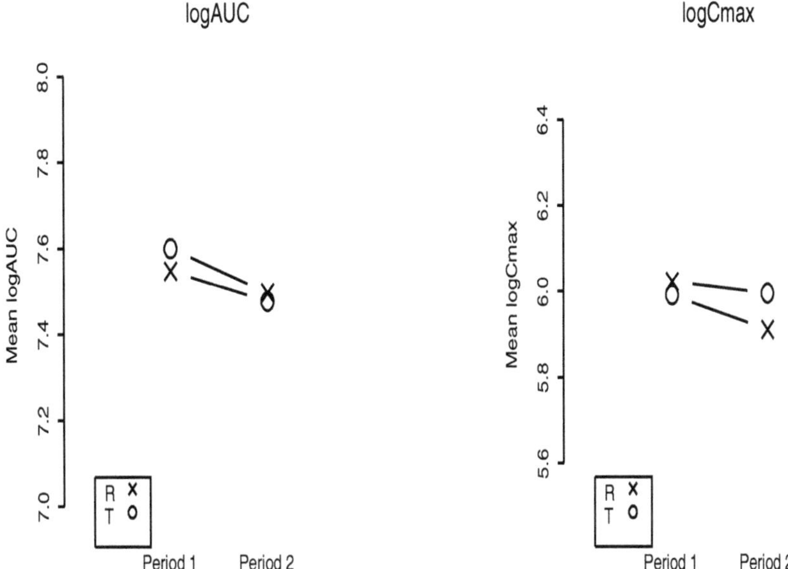

FIGURE 3.8
Example 3.1: Groups-by-Periods Plot

For completeness we show, in Figure 3.8, the groups-by-periods plots for Example 3.1, where the style of Version 1 has been used. Although there is a suggestion of an interaction, it is unlikely that such a small effect, if in fact it is present, could be detected against a background of large between-subject variability. In addition, we have already cautioned against testing for such an interaction. In terms of ABE, although the logCmax means in Period 2 show more of a difference between R and T than the other comparisons, this difference is itself not large.

3.5 Checking Assumptions Made about the Linear Model

No statistical analysis of data is complete without some checks on the assumptions that were made when the model was specified. Our model, it will be recalled, is as defined in (3.1). The main assumptions were that, after allowing for the systematic (i.e., fixed) effects, the between-subject variability and the within-subject variability can be modelled by normal distributions. A simple graphical test of whether a set of values is a sample from a normal distribution is the normal probability (or Q-Q) plot. The values of most interest to us are the within-subject residuals, i.e., the estimates of the ε_{ijk}. We will denote the residual for the kth subject in sequence i and period j as r_{ijk}. It is defined as $r_{ijk} = y_{ijk} - \hat{y}_{ijk}$, where $\hat{y}_{ijk}$ is the value our model predicts (using our given data) for the response of the kth subject in sequence i and period j. Because our model measures everything relative to the grand mean (μ), the two residuals on the same subject add to zero, i.e., ($r_{i1k} + r_{i2k} = 0$). Hence, when testing the residuals for normality, we need only use the residuals from one of the periods.

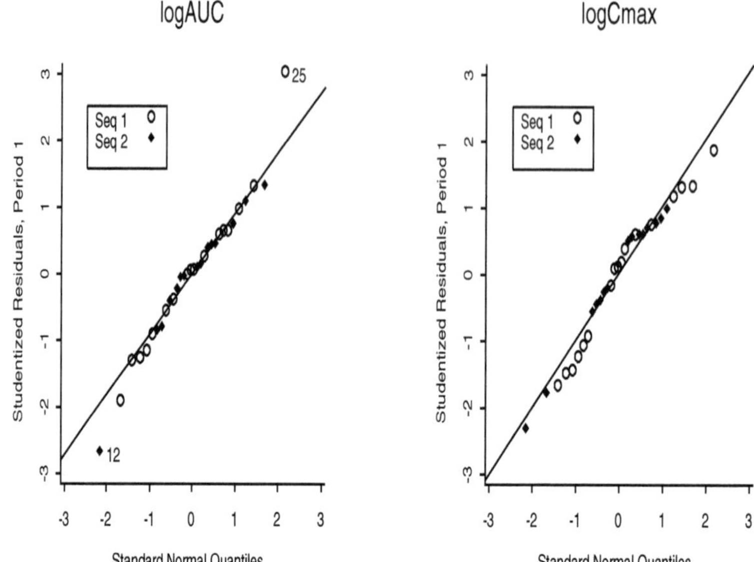

FIGURE 3.9
Example 3.1: Normal Probability Plots

Figure 3.9 displays the Q-Q plots for the studentized residuals corresponding to logAUC and logCmax. Identified on the plots are the two most extreme residuals in each plot. The studentized residuals are the raw residuals (r_{ijk}) divided by their estimated standard error. The standardization is necessary because Var(r_{ijk}) is not a constant. If the plotted data are truly normally distributed, the plotted points should lie on or close to a straight line. We can see that this is mostly true in Figure 3.9, except for the logAUC values of two subjects (12 and 25). A more formal test of normality is one due to Shapiro and Wilk [1135]. For logAUC the p-value for this test is 0.497 and for logCmax it is 0.314. There is no evidence to suggest the studentized residuals are not normally distributed. The responses with the largest studentized residuals (in absolute value) may be outliers. These are values that are typically greater than 3. There is no evidence that our extreme residuals are outliers.

3.6 Power and Sample Size for ABE in the 2×2 Design

In order for an ABE trial to meet its objectives, it should have a good chance of deciding that T and R are average bioequivalent when that is, in fact, the true state of nature. Expressed in statistical terminology, the trial must have sufficient power to reject the two null hypotheses of non-equivalence when T and R are average bioequivalent. Power is the probability of rejecting the two null hypotheses when they are false and is usually chosen to be 0.90. Mathematically, power equals 1 minus the probability of a Type 2 error.

No adjustment is made for multiplicity of endpoints AUC and Cmax [531], and the larger variance of logAUC or logCmax is typically used in the power sample size calculations. It is generally the case that logCmax is more variable than logAUC, as illustrated in the previous example. Practical issues in determining the sample size of ABE trials are considered in more detail in Chapter 5.

As already explained, when using the TOST procedure to determine ABE, we test each of the following two null hypotheses at a significance level of α, where $\Delta = \ln 1.25$. If both are rejected, we conclude that, for the metric being used (logAUC or logCmax), T and R are ABE.

$$\begin{aligned} H_{01} &: \mu_T - \mu_R \leq -\Delta \\ H_{02} &: \mu_T - \mu_R \geq \ \Delta. \end{aligned}$$

In practice, as we have seen, it is convenient to do this using a $100(1-2\alpha)\%$ two-sided confidence interval.

However, in order to calculate the power of the TOST procedure, we will stay within the hypothesis testing framework. The power will be calculated for a 2×2 cross-over trial with $n/2$ subjects in each sequence group. In this case, if $\delta = \mu_T - \mu_R$ and $\text{Var}(\hat{\delta}) = 2\sigma_W^2/n$, the t-statistics for testing each of H_{01} and H_{02} are, respectively, $t_L = (\hat{\delta} + \Delta)/\sqrt{2\hat{\sigma}_W^2/n}$ and $t_U = (\hat{\delta} - \Delta)/\sqrt{2\hat{\sigma}_W^2/n}$, and each has $(n-2)$ degrees of freedom.

Both hypotheses are rejected if $t_L > t_{1-\alpha,n-2}$ and $-t_U > t_{1-\alpha,n-2}$, where $t_{1-\alpha,n-2}$ is the upper $(1-\alpha)$ percentile of the central t-distribution on $n-2$ degrees of freedom.

For given values of n, α, σ_W, and δ_p, where δ_p is a value of δ for which the power is to be calculated, the power function of the TOST procedure can be written (see [856], for example) as

$$\Pi(n, \delta_p, \sigma_W, \alpha) = \int_0^L g(x, \delta_p)\chi_{n-2}(x)dx,$$

where

$$g(x, \delta) = \Phi\left[-Xt + b(\Delta + \delta)\right] + \Phi\left[-Xt + b(\Delta - \delta)\right] - 1,$$

$\Phi\left[.\right]$ is the cumulative distribution function of the standard normal distribution, n is the total sample size, $t = t_{1-\alpha,n-2}/\sqrt{n-2}$, $i = 1, 2$, σ_W is the assumed within-subject standard deviation, $b = \sqrt{(n/2)}/\sigma_W$, $X = \sqrt{(n-2)}\hat{\sigma}_W/\sigma_W$ has a χ distribution with $(n-2)$ degrees of freedom, $\chi_{n-2}(x)$ denotes the density of the χ distribution with $n-2$ degrees of freedom, and $L = \sqrt{n}\Delta/[\sigma_W(\sqrt{2}t)]$.

We note that this is not the first time that such a formula has been presented or discussed. See, for example, [1314], [986], [1145] and [1146].

The power can be conveniently calculated using the R package *PowerTOST* [728]. The functions *power.TOST* and *sampleN.TOST* in this package can be used to calculate the power and sample size, respectively. Both functions take as input the within-subject coefficient of variation, CV, rather than the within-subject standard deviation, σ_W, where $\sigma_W = \sqrt{(\log(1 + CV^2))}$, i.e., $CV = \sqrt{(\exp(\sigma_W^2) - 1)}$. For example, if $\delta_p = \log(0.95)$, $\alpha = 0.05$, and $CV = 0.23$ ($\sigma_W = 0.2270$), the power for $n = 32$ can be calculated by using the following code, which returns a power value of 0.9044.

```
power.TOST(alpha=0.05,logscale=TRUE,theta1=0.8,
           theta2=1.25,theta0=0.95,CV=0.23,
           n=32,design="2x2",method="exact",
           robust=FALSE)
```

If a sample size is needed to achieve a desired power (e.g., 0.9), then this can be obtained from the following code, which returns a value of 32.

```
sampleN.TOST(alpha=0.05,targetpower=0.9,
             logscale=TRUE,theta0=0.95,theta1=0.8,
             theta2=1.25,CV=0.23,design="2x2",
             method="exact",robust=FALSE,print=TRUE,
             details=FALSE,imax=100)
```

These functions have been used to calculate the values displayed in Tables 3.11 and 3.12.

Table 3.11 gives the sample size to achieve a power of 0.8 or 0.9 for values of the true ratio of 0.90, 0.95, and 1, and for values of $CV\%$ ranging from 5% to 100%, where $CV\% = 100CV$.

Table 3.12 gives the corresponding actual powers for the sample sizes in Table 3.11. We note that, for low values of the CV, the actual powers exceed the nominal ones.

TABLE 3.11
Sample Sizes to Achieve Powers of 0.8 or 0.9 for Ratios of 0.9, 0.95, and 1.00

	Power=0.80			Power=0.90		
	Ratios			Ratios		
CV%	0.90	0.95	1.00	0.90	0.95	1.00
5	6	4	4	6	4	4
10	12	8	6	14	8	8
15	22	12	10	30	16	12
20	38	20	16	50	26	20
25	56	28	24	78	38	28
30	80	40	32	108	52	40
35	106	52	42	146	70	52
40	134	66	54	186	88	66
45	166	82	66	230	110	82
50	202	98	80	278	132	100
55	238	116	94	328	156	118
60	276	134	108	382	182	136
65	316	154	124	438	208	156
70	358	174	140	494	234	176
75	400	194	156	554	262	196
80	444	214	172	614	290	218
85	488	236	190	674	320	238
90	532	258	206	734	348	260
95	576	278	224	796	378	282
100	620	300	240	858	406	304

TABLE 3.12
Power Values Corresponding to the Sample Sizes in Table 3.11

	Power=0.80			Power=0.90		
	Ratios			Ratios		
CV%	0.90	0.95	1.00	0.90	0.95	1.00
5	0.95	0.90	0.96	0.95	0.90	0.96
10	0.85	0.92	0.87	0.90	0.92	0.98
15	0.81	0.83	0.84	0.91	0.93	0.92
20	0.82	0.83	0.83	0.90	0.92	0.92
25	0.80	0.81	0.84	0.91	0.91	0.90
30	0.81	0.82	0.82	0.90	0.90	0.91
35	0.81	0.81	0.81	0.90	0.90	0.90
40	0.80	0.81	0.81	0.90	0.90	0.90
45	0.80	0.81	0.81	0.90	0.90	0.90
50	0.80	0.80	0.81	0.90	0.90	0.91
55	0.80	0.80	0.81	0.90	0.90	0.91
60	0.80	0.80	0.80	0.90	0.90	0.90
65	0.80	0.80	0.81	0.90	0.90	0.90
70	0.80	0.80	0.81	0.90	0.90	0.90
75	0.80	0.80	0.80	0.90	0.90	0.90
80	0.80	0.80	0.80	0.90	0.90	0.90
85	0.80	0.80	0.80	0.90	0.90	0.90
90	0.80	0.80	0.80	0.90	0.90	0.90
95	0.80	0.80	0.80	0.90	0.90	0.90
100	0.80	0.80	0.80	0.90	0.90	0.90

3.7 Example in Which Test and Reference Are Not ABE

You may recall in the Introduction to Chapter 2 that Lenny and Denny, the Clinical Pharmacology physician and scientist, were concerned about a particular set of data from a BE trial. These data are given in Table 3.13.

We can see that data has been collected on 49 subjects. Some subjects have missing data points (see Subjects 28 and 46, for example). Before modelling the data, we should understand why these subjects did not produce PK data. In the case of Subject 28, the PK concentrations were too low to produce a quality AUC value, and Subject 46 similarly did not get much drug on board after taking each dose. Subject 35 decided not to participate in the trial and thus had no data.

The subject profiles plots for these data are given in Figure 3.10, where we have included only those subjects that had two data points for either logAUC or logCmax. We can see clearly that for one subject (4 in sequence TR) there is a dramatic change from T to R for both logAUC and logCmax. This subject had particularly low AUC and Cmax values in Period 1, which, though unusual, were quite genuine. We will therefore leave the data for this subject in the set to be analyzed.

The paired-agreement plots are given in Figure 3.11 and do not suggest that there is a significant difference between T and R, although there may be a period difference.

Before we can continue to fit a linear model to the (log-transformed) data, we must decide what to do with the data from those subjects who did not provide a value in both periods. The most precise comparison of T and R is based on the difference of two values on the same subject. Such a comparison is not possible for those subjects with only a single value. If, however, there are two such subjects and one has a value only on T and the other has a value only on R, then a between-subject comparison of T and R is possible by taking the difference of these two single values. However, the precision of such a comparison will be low because the between-subject variation, as we can see from Figure 3.10, is much higher than the within-subject variability. Because we have assumed the subject effects ξ_{ik} are random variables, these between-subject comparisons can be recovered in the analysis if we fit what is known as a mixed model. A full explanation of mixed models is beyond the scope of the present chapter and so we will proceed to analyze the subset of data from those subjects who provided values on both T and R. We will consider mixed models in more detail in Chapter 5. However, the recovery of between-subject information on the comparison of T and R is unlikely to make much difference to the results, and so nothing of significance will be lost by ignoring the data on those subjects who provided only a single value. To justify this assertion, we will also report the results of fitting the mixed model to the complete dataset, but, as already mentioned, a full explanation of how this was done will have to wait until Chapter 5.

TABLE 3.13: Example 3.2

	Sequence RT			
	AUC Period		Cmax Period	
Subject	1	2	1	2
1	58.160	79.340	2.589	2.827
3	69.680	85.590	2.480	4.407
5	121.840	.	5.319	.
8	208.330	377.150	9.634	11.808
10	17.220	14.230	1.855	1.121
11	1407.900	750.790	13.615	6.877
13	20.810	21.270	1.210	1.055
15	.	8.670	0.995	1.084
18	203.220	269.400	7.496	9.618
20	386.930	412.420	16.106	12.536
21	47.960	33.890	2.679	2.129
24	22.700	32.590	1.727	1.853
26	44.020	72.360	3.156	4.546
27	285.780	423.050	8.422	11.167
31	40.600	20.330	1.900	1.247
32	19.430	17.750	1.185	0.910
36	1048.600	1160.530	18.976	17.374
37	107.660	82.700	5.031	6.024
39	469.730	928.050	6.962	14.829
R=Reference, T=Test				

TABLE 3.13: Example 3.2 (continued)

	Sequence RT			
	AUC Period		Cmax Period	
Subject	1	2	1	2
43	14.950	20.090	0.987	2.278
44	28.570	28.470	1.105	1.773
45	379.900	411.720	12.615	13.810
47	126.090	46.880	6.977	2.339
50	75.430	106.430	4.925	4.771
	Sequence TR			
Subject	1	2	1	2
2	150.120	142.290	5.145	3.216
4	36.950	5.000	2.442	0.498
6	24.530	26.050	1.442	2.728
7	22.110	34.640	2.007	3.309
9	703.830	476.560	15.133	11.155
12	217.060	176.020	9.433	8.446
14	40.750	152.400	1.787	6.231
16	52.760	51.570	3.570	2.445
17	101.520	23.490	4.476	1.255
19	37.140	30.540	2.169	2.613
22	143.450	42.690	5.182	3.031
23	29.800	29.550	1.714	1.804
25	63.030	92.940	3.201	5.645
28	.	.	0.531	0.891
29	56.700	21.030	2.203	1.514
30	61.180	66.410	3.617	2.130
33	1376.020	1200.280	27.312	22.068
34	115.330	135.550	4.688	7.358
38	17.340	40.350	1.072	2.150
40	62.230	64.920	3.025	3.041
41	48.990	61.740	2.706	2.808
42	53.180	17.510	3.240	1.702
46	.	.	1.680	.
48	98.030	236.170	3.434	7.378
49	1070.980	1016.520	21.517	20.116
R=Reference, T=Test				

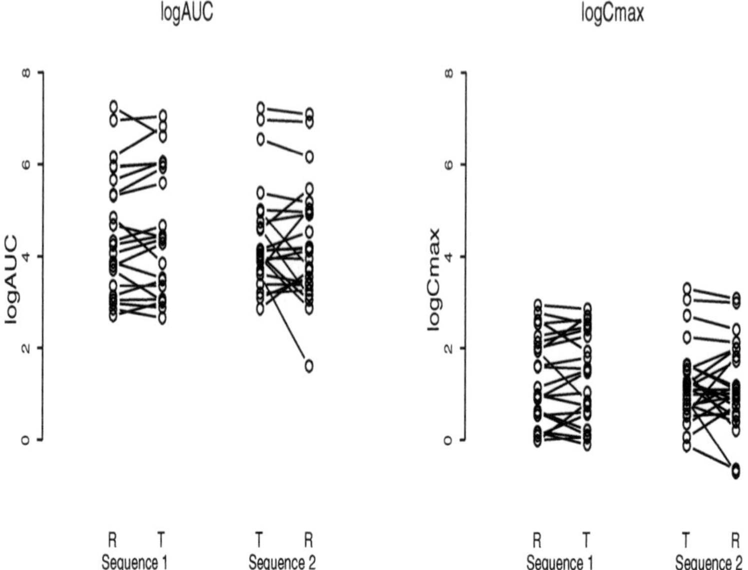

FIGURE 3.10
Example 3.2: Subject Profiles Plot

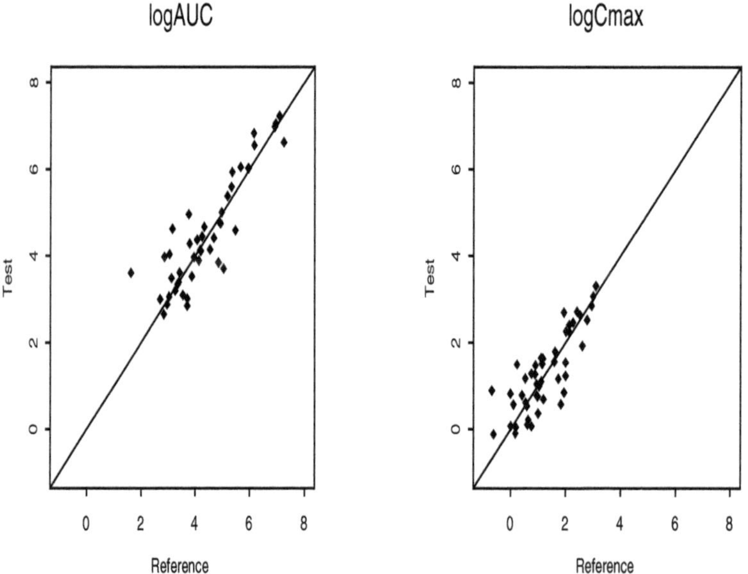

FIGURE 3.11
Example 3.2: Paired-Agreement Plots

The groups-by-periods means for Example 3.2 are given in Table 3.14 and plotted in Figure 3.12. The pattern is similar for both logAUC and logCmax, although there is a larger difference between T and R in the second period for logAUC.

The mean differences versus totals plot is given in Figure 3.13. For logAUC there is a noticeable vertical separation of the centroids, suggesting a possible lack of ABE.

The results of applying the TOST procedure are given in Table 3.15. We can see that the upper limit of the 90% confidence interval for logAUC (and of course AUC) is above the upper boundary for ABE. Therefore, even though ABE is not contradicted when the logCmax data are used, T and R are judged to have failed the FDA criteria for ABE.

The fitted normal densities corresponding to the TOST results are given in Figure 3.14. We can see a large part of the density for logAUC extends to the right of the ABE limit and is consistent with the lack of ABE found by the TOST procedure.

As with our previous example, we look at the normal probability plots to check on our assumptions. These are given in Figure 3.15.

There is very strong evidence that the studentized residuals from the model for logAUC are not normally distributed. The *p*-value from the Shapiro–Wilk test is 0.012 for logAUC and 0.407 for logCmax. This confirms the visual indication that studentized residuals for logAUC are not normally distributed. The largest studentized residual for logAUC is 3.341, from subject 4. This is unusually large in a sample of size 45 from the standard normal distribution and the data value corresponding to this residual is an "outlier" — i.e., a value that is unusual relative to the fitted model. As already noted, this is a subject with a very large drop in value for both logAUC and logCmax over the two periods. Subject 14 has a large increase in both logAUC and logCmax between the periods.

An alternative analysis that does not depend on the assumption that the data are normally distributed is available and we will illustrate this (nonparametric analysis) in the next section. It should be noted, however, that regulatory approval may not be obtained if nonparametric methods are used unless this set of analyses are pre-specified in the protocol and if the Type 1 error rate is adjusted for multiple analyses. Those interested in more information on this topic should consult [732].

TABLE 3.14
Example 3.2: Groups-by-Periods Means (sample size in parentheses)

	logAUC		
Group	Period 1	Period 2	Mean
1(RT)	$\bar{y}_{11.} = 4.55(22)$	$\bar{y}_{12.} = 4.60(22)$	$\bar{y}_{1..} = 4.57$
2(TR)	$\bar{y}_{21.} = 4.43(22)$	$\bar{y}_{22.} = 4.28(22)$	$\bar{y}_{2..} = 4.35$
Mean	$\bar{y}_{.1.} = 4.49$	$\bar{y}_{.2.} = 4.43$	$\bar{y}_{...} = 4.46$
	logCmax		
1(RT)	$\bar{y}_{11.} = 1.33(23)$	$\bar{y}_{12.} = 1.36(23)$	$\bar{y}_{1..} = 1.34$
2(TR)	$\bar{y}_{21.} = 1.27(23)$	$\bar{y}_{22.} = 1.19(23)$	$\bar{y}_{2..} = 1.23$
Mean	$\bar{y}_{.1.} = 1.30$	$\bar{y}_{.2.} = 1.27$	$\bar{y}_{...} = 1.29$

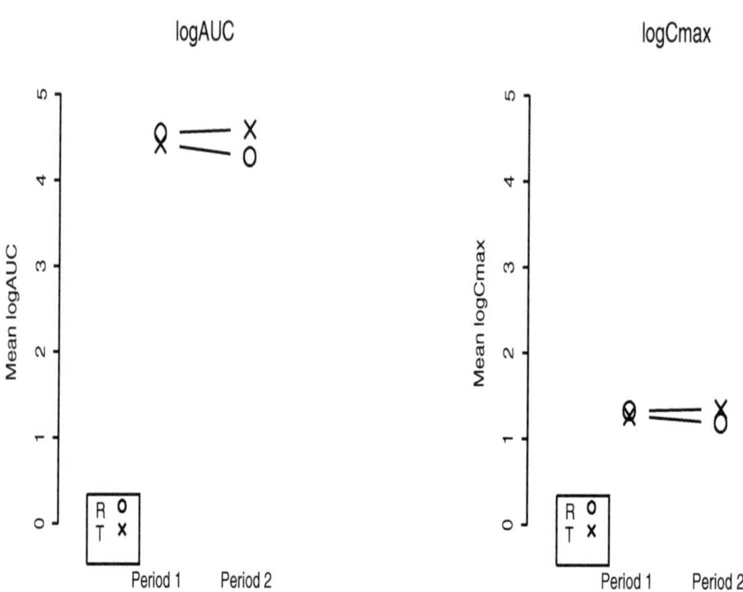

FIGURE 3.12
Example 3.2: Groups-by-Periods Plot

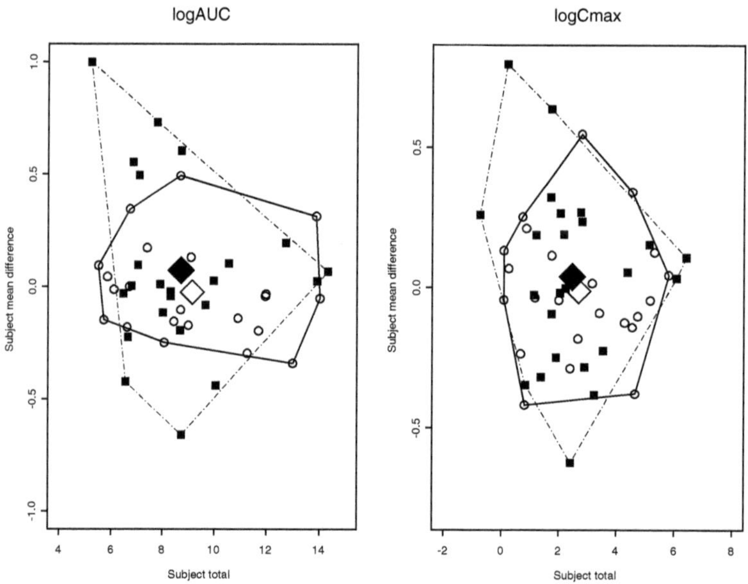

FIGURE 3.13
Example 3.2: Mean Differences versus Totals Plot

TABLE 3.15
Example 3.2: TOST Procedure Results

Endpoint	$\hat{\mu}_T - \hat{\mu}_R$	90% Confidence Interval
logAUC (45 subjects)	0.0970	(-0.0610, 0.2550)
logCmax (47 subjects)	0.0508	(-0.0871, 0.1887)
Endpoint	$\exp(\hat{\mu}_T - \hat{\mu}_R)$	90% Confidence Interval
AUC (45 subjects)	1.10	(0.94, 1.29)
Cmax (47 subjects)	1.05	(0.92, 1.21)

Last, we report the results that are obtained by fitting a mixed model to the complete dataset. These are displayed in Table 3.16 and lead to the same conclusions as were obtained from the data using only those subjects with values in both Period 1 and Period 2.

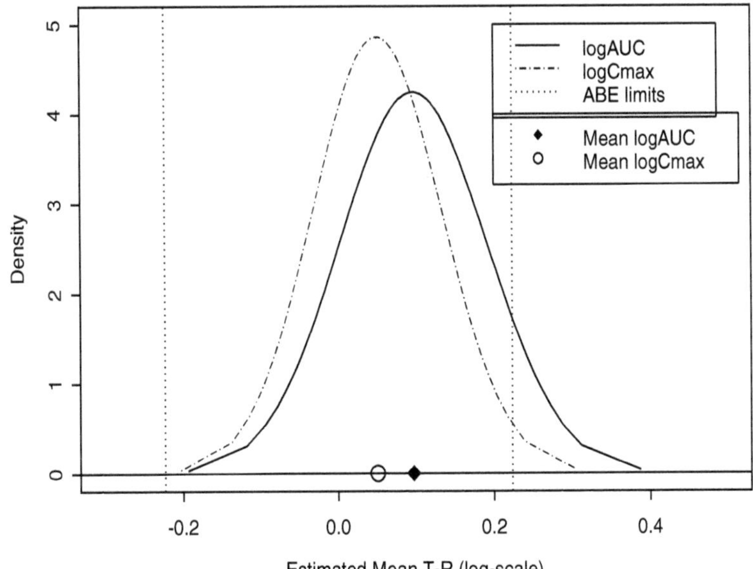

FIGURE 3.14
Example 3.2: Fitted Normal Densities for $\hat{\mu}_T - \hat{\mu}_R$

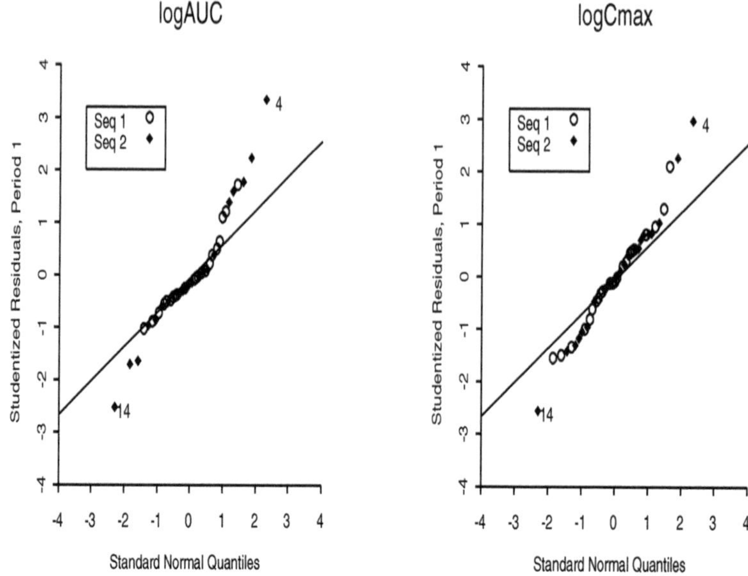

FIGURE 3.15
Example 3.2: Normal Probability Plots

TABLE 3.16
Example 3.2: TOST Procedure Results (all subjects)

Endpoint	$\hat{\mu}_T - \hat{\mu}_R$	90% Confidence Interval
logAUC	0.0940	(-0.0678, 0.2482)
logCmax	0.0468	(-0.0907, 0.1843)
Endpoint	$\exp(\hat{\mu}_T - \hat{\mu}_R)$	90% Confidence Interval
AUC	1.09	(0.93, 1.28)
Cmax	1.05	(0.91, 1.20)

3.8 Nonparametric Analysis

On occasion, in bioequivalence or relative bioavailability studies, there may be a need to analyze unusual endpoints beyond those usually assessed such as logAUC and logCmax. Examples of such endpoints are

1. The ratio Cmax/AUC [325] — an alternative measure of the rate of exposure
2. Partial AUC [330] — an alternative measure of absorption
3. λ (see Equation 1.1, Chapter 1) — a measure of excretion.

Endpoints like these are difficult to assess using models like those introduced up to now, as they are unlikely to be normally distributed. For example, the ratio Cmax/AUC is the ratio of two log-normally distributed variables. Even though it may be possible to derive approximate or exact formulae for the distributions of such endpoints, it is unclear how this would directly benefit the sponsors of such studies or patients. These endpoints are currently viewed as supportive only, and exact quantification of their Type 1 or 2 error rates is not of immediate concern in a regulatory filing.

However, there are statistical procedures available to analyze such (non-normal) data. These procedures are termed "nonparametric" in that they do not assume a particular parametric form (e.g., normal or log-normal) for the endpoint of interest. The nonparametric analysis for the 2×2 cross-over was first described by [705] and later illustrated by [222] in the context of evaluating bioavailability data. An excellent review of nonparametric methods for the analysis of cross-over trials is given by [1263]. See also [1189] and [538]. For a more extensive coverage of the methods covered in this section see [1198].

Such nonparametric analyses should only be utilized when (i) an endpoint is grossly non-normal or (ii) an endpoint cannot be transformed to an endpoint that is normally distributed or (iii) sample size does not permit the application of the central limit theorem. Such an endpoint is Tmax, which is often used to support parametric analysis findings from the analysis of logAUC and logCmax.

Obviously, the interpretation of nonparametric analysis from a regulatory perspective is overshadowed by global regulatory recommendations (see Chapter 2) on provision of adequate sample size to support parametric interpretation. Such nonparametric techniques are generally of interest to sponsors only when small sample sizes are employed and, even then, only when analyzing Tmax or unusual endpoints. If there is evidence that the log-transformed data from an ABE trial are such that it would be unreasonable to assume that they are normally distributed, then the usual two one-sided t-tests (as used in the TOST procedure), can be replaced by Wilcoxon rank-sum tests, or equivalently by Mann–Whitney U-tests. As with normal data, these nonparametric tests are based on within-subject differences.

To illustrate the nonparametric tests, we will use the Tmax values recorded on the subjects in Example 3.1. These are given in Table 3.17.

In order to make a comparison between the parametric and nonparametric procedures, we will first analyze the logTmax values as if they were normally distributed (i.e., on the assumption the Tmax values are log-normally distributed). Although there are no regulatory guidelines on what must be done to determine if T and R are ABE, we will apply the same regulatory hurdles that apply to logAUC and logCmax. In other words, we will apply the usual TOST procedure to logTmax. The results of doing this, along with the back-transformed values, are given in Table 3.18. Applying the familiar regulatory guidelines, T and R cannot be deemed to be ABE, as the upper 90% confidence limit for $\mu_T - \mu_R$, on the logTmax scale, exceeds 0.2231 (and, of course, the upper 90% confidence limit on the Tmax scale exceeds 1.25).

However, we need to check that the assumption that the residuals from our usual linear model (3.1) for logTmax are normally distributed is reasonable. Figure 3.16 displays the histogram of the studentized residuals and a normal probability plot. The studentized residuals look like they can be assumed to be normally distributed. The p-value for the Shapiro–Wilk test for normality is 0.7044, which also gives some assurance that the studentized residuals have a normal distribution. However, a closer inspection of the normal probability plot in Figure 3.16 reveals horizontal bands of residuals, a feature most unlikely to occur if the residuals were normally distributed. Also, of course, the nature of the Tmax variable itself indicates that logTmax will not be normally distributed. The concentrations are only taken at a set of predetermined times, and so Tmax is an inherently discrete random variable.

A further warning sign is that, when Model (3.1) was fitted using PROC MIXED, the estimate of $\hat{\sigma}_B^2$ (not shown) was zero, indicating some instability in the REML fitting procedure for these data. The values in Table 3.18 were therefore calculated using the results of fitting Model (3.1) under the assumption that the subject parameters were fixed rather than random effects. Of course, for a complete dataset like that in Table 3.17, with two values of Tmax for every subject, we should get the same TOST results regardless of whether the subject parameters are fixed or random. The fact that we do not is another indication that a more robust analysis procedure should be used for these data.

When data are log-normal or normal in distribution, it is known that, in most cases, the probability of a Type 2 error is increased when using a nonparametric procedure relative to the parametric procedures discussed in earlier sections [533].

TABLE 3.17: Example 3.1: Tmax

Subject	Sequence	Period	Formulation	Tmax	LogTmax
1	RT	1	R	0.50	-0.693
1	RT	2	T	0.50	-0.693
4	RT	1	R	0.50	-0.693
4	RT	2	T	1.00	0.000
5	RT	1	R	1.50	0.405
5	RT	2	T	0.25	-1.386
8	RT	1	R	1.00	0.000
8	RT	2	T	0.50	-0.693
9	RT	1	R	0.25	-1.386
9	RT	2	T	1.50	0.405
11	RT	1	R	0.50	-0.693
11	RT	2	T	1.00	0.000
16	RT	1	R	1.50	0.405
16	RT	2	T	2.00	0.693
17	RT	1	R	1.50	0.405
17	RT	2	T	1.00	0.000
19	RT	1	R	1.50	0.405
19	RT	2	T	0.50	-0.693
21	RT	1	R	0.50	-0.693
21	RT	2	T	0.50	-0.693
24	RT	1	R	1.00	0.000
24	RT	2	T	0.50	-0.693
25	RT	1	R	1.00	0.000
25	RT	2	T	0.25	-1.386
28	RT	1	R	1.00	0.000
28	RT	2	T	1.50	0.405
29	RT	1	R	1.00	0.000
29	RT	2	T	1.50	0.405
31	RT	1	R	0.50	-0.693

R=Reference, T=Test

TABLE 3.17: Example 3.1: Tmax (continued)

Subject	Sequence	Period	Formulation	Tmax	LogTmax
31	RT	2	T	1.50	0.405
34	RT	1	R	0.50	-0.693
34	RT	2	T	1.50	0.405
36	RT	1	R	0.50	-0.693
36	RT	2	T	1.00	0.000
2	TR	1	T	1.00	0.000
2	TR	2	R	1.00	0.000
3	TR	1	T	0.50	-0.693
3	TR	2	R	0.50	-0.693
6	TR	1	T	1.00	0.000
6	TR	2	R	0.50	-0.693
7	TR	1	T	1.00	0.000
7	TR	2	R	0.25	-1.386
10	TR	1	T	1.50	0.405
10	TR	2	R	1.00	0.000
12	TR	1	T	1.00	0.000
12	TR	2	R	1.00	0.000
15	TR	1	T	0.50	-0.693
15	TR	2	R	1.50	0.405
18	TR	1	T	1.00	0.000
18	TR	2	R	0.50	-0.693
20	TR	1	T	1.00	0.000
20	TR	2	R	0.50	-0.693
22	TR	1	T	2.00	0.693
22	TR	2	R	4.02	1.391
23	TR	1	T	0.50	-0.693
23	TR	2	R	0.50	-0.693
26	TR	1	T	0.50	-0.693
26	TR	2	R	0.25	-1.386
27	TR	1	T	0.50	-0.693
27	TR	2	R	1.00	0.000
30	TR	1	T	0.50	-0.693
30	TR	2	R	1.00	0.000
35	TR	1	T	0.50	-0.693
35	TR	2	R	1.00	0.000
R=Reference, T=Test					

To derive the equivalent of the TOST procedure based on a nonparametric approach, we use the Hodges–Lehmann point estimate and confidence interval for $\mu_T - \mu_R$ [565]. These can be calculated using tables (see [547]), by asymptotic approximation or from software for exact testing such as StatXact [234]. Here we will illustrate the approach that uses the asymptotic approximation.

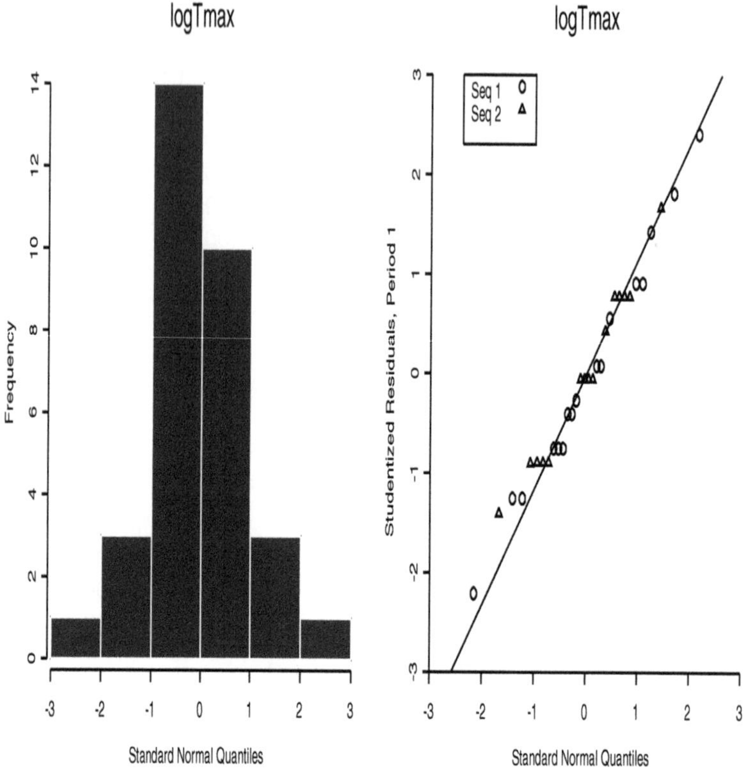

FIGURE 3.16
Example 3.1: Studentized Residuals for Tmax

It will be recalled that the estimate of $\delta = \mu_T - \mu_R$ was obtained previously by comparing the mean period difference from sequence Group 2 with the mean period difference from sequence Group 1:

$$\hat{\delta} = \hat{\mu}_T - \hat{\mu}_R = \frac{1}{2}([\bar{y}_{21.} - \bar{y}_{22.}] - [\bar{y}_{11.} - \bar{y}_{12.}]).$$

The robust estimate of δ is based on similar reasoning, but uses the median rather than the mean.

In order to construct a robust equivalent of the 90% confidence interval used in the TOST procedure, we first calculate for each subject the difference between the logTmax values in Periods 1 and 2 (i.e., $y_{i1k} - y_{i2k}$, for $i = 1, 2$ and $k = 1, 2, \ldots, n_i$).

Let us label the period differences, $y_{11k} - y_{12k}$, in sequence Group 1 as X_i, $i = 1, 2, \ldots, n_1$ and the differences, $y_{21k} - y_{22k}$, in sequence Group 2 as Y_j, $j = 1, 2, \ldots, n_2$. In Example 3.1, $n_1 = 17$ and $n_2 = 15$.

TABLE 3.18
Example 3.1: TOST Procedure Results for Tmax

Endpoint	$\hat{\mu}_T - \hat{\mu}_R$	90% Confidence Interval
logTmax	0.0553	(-0.2021, 0.3126)
Tmax	1.0569	(0.8170, 1.3670)

To calculate the point estimate, we first form the $n_1 \times n_2$ differences $Y_j - X_i$, for $i = 1, 2, \ldots, n_1$ and $j = 1, 2, \ldots, n_2$. The point estimate $\hat{\delta}$ is then half the value of the median of these differences. To obtain the median, the differences are ordered from smallest to largest. To save space, we do not give the list of these ordered differences here. If $n_1 \times n_2$ is odd and equals $2p+1$, say, the median is the $(p+1)$th ordered difference. If $n_1 \times n_2$ is even and equals $2p$, say, the median is the average of the pth and $(p+1)$th ordered differences. For Example 3.1, $n_1 n_2 = 255$ and therefore the median is the 128th ordered difference, which is 0, i.e., $\hat{\delta} = 0/2$.

To obtain a symmetric two-sided confidence interval for δ, with confidence coefficient $1 - \alpha$, we must first obtain an integer, which we will denote by C_α. To get this we use the critical values of the distribution of the Wilcoxon rank-sum test statistic [573], which can be obtained by approximation when n_1 and n_2 are large (i.e., larger than 12) or from Table A.6 of [573] when n_1 and n_2 are small. The Wilcoxon rank-sum test can be considered a nonparametric form of the usual t-test for comparing two independent samples. The rank-sum test uses the ranks of the data rather than the data themselves. We will say more about this test after describing and illustrating the nonparametric form of the TOST procedure.

To obtain C_α when n_1 and n_2 are small (i.e., ≤ 12), we first obtain the value $w(\alpha/2, n_1, n_2)$ from Table A.6. This value is such that, on the null hypothesis of no difference in central location between the two samples under consideration, $\mathrm{P}[W \geq w(\alpha/2, n_1, n_2)] = \alpha/2$, where W is the rank-sum statistic. The value of C_α is then obtained by noting that $[n_2(2n_1 + n_2 + 1)/2] - C_\alpha + 1 = w(\alpha/2, n_1, n_2)$. On the null hypothesis, C_α is the largest integer such that

$$\mathrm{P}\left[\left(\frac{n_2(n_2+1)}{2} + C_\alpha\right) \leq W \leq \left(\frac{n_2(2n_1+n_2+1)}{2} - C_\alpha\right)\right] \geq 1 - \alpha,$$

where $n_1 > n_2$.

For large n_1 and n_2, the integer C_α may, according to Hollander and Wolfe, be approximated by

$$C_\alpha = \frac{n_1 n_2}{2} - z_{\alpha/2}\left[\frac{n_1 n_2(n_1+n_2+1)}{12}\right]^{\frac{1}{2}},$$

where $z_{\alpha/2}$ is the upper $(1 - \alpha/2)$ point of the standard normal distribution.

The $(1-\alpha)$ confidence interval is the $\frac{1}{2}(\delta_L, \delta_U)$, where δ_L is the C_αth ordered difference and δ_U is the $(n_1 n_2 + 1 - C_\alpha)$th ordered difference.

Taking $z_{0.05} = 1.645$, we get $C_\alpha = 84$. That is, the 90% confidence interval is obtained by taking δ_L as the 84th ordered difference and δ_U as the 172nd ordered difference. The resulting 90% confidence interval for δ is $(-0.2027, 0.3466)$. The back-transformed interval is (0.82, 1.41). These are quite similar to those obtained previously, (-0.2021, 0.3126) and (0.82, 1.37), respectively, indicating some robustness of the parametric approach when the sample sizes are relatively large.

The Wilcoxon rank-sum test assumes that the endpoint (logTmax in our case) is expressed on an interval (or metric) scale, so that the same shift on the scale has the same interpretation regardless of its location. Further assumptions made in using this test include randomization of subjects to the groups with random sampling from the same family of distributions with differences between groups only being for location.

To calculate the test statistic, the period differences are ranked, where the ranking is done in terms of the total number of subjects, not separately for each group. Let R_i = [the sum of the ranks of group i], $i = 1, 2$. Under the null hypothesis that $\mu_T = \mu_R$,

$$E[R_1] = n_1(n_1 + n_2 + 1)/2$$

$$E[R_2] = n_2(n_1 + n_2 + 1)/2$$

and

$$\text{Var}[R_1] = \text{Var}[R_2] = n_1 n_2 (n_1 + n_2 + 1 - T)/12,$$

where T is a correction for ties.

If there are no ties, then $T = 0$. If there are v tied sets, with t_s ties in the sth set, where $s = 1, 2, \ldots, v$, then

$$T = \frac{\sum_{s=1}^{v} t_s(t_s^2 - 1)}{[(n_1 + n_2)(n_1 + n_2 - 1)]}.$$

An asymptotic test of the null hypothesis can be based on either R_1 or R_2. For R_1 we calculate

$$z = \frac{R_1 - E[R_1]}{(\text{Var}[R_1])^{\frac{1}{2}}}$$

and compare it with the standard normal distribution. Statistical software, such as `proc npar1way` in SAS, will do the necessary calculations for this test and produce exact P-values for small n_1 and n_2.

In order to apply the nonparametric equivalent of the TOST procedure, we use the mean difference, (Period 1 − Period 2)/2, for each subject. In the analysis we (i) add log(1.25) to the mean differences in Group 2 and apply the Wilcoxon rank-sum test and (ii) subtract log(1.25) from the mean differences in Group 2 and apply the test. The P-values from the exact and asymptotic tests are very similar (0.021 when adding and 0.120 when subtracting, for the exact test) and are not very different from the t-test (0.038 and 0.138). Indeed the conclusions are the same; based on logTmax, T and R are not ABE.

4

BE Studies with More Than Two Periods

Introduction

Denny walked into my office one day after the reports for Example 3.2 came out looking like he had been run over by a bus and dragged over hot coals. He had been (figuratively) when he reviewed the findings with senior management. They obviously did not like the implications for getting together a marketable formulation in time for filing with the FDA.

Nobody ever comes to see you when you release findings they like. That annoyed me when I first started on the job, but after a while I realized it gave one more time to enjoy the moment.

Do take time out to enjoy the good moments on the job. Given the success rate of drugs in clinical development (see Chapter 1), statisticians should expect to be the bearer of bad news on the majority of occasions in their working life. This is ok if you are in an organization that recognizes that failure is far more common in drug development than success, but if you are not, grow a thick skin about such matters, or think about changing jobs. Be careful not to get cynical, though. It is an easy trap to fall into and causes one to not enjoy anything (because you always think about the bad thing that is probably right around the corner and guard against keeping your hopes up). Probabilistically speaking, there will be good moments on the job, and one should maintain one's equanimity so that one can enjoy them.

The question Denny posed to me was simple on the surface — can we explore these data to see if there was any possibility of a follow-up bioequivalence trial being successful?

Note the careful use of the word "we." When a clinician uses "we" with a statistician, it is the royal "we" which can be usually translated as meaning "you."

*I told him that yes, **I** could, but given the findings of Example 3.2, my intuition told me that it was going to be pretty unlikely and that he had better prepare his folks for that message. I would run some programs and get back to him with a quantitative assessment next week. He wanted it sooner, but I told him no.*

I got through to Denny on three of four points here (which is pretty good all things considered). He recognized that I would do the work by next week and that the success of a follow-up study was going to be low, but the idea that he should warn his folks went in one ear and out the other. Maybe clinicians like surprises — I gave up on trying to figure that one out long ago.

Statisticians should also recognize one other truth in drug development which people tend not to mention when they are hiring you. One would think that statisticians would recognize this fact (i.e., we are trained to count), but it seems like it gets by a lot of us. The fact is statisticians are outnumbered in drug development! There are a lot more scientists, clinicians, etc., who need our expertise than there are time or personnel to deliver it.

Hence, an option one sometimes considers as a biostatistician is to go with one's intuition and not spend the time quantifying precisely questions like that posed by Denny. We encourage people not to make the choice to opt out of applying statistical expertise in such situations. It is important to the patients who will be using such medications that we get it right. If worse comes to worse, we recommend taking the time to train the scientists and clinicians to do such work themselves.

4.1 Background

Although the RT/TR design is often the design of choice when testing for ABE, there are situations in which a design with more than two periods is needed. These include

- The drugs to be compared are highly variable;
- Carry-over effects cannot be entirely ruled out due to long half-life, poor metabolism, or other factors inhibiting elimination.

By definition, a drug that is highly variable has a large within-subject variance σ_W^2 (for logAUC or logCmax). Typically this is taken to mean that $\sigma_W^2 \geq 0.09$ for R. Consequently, the estimate of $\mu_T - \mu_R$ will also have a large variance unless many subjects are enrolled. As large ABE trials are unattractive for ethical, statistical, and financial reasons, a better alternative is needed. If more than two periods can be used, then suitable alternative designs are available. The regulatory guidance recommends using four-period, two-sequence designs such as RTRT/TRTR when highly variable drugs are compared.

However, if the time available for the trial does not permit four periods to be used, then a three-period design, with sequences such as RTT/TRR, can be used. We will review and compare these designs in the next section. In Section 4.5 we will review and compare the various four-period designs. In each of these sections we will illustrate the analysis of data and give an example of at least one such trial.

ABE trials are not confined to comparing Test and Reference. Sometimes two alternative versions of Test or Reference are included, leading to the need for designs for three or four formulations. For example, in a confirmatory trial, a 300 mg Test tablet was given either (i) as 3×100 mg tablets or (ii) as a 200 mg tablet plus a 100 mg tablet. This was because, in the early stages of the confirmatory trial, only the 3×100 mg version was available. Later, a 200 mg tablet became available. The commercial formulation of the drug was to be a single 300 mg tablet, and this had to be shown to be ABE to the versions used in the confirmatory trial. A trial with four formulations might arise when both a high and a low dose of Test are to be compared to a high and low dose of Reference. Examples of both of these types of design will be given in Section 4.6. The datasets for each example are given in Section 4.10.

4.2 Three-Period Designs

As already discussed, the need for extra periods usually arises when the drugs being compared are highly variable. Adding an extra period to the RT/TR design is a simple way of increasing the number of responses collected from each subject. In addition, as we shall see, a suitably chosen three-period design can give some protection against the occurrence of (unequal) carry-over effects of T and R.

Here we will only consider designs with two sequences and the only three choices worth considering (see [652], Ch. 3) are the following, where the rows are the sequences and the columns are the periods. We assume that there are $n/2$ subjects assigned to each sequence:

1.	R	T	T	2.	R	T	R	3.	R	R	T
	T	R	R		T	R	T		T	T	R

TABLE 4.1
Expectations of $\bar{y}_{ij.}$ for Design 1

Group	Period		
	1	2	3
1 RTT	$\gamma_1 + \pi_1 + \tau_R$	$\gamma_1 + \pi_2 + \tau_T + \lambda_R$	$\gamma_1 + \pi_3 + \tau_T + \lambda_T$
2 TRR	$\gamma_2 + \pi_1 + \tau_T$	$\gamma_2 + \pi_2 + \tau_R + \lambda_T$	$\gamma_2 + \pi_3 + \tau_R + \lambda_R$

The question now arises as to which one of these should be used. If there are no (differential) carry-over effects, then the three designs are equivalent and any one may be used; the regulatory guidelines express a preference for the RTR/TRT design. However, if differential carry-over effects (i.e., $\lambda_T \neq \lambda_R$) cannot be ruled out, then the first design, RTT/TRR, is preferred, as we will shortly demonstrate.

However, before doing this, let us consider the estimation of $\delta = \mu_T - \mu_R$. As an illustration, we will do this for the first design given above, RTT/TRR.

Let $\bar{y}_{ij.}$ denote the mean of the response (logAUC or logCmax) in period j of sequence group i, where, as already stated, there are $n/2$ subjects in each group. Using an obvious extension of the notation used in Chapter 3, the expectations of the six group-by-period means are given in Table 4.1.

For our illustrative design, the estimator of δ is

$$\hat{\delta} = (-2\bar{y}_{11.} + \bar{y}_{12.} + \bar{y}_{13.} + 2\bar{y}_{21.} - \bar{y}_{22.} - \bar{y}_{23.})/4 \tag{4.1}$$

and $\text{Var}[\hat{\delta}] = 3\sigma_W^2/(2n)$. It is easily confirmed that this is an unbiased estimator:

$$\begin{aligned} E[-2\bar{y}_{11.} + \bar{y}_{12.} + \bar{y}_{13.}] &= -2(\gamma_1 + \pi_1 + \tau_R) + (\gamma_1 + \pi_2 + \tau_T + \lambda_R) \\ &+ (\gamma_1 + \pi_3 + \tau_T + \lambda_T) \\ &= -2\pi_1 + \pi_2 + \pi_3 - 2\tau_R + 2\tau_T + \lambda_R + \lambda_T \end{aligned}$$

and

$$E[-2\bar{y}_{21.} + \bar{y}_{22.} + \bar{y}_{23.}] = -2\pi_1 + \pi_2 + \pi_3 - 2\tau_T + 2\tau_R + \lambda_R + \lambda_T.$$

Taking the second expression away from the first leaves $4(\tau_T - \tau_R)$.

The unbiased estimator of $\lambda_T - \lambda_R$ is

$$\widehat{\lambda_T - \lambda_R} = (-\bar{y}_{12.} + \bar{y}_{13.} + \bar{y}_{22.} - \bar{y}_{23.})/2, \tag{4.2}$$

which again can be easily confirmed. The variance of this estimator is $2\sigma_W^2/n$.

An interesting and important property of the these two estimators is that they have a covariance of zero, which, for normally distributed data, implies they are independent. In other words, if we were to drop the carry-over parameters from the above model, we would get the same estimator of δ as given in (4.1).

We now return to answer the question of which design out of the three possibilities given above is preferred. To compare the designs, it is useful to use the concept of *efficiency*, which is more fully explained in Section 4.9, the Technical Appendix. Defining $\delta = \mu_T - \mu_R$, as before, efficiency is the ratio of $\text{Var}(\hat{\delta})$ in the design under consideration to the value this variance would take in an "ideal" design. In the ideal design the effects of subjects, periods, and carry-over effects can be removed from the estimate of δ. Therefore, in the ideal design, the estimate of δ, using logAUC, for example, would simply be the difference $\bar{y}_T - \bar{y}_R$, where $\bar{y}_T(\bar{y}_R)$ is the mean of all the logAUC values of $T(R)$. If T and R each occurred r times in the design, then $\mathrm{Var}(\bar{y}_T - \bar{y}_R) = 2\sigma_W^2/r = 4\sigma_W^2/(3n)$, as $r = 3n/2$. Such a design may not exist, and its use is merely to provide a lower bound on $\mathrm{Var}(\hat{\delta})$ that may be used as a point of reference when comparing designs. Efficiency is usually expressed as a percentage, so a fully efficient design has a value of 100%. In the presence of differential carry-over effects, the efficiency of the first design is $(4\sigma_W^2/3n)/(3\sigma_W^2/2n) \times 100 = 88.9\%$. The efficiencies of the other designs can be calculated similarly (see Section 4.9) and are 22.2% and 66.7%, respectively. In addition, as already noted, the correlation between $\hat{\delta}$ and $\widehat{\lambda_T - \lambda_R}$ in the first design is zero, whereas in the second and third designs it is 0.87 and 0.50, respectively. In other words, the first design is not only highly efficient in the presence of differential carry-over effects, but is such that the estimator of δ is the same whether or not carry-over effects are entered into the model for the data. Consequently, there is no disadvantage in using this design even if differential carry-over effects are anticipated or cannot be avoided.

4.2.1 Examples of Analysis of BE Trials with Three Periods

Example 4.1

The data in Tables 4.25 and 4.26 are from a trial that used the sequences RTT and TRR. Figure 4.1 shows the corresponding subject profiles plots. The most noteworthy feature in these plots is that, although the between-subject variability is high for both metrics, it is much lower for logCmax compared to logAUC. In addition, the maximum value in each period for logCmax is much lower than the corresponding maximum for logAUC. There is a suggestion for Sequence 2 that the values of R are higher on average than those of T, but this feature is not so evident in Sequence 1. We can also identify a subject in Sequence 2 who only provided two logAUC values.

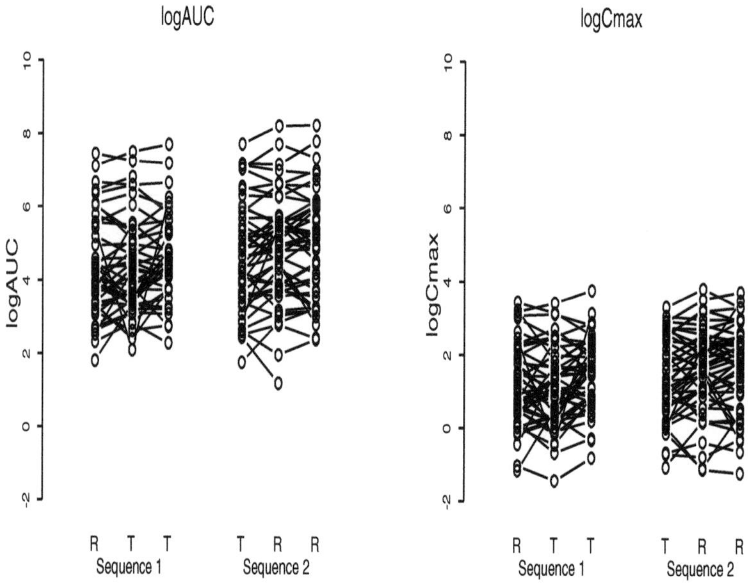

FIGURE 4.1
Example 4.1: Subject Profiles Plot

TABLE 4.2
Example 4.1: Group-by-Period Means (sample size in parentheses)

		logAUC		
Group	Period 1	Period 2	Period 3	Mean
1(RTT)	$\bar{y}_{11.} = 4.35(46)$	$\bar{y}_{12.} = 4.36(45)$	$\bar{y}_{13.} = 4.60(43)$	$\bar{y}_{1..} = 4.43$
2(TRR)	$\bar{y}_{21.} = 4.66(47)$	$\bar{y}_{22.} = 4.88(47)$	$\bar{y}_{23.} = 4.92(47)$	$\bar{y}_{2..} = 4.82$
Mean	$\bar{y}_{.1.} = 4.51$	$\bar{y}_{.2.} = 4.63$	$\bar{y}_{.3.} = 4.77$	$\bar{y}_{...} = 4.63$
		logCmax		
1(RTT)	$\bar{y}_{11.} = 1.18(47)$	$\bar{y}_{12.} = 1.10(47)$	$\bar{y}_{13.} = 1.46(45)$	$\bar{y}_{1..} = 1.24$
2(TRR)	$\bar{y}_{21.} = 1.39(48)$	$\bar{y}_{22.} = 1.60(48)$	$\bar{y}_{23.} = 1.64(48)$	$\bar{y}_{2..} = 1.54$
Mean	$\bar{y}_{.1.} = 1.29$	$\bar{y}_{.2.} = 1.35$	$\bar{y}_{.3.} = 1.55$	$\bar{y}_{...} = 1.40$

The group-by-period means are given in Table 4.2, where, because of the missing data, we have indicated the number of subjects who provided data for each mean. These are plotted in Figure 4.2, where the lower line in each plot refers to Sequence RTT and the upper line to Sequence TRR. Despite the difference in absolute size of the logAUC and logCmax means, there is a similar pattern of formulation differences within each period for both metrics. The only other notable feature is that the means for Sequence 2 are consistently higher than the corresponding means for Sequence 1. To get a graphical impression of the similarity or otherwise of the means of R and T, we can use a version of the mean differences versus totals plot that was used in Chapter 3 for the RT/TR design. In this alternative version of the plot, we replace the within-subject mean difference with a within-subject contrast for the kth subject in sequence group i: $d_{ik} = -(2y_{i1k} - y_{i2k} - y_{i3k})/4$. From Equation (4.1), we can see that $\hat{\delta} = \bar{d}_{1.} - \bar{d}_{2.}$. Instead of the subject totals, we arbitrarily use the mean of each subject, so that we can plot the subject contrasts against the subject means. If the

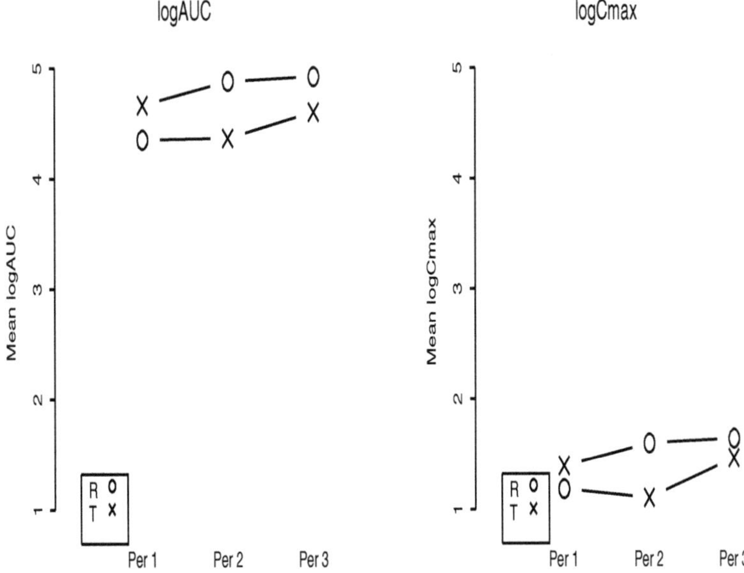

FIGURE 4.2
Example 4.1: Groups-by-Periods Plot

TABLE 4.3
Example 4.1: TOST Procedure Results

log scale		
Endpoint	$\hat{\mu}_T - \hat{\mu}_R$	90% Confidence Interval
logAUC	-0.0270	(-0.1395, 0.0855)
logCmax	-0.0557	(-0.1697, 0.0583)
back-transformed		
Endpoint	$\exp(\hat{\mu}_T - \hat{\mu}_R)$	90% Confidence Interval
AUC	0.97	(0.87, 1.09)
Cmax	0.95	(0.84, 1.06)

contrasts are plotted on the vertical axis, any separation of the groups along this axis is indicative of a lack of equivalence. The resulting plots are given in Figure 4.3. It should be noted that only subjects who have a complete set of three values are included in the plots. As in Chapter 3, we also include the centroids and the convex hulls. From this plot there appears to be little separation of the centroids in the vertical direction. It seems likely that T and R are average bioequivalent.

Of course, to determine if T and R are sufficiently similar to each other to be declared ABE, we must apply the TOST procedure. The results are given in Table 4.3, where subjects have been fitted as fixed effects. We can see that T and R are clearly average bioequivalent.

Example 4.2
The data in Tables 4.27 and 4.28 are from a trial that also used the sequences RTT and TRR. The corresponding subject profiles are given in Figure 4.4. Relatively large between-subject variation is evident, with perhaps a higher variance on the logAUC scale. It is not clear if, on average, T is giving higher or lower values than R.

The group-by-period means are given in Table 4.4, where, because of the missing data, we have again indicated the number of subjects who provided data for each mean. These are plotted in Figure 4.5, where the upper line in each plot refers to Sequence RTT. Even allowing for the difference in absolute size of the logAUC and logCmax means, there is a different pattern of formulation differences within each period for the two metrics. There appears to be more of a difference between the formulations on the logAUC scale. The only other notable feature is that the means for Sequence 1 are consistently higher than the corresponding means for Sequence 2.

A better impression of the difference, if any, between T and R is obtained from a plot of the subject contrasts against the subject means. For Example 4.2, this is given as Figure 4.6. There is a clear separation of the convex hulls for both metrics, suggesting a lack of bioequivalence. In addition, there is clearly more variability in the plotted points from Sequence 2 as compared to Sequence 1.

The results of applying the TOST procedure to these data are given in Table 4.5. Insufficient evidence was present to conclude that T and R are ABE for both AUC and Cmax.

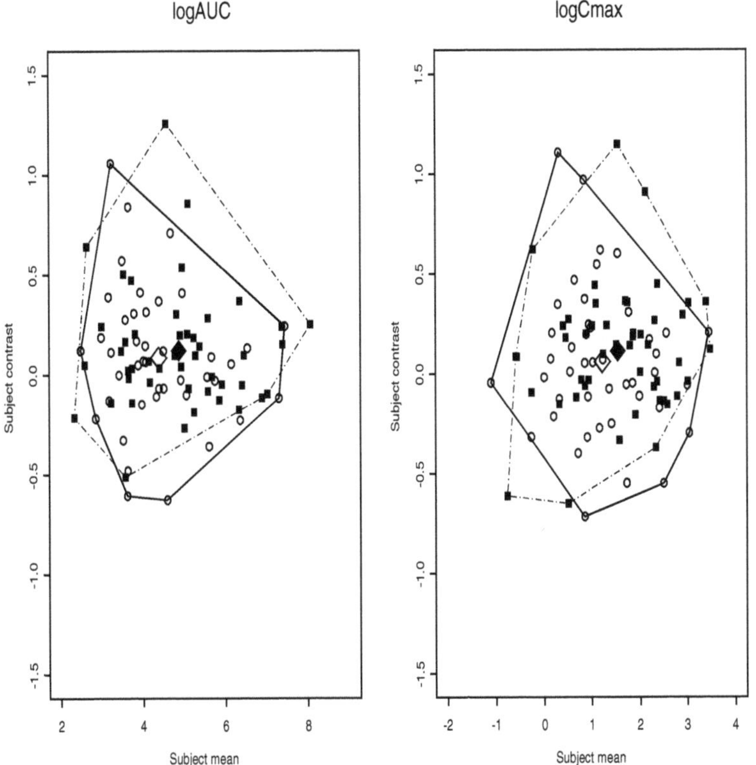

FIGURE 4.3
Example 4.1: Subject Contrasts versus Means Plot

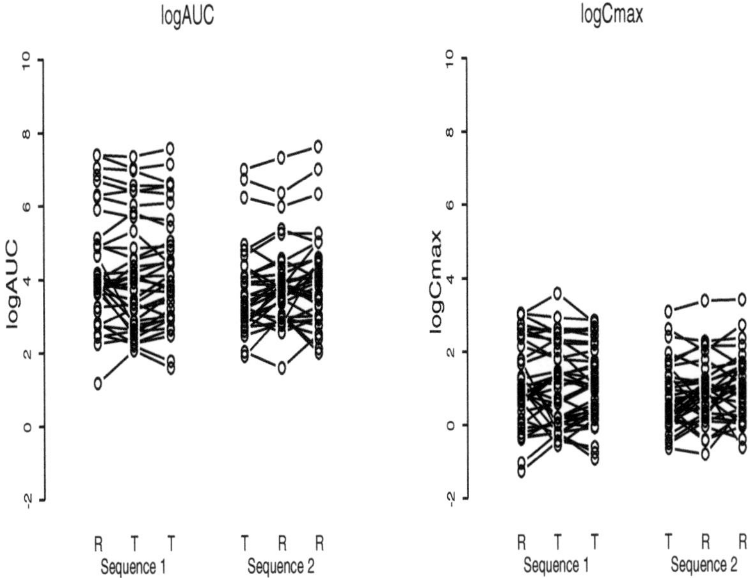

FIGURE 4.4
Example 4.2: Subject Profiles Plot

TABLE 4.4
Example 4.2: Group-by-Period Means (sample size in parentheses)

Group	Period 1	Period 2	Period 3	Mean
		logAUC		
1(RTT)	$\bar{y}_{11.} = 4.30(37)$	$\bar{y}_{12.} = 4.11(38)$	$\bar{y}_{13.} = 4.21(38)$	$\bar{y}_{1..} = 4.21$
2(TRR)	$\bar{y}_{21.} = 3.67(33)$	$\bar{y}_{22.} = 3.83(34)$	$\bar{y}_{23.} = 3.95(35)$	$\bar{y}_{2..} = 3.82$
Mean	$\bar{y}_{.1.} = 4.01$	$\bar{y}_{.2.} = 3.98$	$\bar{y}_{.3.} = 4.08$	$\bar{y}_{...} = 4.02$
		logCmax		
1(RTT)	$\bar{y}_{11.} = 1.13(39)$	$\bar{y}_{12.} = 1.03(39)$	$\bar{y}_{13.} = 1.05(39)$	$\bar{y}_{1..} = 1.07$
2(TRR)	$\bar{y}_{21.} = 0.77(35)$	$\bar{y}_{22.} = 0.88(35)$	$\bar{y}_{23.} = 1.02(35)$	$\bar{y}_{2..} = 0.89$
Mean	$\bar{y}_{.1.} = 0.96$	$\bar{y}_{.2.} = 0.96$	$\bar{y}_{.3.} = 1.04$	$\bar{y}_{...} = 0.98$

TABLE 4.5
Example 4.2: TOST Procedure Results

Endpoint	$\hat{\mu}_T - \hat{\mu}_R$	90% Confidence Interval
logAUC	-0.1719	(-0.2630, -0.0809)
logCmax	-0.1299	(-0.2271, -0.0327)
Endpoint	$\exp(\hat{\mu}_T - \hat{\mu}_R)$	**90% Confidence Interval**
AUC	0.84	(0.77, 0.92)
Cmax	0.88	(0.80, 0.97)

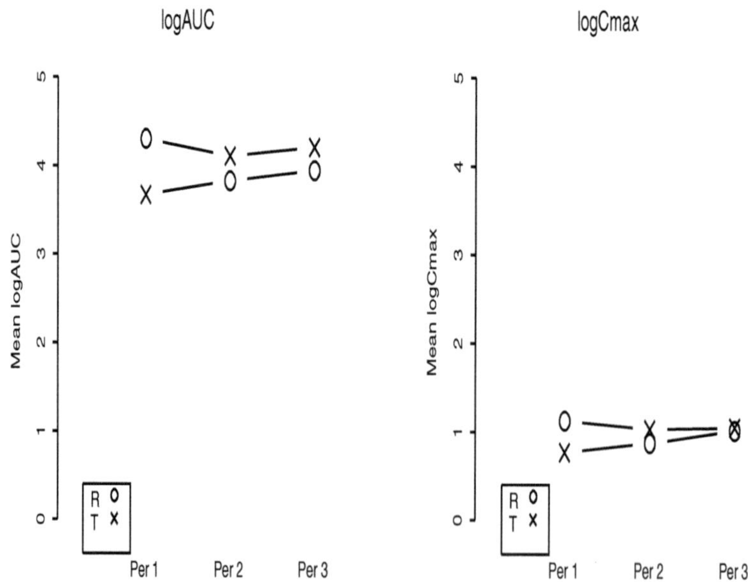

FIGURE 4.5
Example 4.2: Groups-by-Periods Plot

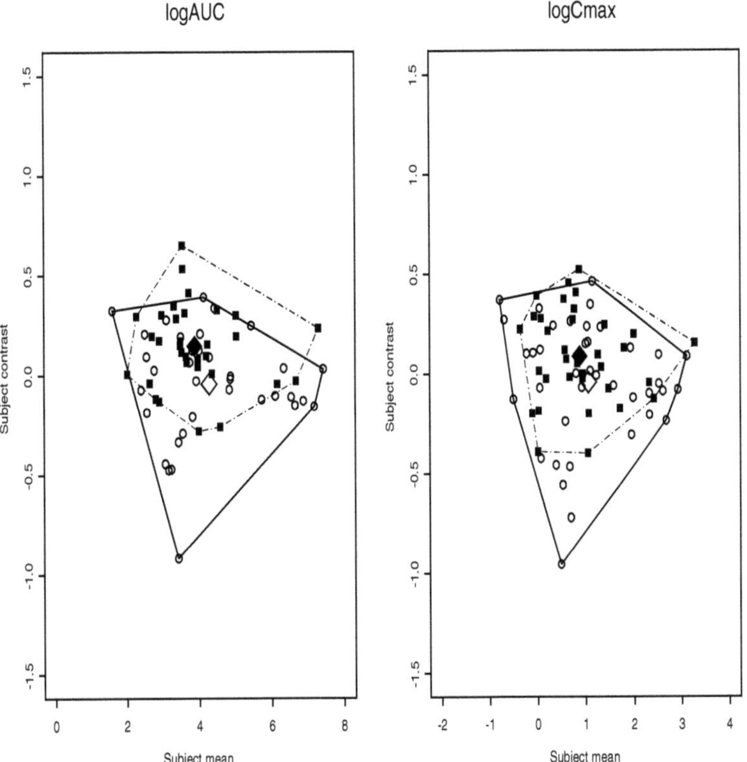

FIGURE 4.6
Example 4.2: Subject Contrasts versus Means Plot

4.3 Within-Subject Variability

It is clear that each of our possible designs for three periods has T repeated in one sequence and R repeated in the other. It is therefore possible to separately estimate the within-subject variance of T and the within-subject variance of R. We will denote these by σ^2_{WT} and σ^2_{WR}, respectively. Let us concentrate on the design that has sequences RTT and TRR. Suppose we want an estimate of σ^2_{WT} for the logAUC values. A simple method of estimation uses only the subjects who have a logAUC value on both occurrences of T. Suppose we denote these values by y_{12k} and y_{13k} for such a subject k in the first sequence group. Then $\text{Var}(y_{12k} - y_{13k}) = 2\sigma^2_{WT}$. To estimate this variance, we first construct the set of differences $y_{12k} - y_{13k}$ and then estimate the variance of the differences. The estimate so obtained, and divided by 2, gives $\hat{\sigma}^2_{WT}$. A similar process can be used to calculate $\hat{\sigma}^2_{WR}$ using the appropriate subjects in the second sequence group. In a 2×2 cross-over a similar procedure is used to calculate $\hat{\sigma}^2_W$ under the assumption that $\sigma^2_{WT} = \sigma^2_{WR} = \sigma^2_W$ [652].

Doing this for Example 4.1, we get, for logAUC, $\hat{\sigma}^2_{WR} = 0.168$ and $\hat{\sigma}^2_{WT} = 0.396$, and for logCmax, $\hat{\sigma}^2_{WR} = 0.214$ and $\hat{\sigma}^2_{WT} = 0.347$.

For Example 4.2, the corresponding values for logAUC are $\hat{\sigma}^2_{WR} = 0.168$, $\hat{\sigma}^2_{WT} = 0.065$, and for logCmax they are $\hat{\sigma}^2_{WR} = 0.201$ and $\hat{\sigma}^2_{WT} = 0.087$.

In both examples, $\hat{\sigma}^2_{WR} > 0.09$ for each metric, indicating that the Reference formulations are highly variable.

In Chapter 5 we will give an alternative method of estimation.

4.4 Robust Analyses for Three-Period Designs

The model assumed for our data (logAUC or logCmax) is as given in (3.1) in Chapter 3:

$$y_{ijk} = \mu_{d[i,j]} + \pi_j + \gamma_i + \xi_{k(i)} + \varepsilon_{ijk}.$$

This makes some strong assumptions about the variance and covariance structure of the repeated measurements on each subject. In particular, it assumes that the variance of each repeated measurement is the same and that the covariance between any two repeated measurements is the same, i.e.,$\text{Var}(y_{ijk}) = \sigma_B^2 + \sigma_W^2$ and

$$\text{Cov}(y_{i1k}, y_{i2k}) = \text{Cov}(y_{i1k}, y_{i3k}) = \text{Cov}(y_{i2k}, y_{i3k}) = \sigma_B^2.$$

If there is any doubt that these assumptions are unlikely to be true, an alternative, robust, analysis is possible. The analysis is robust in the sense that the only assumptions made are that the responses from different subjects are independent, the two groups of subjects are a random sample from the same statistical population, and that the period, treatment, and other effects act additively. The analysis for the sequences RTT and TRR uses the same subject contrasts that were used to construct the subject contrasts versus means plot: $d_{ik} = -(2y_{i1k} - y_{i2k} - y_{i3k})/4$, where it will be recalled that $\hat{\delta} = \bar{d}_{1.} - \bar{d}_{2.}$. The assumptions made in the analysis are then those referring to d_{ik}: the values from different subjects are independent, the values in each group are a random sample from the same statistical population, and finally the only difference, if any, between the groups is a shift in the value of the mean (or median).

Having calculated the values of d_{ik} (for those patients who provided three repeated measurements), the TOST analysis uses the 90% confidence interval based on the t-distribution or, if the data are very non-normal, the Hodges–Lehmann version of the confidence interval.

For the kth subject in Group 1, $k = 1, 2, \ldots, n_1$, we define $d_{1k} = -(2y_{11k} - y_{12k} - y_{13k})/4$ in Group 1 and $d_{2k} = -(2y_{21k} - y_{22k} - y_{23k})/4$ in Group 2. If ${\sigma_d}^2 = \text{Var}[d_{1k}] = \text{Var}[d_{2k}]$, then

$$\text{Var}[\hat{\delta}] = \sigma_d^2 \left[\frac{1}{n_1} + \frac{1}{n_2} \right].$$

To estimate ${\sigma_d}^2$ we use the usual pooled estimator

$${s_p}^2 = \frac{(n_1 - 1)s_1^2 + (n_2 - 1)s_2^2}{(n_1 + n_2 - 2)},$$

where s_1^2 is the sample variance of d_{1k} and ${s_2}^2$ is the sample variance of d_{2k}. To construct the 90% confidence interval for δ we use that fact that, when $\delta = 0$,

$$t = \frac{\bar{d}_{1.} - \bar{d}_{2.}}{\left[s_p^2 \left(\frac{1}{n_1} + \frac{1}{n_2} \right) \right]^{\frac{1}{2}}}$$

has the t-distribution with $(n_1 + n_2 - 2)$ degrees of freedom. It will be noted that the degrees of freedom for the usual TOST interval, based on subjects with all three repeated measurements, is $2(n_1 + n_2) - 3$, as compared to $(n_1 + n_2 - 2)$ for the robust method. Even so, this loss of degrees of freedom rarely has a major effect on the conclusions.

For the data in Example 4.1, $n_1 = 42$, $n_2 = 46$ for logAUC, and $\bar{d}_{1.} = -0.0850$, $\bar{d}_{2.} = -0.1215$ and $\hat{\delta} = -0.0365$. Further, $s_1^2 = 0.1191$, $s_2^2 = 0.0917$, and $s_p^2 = 0.1048$. Based on the t-distribution with 86 degrees of freedom, the TOST 90% confidence is (-0.1514, 0.0783). If the usual analysis (of y_{ijk}) is done, the corresponding interval is (-0.1516, 0.0785), based on the t-distribution with 173 degrees of freedom. The robust interval is a little wider but, in this case at least, the conclusions are the same. For logCmax the robust confidence interval is (-0.1712, 0.0651) on 91 degrees of freedom, as compared to the usual interval of (-0.1685, 0.0623) on 183 degrees of freedom.

For the data in Example 4.2, $n_1 = 35$, $n_2 = 32$ for logAUC and the robust interval is (-0.2880, -0.0897) on 65 d.f. and the usual interval is (-0.2800, -0.0977) on 131 d.f. For logCmax, $n_1 = 39$, $n_2 = 35$ and the robust interval is (-0.2359, -0.0239) on 72 d.f. and the usual interval is (-0.2271, -0.0327) on 145 d.f. Again, the conclusions from both approaches are the same.

An alternative confidence interval that does not rely on the t-distribution is the Hodges–Lehmann point confidence interval described in Chapter 3. In the notation of that chapter, we let $X_k = d_{2k}$ and $Y_k = d_{1k}$. The resulting confidence intervals for Example 4.1 are (-0.1196, -0.0731) for logAUC and (-0.1679, 0.0394) for logCmax. For Example 4.2, the corresponding intervals are $(-0.2635, -0.0771)$ for logAUC and (-0.2042, -0.0071) for logCmax. The conclusions obtained above are not changed for either example. The Hodges–Lehmann confidence intervals can also be constructed using StatXact. For Example 4.1 these are (-0.1199, 0.0734) for logAUC and (-0.1683, 0.0410) for logCmax. For Example 4.2 these are (-0.2635, -0.0771) and (-0.2049, -0.0070), respectively.

4.5 Four-Period Designs

4.5.1 Choice of Design

As already mentioned, four-period designs are recommended by the FDA when the reference drug is highly variable (i.e., $\sigma_W^2 > 0.09$). If we discard the sequences RRRR and TTTT, then there are seven different two-sequence designs and they are

1.	R	R	T	T	2.	R	T	R	T	3.	R	T	T	R
	T	T	R	R		T	R	T	R		T	R	R	T
4.	R	T	R	R	5.	R	R	T	R	6.	R	T	T	T
	T	R	T	T		T	T	R	T		T	R	R	R

and

7.	R	R	R	T
	T	T	T	R

The efficiencies of these designs are given in Table 4.6. In the presence of unequal carry-over effects, only Designs 1 and 3 are worth consideration [652]. It is worth noting that the design recommended by the FDA is Design 2. In the absence of a difference in carry-over effects, Designs 1, 2, and 3 are equally, and fully, efficient.

TABLE 4.6
Efficiencies of Designs 1 through 7

Design	Adjusted for Carry-Over	Unadjusted for Carry-Over
1	90.91	100.00
2	18.18	100.00
3	90.91	100.00
4	54.55	75.00
5	54.55	75.00
6	72.73	75.00
7	66.67	75.00

4.5.2 Examples of Data Analysis for Four-Period Designs

Example 4.3
The data in Table 4.29 are from a trial with four periods that used the sequences RTTR and TRRT. This trial was quite small, with 8 subjects in Group 1 and 9 in Group 2. The subject profiles plots for logAUC and logCmax are given in Figure 4.7. From this plot it is difficult to discern if T and R are ABE. The group-by-period means are given in Table 4.7 and are plotted in Figure 4.8. These seem to indicate that T and R are ABE.

The subject contrasts plots are given in Figure 4.9 and reveal a difference in the centroids, particularly for logCmax, although the actual size of the difference is relatively small. There is also some evidence that there is more variability in the logAUC contrasts for the subjects on sequence TRRT. To clarify matters regarding ABE, we refer to the results of the TOSTs given in Table 4.8, where the fixed-subjects models have been fitted. The evidence is in favor

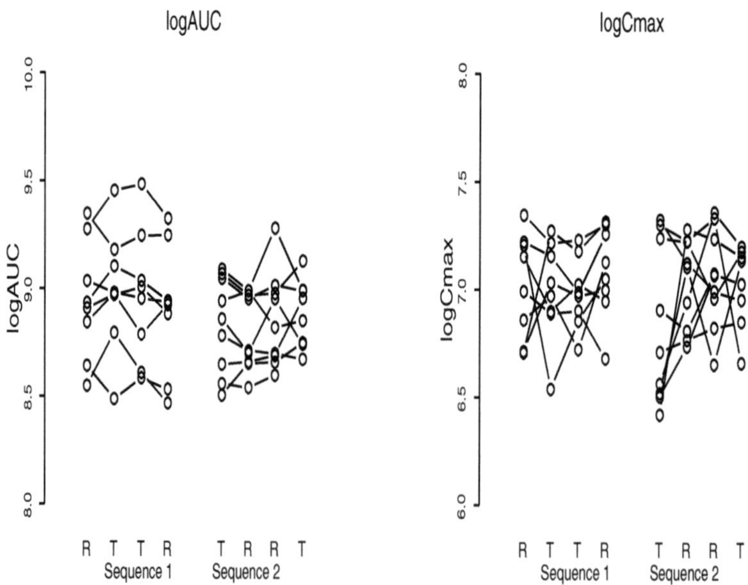

FIGURE 4.7
Example 4.3: Subject Profiles Plot

TABLE 4.7
Example 4.3: Group-by-Period Means (sample size in parentheses)

			logAUC		
Group	Period 1	Period 2	Period 3	Period 4	Mean
1(RTTR)	$\bar{y}_{11.} = 8.94(8)$	$\bar{y}_{12.} = 8.99(8)$	$\bar{y}_{13.} = 8.96(8)$	$\bar{y}_{14.} = 8.91(8)$	$\bar{y}_{1..} = 8.95$
2(TRRT)	$\bar{y}_{21.} = 8.83(9)$	$\bar{y}_{22.} = 8.80(9)$	$\bar{y}_{23.} = 8.85(9)$	$\bar{y}_{24.} = 8.89(8)$	$\bar{y}_{2..} = 8.84$
Mean	$\bar{y}_{.1.} = 8.88$	$\bar{y}_{.2.} = 8.89$	$\bar{y}_{.3.} = 8.91$	$\bar{y}_{.4.} = 8.90$	$\bar{y}_{...} = 8.89$
			logCmax		
1(RTTR)	$\bar{y}_{11.} = 7.02(8)$	$\bar{y}_{12.} = 7.00(8)$	$\bar{y}_{13.} = 6.98(8)$	$\bar{y}_{14.} = 7.08(8)$	$\bar{y}_{1..} = 7.02$
2(TRRT)	$\bar{y}_{21.} = 6.83(9)$	$\bar{y}_{22.} = 7.02(9)$	$\bar{y}_{23.} = 7.06(9)$	$\bar{y}_{24.} = 7.02(8)$	$\bar{y}_{2..} = 6.98$
Mean	$\bar{y}_{.1.} = 6.92$	$\bar{y}_{.2.} = 7.01$	$\bar{y}_{.3.} = 7.02$	$\bar{y}_{.4.} = 7.05$	$\bar{y}_{...} = 7.00$

of concluding that T and R are ABE, although for logCmax the lower end of the confidence interval is close to the lower boundary of -0.2231 (on the log scale). The robust and Hodges–Lehmann exact confidence intervals are (-0.0080, 0.0811) and (-0.0148, 0.0834), respectively, for logAUC and (-0.1786, 0.0038) and (-0.2001, 0.0073), respectively, for logCmax.

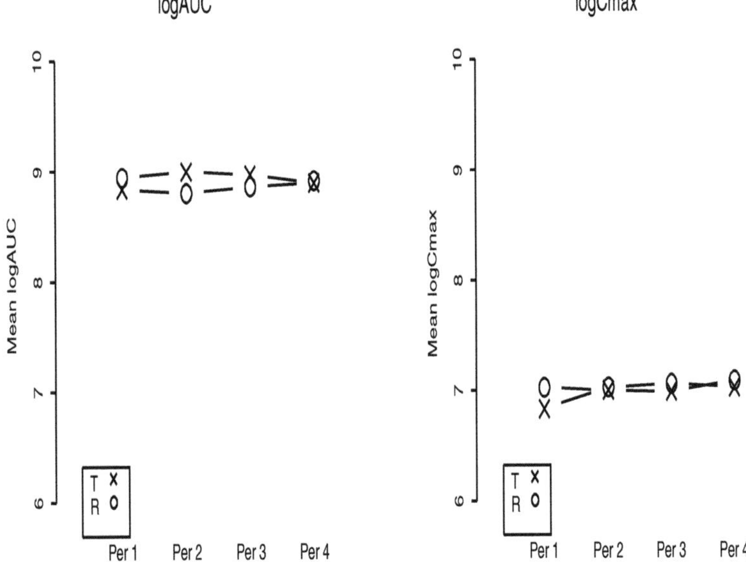

FIGURE 4.8
Example 4.3: Groups-by-Periods Plot

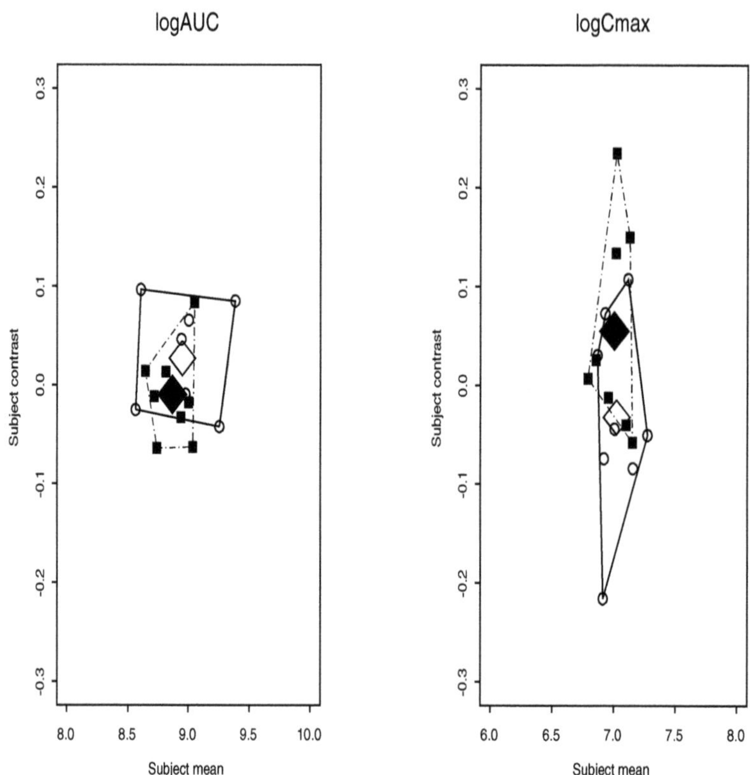

FIGURE 4.9
Example 4.3: Subject Contrasts versus Means Plot

TABLE 4.8
Example 4.3: TOST Procedure Results

Endpoint	$\hat{\mu}_T - \hat{\mu}_R$	90% Confidence Interval
logAUC	0.0352	(-0.0044, 0.0748)
logCmax	-0.0963	(-0.1881, 0.0045)
Endpoint	$\exp(\hat{\mu}_T - \hat{\mu}_R)$	90% Confidence Interval
AUC	1.04	(1.00, 1.08)
Cmax	0.91	(0.83, 1.00)

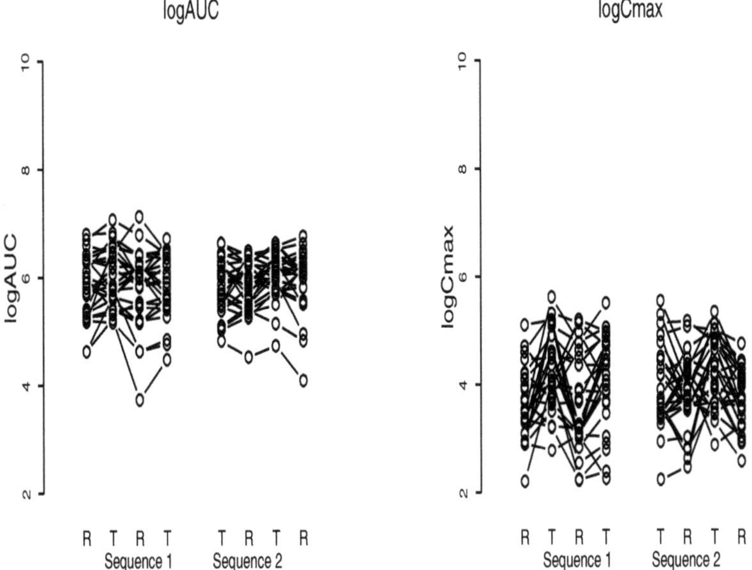

FIGURE 4.10
Example 4.4: Subject Profiles Plot

Example 4.4
The data in Tables 4.30 and 4.31 are from another four-period design, but this time the sequences used were RTRT and TRTR. The subject profiles plots are given in Figure 4.10. The large number of subjects per group makes it difficult to discern much from this plot, other than the relatively large between-subject variation. The group-by-period means are given in Table 4.9 and plotted in Figure 4.11. The picture is clearer now, with a suggestion that for logCmax T and R might not be ABE. The subject contrasts versus means plot is

TABLE 4.9
Example 4.4: Group-by-Period Means (sample size in parentheses)

		logAUC			
Group	Period 1	2	3	4	Mean
1	$\bar{y}_{11.} = 5.80(27)$	$\bar{y}_{12.} = 6.00(27)$	$\bar{y}_{13.} = 5.80(26)$	$\bar{y}_{14.} = 5.85(26)$	$\bar{y}_{1..} = 5.86$
2	$\bar{y}_{21.} = 5.84(27)$	$\bar{y}_{22.} = 5.81(27)$	$\bar{y}_{23.} = 6.04(26)$	$\bar{y}_{24.} = 5.91(26)$	$\bar{y}_{2..} = 5.90$
Mean	$\bar{y}_{.1.} = 5.82$	$\bar{y}_{.2.} = 5.91$	$\bar{y}_{.3.} = 5.92$	$\bar{y}_{.4.} = 5.88$	$\bar{y}_{...} = 5.88$
		logCmax			
1	$\bar{y}_{11.} = 3.63(27)$	$\bar{y}_{12.} = 4.26(27)$	$\bar{y}_{13.} = 3.69(26)$	$\bar{y}_{14.} = 4.09(26)$	$\bar{y}_{1..} = 3.91$
2	$\bar{y}_{21.} = 3.96(27)$	$\bar{y}_{22.} = 3.82(27)$	$\bar{y}_{23.} = 4.26(26)$	$\bar{y}_{24.} = 3.76(26)$	$\bar{y}_{2..} = 3.95$
Mean	$\bar{y}_{.1.} = 3.79$	$\bar{y}_{.2.} = 4.04$	$\bar{y}_{.3.} = 3.97$	$\bar{y}_{.4.} = 3.93$	$\bar{y}_{...} = 3.93$
		Group 1=RTRT; 2=TRTR			

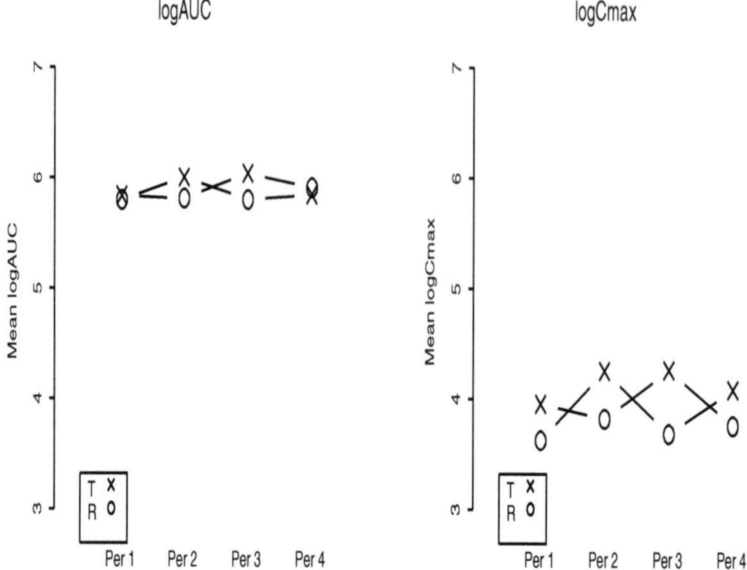

FIGURE 4.11
Example 4.4: Groups-by-Periods Plot

given in Figure 4.12, where it is clear there is a relatively large vertical gap in the centroids for logCmax. This is confirmed from the TOST results given in Table 4.10, where the lower bound of the 90% confidence interval for logCmax is a long way above 0.2231, the upper regulatory limit. The robust and Hodges–Lehmann confidence intervals for logAUC are (0.0311, 1758) and (0.0256, 0.1630), respectively. The corresponding intervals for logCmax are (0.2685, 0.5623) and (0.2681, 0.5626). There is very strong evidence that T and R are not ABE.

TABLE 4.10
Example 4.4: TOST Procedure Results

Endpoint	$\hat{\mu}_T - \hat{\mu}_R$	90% Confidence Interval
logAUC	0.1002	(0.0289, 0.1715)
logCmax	0.4140	(0.2890, 0.5389)
Endpoint	$\exp(\hat{\mu}_T - \hat{\mu}_R)$	90% Confidence Interval
AUC	1.11	(1.03, 1.19)
Cmax	1.51	(1.34, 1.71)

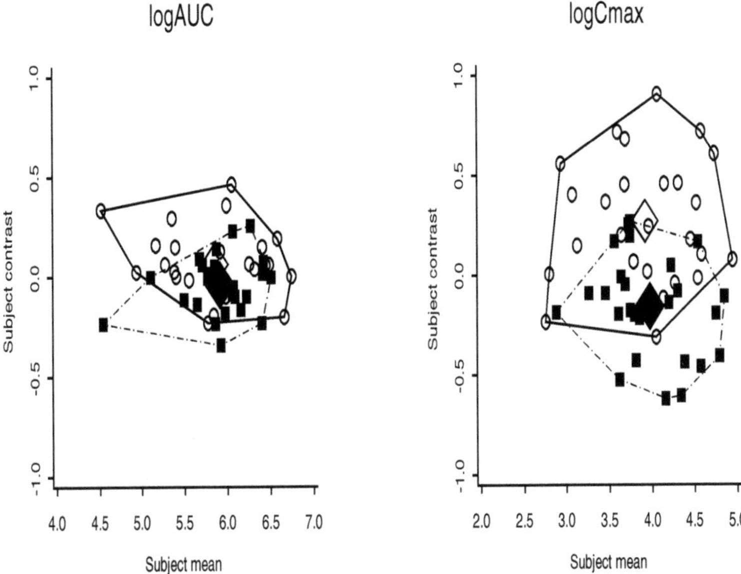

FIGURE 4.12
Example 4.4: Subject Contrasts versus Means Plot

4.6 Designs with More Than Two Treatments

As already mentioned in the Introduction, designs for more than two treatments may be used to show bioequivalence, but these are less common than those for two treatments. Examples 4.5 and 4.6, below are examples where three and four treatments, respectively, were used.

Example 4.5. Trial with Three Treatments
In this trial there were two "reference" formulations, R and S, where R was a dose made up of three 100 mg tablets and S was a dose made up of a 200 mg tablet and a 100 mg tablet. The test formulation was a single 300 mg tablet. Two reference formulations were used because the 200 mg tablet was not available in the early stages of the confirmatory trial when the 3 × 100 mg dose was used. The aim of the trial was to show that T and R were ABE **and** T and S were ABE. The subjects in the trial were randomly allocated to the six sequences: RST, RTS, SRT, STR, TRS, and TSR. The data from this trial are given in Tables 4.32, 4.33, and 4.34. This design is known as a Williams design (see [652], Chapter 4) and is balanced for carry-over effects. In the presence of carry-over effects the variance of any pairwise difference between the formulations is $(5\sigma^2_W)/(12r)$, where r is the number of replications of the complete set of six sequences. In the absence of carry-over effects this variance is $(\sigma^2_W)/(3r)$, which is also the variance in an ideal design. Hence, the efficiency of the Williams design for three formulations is 80% in the presence of carry-over effects and 100% in the absence of carry-over effects. Of course, we do not expect to see any differential carry-over effects and, as we shall see, there is no suggestion from the data that such effects need concern us.

The subject profiles plots are given in Figures 4.13, 4.14, and 4.15. Large between-subject variation is evident and there is a suggestion that S gives a higher response than R or T. The group-by-period means are given in Table 4.11 and are plotted in Figure 4.16.

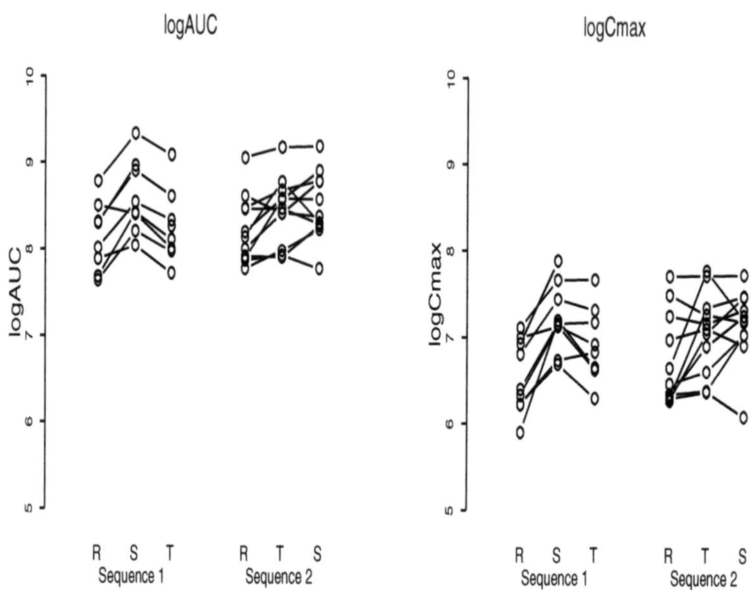

FIGURE 4.13
Example 4.5: Subject Profiles Plot: Sequences 1 and 2

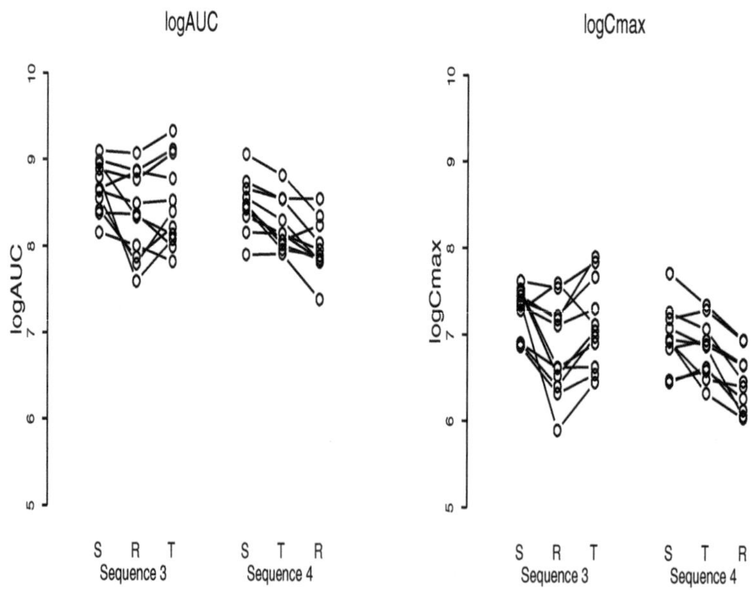

FIGURE 4.14
Example 4.5: Subject Profiles Plot: Sequences 3 and 4

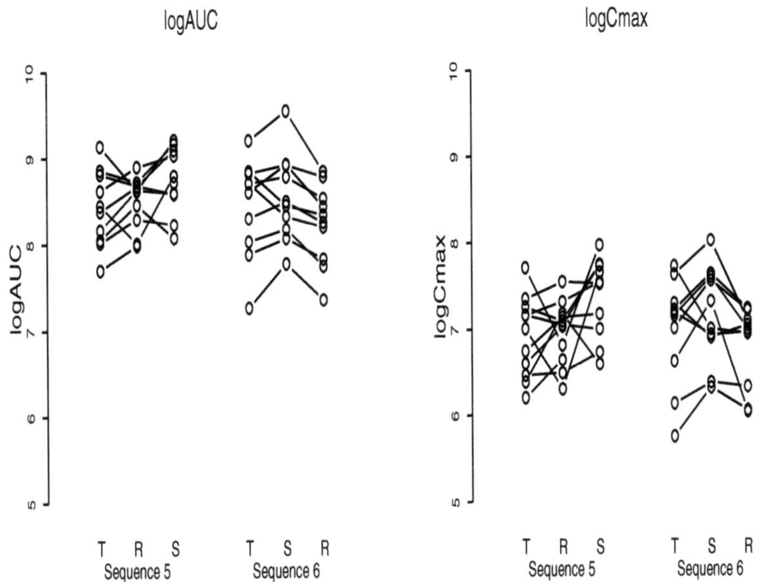

FIGURE 4.15
Example 4.5: Subject Profiles Plot: Sequences 5 and 6

TABLE 4.11
Example 4.5: Group-by-Period Means (sample size in parentheses)

		logAUC		
Group	Period 1	Period 2	Period 3	Mean
1(RST)	$\bar{y}_{11.} = 8.14(8)$	$\bar{y}_{12.} = 8.61(8)$	$\bar{y}_{13.} = 8.27(8)$	$\bar{y}_{1..} = 8.34$
2(RTS)	$\bar{y}_{21.} = 8.23(11)$	$\bar{y}_{22.} = 8.45(11)$	$\bar{y}_{23.} = 8.51(11)$	$\bar{y}_{2..} = 8.40$
3(SRT)	$\bar{y}_{31.} = 8.69(11)$	$\bar{y}_{32.} = 8.37(11)$	$\bar{y}_{33.} = 8.50(11)$	$\bar{y}_{3..} = 8.52$
4(STR)	$\bar{y}_{41.} = 8.49(10)$	$\bar{y}_{42.} = 8.25(10)$	$\bar{y}_{43.} = 8.00(10)$	$\bar{y}_{4..} = 8.25$
5(TRS)	$\bar{y}_{51.} = 8.42(10)$	$\bar{y}_{52.} = 8.50(10)$	$\bar{y}_{53.} = 8.75(10)$	$\bar{y}_{5..} = 8.55$
6(TSR)	$\bar{y}_{61.} = 8.43(10)$	$\bar{y}_{62.} = 8.54(10)$	$\bar{y}_{63.} = 8.23(10)$	$\bar{y}_{6..} = 8.40$
Mean	$\bar{y}_{.1.} = 8.41$	$\bar{y}_{.2.} = 8.45$	$\bar{y}_{.3.} = 8.38$	$\bar{y}_{...} = 8.41$
		logCmax		
1(RST)	$\bar{y}_{11.} = 6.55(9)$	$\bar{y}_{12.} = 7.23(9)$	$\bar{y}_{13.} = 6.94(8)$	$\bar{y}_{1..} = 6.91$
2(RTS)	$\bar{y}_{21.} = 6.74(11)$	$\bar{y}_{22.} = 7.07(11)$	$\bar{y}_{23.} = 7.16(11)$	$\bar{y}_{2..} = 6.99$
3(SRT)	$\bar{y}_{31.} = 7.29(11)$	$\bar{y}_{32.} = 6.82(11)$	$\bar{y}_{33.} = 7.13(11)$	$\bar{y}_{3..} = 7.08$
4(STR)	$\bar{y}_{41.} = 6.99(10)$	$\bar{y}_{42.} = 6.85(10)$	$\bar{y}_{43.} = 6.46(10)$	$\bar{y}_{4..} = 6.77$
5(TRS)	$\bar{y}_{51.} = 6.91(11)$	$\bar{y}_{52.} = 6.97(11)$	$\bar{y}_{53.} = 7.37(10)$	$\bar{y}_{5..} = 7.07$
6(TSR)	$\bar{y}_{61.} = 6.97(10)$	$\bar{y}_{62.} = 7.17(10)$	$\bar{y}_{63.} = 6.79(10)$	$\bar{y}_{6..} = 6.98$
Mean	$\bar{y}_{.1.} = 6.92$	$\bar{y}_{.2.} = 7.01$	$\bar{y}_{.3.} = 6.98$	$\bar{y}_{...} = 6.97$

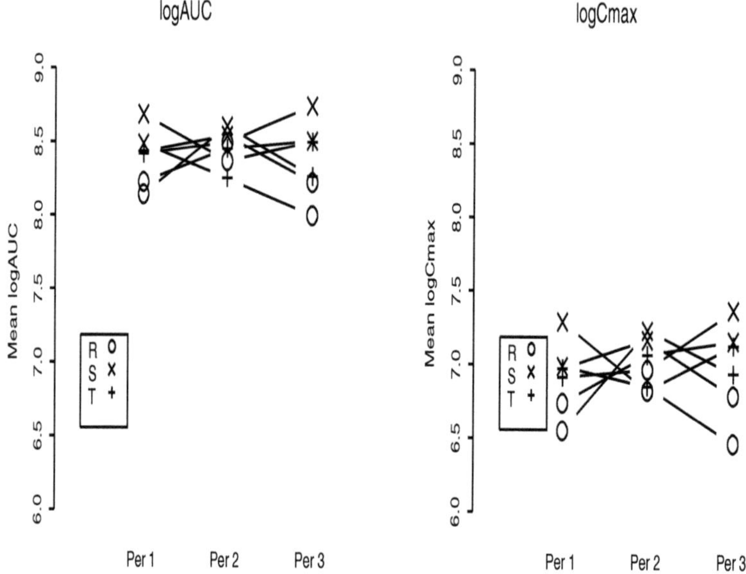

FIGURE 4.16
Example 4.5: Groups-by-Periods Plot

There is a clear ordering within all but one of the periods, with S giving the highest mean response and R the lowest. To determine if each of T and R and T and S are ABE, we use the TOST procedure for each difference and the results are given in Table 4.12. Note that we do not adjust for multiple testing, as we require both pairs to be ABE (across both the AUC and Cmax endpoints and two one-sided tests [1314]). We can conclude that T is

TABLE 4.12
Example 4.5: TOST Procedure Results

		T-R
Endpoint	$\hat{\mu}_T - \hat{\mu}_R$	90% Confidence Interval
logAUC	0.1505	(0.0865, 0.2145)
logCmax	0.2618	(0.1747, 0.3489)
		T-S
Endpoint	$\hat{\mu}_T - \hat{\mu}_S$	90% Confidence Interval
logAUC	-0.1888	(-0.2532, -0.1243)
logCmax	-0.2044	(-0.2921, -0.1167)
		T-R
Endpoint	$\exp(\hat{\mu}_T - \hat{\mu}_R)$	90% Confidence Interval
AUC	1.16	(1.09, 1.24)
Cmax	1.30	(1.19, 1.42)
		T-S
Endpoint	$\exp(\hat{\mu}_T - \hat{\mu}_S)$	90% Confidence Interval
AUC	0.83	(0.78, 0.88)
Cmax	0.82	(0.75, 0.89)

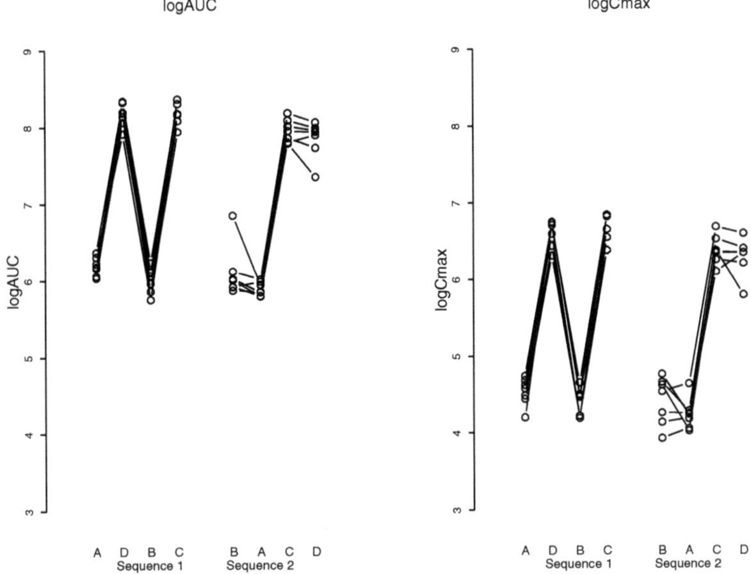

FIGURE 4.17
Example 4.6: Subject Profiles Plot: Sequences 1 and 2

not ABE to R and S. The ordering of the formulation means is, as noted from the previous plots, that S gives a significantly higher response than T, which in turn is significantly higher than R.

Example 4.6. Trial with Four Treatments
In this trial the test formulation could be given as a low or a high dose. Hence, it was necessary to compare these with low and high doses, respectively, of the reference formulation. The four formulations were labelled A, B, C, and D, where A is the Reference, Low dose, B is the Test, Low dose, C is the Reference, High dose, and D is the Test, High dose. The comparisons of interest were therefore B-A and D-C. A Williams design for four periods was used in the trial with sequences ADBC, BACD, CBDA, and DCAB. The efficiency of this design is 90.91% in the presence of differential carry-over effects and 100% in their absence.

The data from this trial are given in Tables 4.35 to 4.38 and the subject profiles plots are given in Figures 4.17 and 4.18. The large changes in the plots occur when moving from a low to a high dose and vice versa. Within a dose there seems relatively good agreement between T and R. The group-by-period means are given in Table 4.13 and are plotted in Figure 4.19, where it will be noted that the symbols for A and C are the circle and triangle, respectively, and the symbols for B and D are the vertical and diagonal crosses, respectively. The large difference between the means values for the two doses (circle and triangle versus vertical and diagonal cross) is clearly displayed, as is the relatively small difference between T and R within doses (circle versus triangle and vertical versus diagonal cross). At first sight, at least, it appears the T and R are ABE at each dose. The results of the TOST procedure are given in Table 4.14, and these confirm the conclusions made from the plots.

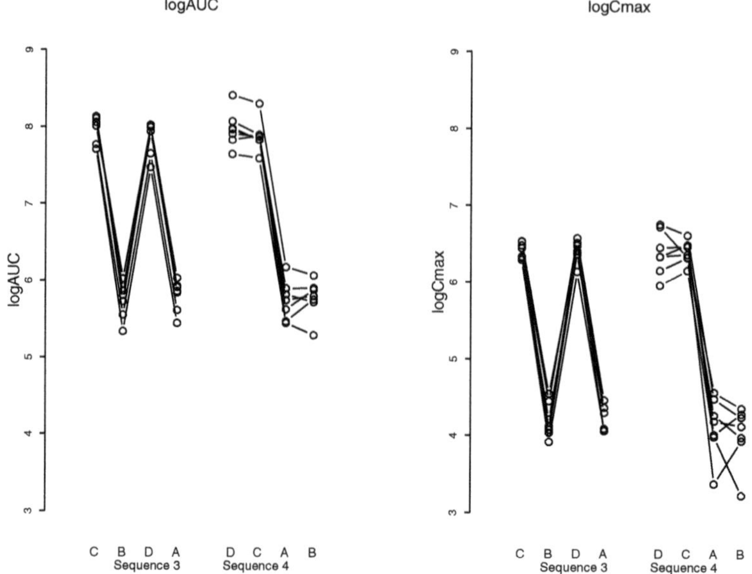

FIGURE 4.18
Example 4.6: Subject Profiles Plot: Sequences 3 and 4

TABLE 4.13
Example 4.6: Group-by-Period Means (sample size in parentheses)

Group	Period 1	Period 2	Period 3	Period 4	Mean
			logAUC		
1(ADBC)	$\bar{y}_{11.} = 6.19(7)$	$\bar{y}_{12.} = 8.17(7)$	$\bar{y}_{13.} = 6.01(7)$	$\bar{y}_{14.} = 8.17(7)$	$\bar{y}_{1..} = 7.14$
2(BACD)	$\bar{y}_{21.} = 6.10(7)$	$\bar{y}_{22.} = 5.89(7)$	$\bar{y}_{23.} = 7.95(7)$	$\bar{y}_{24.} = 7.84(7)$	$\bar{y}_{2..} = 6.95$
1(CBDA)	$\bar{y}_{11.} = 7.99(7)$	$\bar{y}_{12.} = 5.76(7)$	$\bar{y}_{13.} = 7.87(7)$	$\bar{y}_{14.} = 5.81(7)$	$\bar{y}_{1..} = 6.86$
2(DCAB)	$\bar{y}_{21.} = 7.98(7)$	$\bar{y}_{22.} = 7.89(7)$	$\bar{y}_{23.} = 5.74(7)$	$\bar{y}_{24.} = 5.78(7)$	$\bar{y}_{2..} = 6.85$
Mean	$\bar{y}_{.1.} = 7.06$	$\bar{y}_{.2.} = 6.93$	$\bar{y}_{.3.} = 6.90$	$\bar{y}_{.4.} = 6.90$	$\bar{y}_{...} = 6.95$
			logCmax		
1(ADBC)	$\bar{y}_{11.} = 4.54(7)$	$\bar{y}_{12.} = 6.61(7)$	$\bar{y}_{13.} = 4.39(7)$	$\bar{y}_{14.} = 6.64(7)$	$\bar{y}_{1..} = 5.54$
2(BACD)	$\bar{y}_{21.} = 4.41(7)$	$\bar{y}_{22.} = 4.24(7)$	$\bar{y}_{23.} = 6.37(7)$	$\bar{y}_{24.} = 6.29(7)$	$\bar{y}_{2..} = 5.33$
1(CBDA)	$\bar{y}_{11.} = 6.42(7)$	$\bar{y}_{12.} = 4.20(7)$	$\bar{y}_{13.} = 6.41(7)$	$\bar{y}_{14.} = 4.26(7)$	$\bar{y}_{1..} = 5.32$
2(DCAB)	$\bar{y}_{21.} = 6.39(7)$	$\bar{y}_{22.} = 6.39(7)$	$\bar{y}_{23.} = 4.13(7)$	$\bar{y}_{24.} = 4.03(7)$	$\bar{y}_{2..} = 5.23$
Mean	$\bar{y}_{.1.} = 5.44$	$\bar{y}_{.2.} = 5.36$	$\bar{y}_{.3.} = 5.33$	$\bar{y}_{.4.} = 5.30$	$\bar{y}_{...} = 5.36$

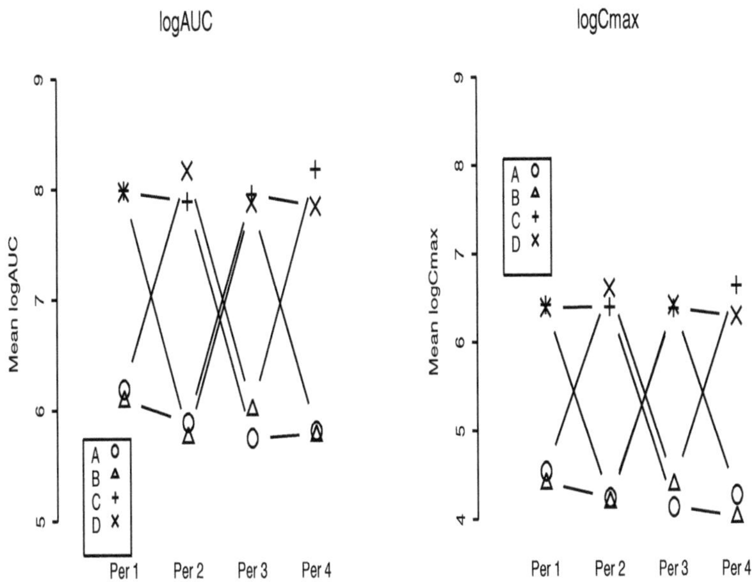

FIGURE 4.19
Example 4.6: Groups-by-Periods Plot

TABLE 4.14
Example 4.6: TOST Procedure Results

		B-A
Endpoint	$\hat{\mu}_B - \hat{\mu}_A$	90% Confidence Interval
logAUC	0.0047	(-0.0544, 0.0638)
logCmax	-0.0355	(-0.1171, 0.0461)
		D-C
Endpoint	$\hat{\mu}_D - \hat{\mu}_C$	90% Confidence Interval
logAUC	-0.0362	(-0.0953, 0.0230)
logCmax	-0.0301	(-0.1117, 0.0515)
		B-A
Endpoint	$\exp(\hat{\mu}_B - \hat{\mu}_A)$	90% Confidence Interval
AUC	1.00	(0.95, 1.07)
Cmax	0.97	(0.89, 1.05)
		D-C
Endpoint	$\exp(\hat{\mu}_D - \hat{\mu}_C)$	90% Confidence Interval
AUC	0.96	(0.91, 1.02)
Cmax	0.97	(0.89, 1.05)

4.7 Adjusting for Multiple Testing

As discussed in Chapter 2, by design, multiple tests are performed to assess bioequivalence using the two one-sided testing procedure. A question often asked is, "Does one need to adjust the TOST (or equivalently the 90% confidence intervals) for multiple tests within a study?"

The sources of multiple tests in bioequivalence are many. Multiple endpoints (AUC, Cmax) are always involved in bioequivalence testing. Also, for example, in studies like Examples 4.5 and 4.6, when more than one test or reference formulation is present, then there may be multiple comparisons of interest across these two endpoints.

To review, in the standard bioequivalence study with only one test and one reference fromulation, the endpoints ln-AUC and ln-Cmax, separately, are tested using the following null hypotheses:

$$H_{01}: \quad \mu_T - \mu_R \leq -\ln 1.25 \tag{4.3}$$

OR

$$H_{02}: \quad \mu_T - \mu_R \geq \ln 1.25 \tag{4.4}$$

where μ_T and μ_R are the means of ln-transformed AUC or Cmax data for test and reference formulations, respectively, versus

$$H_{11}: \quad \mu_T - \mu_R > -\ln 1.25 \tag{4.5}$$

AND

$$H_{12}: \quad \mu_T - \mu_R < \ln 1.25 \tag{4.6}$$

Both null hypotheses must be rejected for ln-AUC **and** for ln-Cmax for average bioequivalence to be demonstrated. The terms "or" and "and" are very important here, as they correspond to the statistical terms $\bigcup$ for union and $\bigcap$ for intersection, respectively.

Within a study, the global null hypothesis for the two one-sided tests across ln-AUC and ln-Cmax become

$$H_0 : H_{01A} \bigcup H_{02A} \bigcup H_{01C} \bigcup H_{02C} \tag{4.7}$$

where H_{01A}, H_{02A} denote the application of the two one-sided tests to A = ln-AUC, H_{01C}, H_{02C} denote the application of the two one-sided tests to C = ln-Cmax, and where $\bigcup$ denotes the union of these null hypotheses. If all null hypotheses are rejected, then one has shown

$$H_1 : H_{11A} \bigcap H_{12A} \bigcap H_{11C} \bigcap H_{12C} \tag{4.8}$$

where H_{11A}, H_{12A} denote the alternative hypotheses for the two one-sided tests to A = ln-AUC, H_{11C}, H_{12C} denote the alternative hypotheses for the two one-sided tests to C = ln-Cmax, and where $\bigcap$ denotes the intersection of these alternative hypotheses.

This approach has been termed the intersection-union test [273] and is protective of type 1 error [1314] at the desired level of 5%, but all four individual null hypotheses must be rejected in order for bioequivalence to be demonstrated. The traditional α-level of 5% (yielding 90% confidence intervals) is not typically adjusted, as the study must reject all null hypotheses and given the findings of [531]. In brief, no adjustment is generally applied for the multiple endpoints AUC and Cmax in bioequivalence testing, as an intersection-union testing procedure is being applied across these two endpoints.

However, what does one do to adjust for multiple tests when a test formulation is compared to multiple reference formulations (e.g., Example 4.5)? What does one do when a high dose is compared to a low dose for a reference and a test formulation (e.g., Example 4.6) in the same study?

What is to be done depends upon the situation. In Example 4.5, multiple reference formulations were used in Phase 3 and the to-be-marketed formulation needed to be shown to be bioequivalent to both of them to support market access, so the equations became

$$H_0 : H(T:R)_{01A} \bigcup H(T:R)_{02A} \bigcup H(T:R)_{01C} \bigcup H(T:R)_{02C} \bigcup$$

$$H(T:S)_{01A} \bigcup H(T:S)_{02A} \bigcup H(T:S)_{01C} \bigcup H(T:S)_{02C}$$

where $H(T:R)_{01A}$, for example, denotes the application of the first two one-sided tests to A = ln-AUC when comparing formulation T to formulation R. If all null hypotheses are rejected, then one has shown

$$H_1 : H(T:R)_{11A} \bigcap H(T:R)_{12A} \bigcap H(T:R)_{11C} \bigcap H(T:R)_{12C} \bigcap$$

$$H(T:S)_{11A} \bigcap H(T:S)_{12A} \bigcap H(T:S)_{11C} \bigcap H(T:S)_{12C}.$$

All comparisons did need to succeed to link the to-be-marketed formulation to the reference formulations. Similarly, in Example 4.6, both the low dose and the high dose were both required to be bioequivalent between formulations. In such circumstances, an α-adjustment is not needed, as the testing procedure being used is an extension to the intersection-union test, and the traditional 90% confidence intervals may be used to support a claim of bioequivalence.

If, however, AUC and Cmax must succeed for only one set of the comparisons of interest (T:R or T:S in Example 4.5, for example), then this would create a subtly different testing problem:

$$H_0 : (H(T:R)_{01A} \bigcup H(T:R)_{02A} \bigcup H(T:R)_{01C} \bigcup H(T:R)_{02C}) \bigcap$$

$$(H(T:S)_{01A} \bigcup H(T:S)_{02A} \bigcup H(T:S)_{01C} \bigcup H(T:S)_{02C})$$

versus the alternative hypothesis

$$H_1 : (H(T:R)_{11A} \bigcap H(T:R)_{12A} \bigcap H(T:R)_{11C} \bigcap H(T:R)_{12C}) \bigcup$$

$$(H(T:S)_{11A} \bigcap H(T:S)_{12A} \bigcap H(T:S)_{11C} \bigcap H(T:S)_{12C})$$

This sort of testing procedure is known as a union-intersection test [273]. To preserve the overall study-wise type 1 error rate at the desired 5%, the individual two one-sided tests for all comparisons of interest should have their individual levels adjusted to a level lower than 5%. To be precise, this test would be termed an intersection-union test for each comparison of interest contained within an overall union-intersection test.

Numerous ways may be used to do this [273], but for simplicity the conservative Bonferroni adjustment is recommended. For example, consider the situation where there was only one reference formulation used in Phase 3, but it is desired to allow for multiple test formulations to be marketed following approval. This would be a Williams square bioequivalence study (as in Example 4.6, sequences ADBC, BACD, CBDA and DCAB), for example, with formulation A being the reference formulation, and formulations B, C, and D being test formulations. If any of B, C, or D showed equivalence to A, then that particular test formulation would be allowed market access. As there are three comparisons of interest, the 5% α usually applied to each two one-sided test would need to be lowered to $\frac{0.05}{3}$ =1.67%

to protect the overall false-positive rate of the study at the level desired by regulators. To do so, one would derive 96.67% confidence intervals instead of the standard 90% confidence intervals for AUC and for Cmax for all the comparisons of interest, B:A, C:A, and D:A. If AUC and Cmax were observed to be bioequivalent using the more stringent α-level for only one comparison of interest (for example, B:A succeeds but not C:A or D:A), one could conclude that formulation B was bioequivalent to A.

One might question how one would power such a study, as multiple correlated tests across multiple correlated endpoints are involved. We will develop simulation for this purpose in Chapter 5. Readers interested in an approximate solution may also wish to consider the approach described in [918].

4.8 Nonparametric Analyses of Tmax

There are a number of alternative approaches to developing a distribution-free or nonparametric analysis of data from cross-over trials with three or more treatments. The simplest and most familiar is an extension of the nonparametric analysis of the design with two treatments and sequences: TR/RT. This can only be applied to a subset of designs and is based on a stratified analysis for two treatments, resulting in the Van Elteren test (see [1113], for example). The particular designs to which this approach is applicable are those that have embedded within them a suitable set of RT/TR designs. We will illustrate such sets for three treatments in the following subsections. For arbitrary designs, confidence intervals can be derived using bootstrap sampling.

The most common need for a nonparametric analysis of bioequivalence data is in the analysis of Tmax. In the following subsections we will analyze Tmax data collected in the trials described in Examples 4.5 and 4.6.

4.8.1 Three Treatments

The data in Tables 4.15, 4.16, and 4.17 are the Tmax values collected in the trial described in Example 4.5. The design is displayed again in Table 4.18. It can be seen that the six sequences have been arranged into three strata. Stratum I includes the two sequences that contain the TR/RT design in Periods 1 and 2, stratum II includes the two sequences that contain the TR/RT design in Periods 1 and 3, and finally stratum III includes the two sequences that contain the TR/RT design in Periods 2 and 3. Within each stratum, T and R can be compared using the Wilcoxon rank-sum test, as described in Section 3.8 of Chapter 3. In particular, the Wilcoxon rank-sum and its variance for each stratum can be calculated. An overall test of T versus R can then be obtained by taking a weighted average of the three rank sums and dividing it by the square root of an estimate of the variances of the weighted average to produce a test statistic. This will be illustrated shortly. A defining characteristic of the parent design is that the pair of sequences in each stratum has T and R in matching periods: 1 and 2 in Stratum I, 1 and 3 in Stratum II and 2 and 3 in Stratum III. This is so that the period effect can be eliminated from the treatment comparison.

To compare T and S, a different arrangement of the design will be needed, as shown in Table 4.19. It can be seen that the sequences in each stratum are a different selection from those used when comparing T and R. At once we can see some disadvantages of this approach: a design containing the appropriate stratification must be available and a new arrangement of sequences is needed for each individual treatment comparison. A general approach applicable to an arbitrary design will be described later.

TABLE 4.15: Example 4.5: Tmax, Williams Design for Three Treatments

	Sequence TRS				Sequence RTS		
	Period				Period		
Subject	1	2	3	Subject	1	2	3
6	4.00	4.00	2.65	2	3.00	3.00	3.00
12	4.00	4.02	3.02	11	2.97	2.00	2.98
17	2.98	3.98	3.98	16	4.00	3.00	3.00
19	3.98	1.50	2.50	20	3.00	2.02	2.50
29	3.02	3.98	4.00	27	2.00	3.98	2.50
32	2.00	1.98	3.00	31	2.48	1.50	1.48
42	3.00	4.00	2.02	40	1.97	1.50	1.53
46	3.00	3.98	2.98	43	4.02	3.98	3.03
49	1.98	2.50	1.52	53	2.50	3.98	3.00
60	1.50	3.98	3.00	59	3.00	3.00	3.98
				61	4.00	2.00	4.00
R=3 × 100mg, S=200mg + 100mg, T=Test							

TABLE 4.16: Example 4.5: Tmax, Williams Design for Three Treatments

	Sequence TSR				Sequence RST		
	Period				Period		
Subject	1	2	3	Subject	1	2	3
4	2.50	2.98	3.02	9	2.98	2.50	2.50
7	2.48	2.50	3.97	13	2.00	2.98	1.50
14	2.98	3.00	3.00	21	2.52	2.50	1.55
23	1.00	2.98	3.00	28	2.50	2.98	2.97
26	4.05	2.98	6.00	33	2.97	1.52	1.02
36	2.98	3.98	3.00	44	4.00	4.00	3.97
39	4.08	4.00	3.98	50	3.98	4.00	4.00
48	1.03	2.00	2.02	58	3.00	4.00	2.48
54	2.48	2.50	2.50				
56	1.50	1.98	2.48				
R=3 × 100mg, S=200mg + 100mg, T=Test							

TABLE 4.17: Example 4.5: Tmax, Williams Design for Three Treatments

	Sequence STR				Sequence SRT		
	Period				Period		
Subject	1	2	3	Subject	1	2	3
5	2.50	1.98	2.55	1	2.50	4.02	3.00
10	1.48	1.50	2.50	8	1.98	1.98	4.00
18	3.00	2.50	2.50	15	1.48	2.50	3.98
22	4.02	3.02	4.02	24	3.00	4.00	4.02
30	4.10	3.02	3.98	25	2.48	3.00	2.98
R=3 × 100mg, S=200mg + 100mg, T=Test							

TABLE 4.17: Example 4.5: Tmax, Williams Design for Three Treatments (continued)

	Sequence STR				Sequence SRT		
	Period				Period		
Subject	1	2	3	Subject	1	2	3
34	4.12	4.00	3.98	35	2.97	3.98	2.50
37	2.98	1.48	4.02	41	3.03	3.05	3.98
47	2.50	3.00	4.00	45	1.53	4.03	3.03
52	3.00	4.00	2.52	51	3.02	6.00	2.52
55	3.00	3.98	2.48	57	3.00	3.98	3.00
				62	2.98	4.00	2.50
R=3 × 100mg, S=200mg + 100mg, T=Test							

Bioequivalence testing is based on the 90% confidence for the Test versus Reference comparison (on the log scale). However, to motivate and explain the construction of the confidence interval, we first start with the construction of the statistic for testing the null hypothesis that the mean treatment difference is zero. We will do this first for a single stratum and then give the generalization.

TABLE 4.18
Williams Design for Three Treatments: Stratified for Comparing T and R

Stratum	Group	Period 1	Period 2	Period 3
I	1	**T**	**R**	S
I	2	**R**	**T**	S
II	3	**T**	S	**R**
II	4	**R**	S	**T**
III	5	S	**T**	**R**
III	6	S	**R**	**T**

TABLE 4.19
Williams Design for Three Treatments: Stratified for Comparing T and S

Stratum	Group	Period 1	Period 2	Period 3
I	1	**T**	R	**S**
I	6	**S**	R	**T**
II	5	**S**	**T**	R
II	3	**T**	**S**	R
III	2	R	**T**	**S**
III	4	R	**S**	**T**

4.8.1.1 Single Stratum

The test statistic is Q, as used by Tudor and Koch [1263] for stratified samples and where the variate is the within-stratum ranks of the responses. We first define Q for a single stratum and show its equivalence to the Wilcoxon rank-sum test. In the process we will also show how the Wilcoxon rank sum can be expressed in terms of U-statistics; this will be useful when we consider the calculation of a confidence interval for the difference of T and R.

For a single stratum we assume that there are two sequences, TR and RT, with T and R in corresponding periods in the two sequences. In addition, we assume that the period 1 to period 2 differences have been calculated and ranked (over the total set of differences). Then

$$Q = \frac{[\bar{R}_1 - \bar{R}_2]^2}{\hat{\text{Var}}(\bar{R}_1 - \bar{R}_2)} = \frac{\frac{n_1 n_2}{n_1+n_2}(\bar{R}_1 - \bar{R}_2)^2}{\sigma_R^2}, \tag{4.9}$$

where $\bar{R}_i = \sum_{k=1}^{n_i} R_{ik}/n_i$, n_i is the number of ranks in sequence $i, i = 1, 2$, $R_{ik}, k = 1, 2, \ldots, n_i$ are the ranks for that sequence and

$$\sigma_R^2 = \frac{\sum_{i=1}^{2}\sum_{k=1}^{n_i}(R_{ik} - \bar{R})^2}{(n_1 + n_2 - 1)}.$$

On the null hypothesis that the distributions of T and R are equal, Q has an asymptotic chi-squared distribution on 1 degree of freedom.

Let $W_1 = \sum_{k=1}^{n_1} R_{1k}$ denote the rank-sum in the first sequence. We will now show that (4.9) is the square of the Wilcoxon rank-sum test statistic. The numerator of this statistic is

$$W_1 - E(W_1) = W_1 - \frac{n_1(n_2 + n_1 + 1)}{2} =$$

$$n_1\bar{R}_1 - \frac{n_1(n_2 + n_1 + 1)}{2} = n_1(\bar{R}_1 - \bar{R}),$$

where $\bar{R} = (\sum_{i=1}^{2}\sum_{k=1}^{n_i} R_{ik})/(n_1 + n_2) = (n_1 + n_2 + 1)/2$. In addition, as $\bar{R}_1 - \bar{R} = \bar{R}_1 - \frac{(n_1\bar{R}_1 + n_2\bar{R}_2)}{n_1+n_2}$, we have

$$W_1 - \frac{n_1(n_2 + n_1 + 1)}{2} = \frac{n_1 n_2(\bar{R}_1 - \bar{R}_2)}{n_1 + n_2}.$$

In the absence of ties,

$$\text{Var}(W_1) = \frac{n_1 n_2(n_1 + n_2 + 1)}{12}.$$

Returning now to Equation (4.9),

$$\sigma_R^2 = \frac{(n_1 + n_2)(n_1 + n_2 + 1)}{12} = \frac{n_1 + n_2}{n_1 n_2}\text{Var}(W_1).$$

Hence,

$$Q = \frac{[W_1 - E(W_1)]^2}{\text{Var}(W_1)}. \tag{4.10}$$

To illustrate this we consider the first stratum in Table 4.18 and first calculate the test statistic in more conventional ways. The calculations are done on the log-scale. Using StatXact, for example, and using asymptotic inference, the Wilcoxon rank-sum test statistic is -1.6922, which is asymptotically $N(0, 1)$ on the null hypothesis. Using SAS `PROC FREQ` to calculate the corresponding Cochran–Mantel–Haenszel statistic with modified ridit scores, the test statistic is 2.8636 ($= 1.6922^2$), which is asymptotically chi-squared on 1 d.f. under the null hypothesis. The corresponding two-sided P-value is 0.0906.

To calculate Q, as defined in (4.10), we note that $\bar{R}_1 = 8.6$, $\bar{R}_2 = 13.1818$, $n_1 = 10$, $n_2 = 11$, and $\sigma_R^2 = 38.40$. Hence, $Q = [(10 \times 11)(8.60 - 13.1818)^2]/38.40 = 2.8636$. In the following we will use the form of the test statistic defined in Equation (4.9).

Before moving on, it is useful to demonstrate one further way of calculating the numerator of the test statistic. Let d_{ik} denote the kth period difference in sequence $i, i = 1, 2$. The $n_1 n_2$ differences defined as $w_{\{k,k'\}} = d_{1k} - d_{2k'}$, where $k = 1, 2, \ldots, n_1$ and $k' = 1, 2, \ldots, n_2$, are known as the Walsh differences. Let s_j denote a weight for stratum j, where $j = 1, 2, 3$. For the moment we are dealing with only one stratum, so we set $s_1 = 1$. For comparison with later equations we will keep s_1 in the following formulae, even though it is unnecessary for the case of a single stratum. We will use d to denote the shift difference between the distributions of d_{1k} and $d_{2k'}$.

The rank-sum for group i can be written as

$$U_i = \sum_{\{w_{k,k'} > d\}} s_1 + 0.5 \sum_{\{w_{k,k'} = d\}} s_1. \tag{4.11}$$

Further, as $U_1 + U_2 = n_1 n_2$ and $U_i = W_i - n_i(n_i + 1)/2$,

$$\sqrt{\frac{n_1 n_2}{n_1 + n_2}} (\bar{R}_1 - \bar{R}_2) = \frac{U_1 - U_2}{2},$$

where $\bar{R}_i = W_i / n_i$. Finally,

$$\frac{U_1 - U_2}{2} = \sum_{\{w_{k,k'} > d\}} s_1 + 0.5 \sum_{\{w_{k,k'} = d\}} s_1 - 0.5 n_1 n_2 s_1.$$

The Wilcoxon rank-sum test statistic can then be expressed as

$$W(d) = \frac{\sum_{\{w_{k,k'} > d\}} s_1 + 0.5 \sum_{\{w_{k,k'} = d\}} s_1 - 0.5\, n_1 n_2\, s_1}{\sqrt{\frac{n_1 n_2}{(n_1 + n_2)}} \sigma_R}. \tag{4.12}$$

Rearranging Equation (4.12) gives

$$W(d) \sqrt{\frac{n_1 n_2}{(n_1 + n_2)}} \sigma_R + 0.5 n_1 n_2 s_1 = \sum_{\{w_{k,k'} > d\}} s_1 + 0.5 \sum_{\{w_{k,k'} = d\}} s_1. \tag{4.13}$$

Solving Equation (4.13) with $W(d) = 0$ gives the median of the Walsh differences (-0.293), and this is (twice) the estimate of δ.

Solving Equation (4.13) with $W(\delta) = \pm 1.645$ gives the positions of the Walsh differences that correspond to (twice) the lower and upper 90% confidence bounds for δ.

For the first stratum,

$$1.645 \sqrt{\frac{n_1 n_2}{(n_1 + n_2)}} \sigma_R + 0.5 n_1 n_2 s_1 = 23.33 + 55 = 78.3.$$

The 79th value in the ordered set of Walsh differences (not shown) is 0.0. For the lower bound we take the $-23.33 + 55 = 31.67$, i.e., the 31st ordered difference, which is -0.629. The 90% confidence interval for δ is therefore (-0.314, 0.000). If we take the limits for bioequivalence to be (-0.223, 0.223) as for AUC and Cmax, then there is clear evidence that T and R are not bioequivalent when Tmax is used as the metric.

For the remaining two strata the estimate and confidence intervals for δ are, respectively, [-0.463, -0.247, -0.098] and [-0.289, -0.143, 0.007]. Again there is strong evidence of a lack of equivalence.

TABLE 4.20
Period Differences for Comparing T and R: Stratum I

Subject	Difference	Difference (log scale)	Stratum	Group	Rank
6	0.00	0.000	I	1	11
12	-0.02	-0.005	I	1	9
17	-1.00	-0.289	I	1	4
19	2.48	0.976	I	1	21
29	-0.96	-0.276	I	1	7
32	0.02	0.010	I	1	14
42	-1.00	-0.288	I	1	5
46	-0.98	-0.283	I	1	6
49	-0.52	-0.233	I	1	8
60	-2.48	-0.976	I	1	1
2	0.00	0.000	I	2	11
11	0.97	0.395	I	2	17
16	1.00	0.288	I	2	16
20	0.98	0.396	I	2	18
27	-1.98	-0.688	I	2	2
31	0.98	0.503	I	2	19
40	0.47	0.273	I	2	15
43	0.04	0.010	I	2	13
53	-1.48	-0.465	I	2	3
59	0.00	0.000	I	2	11
61	2.00	0.693	I	2	20

TABLE 4.21
Period Differences for Comparing T and R: Stratum II

Subject	Difference	Difference (log scale)	Stratum	Group	Rank
4	-0.52	-0.190	II	1	6.0
7	-1.49	-0.470	II	1	4.0
14	-0.02	-0.007	II	1	9.5
23	-2.00	-1.099	II	1	1.0
26	-1.95	-0.393	II	1	5.0
36	-0.02	-0.007	II	1	9.5
39	0.10	0.025	II	1	13.0
48	-0.99	-0.674	II	1	2.0
54	-0.02	-0.008	II	1	8.0
56	-0.98	-0.503	II	1	3.0
9	0.48	0.176	II	2	14.0
13	0.50	0.288	II	2	16.0
21	0.97	0.486	II	2	17.0
28	-0.47	-0.172	II	2	7.0
33	1.95	1.069	II	2	18.0
44	0.03	0.008	II	2	12.0
50	-0.02	-0.005	II	2	11.0
58	0.52	0.190	II	2	15.0

TABLE 4.22
Period Differences for Comparing T and R: Stratum III

Subject	Difference	Difference (log scale)	Stratum	Group	Rank
5	-0.57	-0.253	III	1	9
10	-1.00	-0.511	III	1	3
18	0.00	0.000	III	1	11
22	-1.00	-0.286	III	1	6
44	-0.96	-0.276	III	1	7
34	0.02	0.005	III	1	12
37	-2.54	-0.999	III	1	1
47	-1.00	-0.288	III	1	5
52	1.48	0.462	III	1	17
55	1.50	0.473	III	1	20
1	1.02	0.293	III	2	16
8	-2.02	-0.703	III	2	2
15	-1.48	-0.465	III	2	4
24	-0.02	-0.005	III	2	10
25	0.02	0.007	III	2	13
35	1.48	0.465	III	2	18
41	-0.93	-0.266	III	2	8
45	1.00	0.285	III	2	15
51	3.48	0.867	III	2	21
57	0.98	0.283	III	2	14
62	1.50	0.470	III	2	19

TABLE 4.23
Components of the Stratified Test for Comparing T and R

Statistic	Stratum I	Stratum II	Stratum III
Patients in Each Sequence	(10,11)	(10,8)	(10,11)
Rank-Sum in Each Sequence(W)	(86, 145)	(61, 110)	(91, 140)
$E(W)$	(110,121)	(95,76)	(110,121)
$W - E(W)$	(-24,24)	(-34,34)	(-19,19)
Estimated Variance of Test Statistic	38.40	28.471	38.50
Weight	0.045	0.053	0.045
Rank-Sum Statistic	-1.692	-3.022	-1.338

4.8.1.2 Multiple Strata

The extension of the Wilcoxon rank-sum test statistic to multiple strata is

$$W = \frac{\sum_{i=1}^{q} s_i W_i}{\sqrt{\sum_{i=1}^{q} s_i^2 \operatorname{Var}(W_i)}} = \frac{\sum_{i=1}^{q} s_i W_i}{\sqrt{\sum_{i=1}^{q} s_i^2 \frac{n_{i1}n_{i2}}{n_{i1}+n_{i2}} \sigma_{iR}^2}} , \tag{4.14}$$

where W_i is the rank-sum statistic for the ith single stratum, $\operatorname{Var}(W_i)$ is its variance, s_i is the weight for the ith stratum, σ_{iR}^2 is the variance of the ranks in the ith stratum, and n_{ij} is the number of ranks in sequence group j in stratum i. We will use the weights suggested by Lehmann [754], $s_i = 1/(n_{i1} + n_{i2} + 1)$, which give the Van-Elteren test statistic. However, for our purposes we require the corresponding 90% confidence interval. In a way similar to that described for a single stratum, we can write the numerator of (4.14) as

$$\sum_{i=1}^{q} \sum_{\{w_{ik,ik'} > d\}} s_i + 0.5 \sum_{i=1}^{q} \sum_{\{w_{ik,ik'} = d\}} s_i - 0.5 \sum_{i=1}^{q} n_{i1} n_{i2} s_i . \tag{4.15}$$

Rearranging Equation (4.14), we get

$$\begin{aligned} & W(d)\sqrt{\sum_{i=1}^{q} s_i^2 \frac{n_{i1}n_{i2}}{n_{i1}+n_{i2}} \sigma_{iR}^2} + 0.5 \sum_{i=1}^{q} n_{i1}n_{i2}s_i \\ & = \sum_{i=1}^{q} \sum_{\{w_{ik,ik'} > d\}} s_i + 0.5 \sum_{i=1}^{q} \sum_{\{w_{ik,ik'} = d\}} s_i . \end{aligned} \tag{4.16}$$

As before, we set $W(d) = 0$ and solve to get the estimator of $2d$. Setting $W(d) = \pm 1.645$ gives the positions of the Walsh differences that correspond to (twice) the lower and upper 90% confidence bounds for δ. For T versus R, $\hat{\delta} = 0.192$ with confidence interval (0.136, 0.279) and for T versus S $\hat{\delta} = 0.054$ with confidence interval (-0.005, 0.145).

In summary, there is evidence that T and R are not equivalent but T is equivalent to S.

Bootstrap estimation of confidence intervals

An alternative method of getting a nonparametric estimate of the 90% confidence interval for $\mu_T - \mu_R$ is to use bootstrapping. (See Chapter 5 for a more detailed explanation of the bootstrap.) The method as applied here is to resample with replication from the 60 sets of triples (the three repeated measurements on each subject) and to calculate an estimate of $\mu_T - \mu_R$ from each resample. If this is done a large number of times, say 1000 times, a distribution of the estimator is generated. The 5% and 95% quantiles of this distribution provide a 90% confidence interval for $\mu_T - \mu_R$. The median of this distribution is an estimate of $\mu_T - \mu_R$. There will usually be a choice of estimator to use. Here we have taken the least squares estimator obtained by fitting a linear model with terms for subjects, period, and treatments. The distributions for $\mu_T - \mu_R$ and $\mu_T - \mu_S$ obtained from 1000 resamples are given in Figure 4.20. The quantiles and medians obtained are (0.0889, 0.1811, 0.2670) for $\mu_T - \mu_R$ and (-0.0363, 0.0481, 0.1253) for $\mu_T - \mu_R$. The conclusions obtained are consistent with those obtained from the nonparametric method. The only difference of note is that the lower limits of the bootstrap confidence intervals differ a little from those obtained earlier.

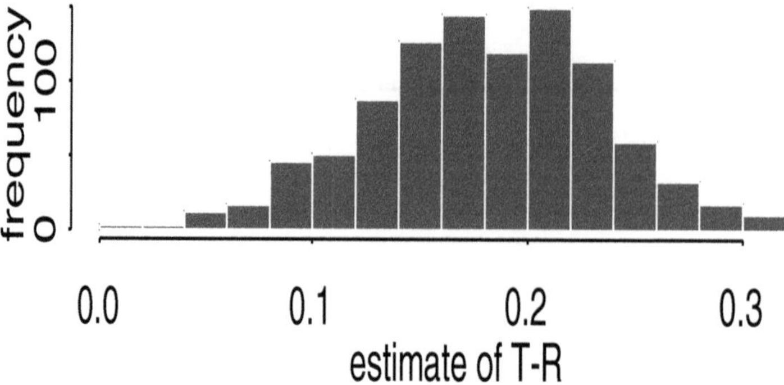

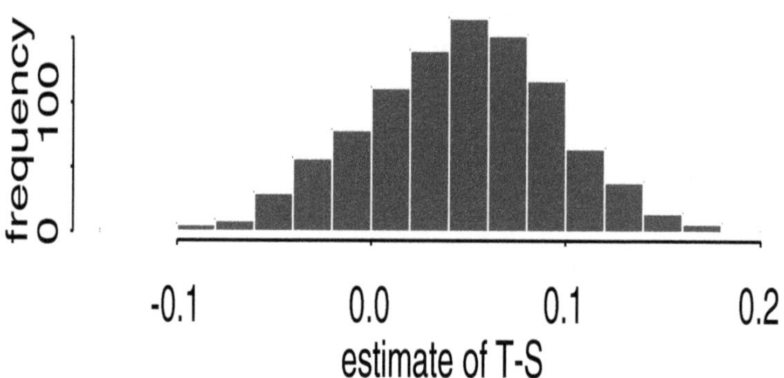

FIGURE 4.20
Example 4.5: Histograms of Bootstrap Distribution of Estimates

4.8.2 Four Treatments

The data in Table 4.39 are the Tmax values obtained in the trial described in Example 4.6. The comparisons of interest were B versus A and D versus C. It is clear from the design of this trial that the sequences cannot be grouped in a way that would allow the nonparametric approach described in the last subsection to be applied. However, we can use the bootstrapping approach. The 90% confidence intervals and medians so obtained are: (-0.2724, -0.0628, 0.1604) for $\mu_B - \mu_A$ and (-0.1062, 0.0703, 0.2554) for $\mu_D - \mu_C$. There is clear evidence of a lack of equivalence for both sets of treatments.

4.9 Technical Appendix: Efficiency

4.9.1 Theory and Illustration

We assume that our model for the response includes terms for a general mean, fixed subject effects, periods, formulations, and carry-over effects. Let the responses, e.g., logAUC, be stored in a random vector $\mathbf{y}$ which is assumed to have mean vector $\mathbf{X}\boldsymbol{\beta}$ and variance-covariance matrix $\sigma_W^2\mathbf{I}$. Here $\mathbf{X}$ is a design matrix with elements that are either 0 or 1, $\boldsymbol{\beta}$ is a vector of unknown subject, period, formulation, and carry-over parameters, and $\mathbf{I}$ is the identity matrix with row and column dimension equal to that of $\mathbf{y}$. The parameters are estimated by ordinary least squares:

$$\hat{\boldsymbol{\beta}} = (\mathbf{X}^T\mathbf{X})^{-1}\mathbf{X}^T\mathbf{Y},$$

with

$$\mathrm{V}(\hat{\boldsymbol{\beta}}) = \sigma_W^2(\mathbf{X}^T\mathbf{X})^{-1}.$$

We assume that any redundant parameters have been removed and $\mathbf{X}^T\mathbf{X}$ is of full rank. This can be achieved, for example, by removing one subject parameter, one period parameter, one formulation parameter and one carry-over parameter. If the design is for n subjects with n of them randomly allocated to each of the two sequences RTT and TRR, there will be $(1 + n - 1 + 1 + 1 + 1 = n + 3)$ parameters. However, we do not need to work with this many parameters to calculate the efficiency. Jones and Kenward [652] show that this can be done using the corresponding design with one subject allocated to each sequence. In other words, we put parameters in the model for sequences instead of subjects. We will illustrate this in the following.

The efficiency of a design compares (1) the variance of the estimated difference between two formulations in the given design to (2) the corresponding variance in an ideal design with the same formulation replication and the same within-subject variance σ_W^2. The ideal design is such that it would completely eliminate the effects of subjects, periods, and carry-over effects from the estimation of the formulation comparison. For example, suppose that T and R each occur r times in the ideal design. The estimate of the formulation difference is $\bar{y}_T - \bar{y}_R$ and its variance is $V_I = 2\sigma_W^2/r$. This is used as the benchmark for other designs.

For the particular cross-over design under consideration, e.g., one with sequences RTT and TRR, and using the particular parametrization given above, the treatment parameter, τ_2 corresponds to the difference between T and R. The variance of this difference is the diagonal element of $\sigma_W^2(X^TX)^{-1}$ that occurs in the position corresponding to τ_2 in the vector of parameters. We will give an example of locating this element below. Let us call this element $V_C = \sigma^2 a_C$.

The efficiency of the cross-over design for the T-R difference is then the percentage:

$$E = 100 \times \frac{V_I}{V_C} = 100 \times \frac{2}{r \times a_C}.$$

Efficiency cannot exceed 100%.

As an example, consider the design with sequences RTT and TRR and $n/2$ subjects per sequence. Suppose we want to allow for a difference in carry-over effects and put these into our model. For the basic calculations we assume $n = 2$, then scale down the variances and covariances according to the true value of n. The design matrix for the model with sequence, period, formulation, and carry-over effects is as follows, where redundant parameters have been removed:

$$\mathbf{X} = \begin{bmatrix} 1 & 0 & 0 & 0 & 0 & 0 \\ 1 & 0 & 1 & 0 & 1 & 0 \\ 1 & 0 & 0 & 1 & 1 & 1 \\ 1 & 1 & 0 & 0 & 1 & 0 \\ 1 & 1 & 1 & 0 & 0 & 1 \\ 1 & 1 & 0 & 1 & 0 & 0 \end{bmatrix}.$$

The columns in this matrix refer to the general mean, Sequence 2, Periods 2 and 3, Formulation T, and the carry-over of T, respectively. Although there is no carry-over effect in the first period, we must include a "dummy" parameter to represent this missing effect if we are to construct the **X** matrix. Our way of doing this is to let the carry-over parameter for T do "double duty" by also taking on the role of this dummy parameter. As long as there are period effects in the model, there is no confusion because the dummy parameter is aliased with the parameter for Period 1 and effectively gets removed correctly in the analysis. The inverse matrix, from which the variances are taken or calculated, is

$$\sigma_W^2(\mathbf{X}^T\mathbf{X})^{-1} = \frac{\sigma_W^2}{4}\begin{bmatrix} 4 & -2 & 2 & -2 & -2 & 0 \\ -2 & 3 & 0 & 0 & 1 & 0 \\ -2 & 0 & 5 & 3 & 0 & -2 \\ -2 & 0 & 3 & 5 & 0 & -2 \\ -2 & 1 & 0 & 0 & 3 & 0 \\ 0 & 0 & -2 & -2 & 0 & 4 \end{bmatrix}.$$

This inverse is for a design with one subject per sequence. To get the correct value of a variance of a comparison of means, we divide the elements of this inverse by the number of responses used in calculating the means. For example, when there are $n/2$ subjects per sequence, the variance of the estimate of T-R, adjusted for carry-over, is $(3\sigma_W^2/4)/(n/2)$, i.e., $a_C = (3/4)/(n/2) = 3/(2n)$, and the variance of the corresponding estimated carry-over difference is $\sigma_W^2/(n/2)$, i.e., $a_C = 2/n$. The required elements of $\sigma_W^2(\mathbf{X}^T\mathbf{X})^{-1}$ are those in the fifth and sixth positions along the diagonal because the parameters that refer to T-R and the carry-over difference are in these positions, respectively, in the vector $\boldsymbol{\beta}$. Because the (5,6)th element of $\sigma_W^2(\mathbf{X}^T\mathbf{X})^{-1}$ is zero, these two estimates are uncorrelated. We are now in a position to calculate the efficiency of the T-R comparison. As each formulation occurs $3n/2$ times in the design, $V_I = 4/3n$ and hence

$$E = 100 \times \frac{2}{r \times a_C} = 100 \times \frac{2}{(3n/2)(3/2n)} = 100 \times \frac{8}{9} = 88.9\%.$$

Although we are not usually interested in the efficiency of the carry-over comparison, we will calculate it for completeness and as a further illustration. Traditionally, the replication for each carry-over effect is taken to be that of the corresponding formulation, e.g., $3n/2$ in the above design. However, as there are no carry-over effects in the first period, this replication is strictly too large. However, we will stick with the traditional approach. Hence, the efficiency of the comparison of the carry-over effects of T and R is

$$E = 100 \times \frac{2}{r \times a_C} = 100 \times \frac{2}{(3n/2)(2/n)} = 100 \times \frac{2}{3} = 66.7.$$

We note that the efficiencies for an arbitrary cross-over design can be calculated using the GenStat statistical analysis system via the procedure XOEFFICIENCY [653].

TABLE 4.24
Efficiencies of Three Alternative Designs

Design	Formulation T-R	Carry-over T-R	Correlation (Formulation, Carry-over)
1. RTT/TRR	88.9	66.7	0.00
2. RTR/TRT	22.2	16.7	0.87
3. RRT/TTR	66.7	16.7	0.50

4.9.2 Comparison of Three Alternative Designs for Three Periods

Here we compare three alternative designs that could be used to compare T and R in a bioequivalence trial. These are

1. R T T   2. R T R   3. R R T
T R R   T R T   T T R .

The efficiencies of the formulation and carry-over comparisons are given in Table 4.24, where we have also included the correlation between the estimators of the formulation and carry-over differences. A major advantage of the first design is that the estimator of the formulation difference does not change if the carry-over parameter is left out of the model, as the correlation is zero. Hence, this design provides some robustness against the presence of a carry-over difference, which, although unexpected, cannot always be ruled out entirely.

4.10 Tables of Data

TABLE 4.25: Example 4.1: Sequence RTT

	Sequence RTT					
	AUC Period			Cmax Period		
Subject	1	2	3	1	2	3
104	37.27	62.18	44.09	2.207	2.901	2.073
105	82.870	24.780	24.700	6.123	1.462	1.468
106	47.800	32.880	124.310	2.586	1.203	6.972
107	88.390	30.850	192.450	4.326	1.589	8.687
108	180.50	108.71	200.57	8.459	5.011	9.104
111	50.59	33.53	100.58	3.133	1.814	7.159
113	634.140	914.900	-	7.154	12.354	8.207
115	420.300	205.740	-	20.221	11.746	-
117	582.260	736.820	784.960	9.819	12.035	17.973
118	45.420	-	70.690	1.636	0.852	1.895
120	437.610	586.470	405.950	9.111	11.708	10.539
R=Reference, T=Test						

TABLE 4.25: Example 4.1: Sequence RTT (continued)

	Sequence RTT					
	AUC Period			Cmax Period		
Subject	1	2	3	1	2	3
121	22.830	13.720	15.750	1.167	0.506	0.756
123	64.58	35.54	65.11	2.949	1.831	2.989
126	15.15	22.35	21.71	0.902	1.234	1.495
128	30.220	27.400	33.190	1.632	0.921	1.221
130	12.420	71.380	62.270	0.636	4.433	4.408
133	39.010	89.410	59.890	1.854	4.091	2.235
136	24.470	42.660	42.390	1.441	2.997	3.070
137	13.840	21.730	41.690	0.846	1.202	2.380
138	28.040	10.970	42.720	1.045	0.629	2.337
139	264.890	243.660	276.540	13.913	9.160	10.632
141	-	-	-	0.355	0.237	0.444
142	227.010	8.080	521.640	11.638	0.655	23.115
147	71.100	16.770	44.080	3.489	1.013	2.434
150	29.660	76.030	60.120	1.439	5.327	4.626
153	1737.430	1416.780	1336.790	21.715	22.405	16.726
154	440.830	163.920	282.290	25.232	6.205	11.416
155	53.830	48.090	78.280	1.715	1.239	2.470
160	41.580	259.550	113.840	2.087	11.067	4.379
161	327.530	210.820	453.230	6.741	3.742	10.083
162	45.570	30.130	83.960	1.876	1.230	6.274
164	142.000	146.630	124.380	5.982	5.288	5.456
168	15.230	31.890	71.680	1.020	1.459	4.637
170	76.490	82.700	114.290	4.224	4.131	6.619
173	87.330	51.370	96.460	5.726	2.431	4.939
174	787.890	737.740	338.520	31.224	23.271	12.711
175	1239.480	1819.440	2232.290	24.013	30.484	43.224
177	29.190	36.580	79.590	1.971	2.296	4.243
179	10.130	16.990	9.820	1.029	1.371	0.718
181	257.590	423.890	224.070	9.964	15.005	6.776
182	51.770	27.630	26.090	3.797	2.312	1.741
184	73.750	90.810	-	2.555	3.242	-
185	49.320	124.000	85.710	1.471	4.079	4.743
186	6.060	28.820	87.630	0.311	1.651	4.870
190	82.780	164.560	213.980	3.889	7.376	7.012
191	98.860	99.020	75.480	4.599	2.969	2.388
194	21.290	46.300	15.410	1.513	2.741	1.411
R=Reference, T=Test						

TABLE 4.26: Example 4.1: Sequence TRR

	Sequence TRR					
	AUC Period			Cmax Period		
Subject	1	2	3	1	2	3
101	12.260	16.190	11.340	0.511	0.688	0.533
102	397.980	267.630	487.550	13.270	7.933	12.952
103	243.810	141.700	198.440	16.771	6.926	9.257
109	182.520	112.340	225.940	8.816	4.921	6.911
110	559.640	533.980	867.750	21.398	19.728	19.909
112	40.020	89.490	20.350	2.568	5.222	0.992
114	-	-	34.810	0.872	0.337	1.558
116	69.380	214.200	193.620	3.543	8.911	5.900
119	68.080	47.190	84.590	2.673	1.501	4.187
122	181.950	259.400	396.260	5.841	10.642	19.245
124	5.820	17.260	25.720	0.347	1.241	1.175
125	39.310	35.660	40.430	2.288	1.786	2.589
127	146.870	319.910	141.860	5.772	10.780	6.768
129	712.110	549.520	459.260	16.116	13.171	10.648
131	2277.520	3726.580	3808.790	18.448	34.145	41.876
132	1278.060	1103.460	1012.040	18.779	17.086	13.170
134	103.320	138.780	170.440	4.974	5.349	8.128
135	21.930	75.290	42.300	1.622	4.791	3.228
140	77.990	104.080	66.860	3.043	5.210	2.625
143	27.210	47.190	25.340	1.170	2.405	1.698
144	296.090	163.310	387.490	10.730	6.443	13.790
145	82.600	247.710	92.940	3.363	9.128	5.311
146	18.010	241.700	205.390	1.011	10.183	9.865
148	123.270	268.090	128.170	4.985	8.893	5.880
149	52.460	201.680	421.550	2.457	6.945	32.983
151	29.830	20.660	24.550	1.691	1.186	1.313
152	414.990	247.580	419.530	14.735	9.851	12.724
156	213.240	87.550	178.660	7.510	2.793	5.323
157	13.580	7.160	10.940	0.496	0.459	0.756
158	172.250	211.290	206.990	7.330	5.667	9.804
159	1161.730	2280.790	1552.490	27.604	45.495	27.220
163	57.260	48.650	89.010	2.691	2.877	6.631
165	350.950	755.270	711.180	7.034	13.040	11.002
166	36.79	41.75	35.39	1.861	2.75	2.784
167	11.57	3.31	-	1.055	0.326	0.296
171	28.440	61.400	25.500	1.246	3.146	1.016
172	1150.280	759.030	1105.080	15.677	15.215	20.192
176	69.630	24.020	26.110	3.971	1.234	0.948
178	179.76	190.89	299.5	4.909	5.374	10.014
180	14.23	22.44	23.70	1.088	1.783	1.733
183	295.690	304.030	277.670	11.125	9.916	10.649
187	34.180	45.140	58.670	1.870	3.055	4.654
188	50.380	87.620	16.460	2.317	4.658	0.719
R=Reference, T=Test						

TABLE 4.26: Example 4.1: Sequence TRR (continued)

	Sequence TRR					
	AUC Period			Cmax Period		
Subject	1	2	3	1	2	3
189	104.08	123.08	129.00	3.73	4.109	6.018
192	17.19	40.01	55.36	1.994	2.786	3.716
193	131.570	156.120	130.480	7.191	12.207	7.532
195	1323.070	1305.500	2464.820	12.897	24.767	27.650
196	654.320	783.530	444.440	12.347	26.041	18.975
R=Reference, T=Test						

TABLE 4.27: Example 4.2: Sequence RTT

	Sequence RTT					
	AUC Period			Cmax Period		
Subject	1	2	3	1	2	3
1	1158.06	1073.74	748.58	15.44	11.93	14.12
4	520.75	410.53	437.96	13.59	9.17	8.85
5	11.44	13.29	14.31	0.70	0.80	0.92
6	-	28.87	19.44	0.68	1.19	1.44
9	51.76	23.75	35.23	2.48	1.20	1.97
10	-	8.93	5.85	0.35	0.79	0.46
15	25.80	27.91	51.47	1.42	1.78	3.24
16	1633.77	1127.82	1267.52	20.18	35.76	16.24
18	105.03	15.61	18.03	5.87	0.81	0.93
19	1635.06	1562.78	1936.28	20.91	18.53	17.17
22	168.29	337.16	227.49	5.82	10.45	5.45
23	3.23	7.84	4.86	0.28	0.64	0.54
25	44.81	12.22	24.56	2.73	0.78	1.53
28	15.54	24.71	29.74	0.91	1.01	1.33
29	48.69	17.61	35.34	3.66	1.22	1.71
32	134.01	204.85	81.73	5.26	7.51	2.91
34	48.15	17.59	20.08	3.60	1.21	1.15
35	39.22	13.58	19.21	5.27	0.99	1.57
36	805.16	602.79	698.12	20.15	12.13	13.05
37	52.97	55.85	44.97	3.46	4.31	2.70
38	23.07	-	39.34	1.02	2.09	1.31
42	46.99	59.85	60.41	2.33	3.54	2.90
47	43.37	50.40	85.98	2.06	2.73	4.02
48	12.25	9.59	11.70	0.72	0.80	0.39
49	15.47	13.90	19.09	0.80	1.04	0.94
50	54.21	93.00	121.17	1.71	3.90	4.77
53	38.92	32.07	61.57	2.78	1.94	3.05
55	947.92	707.40	696.01	11.72	9.97	9.34
57	37.40	78.42	85.38	1.91	4.13	3.55
62	64.95	66.42	91.42	2.74	3.78	5.06
R=Reference, T=Test						

TABLE 4.27: Example 4.2: Sequence RTT (continued)

	Sequence RTT					
	AUC Period			Cmax Period		
Subject	1	2	3	1	2	3
63	9.38	10.95	18.37	1.16	0.77	1.32
67	132.73	128.11	135.28	10.58	5.92	5.56
68	140.46	97.09	153.54	8.52	6.03	7.50
70	366.38	300.67	275.54	13.50	13.41	11.15
71	48.65	40.87	-	2.96	3.08	3.02
73	544.33	617.22	554.04	11.07	13.69	13.11
75	16.69	9.65	13.68	1.90	0.57	1.16
79	60.85	41.24	39.05	2.25	1.76	2.91
80	38.90	61.10	40.88	2.24	3.68	2.50
R=Reference, T=Test						

TABLE 4.28: Example 4.2: Sequence TRR

	Sequence TRR					
	AUC Period			Cmax Period		
Subject	1	2	3	1	2	3
2	17.28	30.30	83.53	1.20	2.23	5.25
3	11.63	16.20	18.23	0.75	1.34	1.27
7	78.03	42.64	148.29	3.80	1.28	5.11
8	6.61	19.83	7.18	0.64	1.22	1.06
11	14.68	16.74	25.73	1.06	1.74	2.89
12	119.77	211.51	148.04	5.07	9.11	4.78
13	36.26	34.02	50.11	2.59	2.29	2.93
14	59.06	94.61	54.46	4.84	5.79	3.03
17	17.47	39.47	31.08	1.41	2.94	2.49
20	1082.90	1497.28	2011.67	21.62	29.04	29.89
24	47.84	46.22	68.04	3.10	3.16	4.48
26	-	19.24	20.01	0.59	1.08	1.54
27	26.30	15.45	88.92	2.15	1.20	4.78
30	23.94	54.15	55.25	1.47	3.07	2.09
31	21.90	18.72	15.20	1.02	1.08	1.02
33	20.20	28.40	44.84	1.52	1.44	2.59
39	59.06	87.12	148.31	2.93	3.50	6.57
40	79.04	31.79	64.29	4.87	1.65	2.93
41	139.30	74.26	92.94	6.96	4.53	5.36
43	503.28	389.44	547.82	10.86	9.53	10.44
45	50.24	52.74	57.02	2.15	2.66	2.32
46	29.35	41.32	33.12	2.02	2.14	1.79
51	-	20.66	8.13	1.25	2.67	0.53
52	26.95	50.10	26.56	1.67	2.74	1.37
54	19.48	12.62	18.78	1.32	0.64	1.30
56	20.27	-	10.64	1.71	0.65	0.94
R=Reference, T=Test						

TABLE 4.28: Example 4.2: Sequence TRR (continued)

	Sequence TRR					
	AUC Period			Cmax Period		
Subject	1	2	3	1	2	3
61	14.57	49.60	58.36	1.06	2.34	2.97
64	56.74	61.83	97.05	3.62	3.12	4.82
65	103.19	187.82	188.43	5.65	8.45	8.41
69	13.12	32.13	18.02	0.94	2.11	0.99
72	14.90	16.00	11.85	1.17	0.94	0.66
74	24.60	39.14	53.98	1.31	2.42	3.63
76	7.50	4.80	12.06	0.52	0.44	1.50
77	828.00	565.73	1085.51	13.37	7.32	14.84
78	33.99	47.96	35.15	2.65	3.17	2.04
R=Reference, T=Test						

TABLE 4.29: Example 4.3: Replicate Design

	Sequence RTTR							
	AUC Period				Cmax Period			
Sub	1	2	3	4	1	2	3	4
1	10671	12772	13151	11206	817	1439	1310	1502
4	7588	8980	8408	7654	823	1133	1065	1095
6	8389	7949	7735	7616	1347	691	949	1153
7	5161	6601	5479	4764	1278	991	1124	1040
9	7399	7873	8153	7211	1547	1361	1380	1485
10	5660	4858	5347	5076	1088	982	995	796
15	6937	7905	6550	7515	953	1065	830	1247
16	11473	9698	10355	10365	1368	1281	1083	1418
	Sequence TRRT							
	AUC Period				Cmax Period			
Sub	1	2	3	4	1	2	3	4
2	6518	6068	5996	5844	1393	1372	1056	1310
3	4939	5728	5760	6313	1481	1377	1529	781
5	7653	8022	10721	8043	709	1035	1571	1342
8	8864	8026	6776	6995	1516	1242	1090	1048
11	8503	7730	8228	8032	999	908	1183	1129
12	7043	6007	7737	6262	679	1220	776	1258
13	5701	5767	5942	7757	822	869	921	947
14	8684	7858	7924	9219	615	1451	1389	1279
18	5210	5120	5420	-	668	842	1176	-
R=Reference, T=Test								

TABLE 4.30: Example 4.4: Replicate Design

	Sequence RTRT							
	AUC Period				Cmax Period			
Sub	1	2	3	4	1	2	3	4
1	812.60	1173.70	889.10	620.10	99.85	204.09	170.94	112.78
3	545.10	542.90	-	-	67.69	41.73	-	-
5	400.00	223.80	173.70	289.70	40.05	25.17	24.48	86.49
6	102.10	185.30	42.00	88.30	28.76	24.83	9.27	10.89
10	304.50	351.50	520.20	335.70	34.35	52.26	142.92	58.48
12	176.10	710.70	409.50	645.50	18.94	161.34	118.89	246.57
15	562.40	490.40	504.70	675.90	28.35	98.50	78.22	140.54
17	207.50	271.60	173.70	240.50	19.18	94.92	21.39	65.45
18	571.30	705.20	619.00	633.60	66.63	134.69	78.10	78.51
21	536.10	595.20	445.50	521.50	42.11	37.82	39.87	116.79
24	449.90	860.40	606.80	577.20	32.53	276.86	118.65	156.33
25	192.50	220.10	233.10	227.00	21.96	38.97	22.26	54.16
28	568.10	321.10	338.30	403.60	110.87	55.64	50.06	84.60
29	735.60	634.50	1244.20	641.90	50.08	58.79	181.53	144.26
31	307.40	481.80	346.60	369.70	87.21	88.75	90.07	132.92
34	292.90	431.00	448.50	267.80	18.07	33.37	21.48	20.87
35	217.20	332.20	103.00	127.50	18.69	174.55	17.06	32.01
39	368.30	292.60	446.10	222.30	52.59	57.88	48.58	47.24
40	193.70	202.80	255.20	244.30	29.30	78.33	21.72	49.27
44	102.00	282.50	245.60	286.20	22.14	63.50	9.38	16.30
46	223.60	645.40	349.00	507.40	27.02	167.28	20.35	121.92
48	615.80	732.10	620.90	665.20	60.94	100.47	26.17	98.08
49	898.40	924.90	398.30	828.30	164.01	180.01	25.21	97.02
50	410.40	329.20	449.40	442.10	59.70	43.65	102.47	40.00
53	332.40	273.60	525.30	293.30	39.96	56.47	42.11	38.75
54	185.20	222.90	182.10	194.10	18.34	16.09	21.50	9.57
57	180.60	174.70	102.90	117.00	9.10	58.44	12.74	18.33
R=Reference, T=Test								

TABLE 4.31: Example 4.4: Replicate Design

	Sequence TRTR							
	AUC Period				Cmax Period			
Sub	1	2	3	4	1	2	3	4
2	216.30	338.00	502.80	398.60	29.06	50.48	35.15	55.71
4	632.60	520.00	716.70	860.40	91.25	43.86	168.78	61.04
7	596.00	659.30	543.80	662.90	257.10	79.04	127.92	81.80
8	402.40	359.80	590.80	444.30	136.27	158.86	148.97	82.41
9	456.70	378.40	477.50	407.90	65.48	87.84	64.57	58.01
11	500.70	323.00	416.30	525.10	31.49	37.07	80.90	33.62
13	160.60	218.00	170.10	124.60	29.61	43.15	27.71	13.11
16	756.00	606.80	477.40	626.80	168.76	174.94	117.31	52.18
R=Reference, T=Test								

TABLE 4.31: Example 4.4: Replicate Design (continued)

	Sequence TRTR							
	AUC Period				Cmax Period			
Sub	1	2	3	4	1	2	3	4
19	511.90	549.70	388.20	141.00	32.23	70.06	32.15	43.11
20	124.00	91.90	113.30	59.50	9.34	11.74	49.23	18.42
22	239.70	265.10	445.90	433.20	38.02	16.79	38.58	83.82
23	609.60	371.60	511.30	432.70	199.07	52.14	118.47	72.04
26	764.40	508.80	757.80	449.40	74.24	35.76	39.27	36.28
27	151.90	194.80	-	-	19.00	20.61	-	-
30	429.10	391.80	316.90	335.10	31.85	74.88	54.88	19.18
32	409.00	514.60	763.10	406.50	30.86	70.84	208.20	65.25
33	271.00	221.00	296.50	463.70	86.01	41.85	67.86	79.81
36	290.80	208.60	243.70	489.80	38.27	40.31	31.56	20.64
37	297.20	502.00	320.40	334.30	49.81	66.64	17.80	25.94
38	163.80	232.10	636.90	434.90	34.56	16.37	114.30	29.58
42	534.10	243.10	418.40	441.90	136.00	33.75	104.12	35.03
43	355.10	415.20	382.70	334.00	64.55	34.04	52.37	41.67
45	320.50	233.90	331.70	260.50	26.35	37.20	76.26	24.60
47	504.50	289.90	550.70	244.20	118.91	49.27	166.61	35.86
52	237.00	505.00	496.30	580.60	30.55	63.90	39.17	40.75
55	246.90	620.90	678.30	752.20	42.20	106.69	150.52	115.15
56	235.40	190.40	318.30	248.40	39.15	13.79	122.03	62.32
R=Reference, T=Test								

TABLE 4.32: Example 4.5: Williams Design for Three Treatments

	Sequence RST					
	AUC Period			Cmax Period		
Subject	1	2	3	1	2	3
9	4089	7411	5513	906	1711	1510
13	2077	3684	2920	504	845	930
21	2665	3113	2263	506	809	543
28	3029	5157	4190	563	1263	759
33	4941	4502	3014	1095	1253	1015
44	2173	4571	3350	366	1341	779
50	-	-	3900	602	1291	1314
58	6555	11351	8895	1229	2138	2144
67	4045	7865	-	1025	2668	-
	Sequence RTS					
	AUC Period			Cmax Period		
Subject	1	2	3	1	2	3
2	3457	6556	4081	776	2387	1355
11	5560	4558	4396	1801	1440	1327
16	3676	5385	5358	544	1556	1776
R=3 × 100mg, S=200mg + 100mg, T=Test						

TABLE 4.32: Example 4.5: Williams Design for Three Treatments (continued)

	Sequence RST					
	AUC Period			Cmax Period		
Subject	1	2	3	1	2	3
20	8636	9750	9892	2238	2256	2277
27	2753	2736	3955	572	593	1142
31	4782	4812	4024	1078	1224	1010
40	2636	2791	2394	546	587	442
43	3011	4544	6587	558	998	1418
53	2685	5335	7454	530	1160	1764
59	4841	5934	6624	1416	1302	1517
61	2392	2947	3779	644	744	1144
R=3 × 100mg, S=200mg + 100mg, T=Test						

TABLE 4.33: Example 4.5: Williams Design for Three Treatments

	Sequence SRT					
	AUC Period			Cmax Period		
Subject	1	2	3	1	2	3
1	7260	6463	8759	1633	1366	2141
8	3504	3011	2501	959	557	697
15	6641	1987	3233	1586	364	633
24	4368	4327	2966	991	748	1001
25	8016	7146	9154	2045	1891	2545
35	7749	4188	3425	1855	757	758
41	8961	8737	11312	1722	1313	2705
45	4537	2633	3723	999	604	1075
51	5658	4904	5077	1539	1227	1490
57	5194	2432	4472	1810	686	1149
62	5787	7069	6530	1461	1995	1236
	Sequence STR					
	AUC Period			Cmax Period		
Subject	1	2	3	1	2	3
5	4250	3487	2891	945	1041	788
10	4839	3064	2582	1051	991	782
18	6317	5175	3123	1432	1184	647
22	3527	3484	2580	656	734	531
30	2717	2743	1625	637	760	463
34	4709	3212	3840	1022	661	609
37	5256	4070	2505	1194	974	432
47	5840	5213	5213	1329	1477	1039
52	4622	2889	2692	1027	562	422
55	8671	6814	4260	2251	1561	1045
R=3 × 100mg, S=200mg + 100mg, T=Test						

TABLE 4.34: Example 4.5: Williams Design for Three Treatments

	Sequence TRS					
	AUC Period			Cmax Period		
Subject	1	2	3	1	2	3
6	6709	5893	5346	1292	1154	1098
12	7026	6134	9520	1417	1207	2312
17	9249	5535	9965	2232	913	2887
19	4664	2998	6592	1103	547	2113
29	5547	7319	8331	1288	1506	1884
32	3500	5611	5394	852	1259	1308
42	4367	5827	8863	736	1135	2288
46	3020	3989	3739	643	660	841
49	-	-	6092	1556	1895	1854
60	3125	4728	3199	594	1317	731
63	2204	2927	-	495	770	-
	Sequence TSR					
	AUC Period			Cmax Period		
Subject	1	2	3	1	2	3
4	4006	4879	3817	1326	1028	1052
7	6924	4674	4183	1475	994	1142
14	6027	6497	5048	1106	1914	1358
23	2642	3178	2496	461	589	561
26	3064	3534	2302	754	1508	419
36	9882	13881	6881	2054	3042	1207
39	1422	2375	1559	316	555	427
48	6029	4114	3625	2261	1097	1038
54	5429	7513	4589	1369	2068	1384
56	6779	7447	6504	1279	1994	1091
R=3 × 100mg, S=200mg + 100mg, T=Test						

TABLE 4.35: Example 4.6: Williams Design for Four Treatments

	Sequence ADBC							
	AUC Period				Cmax Period			
Sub	1	2	3	4	1	2	3	4
2	484	4190	509	4055	108.4	818.0	105.2	914.4
4	584	4134	450	3520	115.0	848.3	90.4	929.8
10	475	3596	350	2809	85.4	550.4	68.0	588.7
15	419	3430	454	3527	66.7	851.1	87.3	772.8
19	504	3635	429	4286	89.1	622.7	67.7	696.3
20	549	2727	314	3565	97.5	729.9	66.0	933.5
25	428	3174	389	3246	101.9	839.9	89.1	589.9
A=Reference Low, B=Test Low, C=Reference High, D=Test High								

TABLE 4.36: Example 4.6: Williams Design for Four Treatments

	Sequence BACD							
	AUC Period				Cmax Period			
Sub	1	2	3	4	1	2	3	4
3	454	409	3571	3167	62.5	65.5	568.2	567.6
7	944	382	2830	2784	93.3	103.4	796.1	730.1
11	370	397	2399	1550	101.6	55.8	586.0	327.5
12	412	346	3010	2848	117.1	69.1	444.4	567.5
17	405	328	2574	2264	70.8	70.2	518.4	495.4
21	354	349	3249	2942	50.6	57.5	572.9	567.4
26	371	329	2427	2667	105.4	72.4	681.9	600.5
A=Reference Low, B=Test Low, C=Reference High, D=Test High								

TABLE 4.37: Example 4.6: Williams Design for Four Treatments

	Sequence CBDA							
	AUC Period				Cmax Period			
Sub	1	2	3	4	1	2	3	4
6	3163	413	3069	345	689.1	94.6	652.1	58.2
8	3410	307	3009	370	554.6	61.5	675.1	87.2
9	3417	352	2975	376	686.6	56.8	606.0	59.8
14	3327	332	2826	350	629.1	86.0	718.8	87.1
18	2223	208	1759	232	563.2	67.7	584.1	74.0
22	2368	257	2104	274	540.2	50.5	464.1	59.2
28	3020	414	3022	419	652.7	59.3	607.2	79.1
A=Reference Low, B=Test Low, C=Reference High, D=Test High								

TABLE 4.38: Example 4.6: Williams Design for Four Treatments

	Sequence DCAB							
	AUC Period				Cmax Period			
Sub	1	2	3	4	1	2	3	4
1	2942	2525	278	359	563.6	658.1	55.6	73.0
5	2740	2634	338	306	565.7	580.3	71.7	53.7
13	2897	2538	313	331	833.4	562.5	96.6	78.6
16	4513	4058	484	434	859.4	745.2	88.9	70.0
23	2095	1987	233	199	388.1	471.6	54.2	25.2
24	3218	2705	365	367	635.6	643.3	66.3	62.1
27	2525	2672	238	316	471.2	557.0	29.4	51.4
A=Reference Low, B=Test Low, C=Reference High, D=Test High								

TABLE 4.39: Example 4.6: Tmax, Williams Design for Four Treatments

	ADBC Period					BACD Period			
Sub	1	2	3	4	Sub	1	2	3	4
2	1.00	1.98	1.05	1.52	3	1.00	0.50	0.52	0.52
4	1.02	1.00	0.57	0.55	7	1.48	0.45	0.53	0.53
10	0.50	1.95	1.02	1.02	11	0.52	1.98	1.45	1.48
15	1.00	0.48	0.48	0.50	12	0.50	0.60	1.47	1.50
19	0.50	1.00	1.45	1.00	17	0.98	1.03	1.00	1.00
20	0.97	0.95	0.48	0.48	21	0.50	1.50	0.48	1.48
25	0.53	0.48	0.47	1.47	26	0.50	0.98	0.50	1.00
	CBDA Period					DCAB Period			
Sub	1	2	3	4	Sub	1	2	3	4
6	0.57	0.50	1.02	0.98	1	0.98	0.48	1.03	0.50
8	1.03	1.02	1.00	0.55	5	0.48	0.48	0.50	0.50
9	0.50	0.48	0.55	1.45	13	0.52	1.02	0.50	0.48
14	0.98	0.48	0.52	0.53	16	0.48	1.00	1.02	0.98
18	0.95	0.97	0.48	1.00	23	0.97	0.95	0.98	3.97
22	0.47	0.95	0.48	1.00	24	1.00	0.97	1.00	1.50
28	1.00	0.48	0.52	0.53	27	3.00	1.50	1.48	1.98
A=Reference Low, B=Test Low, C=Reference High, D=Test High									

Part II

Special Topics in Bioequivalence

5

Dealing with Special BE Challenges

or What one can do when some things that can go wrong, do go wrong...

In business, there is always a lot of talk about challenges and opportunities. These are really the same thing — a demanding task that requires a greater than normal commitment to see through to completion. In "business-speak," when something goes wrong and has to be fixed or changed, this type of thing is typically viewed as a "challenge." A challenge is an opportunity that one does not want to work on, as it has some sort of negative connotation associated with it. In contrast, an opportunity is a challenge that one does want to work on, as it has some sort of positive connotation. It is all a matter of one's perspective on the event in question. Either way, however, statistically speaking, it is probably going to require a lot of work.

When the FDA denies a claim of bioequivalence, there is a great deal of consternation at any given sponsoring company. Everyone usually knows such an event is coming, but it is like getting a big bill requiring immediate payment in the mail — if it came in tomorrow (or even better next week or next month), that would be preferable. My company was no exception, and our senior executives met quickly in one such instance to determine what to do. It was decided to repeat the study "right away" (with some design enhancements). This was definitely referred to from the get-go as a "challenge to the organization."

On top of the dismay among the staff working on the project associated with not having our bioequivalence claim approved, this "right away" action by senior executives generally represents an even greater challenge (and caused even more tangible consternation) among the staff who actually have to do this job. It is advisable not to tell a senior executive that something is impossible (if one values one's job), but often things like this can be very difficult if not impossible.

A human clinical trial of a drug product must have a written protocol (plan for the study) which must be unconditionally approved following review by an independent ethics review committee prior to any subject or patient being screened or dosed. If it involves a new chemical or biologic entity, this entity must be appropriately registered with the local regulatory agency of the appropriate government(s) if required; there is a lot of paperwork involved with these things. In addition, any human volunteer or patient involved in a trial must read and sign an informed consent before being enrolled in a trial and must be screened to ensure they are physically and mentally capable of taking part in the clinical trial. There are contracts with the site that must be reviewed by procurement and legal functions within the sponsoring company prior to signoff, and usually someone who is completely critical to at least one step in this process is on vacation, blissfully unaware of what is going on, until contacted at an inconvenient moment by an extremely stressed person tasked with the "challenge" of tracking them down.

Thus, when something like the above study is to be done "right away," that means the protocol, paperwork, and trial facilities for the study have to have been written and assembled and submitted several days or weeks ***ago*** *in order to get the study started as soon as possible. No one can reasonably be deemed a fortune teller and do such a thing in advance; hence, long hours and long days are the usual result of a challenge to try to have such a trial up and running "Stat."*

Senior executives are also the people responsible for resources at most companies and are often very surprised when they find out how long things really take. The good ones come down and lend a hand until the crisis is past, and we received a lot of senior-level attention on this occasion. Everything that could be done was done (in the space of three weeks), and the trial was good to go on the following Monday. However, we were all so busy working that we forgot to look out the window, an important omission on this occasion.

We finalized the protocol following ethics board review, completed all the regulatory paperwork, and finalized all the contracts. Then we all took a long deep breath and went home for the weekend to recover. Unfortunately, it rained all weekend, as a hurricane was passing through the Caribbean and eastern USA.

We returned to work Monday morning (this was in the days before cell phones and laptops, so work-related communications did not happen, so much, on the weekends) to discover that, despite our best efforts, the trial would not start as desired by our senior executive team. The hurricane had disrupted the shipping of supplies to the site, and we would have to reschedule. We had to delay the trial and resulting regulatory file dates. Some things just cannot be designed into or accounted for in models of bioequivalence trials.

Many other matters, however, can be controlled in design or modelled afterward to assess impact using technologies developed in the 20th century. In this chapter, we describe several such topics and methods for doing so. We hope that readers who find themselves in a "challenging" BE situation find these topics useful.

5.1 Restricted Maximum Likelihood Modelling

The first topic to be considered is that of modelling of pharmacokinetic data using maximum likelihood approaches.

The likelihood is the probability of observing the sample of data obtained in the trial, and is, given these data, a function of a set of specified parameters. For BE testing, the parameters of interest are the formulation, period, and sequence effects and any within- or between-subject variances.

In trials where subjects get repeated exposure to a formulation, i.e., where the design includes sequences such as RTTR and TRRT, it is possible to estimate σ^2_{BT}, σ^2_{BR}, the between-subject variances of T and R, respectively, and the within-subject variances of T and R, σ^2_{WT}, σ^2_{WR}, respectively.

The method of maximum likelihood (ML) determines the parameter estimates to be those values of the parameters that give the maximum of the likelihood. Restricted maximum likelihood estimation (REML) is a form of ML estimation that uses an iterative procedure where within each iteration there are two steps. A simplified description of REML is as follows. Using a first guess or estimate of the parameter values, the procedure keeps the values of the variance parameters fixed and estimates the formulation, period, and sequence effects. This is the first step. The residuals from this model are then calculated and used to reestimate the variance parameters. This is the second step. These steps are repeated until the values of the parameters do not change from one iteration to the next. The "Restricted" in the name of the method arises because, within each step, one set of parameters is fixed while the other set is estimated by maximizing the likelihood under the restriction imposed by the fixed set of parameters.

The usefulness of REML is that it can be used to estimate the between- and within-subject variances. The estimates so obtained are informative for the interpretation of the data, particularly when bioequivalence between T and R is not demonstrated. A second, and less important, property of REML is that it can be used when the dataset is incomplete, i.e., when a complete set of logAUC or logCmax is not obtained from each subject. We illustrated such an analysis in Chapter 3. There, it will be recalled, the REML results were very similar to the results obtained from an analysis that used just those subjects that had a complete set of values. For more information on the properties of REML when the trial has a relatively small number of subjects, see [652].

Some regulatory agencies are not interested in the variance components, as their focus for inference is the mean difference between formulations, and such agencies may require that only fixed effects be fitted in the model [319].

However, even for such agencies, when a trial fails to show bioequivalence it is of interest to determine which factors (i.e., a difference in formulation means, unexpectedly high variability, or both) led to such a circumstance, and REML models may be used to explore data in such a context and in the presence of missing data. The use of REML models is also important in the context of scaled average bioequivalence, and we review the application of such methods in a subsequent chapter.

REML has quite a long history ([118, 514, 740, 961] and has been particulary useful for the analysis of repeated measurements ([652, 699, 881, 1271]). Readers interested in application in the bioequivalence setting should see [967], [970], and [1339].

Obviously, given its iterative nature, REML estimation cannot be done by hand. SAS code to perform these analyses is given in the box below.

For standard two-, three-, and four-period designs such as those found in Examples 3.1, 3.2, 4.5, and 4.6 (i.e., those where no formulation adminstration is replicated), analysis code may be found on the website in `exam1.sas` to `exam4.sas`, respectively. Some `proc mixed` code for Example 4.5 `exam3.sas7bdat` is included here for illustration purposes:

```
proc mixed data=my.exam3
    method=reml ITDETAILS maxiter=200;
    class sequence subject period formula;
    model lnauct=sequence period formula
    /ddfm=KENWARDROGER;
    random subject(sequence);
    estimate 'T-R' formula -1 0 1
    /cl alpha=0.10;
    estimate 'T-S' formula 0 -1 1
    /cl alpha=0.10;
run;
```

Kenward and Roger's [689] denominator degrees of freedom are specified to ensure the correct degrees of freedom are used and that a good estimate of the standard error of $\hat{\mu}_T - \hat{\mu}_R$ is obtained.

Estimates relevant to ABE testing may be found in Table 5.1 for AUC and Cmax on the log scale.

It will be recalled that, while Example 3.1 demonstrated bioequivalence, Example 3.2 did not (see Chapter 3) due to reasons discussed later in this chapter. In Example 4.5, formulation T was not equivalent to R or S, with results indicative of a potentially bioinequivalent new formulation. In Example 4.6, bioequivalence was demonstrated at both high and low doses of drug product.

We have provided two additional datasets, `exam5.sas7bdat` and `exam6.sas7bdat`, on the website that were obtained from trials that used the sequences (RTTR/TRRT) and (RTRT/TRTR), respectively. FDA-recommended code to analyze these [369] may be found in `exam5.sas` and `exam6.sas`, respectively. The `proc mixed` code for `exam5` is given in the box below. The AUC and Cmax data for `exam6` are given in Table 5.4, where we consider other interesting features of these data.

```
proc mixed data=my.exam5
    method=reml ITDETAILS maxiter=200;
    class sequence subject period formula;
    model lnauct=sequence period formula
    /ddfm=KENWARDROGER;
    random formula/type=FA0(2) subject=subject;
    repeated/group=formula subject=subject;
    estimate 'T-R' formula -1 1/CL ALPHA=0.1;
run;
```

Here, as before, the procedure `mixed` is called in SAS and estimates of the test and reference formulations differences are again computed using the `estimate` statement. Note, however, that different specifications are included for the `random` and `repeated` statements (cf., [369]). These are used, as the replication of treatments within each subject permits the estimation of between- and within-subject variances for each formulation.

The `random` statement specifies that a particular choice for the variance structure should be assumed for σ^2_{BT} and σ^2_{BR} (Factor Analytic [1073]) and that the variance associated with subject-by-formulation interaction,

$$\sigma^2_D = \sigma^2_{BT} + \sigma^2_{BR} - 2\rho\sigma_{BT}\sigma_{BR},$$

should be derived, where ρ is the between-subject correlation between the formulations. Estimates of these may be found in Table 5.2.

The `repeated` statement specifies that within-subject variance estimates should be derived for T and R formulations separately.

Average bioequivalence was demonstrated for `exam5` with no evidence of a subject-by-formulation interaction ($\hat{\sigma}_D$ of 0.03 for AUC and 0.02 for Cmax). Test and reference formulations were equivalent for AUC in `exam6` with no evidence of a subject-by-formulation

TABLE 5.1
REML Results from PROC MIXED for Standard Bioequivalence Designs

Example	Dataset	Endpoint	$\hat{\mu}_T - \hat{\mu}_R$	90% CI	$\hat{\sigma}^2_W$
3.1	exam2	$\log AUC(0-\infty)$	-0.0166	-0.0612, 0.0280	0.0110
		$\log AUC(0-t)$	-0.0167	-0.0589, 0.0256	0.0099
		logCmax	-0.0269	-0.1102, 0.0563	0.0384
3.2	exam1	$\log AUC(0-\infty)$	0.0940	-0.0678, 0.2482	0.1991
		logCmax	0.0468	-0.0907, 0.1843	0.1580
4.5	exam3	$\log AUC(0-t)$	$T-R=0.1497$	0.0859, 0.2136	0.0440
			$T-S=-0.1912$	-0.2554, -0.1270	
		logCmax	$T-R=0.2597$	0.1726, 0.3468	0.0846
			$T-S=-0.2088$	-0.2964, -0.1212	
4.6	exam4	$\log AUC(0-\infty)$	$B-A=0.0047$	-0.0545, 0.0638	0.0177
			$D-C=-0.0362$	-0.0953, 0.0230	
		logCmax	$B-A=-0.0355$	-0.1171, 0.0461	0.0336
			$D-C=-0.0301$	-0.1117, 0.0515	

B, D, T = Test Formulations
A, C, R, S = Reference Formulations

TABLE 5.2
REML Results from PROC MIXED for Chapter 5 Examples of Replicate Designs

Dataset	Endpoint	$\hat{\mu}_T - \hat{\mu}_R$	90% CI	$\hat{\sigma}_D$	$\hat{\sigma}^2_{Wi}$
`exam5`	$\log\text{AUC}(0-\infty)$	0.0357	0.0130, 0.0583	0.03	$R = 0.0065$
					$T = 0.0117$
RTTR/TRRT	logCmax	-0.0918	-0.1766, -0.0070	0.02	$R = 0.0404$
					$T = 0.0587$
`exam6`	$\log\text{AUC}(0-t)$	0.1004	0.0294, 0.1714	0.04	$R = 0.1202$
					$T = 0.0756$
RTRT/TRTR	$\log\text{AUC}(0-t')$	0.1043	0.0326, 0.1760	0.02	$R = 0.1212$
					$T = 0.0818$
	logCmax	0.4120	0.2948, 0.5292	0.21	$R = 0.3063$
					$T = 0.2689$
T = Test Formulation R = Reference Formulation					

interaction. Note that, for Cmax in dataset `exam6`, however, in addition to a large increase in mean rate of exposure for the test formulation (0.4120, definitely indicative of bioinequivalence), there was evidence of a subject-by-formulation interaction, as indicated by $\hat{\sigma}_D = 0.21$ (making it even more difficult to demonstrate bioequivalence, as the confidence intervals will be wider by a factor directly proportional to this value). The data in `exam6` had other aspects making it interesting statistically, and we will consider this dataset in more detail later in the chapter.

5.2 Failing BE and the DER Assessment

For some drug products, even if one tries time and time again to demonstrate bioequivalence, it may be that it just cannot be done. A common misconception is that this means the test and reference formulations are "bioinequivalent," in that they deliver different pharmacokinetic profiles causing different pharmacodynamic response. This is not necessarily the case.

An example of a potentially bioinequivalent test product is presented in Figure 5.1. The important thing to note is that the measure of centrality in addition to the bulk of the distribution falls outside the average bioequivalence confidence limit for logAUC. Implicitly, for a product to demonstrate bioequivalence, its true measure of centrality must fall within the limits. Otherwise, it will be next to impossible (or a Type 1 error) for such a product to demonstrate bioequivalence. In this case, the estimated $\mu_T - \mu_R$ tells us that it is most unlikely we will ever be able to demonstrate bioequivalence.

Contrast this with the fitted normal densities of Example 3.2 in Chapter 3. Here the measure of centrality lies within the average bioequivalence acceptance limits, but slightly too much of the distribution lies outside to conclude the test and reference formulations are bioequivalent. These formulations are not bioinequivalent, but insufficient evidence has been provided to show that they are.

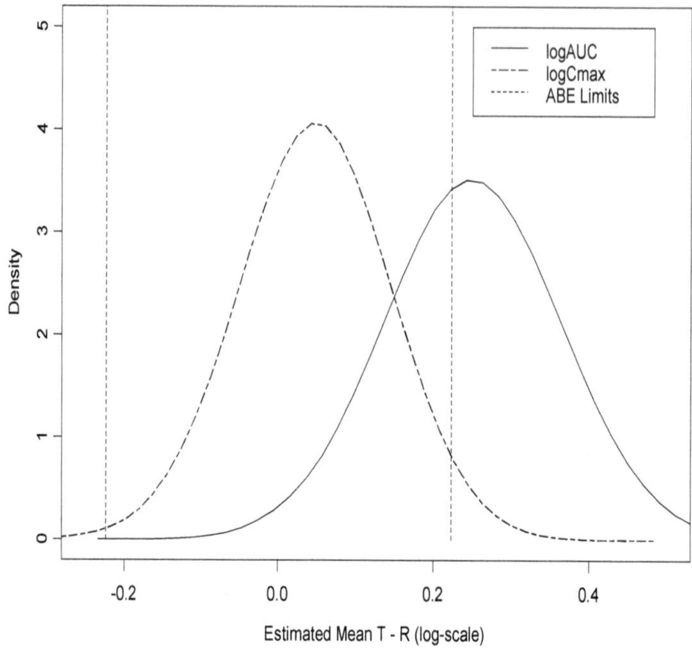

FIGURE 5.1
A Potentially Bioinequivalent Test and Reference Product: Fitted Normal Densities for $\hat{\mu}_T - \hat{\mu}_R$

Formulations may fail to show bioequivalence for several reasons:

1. The estimated $\mu_T - \mu_R$ lies too far from zero,
2. Variation is greater than expected, resulting in too wide a confidence interval for $\mu_T - \mu_R$,
3. Insufficient sample size is used (also yielding too wide a confidence interval for $\mu_T - \mu_R$),
4. Or some combination of these.

In Example 3.2 of Chapter 3, all three factors combine to contribute to the failure to demonstrate bioequivalence. The difference in formulation means, $\hat{\mu}_T - \hat{\mu}_R$, was estimated to be approximately 0.1 for logAUC (on the natural scale, 1.1) while the study had been designed under the assumption that $\mu_T - \mu_R$ would be no greater than ± 0.05. Also, $\hat{\sigma}_W$ was estimated to be approximately 0.45, while the sample size had been chosen in expectation of a σ_W of 0.3. The combination of these two factors in combination with the a priori choice of sample size resulted in a failure to demonstrate bioequivalence. However, given the observed magnitude of these factors, a better designed follow-up study might be able to show bioequivalence successfully. Some might refer to the study as having been "underpowered," implying that insufficient sample size was utilized; however, all three factors contributed to the failure to demonstrate bioequivalence.

Insufficient sample size can result in confidence intervals that are wide in bioequivalence trials, making it difficult to demonstrate bioequivalence. Note, however, that in such failed trials the confidence interval is quite informative [526]. In the case of a failed bioequivalence trial, the confidence interval may be regarded as expressing a plausible range of values for the true $\mu_T - \mu_R$. In the case of Example 3.2, the confidence interval for AUC (recall this is $exp(\hat{\mu}_T - \hat{\mu}_R))$ was (0.94–1.29) with the probability of any given value of $exp(\mu_T - \mu_R)$ decreasing as it becomes further away from 1.1. It is possible therefore that, if we repeated the trial using the same design and sample size, we would observe $exp(\hat{\mu}_T - \hat{\mu}_R)$ of as low as 0.94 and as high as 1.29! Indeed, in a previous relative bioavailability study (of similar design but lower sample size), an estimate of 0.95 for $exp(\hat{\mu}_T - \hat{\mu}_R)$ had been observed.

Note that, in Example 3.2, as a 2×2 cross-over design was used, hence $\sigma_{WT} = \sigma_{WR} = \sigma_W$. These variances are confounded in this design, and we can neither test nor estimate whether $\sigma_{WT} = \sigma_{WR} = \sigma_W$. If a replicate design had been used, it would be possible to separately model the magnitude of intra-subject and inter-subject variation for each formulation. Such a design and analysis might be desirable if we suspected, for instance, that the new formulation resulted in more intra-subject variation than the reference formulation.

Failure to demonstrate bioequivalence is therefore different but related to bioinequivalence. Only in cases where sample size is very large and point estimates for δ lie outside the acceptance bounds would one definitely conclude bioinequivalence was observed. Bioinequivalence is thus quite rare, but failure to demonstrate bioequivalence can occur quite often. In the latter case, it is generally possible to repeat the study or use a more powerful design to attempt to successfully demonstrate bioequivalence.

Turning now to the implications of failure to demonstrate bioequivalence, successful demonstration is not always necessary in regulatory science to secure approval of a new product. For certain new agents, rate and extent of exposure can change in a new formulation relative to that used in clinical trials. For a new product's first regulatory application (i.e., a product invented by the sponsor representing a new chemical or biological entity's first New Drug Application at the FDA, for example), a drug might not need to clearly demonstrate bioequivalence to the full regulatory standard. The FDA's guidance on this follows:

> Where the test product generates plasma levels that are substantially above those of the reference product, the regulatory concern is not therapeutic failure, but the adequacy of the safety database from the test product. Where the test product has levels that are substantially below those of the reference product, the regulatory concern becomes therapeutic efficacy. When the variability of the test product rises, the regulatory concern relates to both safety and efficacy, because it may suggest that the test product does not perform as well as the reference product, and the test product may be too variable to be clinically useful.
>
> Proper mapping of individual dose-response or concentration-response curves is useful in situations where the drug product has plasma levels that are either higher or lower than the reference product and are outside usual BE limits. In the absence of individual data, population dose-response or concentration-response data acquired over a range of doses, including doses above the recommended therapeutic doses, may be sufficient to demonstrate that the increase in plasma levels would not be accompanied by additional risk. Similarly, population dose- or concentration-response relationships observed over a lower range of doses, including doses below the recommended therapeutic doses, may be able to demonstrate that reduced levels of the test product compared to the reference product are associated with adequate efficacy. In either event, the burden is on the sponsor to demonstrate the adequacy of the clinical trial dose-response or concentration-response data to provide evidence of therapeutic equivalence. In the absence of this

evidence, failure to document BE may suggest the product should be reformulated, the method of manufacture for the test product be changed, and/or the BE study be repeated. [373]

If bioequivalence has not been demonstrated for a new product, the task then is to model exposure's (AUC, Cmax) relationship to efficacy and safety in patients using the reference formulation's clinical data. If therapeutic equivalence can be shown for such an exercise, then approval may be obtained. In the knowledge of the extent to which the test formulation changes exposure (measured in a bioequivalence study or studies), one may *simulate* what change of the magnitude observed for AUC and Cmax for the test formulation would be produced in terms of patient response in clinical use.

We refer to this type of modelling and simulation procedure as the DER (Dose-Exposure-Response) assessment. Modelling of bioequivalence data was covered in Chapters 3 and 4. We will develop the basic ideas behind simulation in the next section.

This simulation-based procedure provides regulators with a technique to assess whether the issue in manufacturing poses a risk to the patients using the new product. Note, however, that the DER assessment is limited in scope of application ***to only new (i.e., innovative) products***. Existing marketed products may not apply such a procedure and must demonstrate average bioequivalence to have access to the market (in most cases). There are always exceptions to such a rule, but such exceptions are very rare.

Bear in mind that regulators use average bioequivalence testing as a tool for measuring manufacturing quality. It is not the only tool which may be applied (see Chapter 2), and the extent of the rigor in its application is dependent on how many people are using the product in the marketplace.

For a new innovator product, relatively few patients (only those volunteering for clinical trials, see Chapter 2) will have received the drug. However, when a drug is allowed marketplace access by regulators, the number of patients exposed to the drug increases exponentially. Small changes in the PK for a new innovator product may not result in increased risk to patients in the marketplace using the drug for the first time, and this is studied using the DER assessment. Regulators therefore are free to use their informed judgment in permitting market access for these innovative products.

When a manufacturer makes changes to a marketed formulation or multiple companies begin to market new formulations (at the innovator's patent expiration), there is little room for such judgment. Many people are presumed to be at risk, and the regulators must ensure that, when the patients use the new formulations, their safety and efficacy are protected. When millions of people are using a drug, even a very small change in exposure for a small percentage of patients may result in many people being placed at risk.

Conservative application of the average bioequivalence standard is therefore the rule once an approved drug is on the market, and regulators have little to no freedom to change bioequivalence limits. With few exceptions [40], rigorous application of the 0.80–1.25 limits has protected public health and individual patients using new formulations.

The rationale for this regulatory conservatism is well documented. Hauck et al. [537] showed that allowing wider than the usual acceptance limits (0.80–1.25) allowed larger changes in rate of exposure. This change could result in a less acceptable safety profile for a new formulation (i.e., more undesirable side effects) than the reference formulation. Anderson and Hauck [23] showed that rigorous application of the ABE acceptance criteria protects public health when multiple new formulations enter the marketplace at patent expiration.

Application of the DER assessment is therefore limited in scope to innovator products entering the market for the first time. We now turn to the topic of simulation in order to develop how one goes about a DER assessment.

5.3 Simulation

We introduce simulation here to develop the concepts behind its use and application in clinical pharmacology research. A full discussion of the topic is beyond the scope of this work, and we refer those interested in more information to [1], [97], [501], [570], [640], [980], [1063], [1319], and [1395].

Simulation can be thought of as a means of creating datasets using a computer without going to the trouble of actually doing a study and collecting observations.

This approach assumes we know the truth about the parameters in which we are interested. In bioequivalence, for example, we might assume we know the true values of μ_T, μ_R, σ_B^2, σ_W^2, and the magnitude of any period and sequence effects. A random data generator can then be used in SAS, for example, to simulate PK data.

For example purposes, assume a bioequivalence study has failed, showing a 10% decrease in the new formulation AUC relative to the reference formulation. An AUC of at least 175 is needed for the product to be efficacious in killing bacteria, and concern might exist that, if a patient were switched from the reference to the new formulation in the marketplace, the product might fail to demonstrate efficacy. The reference product had an average AUC of 200 ($\mu_R = \ln 200$), and the new formulation was observed to have an average AUC of 180 ($\mu_T = \ln 180$). We know from previous experience that between-subject variance for logAUC is 0.18 with a within-subject variance of 0.09.

SAS code (an example of such code may be found on the website accompanying this book) can then be used to generate simulated PK data for simulated subjects. Here we set $\mu_T = \ln 180$, $\mu_R = \ln 200$, $\sigma_B^2 = 0.18$, and $\sigma_W^2 = 0.09$. Period and sequence effects are presumed to be null, but are easy to include if desired. LogAUC data for 2500 simulated subjects for the reference and the new test product are output in an SAS dataset called DER.

In statistics, such simulations are used often in working practice. Simulated data are generated and plugged into various methods of analysis under consideration to assess the properties of the statistics being considered. Statisticians may use such techniques to assess the degree of bias (the degree to which $\hat{\delta} \neq \delta$, for example) and precision ($(\hat{\delta} - \delta)^2$, for example). Statisticians also use such techniques to evaluate "what if" scenarios. For example, the presence of two or three subjects with very unusual data points may easily be included in a simulation to assess their impact on the probability of demonstrating average bioequivalence.

Other branches of clinical pharmacology use simulation for other purposes — e.g., the DER assessment described in the last section. Response data are collected and used to develop models to relate exposure to response (see Chapter 11). In our example, we would evaluate the number of subjects achieving an efficacious response (AUC > 175) on the reference formulation and of these subjects assess how many subsequently showed an efficacious response on the test formulation. In this simulation, 73.7% of those having an efficacious response to the reference formulation also had an efficacious response to the test formulation. Note that these findings might also lead one to wish to increase the dose, as a good percentage of those studied on the reference formulation (40%) did not reach efficacious levels! However, one might be constrained in that an AUC greater than 300 (for example) might be associated with an undesirable side-effect. Consideration of such is left to the reader.

In practice in bioequivalence trials, simulation is not often used. Most modern companies have manufacturing well under control by the time of a regulatory application. Bioinequivalence is quite infrequent, and failed bioequivalence studies are becoming rare with the advent of customization and automation in drug development manufacturing.

This is a simplistic modelling and simulation example, but the concepts may be applied in more complex situations.

Clinical pharmacologists work with statisticians to develop such models and use simulations to predict what might be observed in future trials. This is a powerful tool; however, we need to have a care to monitor the assumptions being made in such an exercise. Results are highly dependent on the chosen model parameters, and life has a way of being more complex than any simple model can hope to describe.

5.4 Data-Based Simulation

The first data exploration technique we will consider is a technique some attribute to R.A. Fisher [500] and developed in great detail in an excellent book by Efron and Tibshirani [294]. We encourage readers interested in application of this technique to explore these and other books [1132] and publications (e.g., [1133, 1134]) on the topic.

In this section, we will dwell on the application of the **bootstrap** in bioequivalence. The reader will note its utility as a general data exploration tool, and it will become very handy in our exploration of other clinical pharmacology data.

The bootstrap is "a computer based method for assigning measures of accuracy to statistical estimates" [294]. Essentially, we recognize that the sample of observed data from any clinical trial is *only* a sample from a far larger population (which we obviously cannot sample exhaustively — it is too big). Additionally, the observed data from each subject is a sample of what we would see if we studied that subject again and again. We could even drill down further and look at each individual period's results for each subject as a sample of what we would see if we repeated each period within each subject again and again. However, for this section, we will choose to apply the bootstrap at the subject level, maintaining the actual number of subjects observed within each sequence in accordance with recent draft guidance on the topic [358].

Bootstrapping is accomplished by randomly sampling, with replication, from the original dataset of n subjects. One picks a subject at random from the dataset, includes that data in the analysis dataset, replaces the subject, picks again, replaces the subject, etc., until one has a new dataset with n subjects. The same subject may appear in the bootstrap dataset more than once.

One does this a large number of times to accumulate a set of r bootstrap datasets. The number r is arbitrary but should be pretty large, in general, at least $r \geq 1000$. The chosen method of analysis is then applied to each of the r bootstrap datasets, and a record of each of the r fitted sets of parameters is kept. For any given parameter, the r sets of estimates may be used to estimate moments of the parameter of interest such as its mean and variance.

Obviously, one cannot bootstrap this set of r datasets by hand, and application of this technique was constrained until modern computing power became available in the 1980s–1990s. Some modern software packages offer automated bootstrapping routines, and bootstrapping is easily accomplished in SAS via use of the `MACRO` SAS language.

An SAS macro used for this purpose may be found on the website accompanying this book. Bootstrap samples are generated by calling the SAS macro `bootstrp` from a chosen dataset. Note that a `seed` value is input. This is a random number chosen to tell SAS where to begin sampling and allows one to reproduce the results if the program needs to be rerun.

TABLE 5.3
Number of Successful BE Trials

Dataset	Comparison	AUC	Cmax	Overall
`exam1.sas7bdat`	T-R	41%	67%	38%
`exam2.sas7bdat`	T-R	100%	99%	99%
`exam3.sas7bdat`	T-R	61%	0%	0%
`exam3.sas7bdat`	T-S	16%	5%	4%
`exam3.sas7bdat`	S-R	0%	0%	0%
`exam4.sas7bdat`	B-A	100%	98%	98%
`exam4.sas7bdat`	D-C	100%	100%	100%
`exam6.sas7bdat`	T-R	88%	0%	0%

If a `seed` is not provided, SAS uses the clock to automatically determine where to start. The `bootstrp` macro then samples from the dataset in the manner described above and outputs datasets $r = 1$ to `nrep` where `nrep` is the number of r bootstrap datasets desired. The number chosen in the examples is r=`nrep`=2000.

One then derives the statistic of interest for each bootstrap dataset. For `exam1 - 6` we will estimate the 90% confidence interval for $\mu_T - \mu_R$ for the purposes of providing an example, though any statistic may be treated in this manner. For this exercise, we will be interested in estimating the proportion of cases among the bootstraps where a conclusion of BE may be made.

Following some data manipulations, the output bootstrap datasets are then each used to estimate a 90% confidence interval for $\mu_T - \mu_R$ using `proc mixed`, as shown in Chapter 3. If the confidence interval falls within $\mp \ln 1.25$ for both $\ln AUC$ and $\ln Cmax$ then an overall "success" is registered for that bootstrap dataset.

We can see that it is unlikely a repeat of the study in Example 3.2 (`exam1.sas7bdat`) would be successful. See Table 5.3. Overall only 38% of bootstrapped datasets resulted in a conclusion of bioequivalence. While the percentage of Cmax datasets being bioequivalent was relatively high (at 67%), only 41% of bootstrapped data sets were successful for AUC.

One could also use this tool to evaluate "what if" scenarios, e.g., what if we changed the sample size to $n = 20$ subjects? One could also run the bootstrap procedure repeatedly to obtain a confidence interval for the odds of a successful repeat of a bioequivalence trial. This sort of exercise is left to the reader.

As a caution, we advise that, when using complex models like those currently employed in bioequivalence testing, users of the bootstrap should take care to ensure that their findings are robust to the incidence of non-convergence in the bootstrapped datasets. Note that the REML model used to examine `exam5.sas7bdat` failed to converge in SAS when bootstrapped on a very large number of occasions due to the issues involving the magnitude of variances described in [967]. Therefore, results should be interpreted with caution and are not presented in Table 5.3. The analysis for `exam6.sas7bdat` also failed to converge on a very limited number of occasions (less than 4% of the bootstraps for AUC, and less than 1% for Cmax). Modification to SAS code (see bootstrap_exam1 – 4.sas) may be necessary to ensure enough computer memory is available to run the model repeatedly or to ensure the model converges adequately.

We note that, while the bootstrap is a nice, easy-to-implement data exploration tool given modern computing power, it is important to note that bootstrap sampling introduces randomness into the results. This randomness has implications. In some cases [970], coverage probability of confidence intervals generated using the bootstrap may be lower than expected, leading to an increased possibility of a Type 1 error (see Chapter 1). Therefore, while it is a useful tool for exploring data, caution should be applied when using any findings for making claims in regulatory submissions. Those doing so should be prepared to ensure regulators that the risk of a Type 1 error is maintained at a level acceptable to the public's health.

Although not utilized here, we further note that the bootstrap is a very powerful tool for model validation [510].

5.5 Carry-Over

When carry-over is mentioned in bioequivalence studies, it refers to the occurrence of a nonzero plasma concentration of drug in a sample prior to dosing. As such, it complicates the analysis of bioequivalence data by aliasing or biasing the assessment of changes between formulations. A washout period (of at least five half-lives) is employed to prevent such occurrences.

Carry-over is very unusual but not unknown in bioequivalence studies and can arise from a variety of factors. Some are

1. Long-half-life drugs (with inadequate, too short, washout duration),
2. Serendipitous inclusion in the trial of subjects who poorly metabolize or eliminate the drug,
3. Random occurrences (possibly due to assay problems).

Statistical tests are available to test for carry-over and to evaluate its impact on these changes in formulation means [652]; however, in keeping with comments made in Chapter 3, and previous findings [1113], we do not recommend that those analyzing data from bioequivalence studies carry out statistical tests for the presence of carry-over ([652, 1114, 1115]). We will therefore confine discussion to practical issues and analyses that may be considered when pre-dose concentrations are detected. This would signal that carry-over was present in the bioequivalence design, and we assume that statistical tests will not be used to assess its impact in keeping with [1114, 1115], and [652].

As a practical matter, even if a more than adequate washout is used, there will be instances where pre-dose concentrations in periods after the first are non-null. The example to be considered was a drug that had been on the market for so long that its development predated pharmacokinetic assessment! The plant where the formulation had been manufactured (for many, many years) was closing, and the machinery that made the drug was packed and shipped to another site to continue manufacture, but the people who ran the machines at the old site retired. Therefore, the job was to prove that manufacturing at the new site by the new people but old equipment was to the same quality as the old (closed) site by use of a bioequivalence study.

In designing this bioequivalence study, the complete lack of pharmacokinetic data was problematic. On this occasion we had no basis on which to decide the length of a sufficient washout period, and there was insufficient time to run a pilot study. At risk, the study was designed based on an educated guess about what washout was needed from pharmacodynamic action of the product, but it turned out our guess undershot the needed duration. The example represents a worst-case scenario in that many pharmacokinetic profiles (for 27 subjects of 54 participating) were identified as having pre-dose concentrations in excess of the pharmacokinetic assay's lower limit of detection. AUC and Cmax data are listed in

Table 5.4 for this replicate design. AUC and Cmax values marked with a C denote those where a pre-dose plasma concentration was non-zero and in excess of the pharmacokinetic assay's lower limit of quantification.

TABLE 5.4: Example 5.1: AUC and Cmax Data from a Replicate Cross-Over Study Design with Test and Reference Formulations and Carry-Over (C)

Subject	Seq	Period 1	Period 2	Period 3	Period 4
AUC					
1	RTRT	812.6	1173.7C	889.1	620.1
2	TRTR	216.3	338	502.8C	398.6
3	RTRT	545.1	542.9C	.	.
4	TRTR	632.6	520C	716.7C	860.4C
5	RTRT	400	223.8C	173.7	289.7C
6	RTRT	102.1	185.3	42	88.3
7	TRTR	596	659.3	543.8	662.9
8	TRTR	402.4	359.8	590.8	444.3
9	TRTR	456.7	378.4	477.5	407.9C
10	RTRT	304.5	351.5C	520.2C	335.7C
11	TRTR	500.7	323C	416.3C	525.1C
12	RTRT	176.1	710.7	409.5	645.5
13	TRTR	160.6	218	170.1	124.6
15	RTRT	562.4	490.4C	504.7	675.9
16	TRTR	756	606.8	477.4	626.8
17	RTRT	207.5	271.6	173.7	240.5
18	RTRT	571.3	705.2	619	633.6
19	TRTR	511.9	549.7	388.2	141
20	TRTR	124	91.9	113.3	59.5
21	RTRT	536.1	595.2	445.5	521.5C
22	TRTR	239.7	265.1C	445.9	433.2
23	TRTR	609.6	371.6C	511.3	432.7C
24	RTRT	449.9	860.4C	606.8	577.2C
25	RTRT	192.5	220.1	233.1	227
26	TRTR	764.4	508.8	757.8	449.4
27	TRTR	151.9	194.8	.	.
28	RTRT	568.1	321.1	338.3	403.6C
29	RTRT	735.6	634.5C	1244.2C	641.9
30	TRTR	429.1	391.8C	316.9	335.1C
31	RTRT	307.4	481.8	346.6C	369.7C
32	TRTR	409	514.6C	763.1C	406.5C
33	TRTR	271	221	296.5	463.7
34	RTRT	292.9	431C	448.5	267.8C
35	RTRT	217.2	332.2	103	127.5
36	TRTR	290.8	208.6	243.7	489.8
37	TRTR	297.2	502	320.4	334.3
38	TRTR	163.8	232.1	636.9	434.9
39	RTRT	368.3	292.6C	446.1	222.3C
R=Reference, T=Test C=Carry-Over Concentration at Baseline					

TABLE 5.4: Example 5.1: AUC and Cmax Data from a Replicate Cross-Over Study Design with Test and Reference Formulations and Carry-Over (C) (continued)

Subject	Seq	Period 1	Period 2	Period 3	Period 4
40	RTRT	193.7	202.8	255.2	244.3
42	TRTR	534.1	243.1	418.4	441.9
43	TRTR	355.1	415.2	382.7	334
44	RTRT	102	282.5C	245.6	286.2C
45	TRTR	320.5	233.9	331.7	260.5
46	RTRT	223.6	645.4	349	507.4C
47	TRTR	504.5	289.9	550.7C	244.2
48	RTRT	615.8	732.1C	620.9	665.2C
49	RTRT	898.4	924.9C	398.3	828.3C
50	RTRT	410.4	329.2	449.4	442.1
52	TRTR	237	505C	496.3	580.6C
53	RTRT	332.4	273.6	525.3	293.3
54	RTRT	185.2	222.9	182.1	194.1
55	TRTR	246.9	620.9C	678.3	752.2C
56	TRTR	235.4	190.4	318.3	248.4
57	RTRT	180.6	174.7	102.9	117
Cmax					
1	RTRT	99.85	204.09C	170.94	112.78
2	TRTR	29.06	50.48	35.15C	55.71
3	RTRT	67.69	41.73C	.	.
4	TRTR	91.25	43.86C	168.78C	61.04C
5	RTRT	40.05	25.17C	24.48	86.49C
6	RTRT	28.76	24.83	9.27	10.89
7	TRTR	257.1	79.04	127.92	81.8
8	TRTR	136.27	158.86	148.97	82.41
9	TRTR	65.48	87.84	64.57	58.01C
10	RTRT	34.35	52.26C	142.92C	58.48C
11	TRTR	31.49	37.07C	80.9C	33.62C
12	RTRT	18.94	161.34	118.89	246.57
13	TRTR	29.61	43.15	27.71	13.11
15	RTRT	28.35	98.5C	78.22	140.54
16	TRTR	168.76	174.94	117.31	52.18
17	RTRT	19.18	94.92	21.39	65.45
18	RTRT	66.63	134.69	78.1	78.51
19	TRTR	32.23	70.06	32.15	43.11
20	TRTR	9.34	11.74	49.23	18.42
21	RTRT	42.11	37.82	39.87	116.79C
22	TRTR	38.02	16.79C	38.58	83.82
23	TRTR	199.07	52.14C	118.47	72.04C
24	RTRT	32.53	276.86C	118.65	156.33C
25	RTRT	21.96	38.97	22.26	54.16
26	TRTR	74.24	35.76	39.27	36.28
27	TRTR	19	20.61	.	.
28	RTRT	110.87	55.64	50.06	84.6C

R=Reference, T=Test
C=Carry-Over Concentration at Baseline

TABLE 5.4: Example 5.1: AUC and Cmax Data from a Replicate Cross-Over Study Design with Test and Reference Formulations and Carry-Over (C) (continued)

Subject	Seq	Period 1	Period 2	Period 3	Period 4
29	RTRT	50.08	58.79C	181.53C	144.26
30	TRTR	31.85	74.88C	54.88	19.18C
31	RTRT	87.21	88.75	90.07C	132.92C
32	TRTR	30.86	70.84C	208.2C	65.25C
33	TRTR	86.01	41.85	67.86	79.81
34	RTRT	18.07	33.37C	21.48	20.87C
35	RTRT	18.69	174.55	17.06	32.01
36	TRTR	38.27	40.31	31.56	20.64
37	TRTR	49.81	66.64	17.8	25.94
38	TRTR	34.56	16.37	114.3	29.58
39	RTRT	52.59	57.88C	48.58	47.24C
40	RTRT	29.3	78.33	21.72	49.27
42	TRTR	136	33.75	104.12	35.03
43	TRTR	64.55	34.04	52.37	41.67
44	RTRT	22.14	63.5C	9.38	16.3C
45	TRTR	26.35	37.2	76.26	24.6
46	RTRT	27.02	167.28	20.35	121.92C
47	TRTR	118.91	49.27	166.61C	35.86
48	RTRT	60.94	100.47C	26.17	98.08C
49	RTRT	164.01	180.01C	25.21	97.02C
50	RTRT	59.7	43.65	102.47	40
52	TRTR	30.55	63.9C	39.17	40.75C
53	RTRT	39.96	56.47	42.11	38.75
54	RTRT	18.34	16.09	21.5	9.57
55	TRTR	42.2	106.69C	150.52	115.15C
56	TRTR	39.15	13.79	122.03	62.32
57	RTRT	9.1	58.44	12.74	18.33
R=Reference, T=Test C=Carry-Over Concentration at Baseline					

The average contribution of the nonzero pre-dose concentrations in these subjects relative to the magnitude of Cmax observed in that period was only 1.5%. Thus, for the majority of subjects the presence of carry-over could be deemed negligible as a practical matter. However, two subjects had concentrations of approximately 5.25% and 5.05% relative to the Cmax observed in that period. For the purpose of this example, Subject 1 (Period 2, pre-dose concentration of 10.7) and Subject 10 (Period 3, pre-dose concentration of 7.2) will be deemed to have had such observed data. Results of such magnitude would lead one to consider whether this could have an impact on inference.

Regulatory guidance is quite clear on how to handle such data. The FDA guidance [373] recommends that

> If the pre-dose concentration is less than or equal to 5 percent of Cmax value in that subject, the subject's data without any adjustments can be included in all pharmacokinetic measurements and calculations. If the predose value is greater than 5 percent of Cmax, the subject should be dropped from all BE study evaluations.

TABLE 5.5
Example 5.1: Adjusted Cmax and AUC Data for Subjects 1 and 10

Subject	Period	Adj. AUC(0-t)	Adj. Cmax
1	2	1045.3	193.39
10	3	433.8	135.72

Europe's guidance is a little more specific [319]:

> If there are any subjects for whom the pre-dose concentration is greater than 5% of the Cmax value for that subject in that period, the statistical analysis should be performed with the data from that subject for that period excluded.

These guidances tacitly assume that the occurrence of carry-over of sufficient magnitude to impact inference is random, in line with recent publications on the topic ([652, 1114, 1115]). Indeed, even in the worst-case scenario of carry-over described above, only two subjects had concentrations of such magnitude, and exclusion of Subjects 1 and 10 and/or the data in the particular periods of interest does not materially affect statistical inference. Confirmation of this finding is left to the reader using the SAS code introduced earlier.

This approach has the benefit of simplicity, and, given the sparsity of the occurrence of relevant carry-over, it is expected that its application will suit most circumstances. We will dwell on an alternative approach for (rare) situations when such might not be suitable. Additionally, the handling of such data by non-FDA and European regulatory bodies, for example, is not standardized in guidance, and other agencies might request other approaches to analysis.

We will consider adjustment of data for pre-dose concentrations where the magnitude is sufficient to warrant concern. Consider Subjects 1 and 10 in the example. As the pre-dose concentration has been assayed, it is reasonable to presume that the effect on subsequent observed plasma concentrations is additive relative to the dose received in the period under study, as drug on board pre-dose is simply in the process of being eliminated from the body. One could "slice" a portion of the concentration data from the pharmacokinetic concentration versus time profile and estimate an adjusted Cmax and AUC for use in analysis. For Example 5.1, these data are presented in Table 5.5.

These adjusted data were derived by subtracting the pre-dose concentration from Cmax and by removing an estimated area from the AUC. For the purposes of this example, the t in AUC(0-t) was defined as occurring at 24 hours post dose, and the area "sliced" from the full AUC was derived according to the equations of Chapter 1 consistent with a half-life of 24 hours. In more complex pharmacokinetic profiles, other calculations might be more appropriate. The changes in the data introduced by "slicing" adjustment did not impact statistical inference (confirmation of this is left to the reader) relative to statistical analysis including their original data.

Data manipulation in such a manner may have two unintended effects on bioequivalence testing. It certainly introduces more variation into our model, as adjustment using "slicing" does not take into account the error implicit in pharmacokinetic measurement (due to assay and within-subject variability).

Additionally, data manipulation may introduce bias, as only some data for subjects in certain periods were adjusted. Note in the example above, subjects with very low pre-dose concentrations were present but were neglected, as their values were minimal (around 1.5% of Cmax), and only data for certain periods were adjusted (see Subject 10). As average bioequivalence is a within-subject assessment (each subject serves as their own control), if a subject experiences carry-over sufficient to warrant adjustment in one session, it is more appropriate to adjust all sessions for any relevant pre-dose concentrations for a given subject regardless of magnitude. In the case of the above example, one should consider adjusting data for Subject 10 in Periods 2 and 4 even though pre-dose concentrations in those sessions were only approximately 1.5% of Cmax. Alternatively, if the FDA "data-reduction" approach [373] is used, all of the subject's pharmacokinetic data should be excluded from analysis to avoid the introduction of bias or increased variation.

Those using such adjustment techniques should be explicit about what adjustments were made and the process followed. Regulatory acceptance of such a procedure is unknown and falls outside the scope of current international guidance (other than the FDA's, cf. [373], where an alternative procedure described above is recommended).

Note also that, while not recommended in bioequivalence testing, statistical models for the assessment of differential carry-over in bioequivalence testing in cross-over designs [652] may detect such "slicing" of the data as a factor consistent with the statistical detection of carry-over from such data. Therefore, further care is recommended if such models and data manipulation are applied.

5.6 Optional Designs

The most common study design applied to bioequivalence testing is the 2×2 design, already described in great detail. In cases where one dosing regimen is to be marketed relative to the multiple formulations used in confirmatory trials (e.g., a 300 mg dose is to be marketed but must be confirmed as bioequivalent to a 200 mg tablet with a 100 mg tablet and to three 100 mg tablets), it may be necessary to extend this design to consider more than two regimens in a BE trial. Other trials might include four periods if bioequivalence was to be evaluated between two formulations at a low and at a higher dose, for example. Such is required by certain nations [141] when dose proportionality (discussed in a subsequent chapter) is not demonstrated.

Such designs are simply an extension of the 2×2 design introduced in Chapter 2 and may be analyzed in straightforward fashion as described in Chapters 3 and 4 and [652] and [1113]. We will refer to them as *standard* bioequivalence cross-over designs. For bioequivalence testing, the same model in SAS is typically utilized to analyze the data as that introduced in Chapter 3 with appropriate modifications for the number of sequences ($s = 1, 2, 3...$), periods ($p = 1, 2, 3...$), and treatments. In SAS, the call to `proc mixed`, the `class` statement, the `model` statement, and the `random` statement are all the same. The `estimate` statement changes to accommodate the comparisons of interest.

An additional alternative design has already been mentioned, the replicate design. It is particularly useful for studying bioequivalence of highly variable drugs. A highly variable drug is defined as a drug with a within-subject CV_W (coefficient of variation) of greater than 30%. The coefficient of variation of a variate is the ratio, expressed as a percentage, of the standard deviation of the variate to its mean. For BE testing we note that $\sigma_W^2 = \ln(CV_W^2 + 1)$, i.e.,

$$CV_W = \sqrt{e^{\sigma_W^2} - 1}.$$

In a replicate cross-over design (see Chapter 4), each subject receives each formulation twice. Eligible subjects are randomized to one of two treatment sequences, e.g., TRTR or RTRT. Thus, each subject is studied in four periods and receives each formulation twice over the course of the study. Similar to the two-period cross-over design described previously, a washout period adequate to the drug under study (at least five half-lives) separates each of the four treatment periods.

Formulation means are estimated with measurement and sampling error in cross-over designs. Replication of measurement within each subject reduces sampling error by a factor equivalent to the number of replications. For example, in a standard cross-over design, the variance of an individual's mean response on i =T (or R) is $\sigma_{Bi}^2 + \sigma_{Wi}^2$ where σ_{Bi}^2 is the inter-subject variance and σ_{Wi}^2 is the intra-subject (i.e., sampling error) variance. In a replicate design, the variance of an individual's mean response is $\sigma_{Bi}^2 + (\sigma_{Wi}^2/2)$. Therefore, where high intra-subject variability is of concern, the replicate design will provide more precise estimates of the true individual response.

For a low-variability product, replication does not improve precision dramatically, as σ_{Wi}^2 contributes little to the magnitude of the above expression; however, for a high variability product, replication more precisely defines the range over which an individual's mean response may vary. Such measurement is also more accurate, as replicate measurement and the derivation of corresponding means converges to the true (and unknown) mean under the central limit theorem with increasing replication [1283]. Such measurement may thus allow for better scrutiny of outliers ([1341, 1342]), but as the comparison of formulation means is of direct concern in the success of average bioequivalence studies, the desirability of such improvement in accuracy and precision is immediately apparent as a practical matter.

The number of subjects required to demonstrate average bioequivalence can be reduced by up to 50% using a replicate design relative to the sample size of a 2×2 cross-over trial. Note that the overall number of doses studied, however, remains similar to a 2×2 cross-over and that the study will be of about twice the duration with twice the blood sampling for each individual subject.

Experience indicates that, although it is theoretically possible to perform a bioequivalence trial with more than four periods, such is rarely utilized. Application of such a trial is not generally limited by logistics (how many subjects can be brought in, length of stay, etc.) but by how much blood can be drawn from a human volunteer in a given time interval! FDA guidance [373] recommends that 12–18 blood samples per subject per period be taken to characterize the PK versus time profile and to derive appropriate estimates of AUC, Cmax, and the other endpoints of interest. A blood collection of 500 mL across the length of a study is the usual limit applied to blood sampling for a human volunteer, and subjects should not have donated blood or plasma for approximately two months prior to being in a study.

Bioequivalence trials must also collect blood samples for purposes other than PK assessment. Such blood sampling for safety assessment (laboratory assessment of liver function, for example) from each volunteer at screening, during the trial, and follow-up in addition to PK sampling limits how much blood can ethically be taken without compromising the safety of volunteers in a given time interval. If this amount is exceeded, this could not only pose a danger to volunteers but also would change the amount of blood available in the circulation and potentially impact the ADME properties of PK measurement (defeating the purpose of collecting it).

We now have an extensive range of options for deciding what type of study design can be applied in a bioequivalence study. These options are applied depending on how many subjects are required to have a good chance of success in demonstrating bioequivalence and the extent of clinical resources. A general algorithm for designing average bioequivalence trials is described below.

***Algorithm 5.1: Planning a Bioequivalence Study** [966]*

1. Determine the number of formulations (and doses) to be studied for bioequivalence.
2. Calculate the sample size for a standard cross-over (i.e., a non-replicate 2×2, three- or four-period) design. The details of how to perform sample size calculations will be discussed in the next section.

3. Consider available clinical resources.
4. For products with low to moderate intra-subject variation ($CV_W < 30\%$) where adequate resources are available, use the standard cross-over design.
5. For highly variable products, where sample size exceeds available resources, consider a replicate cross-over design and reassess sample size. If resources are adequate, use the replicate design.
6. For situations where resources are still too limited to achieve desired power, or in situations where one is very uncertain of the magnitude of intra-subject variation (or other critical assumptions), apply a group-sequential design.

Group sequential designs are a further extension of the designs already discussed. These offer the potential for additional resource savings in bioequivalence designs ([482, 535]). A group sequential design consists of one or more interim analyses, at which point the sponsor can decide to stop the trial with concrete evidence of success or failure or to carry on. Well known in the statistics community [978], such designs are easy and straightforward to implement in practice in this setting and are becoming more common in regulated drug and biological development [394].

A group sequential design approach could be used in cases where there is significant uncertainty about estimates of variability. That is, based on previous data, there is a fairly wide range of estimates, such that choosing a lower estimate might result in an underpowered study and choosing a higher estimate might result in an overpowered study, which in either case is a waste of resources. As such, the group sequential design allows one to conduct an interim look with a sample size that provides reasonable power based on a lower (or optimistic) estimate of variability and the final sample size based on a higher (or less optimistic) estimate of variability. Similarly, if uncertainty in the true ratio of bioavailability is of concern, an interim look might be planned based upon sample size required to provide bioequivalence based on the optimistic estimate, with the final look providing conclusive results should this not be the case.

Lastly, a group-sequential design may be applied if it is undesirable to complete a large study due to resource constraints. Some choice of samples for interim analysis may be chosen (based on clinical feasibility) to facilitate an interim look. The probability of success may be quantified at that stage, and, if results are inconclusive, the study can continue to completion.

The two aspects of a group-sequential design that help determine the probability of stopping early are the alpha-spending function to control the overall Type 1 error rate of the study and the decision rule(s) for stopping at an interim analysis. There are many Type 1 error spending functions and decision rules to choose from, but only those relevant to two-stage group-sequential design for a bioequivalence trial will be discussed in this chapter.

The Type 1 error rate, as previously discussed, was set by regulators at 5% per test for bioequivalence studies and is defined as the probability of a false-positive outcome, or, in the case of bioequivalence trials, declaring two formulations are bioequivalent when they are not in truth. Unlike a fixed sample size trial, where there is only one analysis, a group-sequential trial may have multiple analyses. When data from a fixed sample size trial are analyzed repeatedly during the trial, the overall Type 1 error rate becomes inflated if each look is conducted at the same test level. For example, if two bioequivalence test procedures are conducted (each at the usual 5% level), the overall Type 1 error rate, the probability of a false positive on the first or second test, is 8% (instead of 5%); if three are conducted, the overall rate is 11%; and so on [1325].

As such, to control the overall Type 1 error rate of the study, the Type 1 error rate at each analysis must be some value less than the desired overall Type 1 error rate. In a two-stage group-sequential bioequivalence trial, the Type 1 error is typically divided equally between the two analyses. A simple, but conservative, method is the Bonferroni adjustment, which results in an error rate of 2.5% per two one-sided test [i.e., 95% confidence interval (CI)] at each look, but the resulting overall error rate slightly less than 5%. Another alternative, suggested in [994], is to set the error rate at the two analyses at 2.94% (i.e., approximately 94% CI) at each look, resulting in an overall error rate of approximately 5%.

Note that application of such a group-sequential design in bioequivalence testing is not the norm and is in fact discouraged by some guidance [33]. If it is applied, it is expected that most regulators will prefer the position expressed in [33] such that a conservative adjustment (i.e., the Bonferroni procedure) should be applied. For a standard cross-over design with two looks at the data, 95% confidence intervals would be derived at each look.

The decision rule for stopping early (at the first look) should contain both a rule for stopping early when bioequivalence is clearly demonstrated and a rule for futility when bioequivalence is not expected to be demonstrated. For example, one might define the following rule:

1. If the test formulation is demonstrated to be BE at the interim look (i.e., the 95% CIs for AUC and Cmax are contained in 0.80–1.25), then success has been achieved. Stop the study.
2. If $exp(\hat{\mu}_T - \hat{\mu}_R)$ for AUC or Cmax are not in the range 0.80–1.25, then further study is likely to be futile, and the study should be stopped.
3. Otherwise, continue to the final look.

In the next section, we will consider the calculations which go into deriving a sample size in more detail, and discuss several practical issues impacting the choice of sample size. In the remainder of this section, two other important issues will be discussed: derivation of the variance estimates to be used in bioequivalence sample size calculation, and the length of the washout period.

As discussed in Chapter 1, from the time Phase I starts with the first-time-in-humans study to the time in drug development when one would need to do a bioequivalence study, there is extensive study of pharmacokinetics. In general, AUC, Cmax, and the other PK endpoints are derived in multiple clinical pharmacology studies, resulting in a plethora of estimates for σ_W^2 of AUC and Cmax. Each of these study-specific estimates for σ_W^2 may be regarded as independent under the assumption that subjects participating in a given trial do not participate in the other trials.

When independent variability estimates are available across several studies (here studies are denoted $i = 1, 2, ...$), based on the properties of the chi-squared distribution, a method of pooling data across studies is readily available. In brief, a pooled estimate of within-subject variation ($\hat{\sigma}_{PW}^2$) for σ_W^2 is derived as

$$\hat{\sigma}_{PW}^2 = \frac{\sum_i (n_i - s_i)\hat{\sigma}_{Wi}^2}{\sum_i (n_i - s_i)},$$

where $n_i - s_i$ is the respective d.f. (equal to the sample size n_i less the number of sequences s_i in trial i) for the within-subject variability estimate $\hat{\sigma}_{Wi}^2$ from trial i based on the properties of the chi-squared distribution. These pooled estimates of variation for AUC and Cmax will be utilized in the sample size calculations performed in the next section.

Drugs where no such variability estimates exist for use in calculations are very unusual in the modern pharmaceutical industry, especially for those sponsors who conduct the confirmatory clinical trials and clinical pharmacology programs themselves. Even for drug products where no such in-house data are available, there are a variety of other sources of information (e.g., Physician's Desk Reference, Summary Basis for Approval, etc.) which likely will contain some information on PK variability for use in study design. In the rare event that data are not available, the FDA guidance [373] does make mention of running a pilot study of 6–12 subjects in a cross-over design to estimate variability. Those applying such a technique should ensure that AUC and Cmax data from the pilot study are not pooled with the subsequent confirmatory bioequivalence trial to avoid impacting the Type 1 error rate. Alternatively, a group-sequential analysis plan as described above could be applied.

Estimates of mean and variance for half-life $T_{\frac{1}{2}}$ should also be available across the i trials and can be regarded as independent from one another across trials under the same set of assumptions. One could also pool these estimates to determine an overall mean half-life to define the length of washout period; however, we recommend against such a practice given the importance of an adequate washout in the design of such trials and the interpretation of resulting data.

A key assumption in a cross-over design is that, all else being equal, pharmacology and physiology are stable throughout the length of the trial in any given volunteer. This is why normal healthy volunteers are dosed in bioequivalence trials — to prevent the occurrence of or potential for changing disease state from confounding the assessment of any difference in formulations. Therefore, after giving drug and altering (actually causing) PK to be measurable by means of our endpoints AUC and the rest, the washout is utilized to bring back blood concentrations to basal (i.e., null) level, ensure any impact of the drug on the body is negligible, and allow the normal healthy volunteers' bodies to return to "normal" with respect to blood lost to sampling. They then receive the next formulation in the next period, and so on.

As we have seen in Chapter 3, if concentrations do carry over through the washout period and into the next period (checked via collection of a blood sample prior to dosing), these carry-over effects confound to some extent the interpretation of differences between formulations. We therefore encourage readers to be over-cautious in the choice of washout period duration in bioequivalence. It should be at least five times the average mean half-life (across studies) and should be extended longer if significant within-subject variation is observed in $T_{\frac{1}{2}}$. Readers interested in a more quantitative definition of the upper limit of mean $T_{\frac{1}{2}}$ may wish to consider the application of a prediction interval (see, for example, Chapter 2 of [907] for more details), but we will not dwell further on this issue here.

For drugs with extremely long half-lives, a parallel group design [373] may be employed. In a parallel group design, subjects are randomized to receive either formulation T (Test) or R (Reference) in a single period and are not crossed over. Such studies are quite unusual in bioequivalence testing and will not be discussed further here. Readers interested in such an approach should see [196] and [1314]. Another design in the statistical literature that is sometimes considered is the "partial"-replicate design. This is simply a replicate design with the fourth period removed. Although understood statistically ([198, 617]), this type of design was seldom applied in bioequivalence testing. These designs are being more often used due to emerging regulatory guidance on scaled average bioequivalence and will be discussed later.

5.7 Determining Trial Size

Anyone can run a computer program to calculate how many subjects are needed for a BE study. The actual calculation for determining a sample size is the easiest part of what a statistician does in helping a team design a bioequivalence trial. The calculation itself (see

Chapter 3) is straightforward (see Chapter 3, [985], [258], [260], [196], [1113], and [652] for background). The more complex part of the job is to ensure that an adequate interface occurs between Statistics and Clinical to ensure the design and sample size are appropriate to the needs of the study.

The first question one should ask Clinical in designing a bioequivalence trial is, "How many formulations and doses need to be involved?" This will help determine the number of periods (2, 3, or 4) to be applied in the study, and thereafter the number of sequences of treatment administration. This number of sequences is critical, as it (with n, the number of subjects) will define the degrees of freedom associated with the comparison between formulation means. As sample size is generally small in bioequivalence studies ($n \leq 30$ subjects), an imprecise understanding of the degrees of freedom can lead to an imprecise understanding of the power of a trial and its probability of success.

It is assumed for the purposes of this discussion that within-subject variability estimates are available, for both AUC and Cmax, to determine the trial size. For this purpose the larger of the two pooled estimates is of primary interest in calculations, for obvious reasons (i.e., power will be greater, or alternatively the probability of a Type 2 error will be lower, for the endpoint with smaller variation). However, the degree of this increase should be estimated using appropriate code (just switching the estimate of variability) to ensure adequate overall power for the study, as it is known [918] that

$$Power \geq P_{AUC} + P_{Cmax} - (2 - 1)$$

where P_{AUC} is the estimate of power for AUC and P_{Cmax} is the estimate of power for Cmax. In the event that the overall power falls below the desired level, sample size may be increased to compensate, resulting in the desired level of power. For example, if power for Cmax is 0.90, and for AUC 0.95, the resulting overall study power is at least $0.9 + 0.95 - 1 = 0.85$.

The next question to ask Clinical is, "How many beds does clinical have, and how many subjects can be scheduled?" (also known as, "How many spots are available?"). Once the extent of those clinical resources has been determined (see Algorithm 5.1), the calculation may be carried out using the code given in Chapter 3 to determine power (recall this is 1 minus the probability of a Type 2 error) for the given potential sample size range in a standard 2×2 cross-over design.

If this sample size is too large, alteration of the R code given in Chapter 3 may be applied to determine sample size for a two-sequence replicate design (with adjustment of design parameters as appropriate to the study design chosen). This does double the length of the study, but about the sample size. For example halves

```
sampleN.TOST(alpha=0.05,targetpower=0.9,
             logscale=TRUE,theta0=0.95,theta1=0.8,
             theta2=1.25,CV=0.23,design="2x2x4",
             method="exact",robust=FALSE,print=TRUE,
             details=FALSE,imax=100)
```

For a two-stage group-sequential design (i.e., two looks), the Type 1 error rate (the parameter **a** in the above code) should be reset to 0.025 for the Bonferroni adjustment to determine power for the first look. At the second look, the estimate of the variance (parameter **s**) should also be adjusted for having assessed the variance at the first look in accordance with the findings of [636]. Essentially the variance at the end of the trial is weighted for the relative contribution of degrees of freedom at each look.

We now have a determination of power (probability of success) for our trial for a range of potential sample sizes. However, note that we are ***NOT DONE YET!*** It is important that a sensitivity assessment be carried out to ensure that the power of the trial is not overly influenced by any of our assumptions regarding certain parameters. Additionally, the sample size should ensure that power is sufficient relative to a pre-specified level of random dropouts.

Sensitivity of study outcome to random increases in variability should always be considered by the statistician when providing a sample size estimate. Variation greater than expected will result in less precision (wider than expected confidence intervals) and a drop in power for the study. Some authors [482] recommend derivation of a confidence interval for σ_W^2 for use in sample size calculations with regard to sensitivity analysis, and the authors have found this to be a valuable approach to this issue.

Residual estimates of variability derived from our i studies on the natural logarithmic scale may be considered to be distributed as a chi-squared distribution with degrees of freedom equal to the sum of degrees of freedom associated with the estimates of variability such that

$$\sum_i \frac{(n_i - s_i)\hat{\sigma}_{PW}^2}{\sigma_W^2} \sim \chi^2_{\sum_i n_i - s_i}.$$

Then a $(1-\alpha)100\%$ upper confidence bound for σ_W^2 across trials is

$$\hat{\sigma}_{PW}^2 \frac{\sum_i (n_i - s_i)}{\chi^2_{\sum_i n_i - s_i}(\alpha)}$$

where $\chi^2_{\sum_i n_i - s_i}(\alpha)$ is the α quartile of a chi-squared distribution with $\sum_i n_i - s_i$ degrees of freedom.

The next important factor to consider is whether the true bioavailability of the test formulation is the same as the reference formulation. Often this (parameter **ratio** in our code) will randomly differ slightly from unity. Indeed, for highly variable drugs, it is possible for the estimate of the ratio to randomly fall above unity in one trial, and in a follow-up trial of the same formulations to randomly fall below unity! As such, it is not a bad idea to allow for some wobble in the ratio of bioavailability, and FDA guidance generally recommends that sensitivity analyses consider ratios between 0.95 and 1.05.

It is not unusual for subjects to randomly drop out of a trial due to a variety of issues. Food poisoning-induced emesis, the flu, and a family outing are all examples of random reasons why a subject may not participate in a given session of a trial. As the term "volunteer" implies, subjects have the option to withdraw their consent to participate at any time and are not required to give a reason should they choose not to do so. Such missingness at random in data is easily accommodated by REML modelling but does represent a potential loss in power to the trial, as information of such subjects (sometimes termed "lost to follow up") will not be collected in that period. To compensate, a random dropout rate of 5–10% is generally assumed, and the bioequivalence trial over-enrolls to ensure a sufficient number of subjects complete the trial.

Dosing of subjects at the maximum tolerated dose may also result in dropouts over the course of the study; however, it is important to differentiate the "random" dropouts described above from such a potentially systematic dropout rate related to formulation. If a new formulation is less well tolerated than the reference formulation, this may appear in the dataset as an increase in the dropout rate or in adverse event rate on that formulation relative to the reference formulation. Bioequivalence trials are generally not powered to assess the potential for such effects, and we will consider how to assess safety in clinical pharmacology cross-over designs in a later chapter.

One example of this is emesis. Handling of data under this event is treated as a special case in guidance, and may result in data from a subject experiencing this event not being used at all. FDA guidance calls for the following assessment when emesis occurs:

TABLE 5.6
Example: Variability Estimates for Use in Designing a Bioequivalence Study

Study	d.f.	$\hat{\sigma}_W$
1	14	0.23
2	10	0.28
3	10	0.35
4	8	0.15
5	14	0.2
6	24	0.22

We recommend that data from subjects who experience emesis during the course of a BE study for immediate-release products be deleted from statistical analysis if vomiting occurs at or before 2 times median Tmax. In the case of modified-release products, the data from subjects who experience emesis any time during the labeled dosing interval can be deleted. [373]

We now turn to an example of determining a sample size. It was required that two new formulations (S and T) be demonstrated as bioequivalent to the clinical trials formulation (denoted R). We planned to use a three-period, six-sequence bioequivalence design and 30–50 spots were expected to be available in the clinical pharmacology unit.

Table 5.6 lists the estimates of within-subject variability available at that time from previous studies for use in sample size calculations.

Our overall pooled estimate of within-subject standard deviation (σ_W) across studies is $\hat{\sigma}_{PW} = 0.24$ with an upper 50% confidence bound of 0.28. We have at least 30 spots available and as many as 50, and will run the calculations for $n = 30$ and $n = 48$ (recall n must be a multiple of the number of sequences, 6).

Our power for $n = 30$ is 94% and for $n = 48$ 99%, and under Algorithm 5.1, we conclude that this design will be adequate.

For the sensitivity analysis, we first assess the impact of increased variation up to 0.28 standard deviations. Power for $n = 30$ is 82% and for $n = 48$ 97%. The authors' rule of thumb is that at least 80% power should be maintained under random changes in assumptions.

Second, we assess the impact of a change in relative bioavailability to 0.95 instead of unity. Power for $n = 30$ is 85% and for $n = 48$ 96%.

We assess the impact on power if we are very unlucky and variation increases to 0.28 standard deviations along with a decrease in true bioavailability to 0.95. Power for $n = 30$ is 73% and for $n = 48$ 90%. This last scenario is pretty unlikely, but it does not hurt to check.

Last, the drug was well tolerated at the maximum dose, so over-enrollment on the order of 5% is likely called for, so we would over-enroll one or two subjects to ensure that the minimum desired number complete the study.

In this situation, an n of 30–36 subjects should provide at least 90% power (most likely) and approximately 80% power if the assumptions are not too grossly violated.

It is possible to design and implement studies that incorporate adaptive sample sizing, and this topic may be found in the next chapter. We now turn to the topic of outliers.

5.8 What Outliers Are and How to Handle Their Data

Although not explicitly stated in regulatory bioequivalence guidance (see Chapter 2), there is a very great distinction between an outlier in a statistical sense and in a regulatory sense.

In statistical training, outliers are generally introduced as a topic related to assessment of model fit (see, for example, [907] Chapters 2 and 5). An outlier is defined as a residual that has large value — i.e., the model does not fit the data point well. Various statistical procedures and tests have been devised over the years to identify such outliers. In general, if the absolute residual value corrected for variation (termed "studentized residual") is greater than 2 or 3 (depending on how conservative one is), then a data point may be termed a *statistical* outlier.

In terms of statistical impact, an outlier (or set of outliers) may impact the estimate $\hat{\delta}$ (by influencing its position relative to 0) or inflate the estimate of within-subject variance $\hat{\sigma}_W^2$ (resulting in a wider than expected confidence interval) or both. These effects on either of these parameters implicitly make it more difficult to demonstrate average bioequivalence. The previous section provides a quantitative means of determining the potential impact on power (the probability of a successful BE trial).

This statistical assessment is a purely quantitative approach — providing an objective assessment of whether or not a data point is unusual. Statistical science rarely goes further — i.e., to describe what should be done with such data points. In reporting of BE trials, it is usual for statistical results to be presented with and without the outlying data points to determine if the outlier influences the results. This, however, leaves one in a practical quandary — which analysis is to be believed?

Outliers may not be excluded from a bioequivalence data set on statistical grounds alone. From a regulatory review perspective, handling of such data is very difficult, and the FDA and other regulatory agencies require that such data be looked at quite carefully.

If an outlier is the result of a protocol deviation (for example, the subject drank far too much water or chewed up the pill instead of just swallowing it), then deleting the outlier from the dataset may be justified [373]. However, if evidence of such a deviation does not exist, regulators assume that the cause of the outlier is either product failure (maybe the tablet dissolved in some strange manner) or due to a subject-by-formulation interaction (for example, the new formulation might be more bioavailable than the reference formulation in certain subjects). Admittedly, it may also just be a random event, and there is generally no way to differentiate to which of the three categories a given outlier belongs. Average bioequivalence studies are not designed to assess individual product differences but only to compare the formulations means.

In this context, whether an outlier is a product failure, a subject-by-formulation interaction, or a random event is immaterial. These are confounded, and final inference with regard to bioequivalence (and regulatory approval) is based on the full dataset (i.e., including the outliers). If observations are deleted, it is the sponsor's responsibility to provide a rationale to convince the regulators that such is appropriate.

On a practical level, this essentially means in practice that there is no such thing as an outlier in a bioequivalence dataset, and while we recommend that statisticians always check the assumptions of their model, in this context there is little utility in spending too much time worrying about outliers' impact on the findings. The authors have never seen an instance where a protocol violation has resulted in regulators deeming the deletion of a data point as acceptable; however, the authors have seen many instances where outliers from one to two subjects have resulted in a conclusion that bioequivalence was not demonstrated. Example 3.2 (Chapter 3) could be viewed as an example of this. From the data it was impossible to rule out that product failure, a subject-by-formulation interaction, or just a random occurrence of an outlying data point were involved. This generally results in a follow-up BE trial (of similar design) being done, as was described in the prologue to this chapter.

As the impact of outliers cannot be controlled after the study is completed, the best way to deal with them is to acknowledge that they can happen at random and to protect the study's power for random appearance of outliers at the design stage. To do so, it is recommended that bioequivalence studies be powered at 90% and that such trials have at least 80% power under potential inflation of the variability estimate and for potential changes in δ of up to 5%.

5.9 Bayesian BE Assessment

The approach to statistics thus far described is deductive in that we collect data to test a specific hypothesis or set of hypotheses. We use *observed* data to derive statistics to test specific facts in which we are interested. Statistics are used to quantify the probability that the data collected are consistent with our predetermined hypotheses.

For bioequivalence testing, one could denote the probability of observed data given the hypotheses conditions as

$$p(\underline{y}|H_{01}, H_{02}) \tag{5.1}$$

where $\underline{y}$ denotes the observed data, and H_{01}, H_{02} refer to the two one-sided hypotheses of interest for the difference between formulation means (see Equations (12.5) and (12.6)). This direct, deductive approach to statistics enjoys a very long history [500] and is the most often referred to approach in biopharmaceutical statistics. It is referred to as direct probability assessment, as it deals "directly" with the observed data to draw conclusions.

However, this is not the only way to consider looking at data. One might approach data in an inductive manner. In this case, we have a predetermined (rough) idea of the state of nature, and we collect data to give us a more precise idea of this state. This approach is inductive in that we *assume* we know what is happening or will happen, and data are collected to reinforce the point. This approach to statistics also enjoys a long history and was developed in the late 1700s and early 1800s by Bayes and Laplace [500]. It is referred to as indirect probability assessment, as it deals "indirectly" with the observed data to draw conclusions about the unknown parameters of interest. In average bioequivalence testing, for example, $\delta = \mu_T - \mu_R$, the true (unknown) difference in formulation means is the parameter of most interest.

In biopharmaceutical statistics, indirect probability assessment is not employed as often as direct probability assessment. The reason is quite obvious, given a brief rereading of Chapter 1. When making regulatory claims, it is the sponsor's burden to prove to a regulator's satisfaction that the drug is safe, efficacious, and can be manufactured to good quality. The regulator's presumption is that it is not safe, efficacious, nor of good quality until sufficient data are provided to prove otherwise. Therefore, the application of indirect probability assessment is of limited practical utility in regulated bioequivalence testing. Indirect probability assessment is also deemed subjective in that one must make assumptions regarding the conditions being studied.

Note, however, that, when one is not working in a confirmatory setting but is *exploring* clinical development of a compound (as described in Chapter 1), an inductive approach to statistics adds much value. Under such circumstances, the sponsor is working under the assumption that a drug is reasonably safe, efficacious, and of good quality and wishes to collect data to design and study the drug in confirmatory clinical trials. For example, one might perform trials in clinical development to determine the best tolerated and effective dose to subsequently be used in a confirmatory trial. In such a setting, it is not necessary to demonstrate to regulators that such is the case, but only to provide sufficient evidence to satisfy internal decision makers in the sponsoring company. Use of Bayesian inference offers substantial benefit in terms of data exploration (see [110]). Here we will include a brief discussion on indirect probability assessment in bioequivalence for completeness and to introduce concepts to be used later.

In mathematical terms, we first acknowledge we have some idea of what is happening or will happen with the difference in formulation means (expressed as $p(\delta)$). We again collect data from the BE study and calculate a probability; however, here we are interested in the probability of the conditions for δ given the observed data, which we denote as

$$p(\delta|\underline{y})$$

rather than the probability of observing the data given a hypothetical set of conditions. Note there is no explicitly stated hypothesis in this indirect probability setting.

The derivation of an indirect probability may be extremely complex mathematically, and this was a practical bar to the implementation of such approaches to data analysis until recently. Modern computing software has rendered this complexity manageable. Recent developments in Markov chain Monte Carlo-based methods known as Gibbs sampling (e.g., WINBUGS at http://www.mrc-bsu.cam.ac.uk/software/bugs/, last accessed 9 June 2015) were developed in the late 1980s and 1990s [461] to implement indirect probability assessment in a straightforward fashion. The SAS procedure `proc mcmc` is now also available to implement such methods [652]. We will now consider an example in bioequivalence to illustrate the concepts; further illustration of these methods for normal data models may be found in [446].

One first assumes a functional form for $p(\delta)$ and then derives

$$p(\delta|\underline{y}) = \frac{p(\underline{y}|\delta)p(\delta)}{p(\underline{y})}. \tag{5.2}$$

This expression indicates that the probability in which we are interested ($p(\delta|\underline{y})$) is equal to the probability of the data given the possible values of $\mu_T - \mu_R = \delta$ multiplied by our initial idea about the properties of the situation ($p(\delta)$) divided by the overall probability that one would observe the data ($p(\underline{y})$). Note that the expression $p(\underline{y}|\delta)$ is very similar to Equation (5.1). Under certain conditions, inductive and deductive reasoning will yield similar findings statistically, and we will observe such in this example.

We now turn to the example utilizing the AUC and Cmax data found in Example 3.1. WINBUGS and SAS code for this analysis is provided in [652] and is not reproduced here.

This model assumes we know very little about the true values of the unknown parameters of interest (here, $\mu_T - \mu_R$). In Table 5.7 we choose to present medians and 90% confidence intervals. The median is a statistic derived by taking the value in the distribution where 50% of data falls above and 50% of data falls below the value. In keeping with the findings of Laplace [500], the posterior median is the most appropriate measure of centrality for a distribution when using indirect probability assessment.

The findings of Table 5.7 should seem very familiar. If we review these findings relative to the analyses of Chapter 3, we will find that they are very similar. This is generally the case if one uses a noninformative prior distribution, as the weight introduced by this term into Equation (5.2) is minor.

TABLE 5.7
Statistics for δ and σ_W^2 Inverse Probabilities Given AUC and Cmax Data Observed in Example 3.1

Parameter	Median δ (90% BCI)	median σ_W^2
AUC	-0.0166 (-0.0614, 0.0286)	0.0114
Cmax	-0.0270 (-0.1121, 0.0588)	0.0410
BCI = Bayesian Confidence Interval		
5th and 95th Quartiles of p given observed data		

The key problem with the regulatory application of indirect probability assessment in this setting is this dependence on the assumptions of the prior distributions. For example, if one makes a minor change to the model (assumes, for example, that `delta` has a distribution with different moments, such as a standard deviation of 1), the distribution of $p(\delta|\underline{y})$ may sometimes change dramatically. The extent of such a change depends upon the weight of this term in Equation (5.2) relative to the weight of the observed data. In this example, such is not the case, but changes in the assumptions for smaller datasets can result in a different inference, complicating regulatory interpretation when using such a method ([964, 965]). We leave sensitivity analysis to assess this potential to the reader.

6

Adaptive Bioequivalence Trials

Introduction

One of the things not taught in school is deciding when to fight a battle and when to let people figure it out for themselves. Of their own volition, many people are content to remain as they are, working as they have always done, doing as they are told, collecting their pay at regular intervals, and going home on time to other activities. Of course, there is also a proportion of people who do not do that and work to continuously (or periodically) improve how they do business — e.g. faster, lower cost, more efficient, etc. This puts the folks who do not enhance the way they do business in a difficult position — they have to work harder to keep up (which conflicts with one of their aims), and when they are forced to innovate, generally by economic or management pressure, one can be certain they will not like it.

For example, at one point, early in my career, I was asked to develop an approach to dose-finding using Bayesian statistics for a group working in Phase 1 development. It was an interesting project, and after about a year of research, we were ready to roll the project out to the scientists, nurses, and physicians for alpha-testing (where we essentially get a couple of folks to try it out). My boss and the professor, with whom we had collaborated on the project, decided jointly that the professor should be the one to introduce the business unit concerned to the concept.

I will never forget how shabbily and poorly the people in this unit treated the professor's presentation and the product we had put together for their potential use. The request for a few people to pilot the Bayesian approach was denied, vociferously, and quite nastily. The professor and I were a bit stunned coming out of the meeting, but one of the best scientists stopped by to remind us later that day that "Columbus did not get the funding to discover America in a day." He recommended we pursue the project further and come back when the group was more receptive.

It really puzzled me at the time how this audience could be so hostile. But there was more to this than one perceived at first glance. I found out later that this group had been developing their own software program for data storage and basic statistical analysis. They had paid a great deal of money to have it developed, based on the way they had been doing things for years. Several highly influential people had a vested interest in making sure it came to fruition and was deemed "completed" (i.e., if it did not, their bonus would suffer). Incorporation of any new idea (no matter how good) would hold up completion. Thus Bayesian statistics was a no-go.

In reality, this is frequently how politics are in business and in science, but it is a mistake to ignore innovation. There are always folks with a vested interest in doing things as they are right now. The business unit above kept doing business the way they always had, right up until the business environment became more competitive, and there was a drive to cut costs. Then their unit and its home-grown software program proved to be too expensive to maintain.

6.1 Background

In Chapters 3 to 5 we described how to test for average bioequivalence (ABE) using the two one-sided testing (TOST) procedure [1088]. As this procedure is used after the trial has been completed, its power is entirely dependent on the assumptions made at the planning stage. If any of these assumptions are wrong, e.g., the assumed CV is too small, then there is a risk that ABE will not be shown at the end of the trial.

As will also be recalled, the regulatory requirement is that ABE has to be shown for both AUC and Cmax for the Test formulation to be declared bioequivalent to the Reference formulation. To simplify the following presentation, we will use only one of these metrics in our descriptions of the tests of hypotheses and the sample size re-estimation methods. The metric with the larger CV will usually be used to sample size the trial and typically this will be Cmax. Although there are two metrics, there is no inflation of the Type I error rate caused by the multiple testing of both AUC and Cmax, because both metrics have to be significant when using the TOST procedure.

However, if ABE is not shown at the end of the trial, and the estimated CV is larger than was assumed at the planning stage, then there is a temptation to continue the trial by recruiting additional subjects. ABE is then tested by applying the TOST procedure, a second time, to the combined dataset (i.e., using the data from both the original and additional subjects). This is done in the hope that applying the TOST procedure to the enlarged trial dataset will now result in ABE being declared. However, this approach does not preserve the Type I error rate of the TOST procedure when applied to each of AUC and Cmax.

An approach that does guarantee preserving the Type I error rate at its nominal value will be described in the next section. This approach allows for a preplanned unblinded sample size re-estimation step, embedded within a standard group-sequential design. The new testing procedure employs the weighted normal inverse combination of p-values test [46, 753], a test which we will refer to as the *standard combination test.* We will also introduce a robust version of this test, that we refer to as the *maximum combination test* [856]. In the subsequent sections we will illustrate the application of the standard and maximum combination tests. We will then describe the properties of our approach that combines these tests with a sample size re-estimation step and compare these with those of some previously published sample size re-estimation methods [888, 1000, 1363].

In most sections we will also refer to some example R code to do the necessary calculations.

6.2 Two-Stage Design for Testing for ABE

Here we assume that the design of the study is a 2×2 cross-over trial in two stages, with n_1 subjects in the first stage. At the end of the first stage, the TOST procedure is used to test for ABE based on unblinded estimates of the within-subject CV and geometric mean ratio (GMR) of Test to Reference formulations. The significance levels used in the TOST procedure at the end of each stage will be α_1 and α_2, respectively, where, typically, $\alpha_1 = \alpha_2 < \alpha$.

If ABE is shown, then the trial is stopped. If ABE is not shown, then a decision to continue the trial or not is made (see below for how this is decided). If the trial continues, the sample size is re-estimated using the unblinded data from the first stage. We assume that the re-estimated size of the second stage is n_2. A schematic plan of this design is given in Table 6.1.

As noted in the previous section, for regulatory purposes the interim decision must be based on both AUC and Cmax. If ABE can be declared for both, then the trial can be stopped after the first stage. If ABE is not shown for both of AUC and Cmax, then the sample size re-estimation will be based on the metric with the larger CV, which is typically Cmax. If ABE is shown for one metric but not the other, then the decision to continue or stop will be made on the basis of the metric that failed ABE. In this situation, only this

TABLE 6.1
Schematic Plan of Two-Stage Design

Stage 1	Interim Analysis	Stage 2
n_1 subjects	Stop or Continue	$n_2 \geq 0$ subjects
$n_1/2$ per group	Sample size re-estimation	$n_2/2$ per group

metric needs to be tested a second time at the end of the trial. Obviously, this is also the metric used in the sample size re-estimation.

We will assume that $n_1 = N/2$, where N is the total sample size calculated at the planning stage. For precision, we will also assume that the TOST procedure uses a nominal significance level of $\alpha = 0.05$ and that the initial total sample size is calculated to achieve a power of $1 - \beta = 0.8$ to show ABE. This calculation is done under the assumption that the expected (or planning) difference of means on the log-scale is $\delta = \delta_p$, where $\delta = \mu_T - \mu_R$ and CV takes some particular value. The initial sample size is conveniently calculated using the function *power.TOST* in the R package *PowerTOST* [728]. Some example R code to do these calculations is given in Section 6.11.1.

If ABE is not shown at the end of the first stage, then the power of the TOST procedure, based only on the first stage, is calculated using α_1, the estimated CV, n_1, and δ_p. If this power is lower than 0.8, the sample size re-estimation is done and the trial continues into a second stage. If not, then it is decided that the power of the first stage was high enough to make the decision to stop. This is what is done in Method B of [1000], for example. The size of the second stage is n_2. These decisions are summarized in Table 6.2. In our approach, at the end of the second stage, the combination test or its robust version, the maximum combination test, is used in conjunction with the TOST procedure to test for ABE. Note that the value of α_2 (and α_1) will depend on the type of test used at the end of the second stage.

The new methodology in Sections 6.5, 6.6, and 6.7 rely heavily on [856].

TABLE 6.2
Decisions at the End of the First Stage

ABE shown at end of first stage?	Interim decision
Yes	Stop
No	If power to show ABE based on α_1, n_1, and estimated CV from first stage ≥ 0.8, then stop
No	If power to show ABE based on α_1, n_1, and estimated CV from first stage < 0.8, then re-estimate total sample size based on the estimated CV from the first stage

6.3 TOST Using the Standard Combination Test

In the standard TOST procedure the two null hypotheses H_{01} and H_{02}, defined in Equations (2.3) and (2.4) in Chapter 2, are tested at the end of the trial and provide p-values p_1 and p_2, respectively. If both p-values are less than the nominal level α, then ABE is declared. In the two-stage design, the TOST procedure is applied both at the end of the first stage and, if the trial continues, at the end of the second stage. The p-values for hypotheses H_{01} and H_{02}, obtained from the TOST procedure at the end of the first stage, will be denoted by p_{11} and p_{12}, respectively, and the corresponding p-values obtained at the end of the second stage will be denoted by p_{21} and p_{22}. We emphasize that p_{21} and p_{22} are obtained using only the data from the second stage. The TOST procedure at the end of the trial uses the *standard combination test.*

In the standard combination test ([46, 753]), a weighted average of transformed p-values from stages 1 and 2 is used as the test statistic. When used in conjunction with the TOST procedure, for pre-specified weights, w and $1 - w$ $(0 < w < 1)$, the test statistic at the end of stage 2 for H_{01} is

$$Z_{01} = \sqrt{w}\Phi^{-1}(1 - p_{11}) + \sqrt{1-w}\Phi^{-1}(1 - p_{21}),$$

where $\Phi^{-1}(.)$ is the inverse of the cumulative standard normal distribution, and for H_{02} the test statistic is

$$Z_{02} = \sqrt{w}\Phi^{-1}(1 - p_{12}) + \sqrt{1-w}\Phi^{-1}(1 - p_{22}).$$

It is very important that the weights (w and $1 - w$) are pre-specified before the trial begins. With pre-specified weights, the resulting test guarantees control of the Type I error rate at its nominal level, regardless of any modification, e.g., a re-estimation of the sample size, that is done as a result of the interim analysis. Under their respective null hypotheses, both Z_{01} and Z_{02} are standard normal random variables.

To simplify the notation we will use

$$Z_{11} = \Phi^{-1}(1 - p_{11}), \quad Z_{21} = \Phi^{-1}(1 - p_{21})$$

and

$$Z_{12} = \Phi^{-1}(1 - p_{12}), \quad Z_{22} = \Phi^{-1}(1 - p_{22}).$$

For H_{01} the test statistic at the end of the second stage is

$$Z_{01} = \sqrt{w}Z_{11} + \sqrt{1-w}Z_{21},$$

and for H_{02} the test statistic at the end of the second stage is

$$Z_{02} = \sqrt{w}Z_{12} + \sqrt{1-w}Z_{22}.$$

As already noted, in the two-stage design we assume that at the end of the first stage the hypotheses H_{01} and H_{02} are tested using the usual TOST procedure at a significance level $\alpha_1 < \alpha$. If the trial continues to a second stage, we assume that the two hypotheses will be tested again at level α_2. As in the usual TOST procedure, both null hypotheses must be rejected to declare ABE.

For given choices of α_1 and α, the critical value, z_{α_2}, for the combination test of H_{01} at the end of the second stage can be obtained by using the following equation:

$$P(Z_{11} < z_{\alpha_1} \cap Z_{01} < z_{\alpha_2}) \geq 1 - \alpha$$

where $z_{\alpha_i} = \Phi^{-1}(1 - \alpha_i), i = 1, 2.$

Noting that Z_{11} and Z_{01} are bivariate standard normal random variables with correlation $\sqrt{w}$, the above integral equation can easily be solved using function *pmvnorm* in the R package *mvtnorm* [452]. Some example code to do this is given in Section 6.11.2, where, for simplicity, we will assume that $\alpha_1 = \alpha_2$. For $w = 0.5$, $\alpha_1 = \alpha_2 = 0.0304$ and $z_{\alpha_1} = z_{\alpha_2} = 1.8754$; for $w = 0.25$, $\alpha_1 = \alpha_2 = 0.0277$ and $z_{\alpha_1} = z_{\alpha_2} = 1.9163$.

The values of α_1, α_2, z_{α_1}, and z_{α_2} obtained for H_{01} will also be used to test H_{02}.

We note that, when $\alpha_1 = \alpha_2$, the significance levels of the sequential tests are the same as for a standard group-sequential trial with an interim analysis at information fraction w and using a Pocock-type α-spending function.

6.4 Example of Using the Standard Combination Test

Here we will illustrate the use of the standard combination test to test for ABE in a two-stage design.

At the planning stage it is assumed that the CV of log(Cmax), in percentage terms, is 23% and the ratio, on the natural scale, of the true means of Test and Reference is 0.95. Initially, a single-stage design without an interim analysis is considered, and a sample size that gives a power of 0.8 is required. Under these assumptions, and taking $\alpha = 0.05$, the function *sampleN.TOST* in the R library *PowerTOST* [728] gives a sample size of $N = 24$ to achieve a power of 0.8067. This value of N is, in fact, for a fixed design. For a group-sequential design, without a sample size re-estimation, the power would not be 0.8067, but a bit smaller. Section 6.11.1 gives some example R code to calculate the sample size and power of the TOST procedure.

However, there is some doubt as to the true value of the CV: it could be as large as 30%. If this is the case, then a trial with $N = 24$ gives a power of only 0.5577 and so a two-stage design with a sample size re-estimation at the interim is planned. If the assumption of CV = 23% is correct, and it is decided that the interim will be halfway through the trial, it makes sense to make the planned number of subjects in each stage equal to 12. Given this decision, it is reasonable to take $w = 0.5$ as the weight that will be used for the standard combination test. This is an important decision, as it is based on an expectation that $n_1 = n_2$, which may not be correct. In the next section we will see how to mitigate against an incorrect choice for w. The critical value of the standard combination test and corresponding significance level are 1.87542 and 0.03037, respectively. As already noted, some example R code to calculate these values is given in Section 6.11.2.

We proceed assuming $n_1 = 12$, $\alpha = 0.05$, $w = 0.5$, $\alpha_1 = \alpha_2 = 0.0304$, $\beta = 0.2$, and $\delta_p = log(0.95)$.

The first stage of the trial with a total of 12 subjects is completed and the observed within-subject differences for each sequence group are given in Table 6.3. The unblinded estimates from this first stage are $\hat{\delta} = 0.0331$, $\hat{\sigma} = 0.3574$, and $\widehat{CV} = 36.91\%$. The estimated GMR is exp(0.0331) = 1.034. Some example R code to simulate data for the first stage is given in Section 6.11.3 and code to estimate the parameters, test statistics, and p-values for the first stage is given in Section 6.11.4.

The TOST statistics for H_{01} and H_{01} are, respectively

$$T_1 = \frac{(\hat{\delta} - \log(0.8))}{stderr} = 1.7565$$

TABLE 6.3
Simulated Cmax Data for First Stage of a Two-Stage Design

Subject	Group 1 (RT)	Subject	Group 2 (TR)
1	0.1095	7	0.7758
2	-0.6888	8	-0.3118
3	0.0292	9	0.2005
4	-0.0326	10	-0.6748
5	0.6775	11	-0.1591
6	-0.6688	12	-0.0069

and

$$T_2 = \frac{(\log(1.25) - \hat{\delta})}{stderr} = 1.3022,$$

where $stderr = 0.1459$. The respective p-values, on 10 degrees of freedom, are 0.0548 and 0.1110, and these are each compared to $\alpha_1 = 0.0304$. Clearly, ABE has not been achieved at the interim.

We therefore proceed to consider if a second stage is needed. This depends on whether the achieved power for the first stage is less than 0.80, our pre-defined power requirement to declare ABE. Using the estimated CV of 36.91% and assuming a true ratio of means of 0.95, the achieved power of the first stage is, using *PowerTOST*, 0.0183, for $\alpha_1 = 0.0304$. As this is less than 0.80, we will continue. If it had been 0.80 or higher, we would have accepted the decision made at the interim (i.e., ABE not achieved) as final and stopped. Some R code to make the decision as to whether to stop or continue is given in Section 6.11.5.

The new total sample size of the trial (N') is calculated using the estimated CV, the assumed true ratio of 0.95, and a significance level of $\alpha_2 = 0.0304$. Here we will use the standard sample size calculation obtained from *PowerTOST*. This is $N' = 68$, with an achieved power of 0.8081. Thus, the second-stage sample size, $n_2 = N' - n_1$, is $(68 - 12) = 56$. Some example R code to re-estimate the sample size is also given in Section 6.11.5. In Section 6.7 we will describe and illustrate a more advanced sample size calculation based on conditional power and conditional Type I error rates. However, for the purpose of illustrating the analysis of the two-stage design with a sample size re-estimation, the standard sample size calculation is sufficient for now.

The trial is extended and the additional data are given in Table 6.4. Some example R code to simulate data for the second stage is given in Section 6.11.6.

The unblinded estimates from the second stage are $\hat{\delta} = -0.1118$, $\hat{\sigma} = 0.3415$, and $\widehat{CV} = 35.17\%$. The estimated GMR is $\exp(-0.1118) = 0.8942$.

The TOST statistics for H_{01} and H_{02}, on 54 degrees of freedom, are respectively,

$$T_1 = \frac{(\hat{\delta} - \log(0.8))}{stderr} = 1.7248$$

and

$$T_2 = \frac{(\log(1.25) - \hat{\delta}}{stderr} = 5.1907,$$

where $stderr = 0.0645$. The respective p-values are 0.0451 and 1.6255×10^{-6}. Some example R code to estimate the parameters for the second stage and calculate the TOST statistics is given in Section 6.11.7.

TABLE 6.4
Simulated Cmax Data for Second Stage of a Two-Stage Design

Subject	Group 1 (RT)	Subject	Group 2 (TR)
13	-0.1536	41	0.6286
14	0.1128	42	0.0137
15	0.3096	43	-0.1762
16	1.4555	44	1.0213
17	0.1030	45	-0.4475
18	-0.3317	46	0.3559
19	0.0536	47	-0.3835
20	0.3641	48	-0.0042
21	0.4193	49	-0.1826
22	-0.0716	50	-0.4234
23	-0.1361	51	-0.4085
24	-0.3981	52	-0.2508
25	-0.3934	53	-0.4037
26	-0.0876	54	-0.3587
27	0.1541	55	-0.5949
28	0.5964	56	0.6090
29	-0.6216	57	0.4746
30	-0.2219	58	-0.6212
31	-0.2395	59	0.6777
32	0.8597	60	-0.1294
33	0.5992	61	0.0008
34	-0.0238	62	-0.4009
35	0.3881	63	-0.9945
36	0.2083	64	-0.9417
37	-0.1400	65	0.8338
38	0.3870	66	-0.5862
39	0.0437	67	-0.0480
40	0.5645	68	0.2778

To calculate the standard combination test, we need the component z-statistics. From the first stage these are

$$Z_{11} = \Phi^{-1}(1 - 0.0548) = 1.6004, \qquad Z_{12} = \Phi^{-1}(1 - 0.1110) = 1.2211$$

and from the second stage these are:

$$Z_{21} = \Phi^{-1}(1 - 0.0451) = 1.6939, \qquad Z_{22} = \Phi^{-1}\left(1 - 1.6255 \times 10^{-6}\right) = 4.6543.$$

With $w = 0.5$, the standard combination tests for each of the hypotheses, H_{01} and H_{02}, are, respectively,

$$Z_{01} = \sqrt{w}Z_{11} + \sqrt{1-w}Z_{21} = 2.3294,$$

and

$$Z_{02} = \sqrt{w}Z_{12} + \sqrt{1-w}Z_{22} = 4.1546.$$

These z-statistics are compared to 1.8754, the upper $1 - \alpha_2$ percentile of the standard normal distribution.

Clearly both tests are significant and ABE can be declared for Cmax based on the enlarged trial.

Some example R code that applies the standard combination test is given in Section 6.11.8.

A limitation of the standard combination test is that it requires the weight w to be pre-specified. One way to lessen the dependence on the choice of weight is to use the maximum combination test, which we describe and illustrate in the next section.

6.5 Maximum Combination Test

A potential disadvantage of the standard combination test is its dependence on the choice of weight w. Ideally, the ratio $w : (1-w)$ should equal $n_1 : n_2$, the ratio of the sample sizes of the first and second stages. As the final value of n_2 is unknown at the planning stage, it is difficult to ensure the correct choice of w. If the trial goes as planned, and no sample size re-estimation is needed, then we expect $n_1 = n_2 = N/2$. If a sample size re-estimation is needed, then we would expect $n_2 > n_1$. One way out of this dilemma is to pre-specify two sets of weights, where one set would have $w = 0.5$ and the other would have $w < 0.5$, e.g., $w = 0.25$, and apply the TOST procedure with the weight that gives the largest power to reject H_{01} and H_{02}. Choosing values of $w < 0.5$ gives more weight to the data in the second stage. However, if we use two sets of weights, we must modify the significance levels of the test. This modification of the standard combination test was first introduced in [856] and we closely follow the derivation given there.

Suppose the two pre-specified sets of weights are $(w, 1-w)$ and $(w^*, 1-w^*)$, respectively. At the end of the second stage we construct the standard combination test for each set of weights.

For H_{01}, for example, the two test statistics at the end of the second stage will be $Z_{01} = \sqrt{w}Z_{11} + \sqrt{(1-w)}Z_{21}$ and $Z^*_{01} = \sqrt{w^*}Z_{11} + \sqrt{(1-w^*)}Z_{21}$. The test statistic that gives the larger power is, of course, the larger of Z_{01} and Z^*_{01}. We therefore define the maximum combination test statistic as $Z_{\max} = \max(Z_{01}, Z^*_{01})$.

Assuming that the null hypothesis, H_{01}, is true, we must solve the following equation for given values of α_1 and α to obtain the critical value, $z_{\max}$, that controls the Type I error rate:

$$P(\{Z_{11} < z_{\alpha_1}\} \cap \{Z_{01} < z_{\max}\} \cap \{Z^*_{01} < z_{\max}\}) = 1 - \alpha.$$

The equation can be simplified if, as in our example, we use equal critical values for both stages.

In order to solve this equation, we note that Z_{11}, Z_{01}, and Z^*_{01} are trivariate normal with covariance (correlation) matrix

$$\begin{pmatrix} 1 & \sqrt{w} & \sqrt{w^*} \\ \sqrt{w} & 1 & \rho \\ \sqrt{w^*} & \rho & 1 \end{pmatrix}$$

where $\rho = \sqrt{ww^*} + \sqrt{(1-w)(1-w^*)}$.

In a way similar to that used for the standard combination test, this integral equation can be solved with the aid of function *pmvnorm* in the R package *mvtnorm* [452]. Some example R code to calculate the critical values is given in Section 6.11.9. We will denote the solution as $z_{\max}$. For our chosen example values of $w = 0.5$, $w^* = 0.25$, and $\alpha = 0.05$, $z_{\max} = 1.9374$, corresponding to a nominal level of $\alpha_{\max} = 1 - \Phi(z_{\max}) = 0.0264$. We note that $z_{\max}$ is not normally distributed. Of course, the same reasoning will apply to the maximum combination test for H_{02} and the same value of $z_{\max}$ will be obtained. In the next section we will illustrate the use of the maximum combination test using our example first-stage dataset.

6.6 Using the Maximum Combination Test

In this section we will assume that the trial was planned with the aim of using the maximum combination test. The data obtained at the end of the first stage will still be those given in Table 6.3. As we are to use the maximum combination test at the end of the second stage, we must modify both how we test the null hypotheses at the end of the first stage and how we re-estimate the sample size for second stage. This is because the significance level for the TOST procedure at the end of the first and second stages will change from 0.0304 to the nominal level of 0.0264.

The TOST p-values from the first stage, it will be recalled, were 0.0548 and 0.1110. Compared to the significance level of 0.0264, neither of these is significant. As the power of the first stage, using the revised significance level, is only 0.0140, we continue to re-sample size the second stage. Using the revised significance level, the increased total sample size is $N' = 70$. That is, $n_2 = 58$, a slight increase compared to the sample size using the standard combination test. Some example R code that re-estimates the sample size based on the maximum combination test is given in Section 6.11.10. Some example R code to calculate the power of the first stage, using the significance level of the maximum combination test, is given in Section 6.11.11.

To provide an example dataset for the second stage when using the maximum combination test, we keep the data from Table 6.4 and add data for two additional subjects, to give a second-stage dataset for 58 subjects. The augmented dataset is given in Table 6.5. Some example R code that provides data for the second stage is given in Section 6.11.12.

The unblinded estimates from the second stage are $\hat{\delta} = -0.1196$, $\hat{\sigma} = 0.3428$, and $\widehat{CV} = 35.31\%$. The estimated GMR is $\exp(-0.1196) = 0.8873$. Some example R code to estimate the parameters and TOST statistics is given in Section 6.11.13.

The TOST statistics for H_{01} and H_{02}, on 58 degrees of freedom, arem respectively,

$$T_1 = \frac{(\hat{\delta} - \log(0.8))}{stderr} = 1.6270$$

and

$$T_2 = \frac{(\log(1.25) - \hat{\delta}}{stderr} = 5.3849,$$

where $stderr = 0.0636$. The respective p-values are 0.0547 and 7.4294×10^{-7}.

To calculate the standard combination test, we need the component z-statistics. From the first stage these are

$$Z_{11} = 1.6004, \quad Z_{12} = 1.2211$$

and from the second stage these are

$$Z_{21} = 1.6011, \quad Z_{22} = 4.8131.$$

TABLE 6.5
Simulated Cmax Data for Second Stage of a Two-Stage Design when Using Maximum Combination Test

Subject	Group 1 (RT)	Subject	Group 2 (TR)
13	-0.1536	41	0.6286
14	0.1128	42	0.0137
15	0.3096	43	-0.1762
16	1.4555	44	1.0213
17	0.1030	45	-0.4475
18	-0.3317	46	0.3559
19	0.0536	47	-0.3835
20	0.3641	48	-0.0042
21	0.4193	49	-0.1826
22	-0.0716	50	-0.4234
23	-0.1361	51	-0.4085
24	-0.3981	52	-0.2508
25	-0.3934	53	-0.4037
26	-0.0876	54	-0.3587
27	0.1541	55	-0.5949
28	0.5964	56	0.6090
29	-0.6216	57	0.4746
30	-0.2219	58	-0.6212
31	-0.2395	59	0.6777
32	0.8597	60	-0.1294
33	0.5992	61	0.0008
34	-0.0238	62	-0.4009
35	0.3881	63	-0.9945
36	0.2083	64	-0.9417
37	-0.1400	65	0.8338
38	0.3870	66	-0.5862
39	0.0437	67	-0.0480
40	0.5645	68	0.2778
69	0.8517	70	0.1783

With $w = 0.5$, the standard combination tests for each of the hypotheses, H_{01} and H_{02}, are, respectively,

$$Z_{01} = 2.2638, \quad Z_{02} = 4.2669,$$

and for $w^* = 0.20$, respectively,

$$Z^*_{01} = 2.1868, \quad Z^*_{02} = 4.7789.$$

For H_{01}, $Z^1_{\text{max}} = \max(Z_{01}, Z^*_{01}) = 2.2638$ and for H_{02}, $Z^2_{\text{max}} = \max(Z_{02}, Z^*_{02}) = 4.7789$. These z-statistics are compared to z_{max}=1.9374, as noted above.

Clearly both tests are significant and ABE can be declared for Cmax.

Some example R code that applies the maximum combination test is given in Section 6.11.14.

6.7 Conditional Errors and Conditional Power

Previously, in the sample size re-estimation step we used the standard power calculation for the TOST procedure as implemented in *PowerTOST*. Also, the significance thresholds for the second stage depended on whether the standard or maximum combination test was used (i.e., on either z_{α_2} or $z_{\max}$). In doing this we ignored any information available from the first stage that could be used to modify the significance level for the second stage and any information on the remaining power that has to be achieved in the second stage.

Let us first consider the significance level to be used at the end of the second stage for the null hypothesis H_{01} using the standard combination test with weight w.

The standard combination test can be written as a test on the second-stage data given the p-values obtained in the first stage. For H_{01}, the conditional error rate of this test is $\alpha_1^c = P(Z_{21} > z_{\alpha_2} \mid p_{11} \text{ and } H_{01} \text{ true})$.

To obtain α_1^c, we first note that the Type I error rate of the standard combination test for H_{01} is

$$Pr(\sqrt{w}Z_{11} + \sqrt{1-w}Z_{21} > z_{\alpha_2} | H_{01} \text{ true}).$$

As shown in [856], this expression can be rearranged to give

$$\alpha_1^c = 1 - \Phi\left(\frac{1}{\sqrt{1-w}}(z_{\alpha_2} - \sqrt{w}Z_{11})\right).$$

Similarly, for H_{02}, it can be shown that

$$\alpha_2^c = 1 - \Phi\left(\frac{1}{\sqrt{1-w}}(z_{\alpha_2} - \sqrt{w}Z_{12})\right).$$

Hence, for a given value of n_2, ABE can be declared at the end of the second stage if the TOST statistics for the second-stage only are such that $T_{21} > t_{n_2-2,\alpha_1^c}$ and $T_{22} > t_{n_2-2,\alpha_2^c}$.

Some example R code to calculate these conditional errors is given in Section 6.11.15.

Using this property, and for a given value of n_2, the power of the second stage (and hence the power of the standard combination test) can be calculated using the non-central bivariate t-distribution, by integrating over the rejection region of the two one-sided tests. Some example R code that calculates the power for a given value of n_2 using the function *pmvt* in library *mvtnorm* is given in Section 6.11.16.

To illustrate the calculation of the adjusted significance levels for the standard combination test, we recall that $Z_{11} = 1.6004$ and $z_{\alpha_2} = 1.8754$. Hence for $w = 0.5$, $\alpha_1^c = 1 - \Phi(1.0519) = 0.1464$. Similarly, using $Z_{12} = 1.2211$, $\alpha_2^c = 0.0762$.

For $n_2 = 38$, for example, the R code in Section 6.11.16 gives a conditional power of 0.8170 for the second stage to reject H_{01}, assuming $\alpha_1^c = 0.1464$ and $\alpha_2^c = 0.0762$. For $n_2 = 36$, the conditional power is 0.7965.

However, when calculating n_2 to achieve a certain level of power for the final tests of H_{01} and H_{02}, we should also take account of the estimated power achieved in the first stage, as this may reduce the number of subjects needed for the second stage. Using the estimated CV from the first-stage data, and given the values of n_1, α_1, and the assumed true value of the ratio of means, the estimated power of the first stage can be calculated using *PowerTOST*, as previously illustrated in Section 6.4. Let us denote this estimated power by $(1 - \hat{\beta}_1)$.

Further, let us denote the conditional power of the second stage by $1 - \beta^c$. To derive an expression for this, we follow the derivation in [856] and define R_i as the event that ABE is declared at the end of stage $i, i = 1, 2$. Also, we define R as the event that ABE is declared at the end of the trial where $R = R_1 \cup R_2$. Denoting the complement of R_i as $\bar{R}_i$, the power to declare ABE at the end of the trial is $Pr(R) = 1 - \beta = 1 - Pr(\bar{R}_1 \cap \bar{R}_2)$. In addition, the conditional power of the second stage can be expressed as $1 - \beta^c = Pr(R_2|\bar{R}_1)$.

Further, expressing $P(R)$ in an alternative way, we have

$$Pr(R) = Pr(R_1) + Pr(\bar{R}_1 \cap R_2) = Pr(R_1) + Pr(R_2|\bar{R}_1)Pr(\bar{R}_1).$$

Hence

$$1 - \beta = (1 - \hat{\beta}_1) + (1 - \beta^c)\hat{\beta}_1$$

and

$$1 - \beta^c = \frac{\hat{\beta}_1 - \beta}{\hat{\beta}_1}.$$

Some example R code to calculate the conditional power is given in Section 6.11.17.

Returning to our example dataset from the first stage, the estimated CV was 36.9112%. For $n_1 = 12$, $\delta_p = 0.95$, and $\alpha_2 = 0.0304$, the estimated power of the first stage is $(1 - \hat{\beta}_1) = 0.0183$, giving a conditional power of $1 - \beta^c = 0.7963$ for the second stage. Given the conditional error rates of $\alpha_1^c = 0.1464$ and $\alpha_2^c = 0.0762$ and using the R code in Section 6.11.16, the value of n_2 needed to achieve a power of 0.7963 is, as noted above, $n_2 = 36$, with a power of 0.7965.

With some modifications, the above logic can be applied to the maximum combination test, to give corresponding expressions for the conditional errors and conditional power. As shown in [856], for H_{01}, the conditional error, $\alpha_{\max_1}$, is

$$\alpha_{\max_1} = 1 - \Phi\{\min[(z_{\max} - \sqrt{w}Z_{11})/\sqrt{1-w}, (z_{\max} - \sqrt{w^*}Z_{11})/\sqrt{1-w^*}]\}.$$

For H_{02}, the conditional error is

$$\alpha_{\max_2} = 1 - \Phi\{\min[(z_{\max} - \sqrt{w}Z_{12})/\sqrt{1-w}, (z_{\max} - \sqrt{w^*}Z_{12})/\sqrt{1-w^*}]\}.$$

As for the standard combination test, the conditional power of the maximum combination test can be calculated using the conditional errors $\alpha_{\max_1}$ and $\alpha_{\max_2}$. Some example R code to calculate the conditional errors and conditional power of the maximum combination test is given in Section 6.11.18. The conditional errors are $\alpha_{\max_1} = 0.1272$ and $\alpha_{\max_2} = 0.0644$. The power of the first stage based on $\widehat{CV} = 36.91\%$ and $\alpha_{\max} = 0.0264$ is 0.0140, giving a conditional power of 0.7972 for the second stage.

6.8 Algorithm for Sample Size Re-Estimation

Here we will put all the ideas presented in the previous sections into a single algorithm that gives the steps in our recommended approach to the design and analysis of a two-stage design that includes an interim sample size re-estimation step. In the next section we will compare the properties of this algorithm with Method B of [1000] using a simulation study.

We assume that, if a second stage is required, the maximum combination test will be used in the final data analysis.

At the planning stage, the sample size, N, for a single-stage 2×2 cross-over trial for ABE is calculated using chosen values of $1 - \beta$, CV, δ_p, and α for the metric (AUC or Cmax) of interest. This calculation will use a significance level of $\alpha = 0.05$ and can be done using *PowerTOST*. The number of subjects in the first stage is then $n_1 = N/2$, divided equally between two sequence groups (RT and TR).

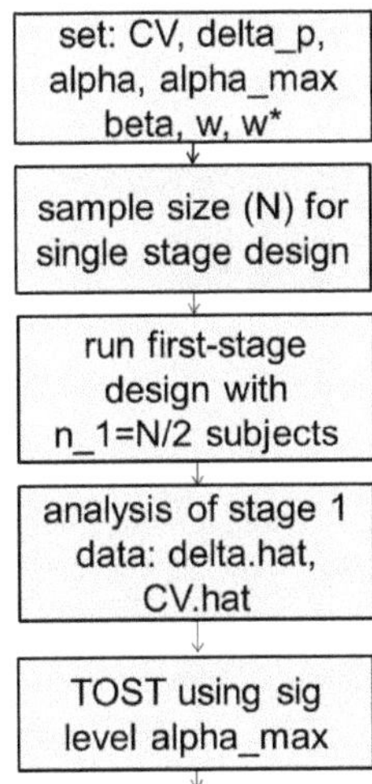

FIGURE 6.1
Planning and Analysis of First Stage

The first steps in our algorithm are given in Figure 6.1. First, the parameters (CV, α, β, δ_p, w, w^*, and α_{max}) needed for the sample size calculations and significance testing are specified. Then the sample size is calculated and the first stage design is run. The TOST procedure using α_{max} is then applied to the data obtained. Initially we set $\delta_p = \log(0.95)$.

The next steps are shown in Figure 6.2 where decisions are made depending on the result of the TOST procedure and the power achieved at the end of the first stage. As explained in [856], it is important in the sample size re-estimation calculation that the sign attached to δ_p in the calculation is the same as the sign of $\hat{\delta}$. We refer to this alignment of signs as the *adaptive planning step*. Assuming that the decision is made to add a second stage, the conditional errors and conditional power as defined in Section 6.7 are calculated in preparation for the sample size re-estimation.

These calculations, the sample size re-calculation step, and the running of the second stage are shown in Figure 6.3. The size of the second stage is n_2. We ensure $n_2 \geq 4$ in order the there are least 2 degrees of freedom to estimate the variance.

The final steps are shown in Figure 6.4 where the TOST procedure is applied using the maximum combination test and the final decision regarding ABE is made.

For our example, we give in Table 6.6 the results of each step of the analysis when the maximum combination test is used and the sample size re-estimation is based on the conditional errors and conditional power. The sample size re-estimation step used conditional errors of $\alpha_{\max_1} = 0.1272$ and $\alpha_{max_2} = 0.0644$, and the size of the second stage was chosen to achieve a conditional power of 0.7972. Section 6.11.19 has example R code to re-estimate the sample size of the second stage. In this situation $n_2 = 50$. The data for the second stage were then taken from the first 25 subjects in each group as given in Table 6.4. As with the previous analyses, the final conclusion is that ABE is achieved for the Cmax endpoint.

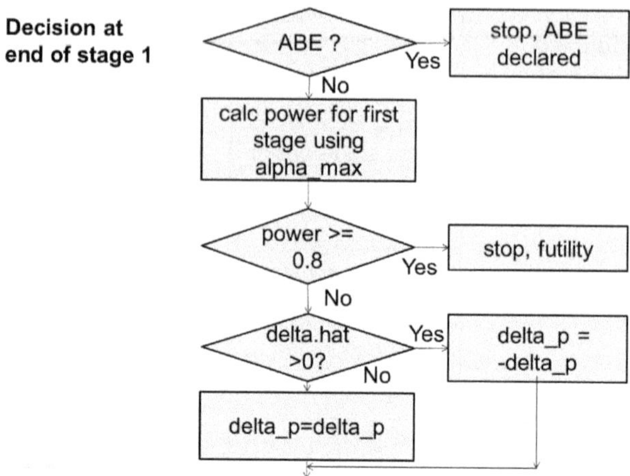

FIGURE 6.2
Decisions Made at the End of the First Stage

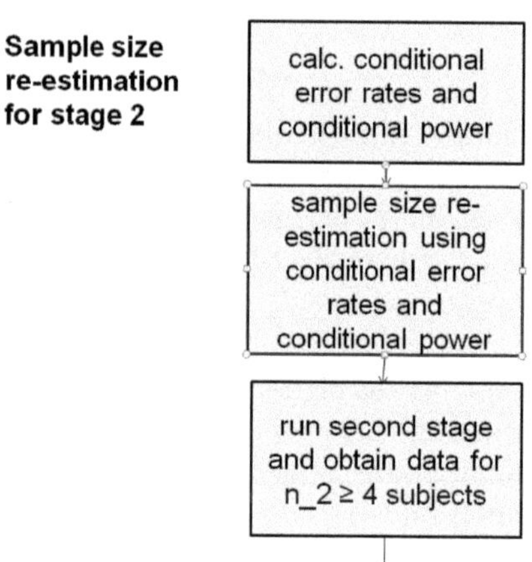

FIGURE 6.3
Sample Size Re-Estimation

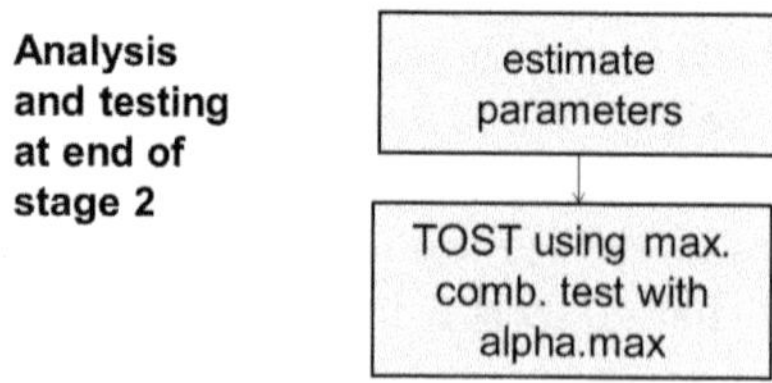

FIGURE 6.4
Analysis at End of Trial

TABLE 6.6
Summary of Steps in Analysis of a Two-Stage Design, Using the Maximum Combination Test

Set initial parameters	$CV = 23\%$, $\alpha = 0.05$, $\delta_p = log(0.95)$, $1-\beta = 0.8$, $w = 0.5$, $w^* = 0.25$, $\alpha_{max} = 0.0264$
Calculate sample size for first stage	$\alpha = 0.05$, $N = 24$, $n_1 = N/2 = 12$
Interim analysis of first-stage data	$\hat{\delta} = 0.0331$, $\hat{CV} = 36.91\%$, $T_1 = 1.7565$, $T_2 = 1.3022$, $df = 10$, $\alpha_{max} = 0.0264$, $p_{11} = 0.0548$, $p_{12} = 0.1110$, $Z_{11} = 1.6004$, $Z_{12} = 1.2211$
Decision after first stage	ABE not declared, achieved power $= 0.0140$, decision $=$ continue to second stage
Achieved power, conditional power, conditional error rates	$1-\hat{\beta}_1 = 0.0140$ $1-\beta^c = 0.7972$ $\alpha_{\max_1} = 0.1272$, $\alpha_{max_2} = 0.0644$
Sample size re-estimation with adaptive planning	$\hat{\delta} > 0$, hence $\delta_p = -log(0.95)$, $n_2 = 50$
Analysis of second-stage data (using first 25 subjects in each group of simulated data in Table 6.4)	$\hat{\delta} = -0.0982$, $\hat{CV} = 36.39\%$, $T_1 = 1.7710$, $T_2 = 4.5560$, $df = 48$, $\alpha_{max} = 0.0264$, $p_{21} = 0.0414$, $p_{22} = 1.7947 \times 10^{-5}$, $Z_{21} = 1.7341$, $Z_{22} = 4.1324$
Maximum combination test	$Z_{01} = 2.3578$, $Z_{02} = 3.7856$, $Z^*_{01} = 2.3019$, $Z^*_{02} = 4.1894$, $Z^1_{\max} = 2.3578$, $Z^2_{\max} = 4.1894$, $z_{\max} = 1.9374$
Decision at end of trial	$Z^1_{\max} \geq z_{\max}$ and $Z^2_{\max} \geq z_{\max}$ ABE achieved

6.9 Operating Characteristics

The previous section described an algorithm based on the maximum combination test, adaptive planning, conditional error rates, and conditional power. The steps in this algorithm are repeated in the flow diagram given in Figure 6.5. We note from this figure that the algorithm allows a stop of the trial after the interim analysis for either success (ABE declared) or futility (failure to declare ABE at the end of the first stage but the estimated power of the first stage is at least 0.80). If we continue, then the total sample size is re-estimated using the estimated CV from the first stage. We know this will not inflate the Type I error rate above its nominal level of 5%, but it is of interest to learn about the sample sizes produced by the algorithm and the level of power achieved at the end of the trial. We will do this using a simulation exercise.

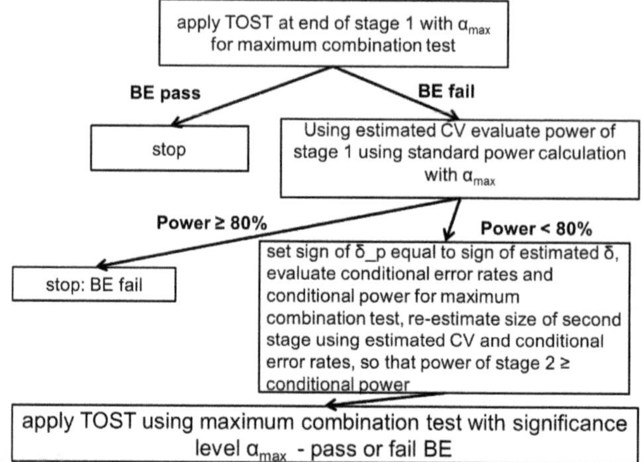

FIGURE 6.5
Flow Diagram for the Method of Maurer et al. [856]

Before we do that, however, we briefly describe a different sample size re-estimation algorithm that has been published in the literature (Method B of [1000]). The flow diagram for this algorithm is given in Figure 6.6.

We note some similarities between the flow diagrams, e.g., the stop for futility, but also some important differences. The major difference is that the algorithm described in Figure 6.6 cannot guarantee to control the Type I error rate at or below its nominal level of 5%. This is because the analysis of the second stage involves pooling the data from both stages and applying the TOST procedure to this combined dataset. Also, the sample size re-estimation step uses the standard sample size calculation (e.g., as given by *PowerTOST*) to re-sample size the whole trial (and not directly the second stage). In addition, adaptive

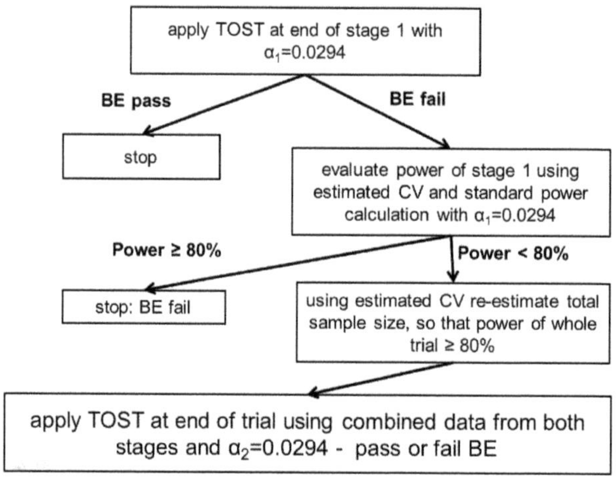

FIGURE 6.6
Flow Diagram for Method B of Potvin et al. [1000]

planning, conditional error rates, and conditional power are not used in the calculations. Of course, the conservatism of the TOST procedure may limit the amount of inflation of the Type I error rate, but this inflation cannot be entirely removed. From a regulatory perspective, this is clearly undesirable, as the false positive rate cannot be controlled (with certainty) at its nominal level and the actual amount of inflation is unknown in general. We note that four algorithms were described by [1000], with Methods B and C having similar properties and Method C being recommended. However, in [888] Method D was recommended when the true ratio of means is 0.90 and not 0.95. Method D is a variation on Method C where the significance level of the TOST procedure at the end of the trial is reduced slightly. Both papers reported the results of a simulation exercise to estimate the Type I error rate and power of each method. The results reported in [888] demonstrate that the Type I error rate can be inflated (between 0.0522 and 0.0547) for Methods B and C. The new algorithm described in this chapter ensures that the Type I error rate is not inflated whatever the value of the ratio.

Given its similarity, we will compare the operating characteristics of the algorithm proposed in this chapter with Method B of [1000]. By operating characteristics we mean simulation-generated metrics such as the achieved Type I error rate, the achieved power to declare ABE at the end of the trial, and the average total sample size. We will also use the same configuration of simulation scenarios considered by [1000], which consists of all combinations of $n_1 = (12, 24, 36, 48, 60)$ and $CV = (10, 20, \ldots, 90, 100)$. Note that here the values of n_1 and CV do not depend on each other: we have just chosen a grid of values to use in the simulation exercise. When calculating the sample size, we always assume $\delta_p = 0.95$ for the planned value of the true ratio. Each of the combinations of n_1 and CV was also run with simulated data that were generated under the assumption that the true ratio of means was either 0.95 or 1.25. The latter ratio was used to assess the Type I error rate. We could, of course, have used 0.80 for this latter ratio and obtained equivalent results to when the ratio is 1.25. For our algorithm we will use $w = 0.50$ and $w^* = 0.25$ for the maximum combination test.

In each simulation, the value of the ratio of means (0.95 or 1.25) was chosen and the values of n_1 and CV were fixed to one of the 50 combinations described above. Then a million trial datasets for this set of values were simulated and the new algorithm and Method B of [1000] applied. The results were then summarized by counting the number of times ABE was declared at the end of either the first or second stages. When expressed as a proportion out of the total number of simulated trials, this gives an estimate of power (if the ratio = 0.95) or Type I error rate (if the ratio = 1.25). In addition, the final sample size of each trial was recorded, and the average sample size over the total number of simulations was calculated. To maintain comparability with the results of [1000], we put a very large upper limit ($N = 4000$) on the allowed total sample size. In practice, of course, an upper limit on the total sample size will be imposed by practical constraints. We will consider such a situation later in this section.

Table 6.7 shows the simulation-based estimates of the power to declare ABE when using Method B of [1000]. These values are also plotted in Figure 6.7, where each solid point shows the power achieved at a particular pair of values of n_1 and CV. To aid the visual interpretation of the plot, we have joined these discrete points by lines. So, for example, the solid line is for $n_1 = 12$ and the points on it are the powers achieved for CV = 10, 20, ..., 100. We can see that for $n_1 = 12$ the power is below 0.80 for all CV values larger than 20. A similar pattern is observed for $n_1 = 24$ (the line with short dashes), except that the power drops below 0.8 after CV = 40. Generally speaking, Method B of [1000] fails to ensure that the achieved power of the trial is greater or equal to the desired value of 0.8 over the whole range of values of n_1 and CV.

TABLE 6.7
Simulation-Based Estimates of Power for Method B When True Ratio = 0.95

CV%	$n_1 = 12$	$n_1 = 24$	$n_1 = 36$	$n_1 = 48$	$n_1 = 60$
10	0.98	1.00	1.00	1.00	1.00
20	0.84	0.88	0.95	0.99	1.00
30	0.78	0.83	0.84	0.86	0.90
40	0.75	0.80	0.82	0.83	0.83
50	0.73	0.78	0.80	0.82	0.82
60	0.73	0.77	0.79	0.80	0.81
70	0.72	0.77	0.78	0.79	0.80
80	0.72	0.77	0.78	0.79	0.79
90	0.72	0.77	0.78	0.79	0.79
100	0.72	0.77	0.78	0.79	0.79

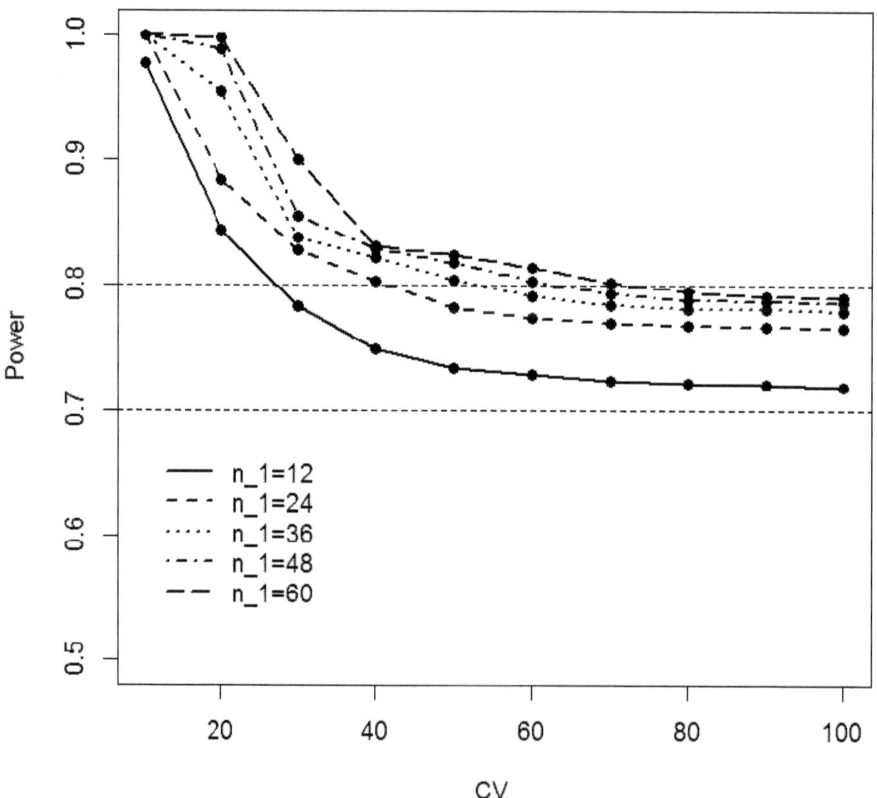

FIGURE 6.7
Simulation-Based Power Estimates for Method B when True Ratio = 0.95

TABLE 6.8
Simulation-Based Estimates of Power for Algorithm that Uses the Maximum Combination Test ($w = 0.5, w^* = 0.25$) When True Ratio = 0.95

CV%	$n_1 = 12$	$n_1 = 24$	$n_1 = 36$	$n_1 = 48$	$n_1 = 60$
10	0.98	1.00	1.00	1.00	1.00
20	0.85	0.88	0.95	0.99	1.00
30	0.81	0.83	0.83	0.85	0.89
40	0.80	0.83	0.83	0.83	0.82
50	0.80	0.83	0.83	0.83	0.83
60	0.80	0.83	0.83	0.83	0.84
70	0.79	0.83	0.84	0.84	0.84
80	0.79	0.83	0.84	0.84	0.84
90	0.79	0.83	0.84	0.84	0.84
100	0.79	0.83	0.84	0.84	0.84

Table 6.8 shows the simulation-based estimates of the power to declare ABE when using the algorithm based on adaptive planning, conditional error rates, conditional power, and the maximum combination test. These values are also plotted in Figure 6.8. We see that, apart from some values for $n_1 = 12$, the powers are all above 0.8, as required. The remaining values for $n_1 = 12$ are only slightly below 0.8.

Of some importance is the average sample size needed to achieve or exceed the target power. The average sample sizes for each of the two methods are given in Tables 6.9 and 6.10, respectively. The differences (rounded) in the sample sizes are displayed in Table 6.11. Clearly there is a price to pay if the desired target power is to be achieved, but this is moderate for low values of CV and high n_1. A poor choice of n_1, when the true CV is high, requires a large final sample size to compensate. However, this is a logical consequence of correctly requiring that the target power is maintained.

The final sample size is also of importance when the null hypothesis is true, i.e., when the true ratio is 0.8 or 1.25. Large sample sizes under this scenario are clearly undesirable. Tables similar to those above, but obtained under the null hypothesis, reveal similar sample sizes for Method B of [1000] and slightly larger sample sizes for the alternative algorithm presented here (see Table 6.12). Clearly, it is desirable to stop trials going into a second stage if the evidence for ABE is weak (i.e., when it is more likely that the null hypothesis is true). Some form of futility rule is therefore desirable, and we consider some possibilities next.

Although both Method B and the current method allow stopping after the first stage if ABE is not declared and the estimated power from the first stage is 0.8 or greater, we can increase the chance of stopping if we introduce an additional futility rule. An example of such a rule is given by [1363] in their update of the methods first introduced in [1000]. This futility rule is based on an optimization algorithm and depends on the size of the assumed CV and which of their Methods E and F is used. To see the effect of using such a rule, we have chosen a stand-alone futility rule that is independent of the method used and the size of the CV. The rule is to stop the trial after the interim analysis if the 90% confidence interval for the true ratio of Test to Reference is totally outside the limits of $(0.95, 1.05)$.

Table 6.13 gives the simulation-based stopping rates under the assumptions of the null hypothesis (true ratio = 0.8, as in [1363]) when the maximum combination test algorithm is used with $w = 0.5$ and $w^* = 0.25$. These results are for an extreme situation and are a good test of the futility rule. We can see that the chance of stopping is clearly related to the precision of estimation of the confidence interval, with large n_1 or small CV increasing the

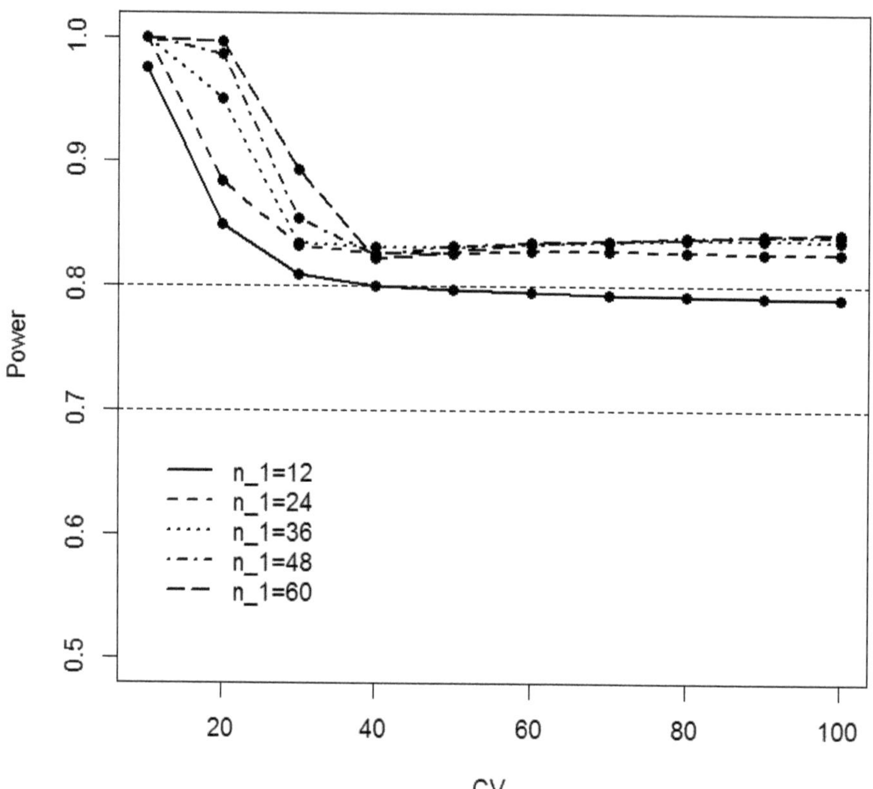

FIGURE 6.8
Simulation-Based Power Estimates for Maximum Combination Test ($w = 0.5, w^* = 0.25$) when True Ratio = 0.95

chance of stopping. The corresponding average final sample sizes are given in Table 6.14. The values in this table when compared with those in Table 6.12 show that the futility rule is effective in stopping the trial and saving sample size, especially when n_1 is large. The achieved Type I error rates are also of some interest and these are plotted in Figure 6.9. We can see that the use of the futility bound has introduced some conservatism into the error rates. This is not unexpected given that the impact of the futility bound should be to reduce the number of trials going into the second stage that would erroneously pass ABE at the end of the trial.

Of equal interest is how the futility rule performs when ABE is very likely to be declared, e.g., when the true ratio = 0.95. The stopping rates in this situation are given in Table 6.15 and can be seen to be about 0.05 or less. The average sample sizes in this situation are given in Table 6.16 and can be seen to be comparable to or smaller than those given in Table 6.10, which are for the situation when the futility rule is not used. In addition, the power is not too adversely affected by applying the futility rule, as can be seen in Figure 6.10. In fact, the use of the futility rule has ensured that the achieved powers for $n_1 > 12$ are closer to 0.8.

TABLE 6.9
Average Total Sample Sizes for Method B When True Ratio = 0.95

CV%	$n_1 = 12$	$n_1 = 24$	$n_1 = 36$	$n_1 = 48$	$n_1 = 60$
10	12.02	24.00	36.00	48.00	60.00
20	20.64	24.62	36.00	48.00	60.00
30	46.35	39.87	40.73	48.90	60.06
40	78.92	76.05	67.19	63.98	67.40
50	117.32	116.93	112.56	102.29	95.37
60	160.83	160.54	159.85	154.95	144.01
70	207.51	207.49	207.45	206.50	201.56
80	256.83	256.73	256.71	256.74	255.62
90	307.42	307.52	307.38	307.38	307.29
100	358.76	358.88	358.69	358.76	358.74

TABLE 6.10
Average Total Sample Sizes for Maximum Combination Test ($w = 0.5, w^* = 0.25$) When True Ratio = 0.95

CV%	$n_1 = 12$	$n_1 = 24$	$n_1 = 36$	$n_1 = 48$	$n_1 = 60$
10	12.05	24.00	36.00	48.00	60.00
20	21.13	24.78	36.01	48.00	60.00
30	50.60	40.76	40.89	49.04	60.10
40	92.42	81.14	69.29	64.42	67.33
50	143.94	131.72	120.24	106.64	97.27
60	204.06	188.63	177.83	166.34	151.67
70	270.07	251.36	239.27	228.91	217.46
80	340.88	318.40	304.14	293.24	282.97
90	414.34	388.95	371.62	359.27	349.13
100	489.79	461.15	441.47	427.36	415.83

TABLE 6.11
Difference in Average Total Sample Sizes for the Two Methods When True Ratio = 0.95

CV%	$n_1 = 12$	$n_1 = 24$	$n_1 = 36$	$n_1 = 48$	$n_1 = 60$
10	0.02	0.00	0.00	0.00	0.00
20	0.50	0.16	0.01	0.00	0.00
30	4.25	0.89	0.16	0.14	0.04
40	13.50	5.09	2.09	0.44	-0.07
50	26.62	14.80	7.68	4.36	1.90
60	43.22	28.08	17.98	11.39	7.65
70	62.56	43.86	31.82	22.41	15.89
80	84.05	61.67	47.44	36.50	27.35
90	106.92	81.43	64.24	51.90	41.84
100	131.03	102.27	82.78	68.61	57.09

TABLE 6.12
Average Total Sample Sizes for Maximum Combination Test ($w = 0.5, w^* = 0.25$) When True Ratio = 0.80

CV%	$n_1 = 12$	$n_1 = 24$	$n_1 = 36$	$n_1 = 48$	$n_1 = 60$
10	12.38	24.00	36.00	48.00	60.00
20	34.98	30.06	36.12	48.00	60.00
30	70.31	70.89	64.75	58.49	61.34
40	114.48	120.49	119.96	114.94	107.91
50	167.39	175.04	180.27	179.86	175.60
60	228.47	234.61	242.46	247.67	247.71
70	295.22	299.64	307.08	314.81	320.35
80	366.20	368.16	374.63	382.81	391.11
90	440.73	439.80	444.76	452.08	460.56
100	515.83	512.96	516.22	522.45	530.63

TABLE 6.13
Stopping Rates When the Maximum Combination Test Is Used and the Futility Rule is Applied after the First Stage When True Ratio = 0.80

CV%	$n_1 = 12$	$n_1 = 24$	$n_1 = 36$	$n_1 = 48$	$n_1 = 60$
10	0.97	1.00	1.00	1.00	1.00
20	0.52	0.84	0.96	0.99	1.00
30	0.29	0.53	0.71	0.83	0.90
40	0.19	0.35	0.49	0.61	0.70
50	0.14	0.25	0.36	0.45	0.53
60	0.12	0.20	0.28	0.35	0.42
70	0.11	0.17	0.23	0.29	0.34
80	0.09	0.14	0.19	0.24	0.29
90	0.09	0.13	0.17	0.21	0.25
100	0.08	0.12	0.15	0.19	0.22

TABLE 6.14
Average Total Sample Sizes for Maximum Combination Test ($w = 0.5, w^* = 0.25$) When True Ratio = 0.80 and Futility Rule Applied

CV%	$n_1 = 12$	$n_1 = 24$	$n_1 = 36$	$n_1 = 48$	$n_1 = 60$
10	12.04	24.00	36.00	48.00	60.00
20	22.36	24.89	36.01	48.00	60.00
30	51.34	41.56	41.63	49.14	60.10
40	91.87	78.06	68.83	65.62	68.13
50	141.39	124.53	112.96	103.47	97.54
60	198.71	178.23	165.08	154.14	144.10
70	261.05	236.95	221.84	210.16	199.64
80	328.59	299.97	282.59	269.16	258.12
90	397.92	365.88	345.92	330.66	318.53
100	468.74	433.37	410.74	393.88	380.07

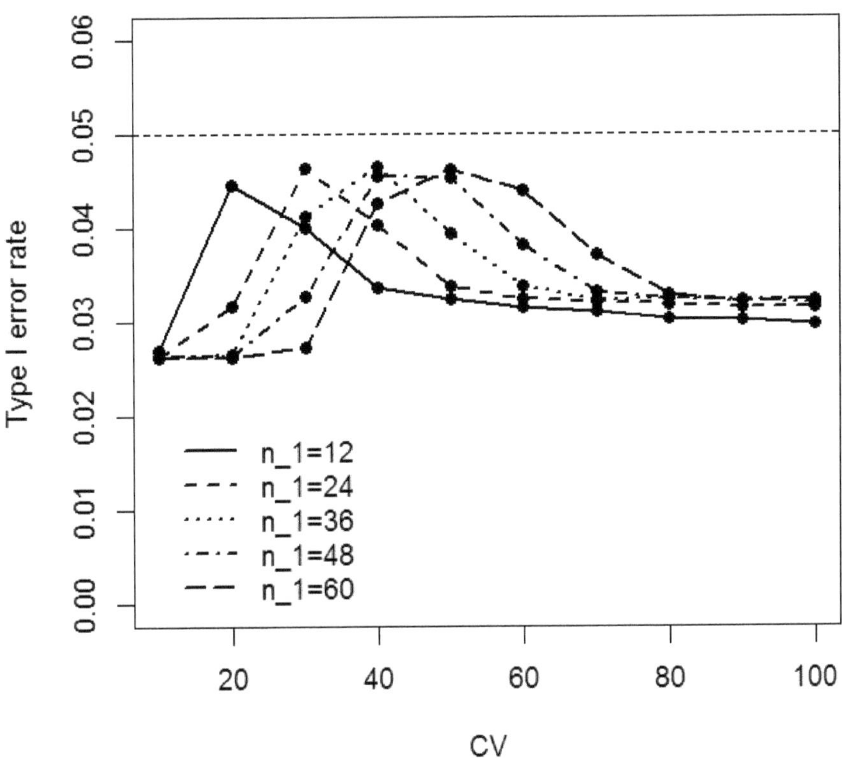

FIGURE 6.9
Simulation-Based Type I Error Rate Estimates for Maximum Combination Test ($w = 0.5, w^* = 0.25$) when True Ratio = 0.80 and Futility Rule Applied

We said earlier that in practice there will be a limit on the total sample size. This will be due to budget and time constraints. As an example, we consider applying an upper limit equal to four times the size of the first stage in addition to the futility bound already discussed. Table 6.17 gives the achieved average total sample sizes when both limits are enforced. The rightmost column gives the sample size (N_s) needed for a single-stage design to achieve a power of 0.80 for the corresponding value of the CV. Table 6.18 gives the simulation-based powers corresponding to the average samples sizes in Table 6.17. Obviously, when the sample size is allowed to equal or exceed the planned sample size, a power of 0.80 or higher is achieved. If the re-estimated total sample size is greater than $4n_1$, it is clearly sensible to stop the trial after the first stage.

TABLE 6.15
Stopping Rates When the Maximum Combination Test Is Used and the Futility Rule Is Applied after the First Stage When True Ratio = 0.95

CV%	$n_1 = 12$	$n_1 = 24$	$n_1 = 36$	$n_1 = 48$	$n_1 = 60$
10	0.03	0.03	0.03	0.03	0.03
20	0.03	0.03	0.03	0.03	0.03
30	0.03	0.03	0.03	0.03	0.03
40	0.04	0.03	0.03	0.03	0.03
50	0.04	0.04	0.03	0.03	0.03
60	0.04	0.04	0.03	0.03	0.03
70	0.04	0.04	0.04	0.03	0.03
80	0.04	0.04	0.04	0.04	0.03
90	0.05	0.04	0.04	0.04	0.04
100	0.05	0.04	0.04	0.04	0.04

Finally, we revisit the choice of weights for the maximum combination test. All our previous results were for the case where $w = 0.50$ and $w^* = 0.25$. Tables 6.19 and 6.20 give, respectively, the simulation-based power and average sample size for the algorithm that uses the maximum combination test in conjunction with conditional error rates and conditional power, for weights $w = 0.40$ and $w^* = 0.20$. Here we have not enforced any limit on the sample size or used a futility boundary.

TABLE 6.16
Average Total Sample Sizes for Maximum Combination Test ($w = 0.5, w^* = 0.25$) When True Ratio = 0.95 and Futility Rule Applied

CV%	$n_1 = 12$	$n_1 = 24$	$n_1 = 36$	$n_1 = 48$	$n_1 = 60$
10	12.05	24.00	36.00	48.00	60.00
20	20.74	24.73	36.01	48.00	60.00
30	49.01	39.56	40.37	48.90	60.09
40	88.96	77.90	66.78	62.73	66.30
50	138.11	125.87	115.03	102.33	93.77
60	195.16	179.55	169.56	158.64	144.98
70	257.81	238.66	227.46	217.90	207.27
80	325.05	301.62	288.26	278.28	269.23
90	395.14	367.49	351.77	340.27	331.07
100	466.38	435.53	417.05	403.71	393.43

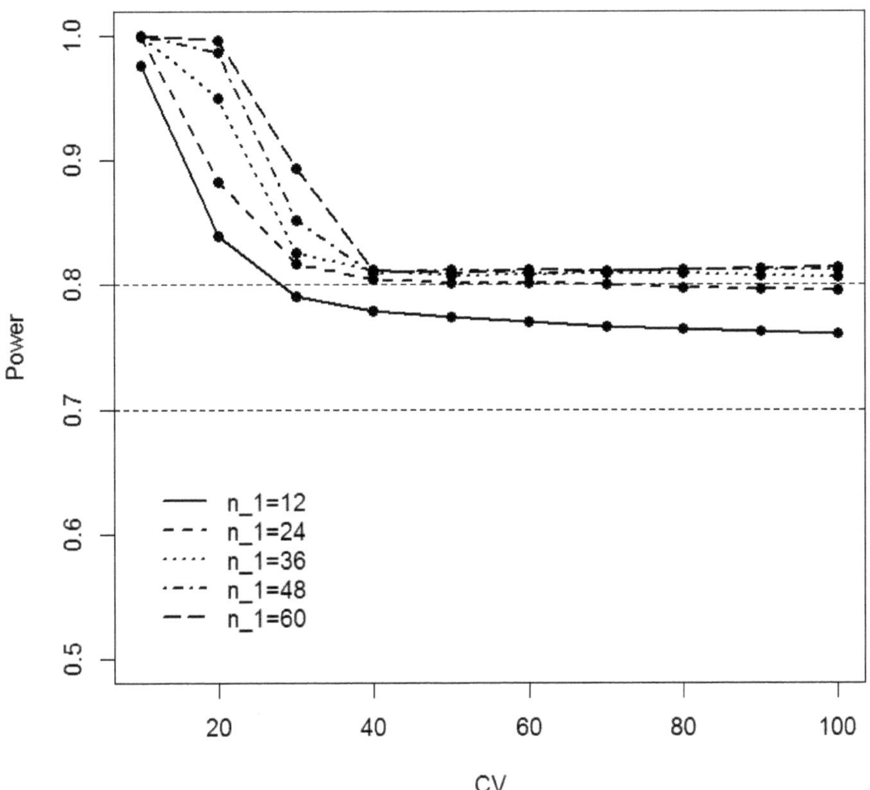

FIGURE 6.10
Simulation-Based Power Estimates for Maximum Combination Test ($w = 0.5, w^* = 0.25$) when True Ratio = 0.95 and Futility Rule Applied

TABLE 6.17
Average Total Sample Sizes for Maximum Combination Test ($w = 0.5, w^* = 0.25$) When True Ratio = 0.95, Futility Rule and Maximum Sample Size Limit ($n_{max} = 4n_1$) Applied

	$n_1 = 12$	$n_1 = 24$	$n_1 = 36$	$n_1 = 48$	$n_1 = 60$	
CV%	$n_{max} = 48$	$n_{max} = 96$	$n_{max} = 144$	$n_{max} = 192$	$n_{max} = 240$	N_s
10	12.05	24.00	36.00	48.00	60.00	8
20	20.57	24.73	36.01	48.00	60.00	20
30	38.39	39.48	40.37	48.90	60.09	40
40	44.89	70.75	66.49	62.73	66.30	66
50	46.17	87.90	106.69	101.45	93.69	98
60	46.41	92.25	130.42	146.98	142.87	134
70	46.42	93.02	137.92	173.68	190.48	174
80	46.39	93.12	139.53	183.45	217.69	214
90	46.36	93.05	139.78	185.97	228.82	258
100	46.34	92.99	139.74	186.41	232.30	300

N_s = planned sample size (for single stage) to achieve power of at least 0.8.

TABLE 6.18
Simulation-Based Estimates of Power for Maximum Combination Test ($w = 0.5, w^* = 0.25$) When True Ratio = 0.95, Futility Rule and Maximum Sample Size Limit ($n_{max} = 4n_1$) Applied

	$n_1 = 12$	$n_1 = 24$	$n_1 = 36$	$n_1 = 48$	$n_1 = 60$
CV%	$n_{max} = 48$	$n_{max} = 96$	$n_{max} = 144$	$n_{max} = 192$	$n_{max} = 240$
10	0.98	1.00	1.00	1.00	1.00
20	0.84	0.88	0.95	0.99	1.00
30	0.73	0.82	0.83	0.85	0.89
40	0.51	0.78	0.81	0.81	0.81
50	0.26	0.68	0.79	0.81	0.81
60	0.08	0.52	0.72	0.79	0.81
70	0.02	0.36	0.61	0.73	0.78
80	0.00	0.21	0.49	0.65	0.74
90	0.00	0.10	0.37	0.55	0.67
100	0.00	0.03	0.26	0.46	0.59

Comparing these tables with Tables 6.8 and 6.10, we can see that almost identical power is achieved for all combinations of CV and n_1, but there is a saving in average sample size for most CV values greater than 50. For CV values lower than 50, there is either no or a very slight increase in average sample size. This suggests that, when the true CV is large, a choice of w and w^* that gives more weight to the second stage is beneficial.

TABLE 6.19
Simulation-Based Estimates of Power for Algorithm That Uses the Maximum Combination Test ($w = 0.40, w^* = 0.20$) and True Ratio = 0.95

CV%	$n_1 = 12$	$n_1 = 24$	$n_1 = 36$	$n_1 = 48$	$n_1 = 60$
10	0.98	1.00	1.00	1.00	1.00
20	0.85	0.88	0.95	0.99	1.00
30	0.80	0.83	0.83	0.85	0.89
40	0.80	0.82	0.83	0.82	0.82
50	0.79	0.82	0.83	0.83	0.83
60	0.79	0.82	0.83	0.83	0.83
70	0.79	0.83	0.83	0.83	0.83
80	0.79	0.83	0.83	0.84	0.83
90	0.79	0.82	0.83	0.84	0.84
100	0.79	0.82	0.83	0.84	0.84

TABLE 6.20
Average Total Sample Sizes for Maximum Combination Test ($w = 0.40, w^* = 0.20$) and True Ratio = 0.95

CV%	$n_1 = 12$	$n_1 = 24$	$n_1 = 36$	$n_1 = 48$	$n_1 = 60$
10	12.05	24.00	36.00	48.00	60.00
20	21.39	24.82	36.01	48.00	60.00
30	50.45	41.25	41.14	49.09	60.11
40	90.69	81.44	70.18	65.10	67.70
50	140.08	130.37	120.75	107.92	98.40
60	196.80	185.09	176.62	167.03	153.33
70	259.47	245.01	235.59	227.70	218.05
80	326.46	309.01	297.65	289.34	281.64
90	395.73	375.51	362.58	352.75	344.77
100	466.55	443.97	428.96	417.61	408.79

6.10 Conclusions

We have seen that a sample size re-estimation after the first stage can be beneficial in recovering power that might otherwise have been lost. The new algorithm described in this chapter has the strong advantage that it ensures that the Type I error rate is not inflated above its nominal level while preserving the desired level of power. Some robustness to the choice of weights is possible by using the new maximum combination test. Indeed, more than two sets of weights could be used, although this is probably unnecessary in the present setting of testing for ABE. For situations where ABE is unlikely to be shown, futility rules at the interim analysis can be beneficial in stopping failed trials and saving sample size. For situations where it might turn out that the true (but unknown) CV is much larger than expected, giving even more weight to the second stage can be beneficial in terms of reducing sample size.

6.11 Technical Appendix: R code

6.11.1 Power and sample size for single-stage design

```
library(mvtnorm)
library(PowerTOST)

############################################################
## example code for chapter on adaptive two-stage designs
############################################################

############################################################
## Warning: this code comes without any guarantee that
## it is correct and does as it is intended to.
## Use of it is at own risk.
############################################################
```

```
##########################################################
##########################################################
## sample size and power calculations for a single stage
## design
##########################################################
##########################################################

##########################################################
## ABE limits (on ratio scale)
theta1=0.8
theta2=1.25

## assumed true ratio of Test to Reference
theta0=0.95

## significance level
alpha=0.05

## planned power
power.min=0.8

## assumed true CV (%)
CV=23 # for example

## sample size calculation for CV=23, alpha=0.05 and
## target power=0.8
sampleN.TOST(alpha=alpha,targetpower=power.min,
             logscale=TRUE,theta0=theta0,theta1=theta1,
             theta2=theta2, CV=CV/100,design="2x2",
             method="exact",robust=FALSE,print=TRUE,
             details=FALSE,imax=100)

## sample size calculation for CV=30, alpha=0.05 and
## target power=0.8
CV=30 # for example
sampleN.TOST(alpha=0.05,targetpower=power.min,
             logscale=TRUE,theta0=theta0,theta=theta1,
             theta2=theta2,CV=CV/100,design="2x2",
             method="exact",robust=FALSE,print=TRUE,
             details=FALSE,imax=100)

#####################################################

##power calculation for n.planned=24, CV=23 and
## alpha=0.05
## assumed true CV (%)
CV=23 # for example
n.planned=24
power.TOST(alpha=alpha,logscale=TRUE,theta1=theta1,
           theta2=theta2,theta0=theta0,CV=CV/100,
```

```
          n=n.planned,design="2x2",method="exact",
          robust=FALSE)

CV=30 # for example
n.planned=24
power.TOST(alpha=alpha,logscale=TRUE,theta1=theta1,
          theta2=theta2,theta0=theta0,CV=CV/100,
          n=n.planned,design="2x2",method="exact",
          robust=FALSE)

####################################################
```

6.11.2 Critical values for standard combination test

```
####################################################
####################################################
## critical values for the standard
## combination test
####################################################
####################################################

####################################################
## choice of weight for standard combination test
####################################################
w1=0.5 # for example
w2=1-w1

####################################################
## this version assumes that the same alpha is
## used in both stages but the choice of weights
## need not be w1=w2=0.5
####################################################
###################
## set parameters #
###################

## true ratio of Test to Reference
## (for simulating data)
true.BE.ratio=0.95 # for example

## true CV (%)
CV=30 # for example

## overall significance level
alpha=0.05

####################################################
## significance level for standard combination
## test at end of stages 1 and 2
####################################################
## chosen to be equal here
```

```
##(see directly below for code to do calculations)
####################################################
## alpha.stage.1=0.03037   # for weight = 0.5
## alpha.stage.2=0.03037
## z.crit.stage.1=1.87542
## z.crit.stage.2=1.87542
####################################################

####################################################
## correlation matrix for bivariate normal
####################################################
corr=diag(1,2,2)
corr[1,2]=sqrt(w1)
corr[2,1]=corr[1,2]

####################################################
## function to solve for critical value
## (equal alphas in stages 1 and 2)
####################################################
f <- function (x)(pmvnorm(lower=rep(-Inf,2),
     upper=c(x,x),mean=rep(0,2),corr=corr,
     abseps=0.0000001)-(1-alpha))
####################################################

####################################################
## get critical value of standard
## combination test
####################################################
z.crit.stage.1=uniroot(f, c(0, 5),
tol=0.0000000001)$root

####################################################
## convert this to a significance level
####################################################
alpha.stage.1=1-pnorm(z.crit.stage.1)
z.crit.stage.2=z.crit.stage.1
alpha.stage.2=alpha.stage.1
####################################################

####################################################
## critical value for z-test first and
## second stages (weight w1)
####################################################
print(c("weight = ",w1,"alpha stage 1 =
",alpha.stage.1,"z.crit.stage.1 = ",z.crit.stage.1))
```

6.11.3 Simulation of data for first stage and application of TOST at interim

```
####################################################
####################################################
## simulate data (within-subject differences)
## for first stage, estimate model parameters,
## apply TOST procedure and
## calculate achieved power of first stage
####################################################
####################################################
## size of stage
n.stage.1=12
## true CV (%)
CV=30
## true sigma
true.sigma=sqrt(log(1+(CV/100)^2))
## true ratio
true.BE.ratio=0.95
## true delta
true.delta=log(true.BE.ratio)

diff.11=rnorm(n.stage.1/2,-true.delta,sqrt(2)*true.sigma)
diff.12=rnorm(n.stage.1/2, true.delta,sqrt(2)*true.sigma)

####################################################
## simulated data for first stage in book example
####################################################
data.first=matrix(c(
 0.1095,  0.7758,
-0.6888, -0.3118,
 0.0292,  0.2005,
-0.0326, -0.6748,
 0.6775, -0.1591,
-0.6688, -0.0069),nrow=6,byrow=TRUE)

diff.11=data.first[,1]
diff.12=data.first[,2]
```

6.11.4 Application of TOST at interim

```
####################################################
## estimate of mean difference
delta.hat.stage.1=(mean(diff.12)-mean(diff.11))/2
## unblinded estimate of variance
errdf.stage.1=n.stage.1-2
var.hat.stage.1=0.5*((n.stage.1/2-1)*var(diff.11) +
(n.stage.1/2-1)*var(diff.12))/errdf.stage.1
CV.hat.stage.1=sqrt(exp(var.hat.stage.1)-1)
sigma.hat.stage.1=sqrt(var.hat.stage.1)
```

```
##########################################################
print(delta.hat.stage.1)
print(exp(delta.hat.stage.1))
print(var.hat.stage.1)
print(sqrt(var.hat.stage.1))
print(CV.hat.stage.1)

########################################################
## standard error of treatment difference on log scale
stderr.stage.1=sqrt(2*var.hat.stage.1/n.stage.1)
########################################################
print(stderr.stage.1)

###########################################################
## test statistics for stage 1
T1.stage.1=(delta.hat.stage.1 - log(0.8))/stderr.stage.1
T2.stage.1=(log(1.25) - delta.hat.stage.1)/stderr.stage.1
###########################################################
print(c(T1.stage.1,T2.stage.1))

##################################################
## p-values for stage 1 (based on t-tests)
p.val.T1.stage.1=1-pt(T1.stage.1,errdf.stage.1)
p.val.T2.stage.1=1-pt(T2.stage.1,errdf.stage.1)
###################################################
print(c(p.val.T1.stage.1,p.val.T2.stage.1))

###################################################
## convert these into z-statistics
## to use in combination test
###################################################
Z1.stage.1=qnorm(1-p.val.T1.stage.1)
Z2.stage.1=qnorm(1-p.val.T2.stage.1)
###########################################
print(c(Z1.stage.1,Z2.stage.1))

#################################################################
## TOST for first stage using z-statistics and z critical value
## based on alpha.stage.1
#################################################################
# can null hypothesis be rejected at left side?
z.nrejlow.stage.1 = (Z1.stage.1 >= z.crit.stage.1)
## can null hypothesis be rejected at right side?
z.nrejupp.stage.1 = (Z2.stage.1 >= z.crit.stage.1)
## can reject null hypothesis at both sides?, i.e., ABE accepted
z.nABE.passed.stage.1 = (z.nrejlow.stage.1 & z.nrejupp.stage.1)
## print if pass ABE (TRUE) or not (FAIL)
print(z.nABE.passed.stage.1)
###################################################################
```

6.11.5 Decision at interim and sample size re-estimation

```
#######################################################
## achieved power of first stage
## for standard combination test with weight  = 0.5
#######################################################
alpha.stage.1=0.0304
planned.BE.ratio=0.95
power.abe.stage.1=power.TOST(
             alpha=alpha.stage.1,
             logscale=TRUE,theta1=theta1,
             theta2=theta2,theta0=planned.BE.ratio,
             CV=CV.hat.stage.1,n=n.stage.1,design="2x2",
             method="exact",robust=FALSE)
print(power.abe.stage.1)

#######################################################
## stop trial if fail ABE and futile at interim
#######################################################
## set default values to be updated later
stop.at.stage.1.abe=0  # stop for ABE,       0 = FALSE
stop.at.stage.1.fut=0  # stop for futility, 0 = FALSE

if(z.nABE.passed.stage.1==FALSE)
{
## if power at first stage is >= power.min then stop
if(power.abe.stage.1 >= power.min)
{
new.n.final.stage.1=n.stage.1
power.abe.final.stage.1=power.abe.stage.1
stop.at.stage.1.fut=1
}
}

########################################################
## stop trial if pass ABE at interim for alpha.stage.1
########################################################
if(z.nABE.passed.stage.1==TRUE)
{
stop.at.stage.1.abe=1
new.n.final.stage.1=n.stage.1
power.abe.final.stage.1=power.abe.stage.1
}

print(c(stop.at.stage.1.fut,stop.at.stage.1.abe))

if(stop.at.stage.1.fut==0 & stop.at.stage.1.abe==0)
{
print("decision is to continue to second stage")
}
```

```
if(stop.at.stage.1.fut!=0 | stop.at.stage.1.abe!=0)
{
print("decision is to stop after first stage")
}

#######################################################
## assume here that decision is to continue to
## stage 2 and re-sample size
#######################################################

#############################
## sample size re-estimation
#############################
nmax=4000
n.planned=24
n.increase=n.planned
power.abe.increase=power.TOST(alpha=alpha.stage.1,
                   logscale=TRUE,
                   theta1=theta1,theta2=theta2,
                   theta0=planned.BE.ratio,
                   CV=CV.hat.stage.1,n=n.increase,
                   design="2x2",
                   method="exact",robust=FALSE)
repeat
{
n.increase=n.increase+2
power.abe.increase=power.TOST(alpha=alpha.stage.1,
                   logscale=TRUE,
                   theta1=theta1,
                   theta2=theta2,
                   theta0=planned.BE.ratio,
                   CV=CV.hat.stage.1,n=n.increase,
                   design="2x2",
                   method="exact",robust=FALSE)
if(power.abe.increase>=power.min |
n.increase>=nmax) {break}
} #end of repeat loop
n.final.stage.1=n.increase
new.n.stage.2=n.final.stage.1-n.stage.1
power.abe.final.stage.1=power.abe.increase

print(c(new.n.stage.2,n.final.stage.1,
power.abe.final.stage.1))
```

6.11.6 Simulation of data for second stage

```
#####################################################
#####################################################
## simulation of second-stage data and application
## of TOST using the standard combination test
```

```
########################################################
########################################################

########################################################
## simulate data for second stage
########################################################
diff.21=rnorm(new.n.stage.2/2,-true.delta,sqrt(2)*true.sigma)
diff.22=rnorm(new.n.stage.2/2, true.delta,sqrt(2)*true.sigma)

########################################################
## below are the simulated data for second stage
## in the book example
########################################################
data.second=matrix(c(
-0.1536,  0.6286,
 0.1128,  0.0137,
 0.3096, -0.1762,
 1.4555,  1.0213,
 0.1030, -0.4475,
-0.3317,  0.3559,
 0.0536, -0.3835,
 0.3641, -0.0042,
 0.4193, -0.1826,
-0.0716, -0.4234,
-0.1361, -0.4085,
-0.3981, -0.2508,
-0.3934, -0.4037,
-0.0876, -0.3587,
 0.1541, -0.5949,
 0.5964,  0.6090,
-0.6216,  0.4746,
-0.2219, -0.6212,
-0.2395,  0.6777,
 0.8597, -0.1294,
 0.5992,  0.0008,
-0.0238, -0.4009,
 0.3881, -0.9945,
 0.2083, -0.9417,
-0.1400,  0.8338,
 0.3870, -0.5862,
 0.0437, -0.0480,
 0.5645,  0.2778),nrow=28,byrow=TRUE)

diff.21=data.second[,1]
diff.22=data.second[,2]
new.n.stage.2=2*length(diff.21)
```

6.11.7 Estimation and TOST for second stage

```
#####################################################
#####################################################
## Estimation and TOST for second stage
## using the standard combination test
#####################################################
#####################################################

#####################################################
## df for second stage
errdf.stage.2=new.n.stage.2-2
#####################################################

#####################################################
## estimate parameters
#####################################################
delta.hat.stage.2=(mean(diff.22)-mean(diff.21))/2
## unblinded estimate of variance
var.hat.stage.2=0.5*((new.n.stage.2/2-1)*var(diff.21)+
                     (new.n.stage.2/2-1)*var(diff.22))/
                     errdf.stage.2
CV.hat.stage.2=sqrt(exp(var.hat.stage.2)-1)
######################################################
print(delta.hat.stage.2)
print(exp(delta.hat.stage.2))
print(var.hat.stage.2)
print(sqrt(var.hat.stage.2))
print(CV.hat.stage.2)

##########################################################
## standard error of treatment difference for stage 2 only
stderr.stage.2=sqrt(2*var.hat.stage.2/new.n.stage.2)
##########################################################
print(stderr.stage.2)

##########################################################
## one-sided t-test values for stage 2
T1.stage.2=(delta.hat.stage.2 - log(0.8))/stderr.stage.2
T2.stage.2=(log(1.25) - delta.hat.stage.2)/stderr.stage.2
##########################################################
print(T1.stage.2)
print(T2.stage.2)

## p-values for stage 2
p.val.T1.stage.2=1-pt(T1.stage.2,errdf.stage.2)
p.val.T2.stage.2=1-pt(T2.stage.2,errdf.stage.2)
##########################################################
print(p.val.T1.stage.2)
print(p.val.T2.stage.2)
```

```
###########################################################
## convert these into z-statistics
## for use in the combination test
###########################################################
Z1.stage.2=qnorm(1-p.val.T1.stage.2)
Z2.stage.2=qnorm(1-p.val.T2.stage.2)
###########################################################
print(Z1.stage.2)
print(Z2.stage.2)
###########################################################
```

6.11.8 Application of the standard combination test

```
###########################################################
###########################################################
## application of the standard combination test
## for weight = 0.5
###########################################################
###########################################################
w1=0.5
w2=1-w1
###########################################################
alpha.stage.2=0.03037
z.crit.stage.2=1.87542
###########################################################

###########################################################
## z-statistics
###########################################################
Z1=sqrt(w1)*Z1.stage.1 + sqrt(w2)*Z1.stage.2
Z2=sqrt(w1)*Z2.stage.1 + sqrt(w2)*Z2.stage.2
###########################################################
print(Z1)
print(Z2)

###########################################################
## test for ABE using combination test
###########################################################
## reject null hypothesis at left side?
nrejlow.comb = (Z1 >= z.crit.stage.2)
## reject null hypothesis at right side?
nrejupp.comb = (Z2 >= z.crit.stage.2)
## reject null hypothesis at both sides?, i.e.,
## is ABE accepted?
nABE.passed.comb = (nrejlow.comb & nrejupp.comb)
## print if pass ABE (TRUE) or not (FAIL)
print(nABE.passed.comb)
###########################################################
```

6.11.9 Critical values for maximum combination test

```
##############################################################
##############################################################
## calculation of critical values for
## maximum combination test
##############################################################
##############################################################

##############################################################
## set up what is needed for trivariate normal
## calculations to get critical value for maximum
## combination test (assuming equal alpha levels for
## each stage)
##############################################################

##############################################################
# choice of weights
##############################################################
w1=0.5
w2=1-w1
w1.star=0.25
w2.star=1-w1.star
##############################################################
## correlation matrix for trivariate normal
##############################################################
rho=sqrt(w1*w1.star) + sqrt(w2*w2.star)
corr=diag(1,3,3)
corr[1,2]=sqrt(w1)
corr[1,3]=sqrt(w1.star)
corr[2,1]=corr[1,2]
corr[3,1]=corr[1,3]
corr[2,3]=rho
corr[3,2]=corr[2,3]

##############################################################
## function uses in uniroot to solve for critical value
## of maximum combination test
##############################################################

##############################################################
f <- function (x)(pmvnorm(lower=rep(-Inf,3),
                  upper=c(x,x,x), mean=rep(0,3),corr=corr,
                  abseps=0.0000001)-(1-alpha))
##############################################################
## get critical value of robust combination test for
## Z.max.1 and Z.max.2
z.crit.max=uniroot(f, c(0, 5),tol=0.0000000001)$root
##############################################################
alpha.max= 1-pnorm(z.crit.max)
##############################################################
```

```
## critical value for z.max test
#########################################################
print(c("alpha.max = ",round(alpha.max,5),
"z.crit.max = ", round(z.crit.max,5)))
#########################################################
```

6.11.10 Sample size re-estimation using the maximum combination test

```
##########################################################
##########################################################
## sample size re-estimation for
## maximum combination test
##########################################################
##########################################################

nmax=4000
n.increase=n.planned
power.abe.increase=power.TOST(alpha=alpha.max,
                   logscale=TRUE,
                   theta1=theta1,theta2=theta2,
                   theta0=planned.BE.ratio,
                   CV=CV.hat.stage.1,n=n.increase,
                   design="2x2",
                   method="exact",robust=FALSE)
repeat
{
n.increase=n.increase+2
power.abe.increase=power.TOST(alpha=alpha.max,
                   logscale=TRUE,
                   theta1=theta1,
                   theta2=theta2,
                   theta0=planned.BE.ratio,
                   CV=CV.hat.stage.1,n=n.increase,
                   design="2x2",
                   method="exact",robust=FALSE)
if(power.abe.increase>=power.min |
n.increase>=nmax) {break}
} #end of repeat loop
n.final.stage.1=n.increase
new.n.stage.2=n.final.stage.1-n.stage.1
power.abe.final.stage.1=power.abe.increase


print(c(new.n.stage.2,n.final.stage.1,
power.abe.final.stage.1))
```

6.11.11 Power of first stage using the maximum combination test

```
#####################################################
#####################################################
## power for a given first stage sample size,
## using the adjusted alpha levels
## for the maximum combination test
#####################################################
#####################################################

## first stage sample size
n.stage.1=12
planned.BE.ratio=0.95
alpha.max=0.0264
power.planned.alpha.max=power.TOST(
             alpha=alpha.max,
             logscale=TRUE,theta1=theta1,
             theta2=theta2,theta0=planned.BE.ratio,
             CV=CV.hat.stage.1,n=n.stage.1,design="2x2",
             method="exact",robust=FALSE)
print(power.planned.alpha.max)
```

6.11.12 Simulation of data for second stage when maximum combination test is used

```
##########################################################
##########################################################
## second-stage data for the book example that uses the
## maximum combination test and a sample size
## re-estimation that does not make use of conditional
## errors and conditional power
##########################################################
##########################################################
##########################################################
## use these data
##########################################################
data.second.max=matrix(0,29,2)
data.second.max[1:28,]=data.second[1:28,]
data.second.max[29,]=c( 0.8517,  0.1783)
diff.21=data.second.max[,1]
diff.22=data.second.max[,2]
new.n.stage.2=2*length(diff.21)

#########################################################
## second-stage data for book example when
## using the maximum combination test and
## sample size re-estimation is based on conditional
## errors and conditional power
#########################################################
```

```
##############################################################
data.second.max=matrix(0,25,2)
data.second.max[1:25,]=data.second[1:25,]
diff.21=data.second.max[,1]
diff.22=data.second.max[,2]
new.n.stage.2=2*length(diff.21)
#####################################
```

6.11.13 Estimation and TOST for second stage when maximum combination test is used

```
##############################################################
##############################################################
## TOST using the maximum combination test
##############################################################
##############################################################

##############################################################
## df for second stage
errdf.stage.2=new.n.stage.2-2
##############################################################

##############################################################
## estimate parameters
##############################################################
delta.hat.stage.2=(mean(diff.22)-mean(diff.21))/2
## unblinded estimate of variance
var.hat.stage.2=0.5*((new.n.stage.2/2-1)*var(diff.21) +
                      (new.n.stage.2/2-1)*var(diff.22))/
                       errdf.stage.2
CV.hat.stage.2=sqrt(exp(var.hat.stage.2)-1)
##############################################################
print(delta.hat.stage.2)
print(exp(delta.hat.stage.2))
print(var.hat.stage.2)
print(sqrt(var.hat.stage.2))
print(CV.hat.stage.2)

##############################################################
## standard error of treatment difference for stage 2 only
stderr.stage.2=sqrt(2*var.hat.stage.2/new.n.stage.2)
##############################################################
print(stderr.stage.2)

##############################################################
## one-sided t-test values for stage 2
T1.stage.2=(delta.hat.stage.2 - log(0.8))/stderr.stage.2
T2.stage.2=(log(1.25) - delta.hat.stage.2)/stderr.stage.2
##############################################################
print(T1.stage.2)
print(T2.stage.2)
```

```
## p-values for stage 2
p.val.T1.stage.2=1-pt(T1.stage.2,errdf.stage.2)
p.val.T2.stage.2=1-pt(T2.stage.2,errdf.stage.2)
##########################################################
print(p.val.T1.stage.2)
print(p.val.T2.stage.2)

##########################################################
## convert these into z-statistics
## for use in the combination test
##########################################################
Z1.stage.2=qnorm(1-p.val.T1.stage.2)
Z2.stage.2=qnorm(1-p.val.T2.stage.2)
##########################################################
print(Z1.stage.2)
print(Z2.stage.2)
##########################################################
```

6.11.14 Apply maximum combination test

```
############################################################
w=0.5
w.star=0.25
##################################################
## get z-statistics
############################################################
print(c(Z1.stage.1,Z2.stage.1))
print(c(Z1.stage.2,Z2.stage.2))
Z1.w=sqrt(w)*Z1.stage.1 + sqrt(1-w)*Z1.stage.2
Z2.w=sqrt(w)*Z2.stage.1 + sqrt(1-w)*Z2.stage.2

Z1.w.star=sqrt(w.star)*Z1.stage.1 + sqrt(1-w.star)*Z1.stage.2
Z2.w.star=sqrt(w.star)*Z2.stage.1 + sqrt(1-w.star)*Z2.stage.2

print(c(Z1.w,Z2.w))
print(c(Z1.w.star,Z2.w.star))

Z1.max=max(Z1.w,Z1.w.star)
Z2.max=max(Z2.w,Z2.w.star)
print(c(Z1.max,Z2.max))

#######################################################
## test for ABE using maximum combination test
#######################################################

## reject null hypothesis at left side?
nrejlow = (Z1.max >= z.crit.max)
## reject null hypothesis at right side?
nrejupp = (Z2.max >= z.crit.max)
## reject null hypothesis at both sides?, i.e., is ABE accepted?
```

```
z.passed = (nrejlow & nrejupp)
print(z.passed)
############################################################
```

6.11.15 Conditional errors for second stage

```
############################################################
w1=0.5
w2=1-w1
## critical value for combination tests
#z.crit.stage.2=1.9374 #  maximum comb test
z.crit.stage.2=1.87542 #  standard comb test
############################################################

############################################################
## values for H_{01}
############################################################
## calculate value within Phi function
############################################################
val.1=(z.crit.stage.2 - sqrt(w1)*Z1.stage.1)/sqrt(w2)
############################################################
## conditional error at interim
############################################################
alpha.c.1=1-pnorm(val.1)
print(alpha.c.1)
############################################################
## critical value for t-test for second stage t-test
#errdf=54  # standard combination test
errdf=48   # maximum combination test
t.crit.1=qt((1-alpha.c.1),errdf)
print(t.crit.1)
############################################################

############################################################
## values for H_{02}
############################################################
############################################################
## calculate value within Phi function
############################################################
val.2=(z.crit.stage.2 - sqrt(w1)*Z2.stage.1)/sqrt(w2)
############################################################
## conditional error at interim
############################################################
alpha.c.2=1-pnorm(val.2)
print(alpha.c.2)
############################################################
############################################################
## critical value for t-test for second stage t-test
errdf=54   # standard combination test
errdf=48   # maximum combination test
t.crit.2=qt((1-alpha.c.2),errdf)
```

```
print(t.crit.2)
##########################################################
```

6.11.16 Power of second stage using conditional errors

```
##########################################################
##########################################################
## conditional power function for given value (n)
## of second-stage sample size using function pmvt
## in library mvtnorm
##########################################################
##########################################################

##########################################################
## parameters for mvtnorm
##########################################################
#sigma.hat.stage.1 = 0.3574
#alpha.c.1 = 0.1272 # for maximum combination test
#alpha.c.2 = 0.0644 # for maximum combination test
alpha.c.1 = 0.1464 # for standard combination test
alpha.c.2 = 0.0762 # for standard combination test
planned.BE.ratio=0.95
delta=log(planned.BE.ratio)
Delta=log(1.25)
corr <- c(1, -1, -1, 1)
corr <- matrix(corr, ncol =2)

##########################################################
Power <- function(n2)(
pmvt(
     lower = c(qt(1-alpha.c.1, n2-2),
              qt(1-alpha.c.2, n2-2)),
     upper = c(Inf,Inf),
     delta = c((delta+Delta) /
            (sigma.hat.stage.1*sqrt(2/n2)),
              (Delta-delta) /
            (sigma.hat.stage.1*sqrt(2/n2))),
df = n2-2, corr = corr) )
##########################################################

##########################################################
## power of second-stage for given value of n2
##########################################################
n2=38
power.n2=Power(n2)[1]
print(power.n2)
############################################
```

6.11.17 Conditional power at interim

```
##################################################
##################################################
## conditional power at interim
##################################################
##################################################
planned.beta=1-power.min
alpha.stage.1=0.0304  # standard combination test
#################################################
## power for first stage based on alpha.stage.1
#################################################
power.abe.stage.1=power.TOST(alpha=alpha.stage.1,
                  logscale=TRUE,theta1=theta1,
                  theta2=theta2,theta0=planned.BE.ratio,
                  CV=CV.hat.stage.1,n=n.stage.1,
                  design="2x2",method="exact",
                  robust=FALSE)
print(power.abe.stage.1)

beta.1.hat=1-power.abe.stage.1

cond.power=(beta.1.hat-planned.beta)/beta.1.hat
print(cond.power)
################################################
```

6.11.18 Conditional errors for maximum combination test

```
w2=1-w1
w2.star=1-w1.star

#################################################################
## power for first stage,using the adjusted alpha levels
## for the maximum combination test
#################################################################

## first stage sample size
n.stage.1=12

## df for TOST at interim
errdf.stage.1=n.stage.1-2

## power of planned trial (using alpha from standard combination test)
planned.BE.ratio=0.95
power.abe.stage.1.max=power.TOST(alpha=alpha.max,logscale=TRUE,
                      theta1=theta1,theta2=theta2,theta0=planned.BE.ratio,
                      CV=CV.hat.stage.1,n=n.stage.1,design="2x2",
                      method="exact",robust=FALSE)
print(power.abe.stage.1.max)
```

```
################################################
beta.1.hat=1-power.abe.stage.1.max
################################################

################################################
## calculate value within Phi function
############################################################
val.11=(z.crit.max - sqrt(w1)*Z1.stage.1)/sqrt(w2)
val.12=(z.crit.max - sqrt(w1.star)*Z1.stage.1)/sqrt(w2.star)
val.min=min(val.11,val.12)
###########################################################

################################################
## conditional error at interim based on
## maximum combination test
################################################
alpha.c.1.max=1-pnorm(val.min)
print(alpha.c.1.max)
################################################

################################################
## calculate values within Phi function
############################################################
val.21=(z.crit.max - sqrt(w1)*Z2.stage.1)/sqrt(w2)
val.22=(z.crit.max - sqrt(w1.star)*Z2.stage.1)/sqrt(w2.star)
val.min=min(val.21,val.22)
############################################################

################################
## conditional error at interim
################################
alpha.c.2.max=1-pnorm(val.min)
print(alpha.c.2.max)
################################

####################################
## conditional power at interim
################################################
planned.beta=1-power.min
cond.power=(beta.1.hat-planned.beta)/beta.1.hat
print(cond.power)
################################################
```

6.11.19 Sample size for maximum combination test using conditional errors

```
#########################################################
#########################################################
## conditional power function for given value (n2)
## and conditional errors for maximum combination test
## of second-stage sample size using function pmvt
```

```
## in library mvtnorm
############################################################
############################################################

############################################################
## parameters for mvtnorm
############################################################
#planned.BE.ratio=0.95
planned.BE.ratio=1/0.95 # adaptive planning
delta=log(planned.BE.ratio)
Delta=log(1.25)
corr <- c(1, -1, -1, 1)
corr <- matrix(corr, ncol =2)

############################################################
Power <- function(n2)(
pmvt(
     lower = c(qt(1-alpha.c.1.max, n2-2),
               qt(1-alpha.c.2.max, n2-2)),
     upper = c(Inf,Inf),
     delta = c((delta+Delta) /
            (sigma.hat.stage.1*sqrt(2/n2)),
               (Delta-delta) /
            (sigma.hat.stage.1*sqrt(2/n2))),
df = n2-2, corr = corr) )
############################################################

############################################################
## power of second-stage for given value of n2
############################################################
n2=38
power.n2=Power(n2)[1]
print(power.n2)
n2=40
power.n2=Power(n2)[1]
print(power.n2)
n2=48
power.n2=Power(n2)[1]
print(power.n2)
n2=50
power.n2=Power(n2)[1]
print(power.n2)
```

7

Scaled Average Bioequivalence Testing

Introduction

A few years later, I was asked to attend a meeting in Hilton Head, South Carolina, where bioequivalence was one of the topics of discussion. There were presentations by several statisticians from the FDA, academia, and industry on the topic. I regarded this as somewhat of a pain — there was a lot of work to do, I had a date that weekend, and I could not see where flying off to Hilton Head was going to be helpful to anyone at all. Plus I had a cold, and flying on the puddle jumpers one takes to Hilton Head with a head cold is a bad idea....

My boss, however, said I had to go. It was expected that I would attend (and eventually participate in) such conferences as a matter of professional development, representing the company and the discipline of statistics (etc., etc.). Also, she did not have time to go. So I dutifully packed my bags and headed down. One of the reasons I had gone to work was that I was tired of sitting through lectures, but I left secure in the knowledge that at least maybe I could possibly play golf while down there.

When the conference was over, I came back and reported on the upcoming new FDA proposals about assessing bioequivalence. I was still pretty new to the company and industry at this point, so how bioequivalence testing was done did not really bother me one way or the other. As long as I knew what to do with the data and how to design the studies, I was holding up my end. The FDA was planning to issue a draft guidance on the topic later that year. I did not get to play golf, and the puddle jumpers made my cold worse. My doctor did not even want to see me and prescribed antibiotics.

The reaction I received after sharing what I had heard at the conference was kind of like the reaction one gets when accidently knocking over a bees' nest — the bees are very surprised, kind of annoyed, do not like it, and may be less than friendly. My boss was very surprised by the information I brought back and, to be blunt, did not believe me. I argued about it with her for a while, showed her my notes, and pointed out that if she did not like the message, it was not my fault as I was just reporting what I had heard. In the end, I had her invite one of the local academic statisticians who had given a talk at the meeting to come to "the Unit" to discuss the upcoming FDA proposals.

If she did not believe me, I figured she would believe him. It is amazing how often this type of thing happens in industry (the inviting of external people to make a point). I have had to do this type of thing several times since then. You may know exactly what is going on for a particular issue, but very often people at the company want to hear it themselves from someone else external to the company before they will believe that they really have to do anything about it. It has been pointed out that we have to pay these people to come talk to us (i.e., this approach is not really cost effective), but that is how business is often done.

After the external academician came in and spoke with us, my boss believed me, and there was a great deal of discussion at the company about the possible implications of this proposal (nobody knew) and when it would come into effect (no one knew that either). In the end, my boss asked that I go down to Washington, DC, with her the following winter after the draft guidance was issued [358] for a special FDA Advisory Board meeting on the topic. These are meetings of experts (external to the FDA) on a particular topic who advise the FDA on how to protect public health.

In the end, this resulted in my spending the next approximately five years working on this area of bioequivalence, doing extensive research and presenting at various meetings here, there, and everywhere on the topic and its implications for public health. It was important and also interesting research, and I saw most of the airports in North America (and beyond).

The lessons of this experience are

1. *Conference attendance (even if one is not presenting a paper or poster) is actually important. It keeps one on the cutting edge at work.*
2. *In the modern world, it is not enough to just do your day job. Working folks should engage in research that benefits them professionally at their company and also externally.*
3. *All that said, five years of research is a long time and a lot of research. Be careful what conferences you choose to attend.*

7.1 Background

As discussed in greater detail in Chapter 2, in the late 1990s, the US Food and Drug Administration (FDA) considered switching to newer techniques for bioequivalence assessment, known as individual bioequivalence and population bioequivalence. It was eventually decided that these particular approaches would not proceed, but their development did lead to what is known as scaled average bioequivalence.

Individual bioequivalence was to be assessed using the following aggregate statistic [358]:

$$\frac{(\mu_T - \mu_R)^2 + \sigma_D^2 + \sigma_{WT}^2 - \sigma_{WR}^2}{max(0.04, \sigma_{WR}^2)} \tag{7.1}$$

where μ_T and μ_R are the means of ln-transformed AUC or Cmax data for test and reference formulations, respectively, σ_D^2 is the variance associated with subject-by-formulation interaction, and σ_{WT}^2 and σ_{WR}^2 are the within-subject variances for the test and reference formulations, respectively. The derivation of such estimates is discussed in Chapter 5.

Because the within-subject variance of each formulation cannot be separately estimated from between-subject variance estimates in most two-period cross-over designs of the form (TR, RT), a replicate design (see Chapters 4 and 5) was generally required for individual bioequivalence assessment [358].

This individual bioequivalence approach was abandoned by the FDA following debate (see Chapter 2) for a number of reasons. However, theoretical issues remained with certain classes of drug (which individual bioequivalence was in part attempting to address). Highly variable drugs, and also narrow therapeutic index drugs, have been the subject of debate at various times, as it was thought that the 0.80–1.25 average bioequivalence acceptance range was too stringent (in the former case), requiring "large" trials, and might be too wide, not protecting public health in the latter case.

The threshold for declaring a drug's ln-AUC and ln-Cmax to be highly variable is generally set at an approximate threshold for $\sigma_{WR} > 0.3$ as a rule of thumb, making the identification of a highly variable drug straightforward. Precisely stated, a highly variable drug is one in which $\sigma_W \geq 0.294$ corresponding to an intra-subject coefficient of variation of at least 30%. Recall that $CV_W = \sqrt{e^{\sigma_W^2} - 1}$, as discussed in Chapter 5. Earlier proposals had considered an intra-subject coefficient of variation of 25% (a natural-log scale within-subject SD of 0.2462) as highly variable [90].

Examples of narrow therapeutic drugs are digoxin and warfarin — a small change in dose or exposure can result in a large change in safety and efficacy. Narrow therapeutic index drugs generally exhibit low levels of within-subject variability but are not identified as narrow therapeutic index drugs by their variability estimates alone.

In the middle years of the 2000 decade, the FDA and the European regulatory agency (EMEA) devoted further attention to such products. They arrived at different testing approaches for highly variable drugs, and we will study each approach in subsequent sections of this chapter. First we will study a general approach to scaled average bioequivalence using a standard 2×2 bioequivalence design.

This approach advocates the *scaling* (i.e., widening) of the acceptance limits (traditionally $\pm \ln 1.25$ for average bioequivalence) for reference product intra-subject variation in excess of a coefficient of variation (CV) of 30% for highly variable drugs and will be referred to as scaled average bioequivalence (SABE). In essence, an acceptance value greater than $\ln 1.25$ would be used (depending on the observed variability) to determine bioequivalence. As with average bioequivalence, AUC and Cmax are the endpoints of interest and are ln transformed for analysis.

In most publications and guidance on these topics, narrow therapeutic index drugs were not to be held to a stricter standard than the traditional average bioequivalence acceptance limits $\mp \ln 1.25$ (see, for example, [358], [373]); however, this may be reconsidered by regulators, as evidenced by [244, 319, 339, 793] when circumstances warrant. In this chapter, we will not discuss narrowing (i.e., lowering) the acceptance limit from the traditional acceptance limit $\ln 1.25$, but in theory, the methods discussed hereafter for scaling for highly variable drugs are readily applicable to such an exercise.

Tothfalusi and Endrenyi [1246] provide an excellent review of the scaled average bioequivalence topic, expanding on their consideration of the topic in [1245], and review the state of the topic in [336, 337]. In essence, scaled average bioequivalence may be viewed as a special case of individual bioequivalence where $\sigma^2_{WT} = \sigma^2_{WR} = \sigma^2_W$ and $\sigma^2_D = 0$.

As such, the statistic of interest becomes

$$\frac{(\mu_T - \mu_R)^2 + \sigma^2_D + \sigma^2_{WT} - \sigma^2_{WR}}{max(0.04, \sigma^2_{WR})} = \frac{(\mu_T - \mu_R)^2 + 0 + \sigma^2_W - \sigma^2_W}{max(0.04, \sigma^2_W)} \tag{7.2}$$

reducing to

$$\frac{(\mu_T - \mu_R)^2}{\sigma^2_W}. \tag{7.3}$$

Note that, in the denominator of this expression (7.3), $max(0.04)$ is not included, as it was in individual bioequivalence testing. This is in keeping with the description of [1246]. For drugs with low to moderate variability ($\sigma_W < 0.294$), the traditional average bioequivalence tests (see previous chapters) are used [1246].

For high variation drugs, the two one-sided tests then become

$$H_{01}: \quad \frac{\mu_T - \mu_R}{\sigma_W} \leq -\eta \tag{7.4}$$

versus the alternative

$$H_{11}: \quad \frac{\mu_T - \mu_R}{\sigma_W} > -\eta$$

and

$$H_{02}: \quad \frac{\mu_T - \mu_R}{\sigma_W} \geq \eta \tag{7.5}$$

versus the alternative

$$H_{12}: \quad \frac{\mu_T - \mu_R}{\sigma_W} < \eta.$$

The observed difference in means $\hat{\mu}_T - \hat{\mu}_R$ is assessed relative to (i.e., divided by) the observed within-subject standard deviation $\hat{\sigma}_W$ — hence *scaled* average bioequivalence (SABE).

The scaled average bioequivalence acceptance criteria η is a pre-defined regulatory acceptance criteria. Values of η discussed in the literature range from ± 0.7 to ± 1.1 versus the traditional average bioequivalence limits of $\pm \ln 1.25 = \pm 0.223$. As with individual bioequivalence and population bioequivalence, acceptance criteria would to some extent still be design dependent — in that running a "dirty" study (i.e., a poorly controlled study) would yield higher variability, making it easier to demonstrate scaled average bioequivalence.

As with average bioequivalence, in a 2×2 cross-over, this scaled average bioequivalence two one-sided test procedure may be assessed using a confidence interval. Tothfalusi and Endrenyi [1246] stated that

$$[t_{0.05}(\lambda, n-2), t_{0.95}(\lambda, n-2)]$$

is a 90% confidence interval for $\frac{\mu_T - \mu_R}{\sigma_W}$ where t_α denotes the α quartile of a noncentral t distribution with noncentrality parameter $\lambda = \frac{(\hat{\mu}_T - \hat{\mu}_R)\sqrt{n/2}}{\hat{\sigma}_W}$ with $n-2$ degrees of freedom (n being the overall sample size of the study).

If these limits lie between $-\eta\sqrt{n/2}$ and $\eta\sqrt{n/2}$, then scaled average bioequivalence is demonstrated.

Consider Example 3.1 from Chapter 3. The statistics of interest may be derived by entering the appropriate values into the following SAS code. We utilize $\eta = 0.795$ for the purposes of this example.

```
data sabe_auc;
eta=0.795;n=32;d=-0.01655;s2=0.01100;
lambda=(d*((n/2)**(0.5)))/(s2**0.5);
t_05=TINV(0.05,30,lambda);
t_95=TINV(0.95,30,lambda);
ll=-eta*((n/2)**(0.5));ul=eta*((n/2)**(0.5));
run;
proc print data=sabe_auc noobs;
var ll t_05 t_95 ul;run;

data sabecmax;
eta=0.795;n=32;d=-0.02694;s2=0.03835;
lambda=(d*((n/2)**(0.5)))/(s2**0.5);
t_05=TINV(0.05,30,lambda);
t_95=TINV(0.95,30,lambda);
ll=-eta*((n/2)**(0.5));ul=eta*((n/2)**(0.5));
run;
proc print data=sabecmax noobs;
var ll t_05 t_95 ul;run;
```

In this analysis of Example 3.1, the lower limits of interest are -2.37 and -2.28, and the upper limits are 1.04 and 1.12 for ln-AUC and ln-Cmax, respectively, indicating that scaled average bioequivalence was demonstrated, as these fall within the limits (-3.18 and 3.18).

Individual bioequivalence was initially proposed for assessment using the bootstrap [358]. Thereafter, an approximation procedure was developed by Hyslop et al. ([616, 617]) (not requiring the bootstrap) and subsequently adopted in FDA guidance [369]. Interested readers should also see [1245] for more information on extension of the Hyslop et al. procedure as applied to scaled average bioequivalence testing. We will consider the Hyslop et al. procedure as applied in the approach adopted by the FDA for scaled average bioequivalence testing in a subsequent section.

Equation (7.3) is also interesting in a more purely statistical sense. If all variance terms are assumed to be homogeneous across formulations (i.e., $\sigma^2_{BT} = \sigma^2_{BR} = \sigma^2_B$ and $\sigma^2_{WT} = \sigma^2_{WR} = \sigma^2_W$) and subject-by-formulation variance is assumed to be negligible ($\sigma^2_D = 0$), an alternative expression for the distance between the distribution of responses between formulations reduces to ([34, 281])

$$\frac{(\mu_T - \mu_R)^2}{\sigma^2} \tag{7.6}$$

where $\sigma^2 = \sigma^2_B + \sigma^2_W$. This expression (7.6) is the Kullback–Leibler divergence [726] — a measure of the discrepancy between test and reference formulation distributions.

This is the concept that regulators are really interested in assessing — i.e., are the ln-AUC and ln-Cmax **distributions** of the test and reference formulations the same (within acceptable limits), accounting for each subject as their own control? However, statistical science and regulatory science are not switchable or interchangeable, especially when one factors in other sciences, including medical science and pharmacology. Therefore, regulatory agencies have introduced approaches which are a slight variation on these general approaches to scaled average bioequivalence, consistent with their local regulatory needs and expert opinions concerning the protection of public health.

For example, the Canadian regulatory authority takes a very practical attitude toward such highly variable products and only requires that the point estimate $exp(\hat{\mu}_T - \hat{\mu}_R)$ fall in the interval 0.80–1.25 for Cmax ([140, 141]).

We now turn to the statistics and study designs used for scaled average bioequivalence testing implemented in Europe by the EMEA followed by those of the FDA. Each will consider the conditions under which scaled average bioequivalence may be applied, describe the model and procedure to be used for testing with application to a dataset, and end with a discussion of sample size requirements for testing. These sections are followed by a general discussion of some issues with the practical application of scaled average bioequivalence.

7.2 Scaled Average Bioequivalence in Europe

Comprehensive reviews of the European bioequivalence guidance [319] are given in [440, 890, 1268]. In this section, we will consider only the elements of the guidance specifically relating to the statistics of scaled average bioequivalence.

To review, the traditional two one-sided testing procedure tests have been used for some time to test for average bioequivalence. The endpoints ln-AUC and ln-Cmax, separately, are tested using these null hypotheses:

$$H_{01}: \quad \mu_T - \mu_R \leq -\ln 1.25 \tag{7.7}$$

or

$$H_{02}: \quad \mu_T - \mu_R \geq \ln 1.25 \tag{7.8}$$

where μ_T and μ_R are the means of ln-transformed AUC or Cmax data for test and reference formulations, respectively. Both null hypotheses must be rejected for ln-AUC and for ln-Cmax for average bioequivalence to be demonstrated. To meet the European requirements, a sample size of $n \geq 12$ subjects should be used in the study.

The European bioequivalence guidance [319] allows for the modification of the traditional average bioequivalence null hypotheses for ln-Cmax (only) to be

$$H_{01}: \quad \frac{\mu_T - \mu_R}{\sigma_{WR}} \leq -0.76 \tag{7.9}$$

or

$$H_{02}: \quad \frac{\mu_T - \mu_R}{\sigma_{WR}} \geq 0.76 \tag{7.10}$$

where σ^2_{WR} is the within-subject variance of the reference formulation, and when

1. such is clinically justified,
2. under specific conditions regarding the observed variability (discussed in the following),
3. where this is specified in the protocol,
4. and where a partial replicate (a three-period design with sequences RRT, RTR, TRR) or replicate design (a four-period design with sequences such as RTRT, TRTR) is used such that an estimate for σ_{WR} is obtained in $n \geq 12$ subjects.

Both null hypotheses (Equations (7.9) and (7.10)) must be rejected for ln-Cmax for scaled average bioequivalence to be demonstrated under this guidance [319]. The traditional two one-sided tests (Equations (7.7) and (7.8)) must also be rejected for ln-AUC to conclude that the study is successful.

The guidance implies that the observed within-subject standard deviation for the reference formulation for ln-Cmax must have a history of observed high variability $\hat{\sigma}_{WR} \geq 0.294$ and must be observed to do so in the study without undue influence from outliers (for more on outliers, see Chapter 5).

As a practical matter, then, if the 90% confidence intervals for $\hat{\mu}_T - \hat{\mu}_R = \hat{\delta}$ fall within the acceptance boundaries $-\ln 1.25, \ln 1.25$ as traditionally done for ln-AUC and within the scaled acceptance boundaries of $-0.76(\hat{\sigma}_{WR}), 0.76(\hat{\sigma}_{WR})$ for ln-Cmax, then scaled average bioequivalence is successfully demonstrated under the European approach.

Certain caveats to the scaled average bioequivalence two one-sided hypothesis tests for ln-Cmax are applied. If $\hat{\sigma}_{WR} > 0.4723$, then σ_{WR} is set to 0.4723 in the null hypotheses for ln-Cmax. This choice of limit (0.4723) appears to be based upon constraint to allow for widening of acceptance criteria to correspond to 50% CVw but no farther. For example, if, for ln-Cmax $\hat{\sigma}_{WR} = 0.48$, then the 90% confidence interval for $\mu_T - \mu_R = \delta$ should fall within the limits $\pm 0.76(0.4723)$ NOT $\pm 0.76(0.48)$ to declare scaled average bioequivalence. Last, if scaled average bioequivalence is used, $0.80 < e^{\hat{\delta}} < 1.25$ must also be shown for Cmax in the study.

In effect, this allows for widening of the acceptance criteria from $\mp \ln 1.25$ up to a maximum of $\mp \ln 1.4319$ for ln-Cmax based on observed reference formulation variability, subject to caveats that there is prior clinical justification, previous observation of high variability, pre-specification of the testing procedure in the study protocol, actual observation of high variability, and an acceptable observed point estimate for ln-Cmax. For clarity again, none of this applies to ln-AUC. That endpoint must meet the traditional average bioequivalence acceptance criteria. If the observed estimate for within-subject reference formulation standard deviation $\hat{\sigma}_{WR} < 0.294$ in the study for ln-Cmax, then the traditional average bioequivalence testing approach is also used to test ln-Cmax.

The European guidance also requires that a certain set of models be used for analysis ([319, 322]). The fixed effect model of interest in the guidance is described in Chapters 3 and 4, and so will not be discussed further here. We will explore these using the data of

Chapter 4, Example 4.4, using SAS code. These data and code may also be found on the website. For the comparison of the reference formulation to test formulation to derive a 90% confidence interval for $\mu_T - \mu_R$, the code to fit the desired model is ([322]):

```
proc glm data=four;
class formula subject period sequence;
model ln_auc=sequence subject(sequence) period
 formula;
test h=sequence e=subject(sequence);
lsmeans formula/adjust=t pdiff=control("R") CL
ALPHA=0.1;
run;
proc glm data=four;
class formula subject period sequence;
model ln_cmax=sequence subject(sequence) period
formula;
test h=sequence e=subject(sequence);
lsmeans formula/adjust=t pdiff=control("R") CL
ALPHA=0.1;
run;
```

This model is the same as that utilized in Chapters 3 and 4 for complete datasets. The within-subject variability estimate obtained from the model and used to estimate the confidence interval is assumed to be homogeneous across formulations (i.e., $\sigma^2_{WR} = \sigma^2_{WT} = \sigma^2_W$). Where there is missing data, however, no imputation method is used to recover information (see Chapter 5 and [652] for more information). Hence results using `proc glm` may differ from `proc mixed` in datasets with missing data, but match for complete datasets. This particular data set has missing data, and readers may explore the difference between application of a fixed effect model relative to a mixed effect model using the data and code on the website.

The rationale for the preference for use of `proc glm` in this guidance versus `proc mixed` is described in detail in [322]. To summarize, as only the 90% confidence interval for $\mu_T - \mu_R$ and σ^2_{WR} for ln-Cmax are of interest in this setting for formal bioequivalence hypothesis testing, the guidance focuses consideration of potential models to estimate only the specific parameters that are needed for inference to simplify data interpretation. The use of this particular fixed effect model should be stated in the protocol to meet European requirements ([319]).

Readers may verify that the estimates of $\hat{\delta}$ (90% CI) are 0.1002 (0.0289, 0.1715) for ln-AUC and 0.4140 (0.2890, 0.5389) for ln-Cmax using the data for Example 4.4 and code on the website. Clearly, average bioequivalence is not demonstrated for ln-Cmax, and we can already tell that scaled average bioequivalence for ln-Cmax is not possible as the point estimate for $e^{\hat{\delta}} > 1.25$.

However, to formally evaluate scaled average bioequivalence for ln-Cmax, an estimate for σ_{WR} is needed. The estimate of variability for the reference formulation for ln-Cmax is to be obtained using the following code ([322]):

```
data var;set four;
if formula='R';run;

proc glm data=var;
class subject period sequence;
model ln_cmax=sequence subject(sequence) period;
run;
```

The resulting mean squared error parameter is the estimate for $\hat{\sigma}^2_{WR}$, and here it is 0.3097 such that $\hat{\sigma}_{WR}$ is 0.5565, which is clearly a highly variable finding. This estimate is used to determine the scaled average bioequivalence acceptance region for ln-Cmax. In this setting, the null hypotheses would then be constrained to

$$H_{01}: \quad \frac{\mu_T - \mu_R}{0.4723} \leq -0.76 \tag{7.11}$$

or

$$H_{02}: \quad \frac{\mu_T - \mu_R}{0.4723} \geq 0.76 \tag{7.12}$$

as $\hat{\sigma}_{WR} = 0.5565 > 0.4723$, and the acceptance region for ln-Cmax would therefore be the 90% confidence interval falling within $\pm 0.76(0.4723) = \mp 0.3589$.

As H_{02} is not rejected for ln-Cmax, with the upper 90% confidence bound falling above 0.3589, scaled average bioequivalence is not demonstrated.

The required sample sizes to achieve the European scaled average bioequivalence requirement for ln −Cmax may be found in [1249] and are reproduced with the kind permission of Professor Endrenyi in Tables 7.1 and 7.2 for partial replicate (three-period) and replicate (four-period) designs, respectively. Readers should note that SAS code for sample size derivations to determine the number of subjects required for ln-AUC using the traditional average bioequivalence approach is given in Chapter 5.

So, to design a European scaled average bioequivalence study, estimates of δ and of σ^2_W are required for ln-AUC and of δ and of σ^2_{WR} are required for ln-Cmax. We will use the estimates from Example 4.4 for illustrative purposes. Using the desired European model, the resulting estimates are $\hat{\delta} = 0.1002$ and $\hat{\sigma}^2_W = 0.0984$ for ln-AUC and $\hat{\delta} = 0.4140$ and $\hat{\sigma}^2_{WR} = 0.3097$ for ln-Cmax. It should be noted that ln-AUC is also highly variable in this example given the definition currently in use; however, the European guidance explicitly requires that bioequivalence for ln-AUC be demonstrated using the traditional average bioequivalence approach [319].

The CV_{WR} for Cmax is estimated as:

$$CV_{WR} = \sqrt{e^{0.3097} - 1} = 60.3\%.$$

For the purposes of this illustrative sample size derivation, we will assume that the $\hat{\delta}$ observed in Example 4.4 for ln-AUC and ln-Cmax were mistaken and apply a $\delta = 0$ for uniformity across endpoints. This corresponds to a GMR (see Tables 7.1 and 7.2) of $e^0 = 1$. In practice one would assume this would vary by at least 5% (see Chapter 5), but we will neglect that aspect for this example.

From Tables 7.1 and 7.2, we see that $n = 41$ subjects are required for scaled average bioequivalence testing of ln-Cmax using a three-period design (with sequences RRT, RTR, TRR) for 90% power and that $n = 29$ subjects are required for scaled average bioequivalence testing using a four-period replicate design (with sequences RTRT, TRTR) for 90% power. As more periods are required for the three-period design, it is likely that the replicate design would be applied. As such, we need to confirm that the sample size of $n = 29$ is adequate for average bioequivalence testing of ln-AUC based on the variability estimate and applying a replicate design. This is left as a exercise for interested readers (note that modification to the code given in Chapter 5 should be applied), and it is found that at least 90% power is provided for ln-AUC using the above design assumptions.

We now turn to the FDA alternative proposal for scaled average bioequivalence testing.

TABLE 7.1: Sample Sizes for the European Scaled Average Bioequivalence Requirements in Three-Period Studies

	GMR							
CV_{WR}	0.85	0.90	0.95	1.00	1.05	1.10	1.15	1.20
80% Power								
30%	194	53	27	22	26	45	104	>201
35%	127	51	29	25	29	45	84	>201
40%	90	44	29	27	30	42	68	139
45%	77	40	29	27	29	37	57	124
50%	75	40	30	28	30	37	53	133
55%	81	42	32	30	32	40	56	172
60%	88	46	36	33	36	44	63	>201
65%	99	53	40	37	40	50	71	>201
70%	109	58	45	41	45	56	80	>201
75%	136	67	50	46	50	62	89	>201
80%	144	72	54	51	55	68	97	>201
90% Power								
30%	>201	74	36	28	36	62	147	>201
35%	181	70	39	32	39	63	117	>201
40%	130	61	38	33	39	57	94	>201
45%	132	55	37	33	38	51	85	>201
50%	158	55	39	34	38	51	84	>201
55%	178	59	41	37	41	53	97	>201
60%	199	64	45	41	46	60	112	>201
65%	>201	72	51	46	51	67	125	>201
70%	>201	82	57	52	57	76	141	>201
75%	>201	93	66	58	64	85	161	>201
80%	>201	100	70	63	71	93	176	>201
CV: Coefficient of variation; GMR: Ratio of geometric means								
Reproduced with permission from [1249] Table A1								

TABLE 7.2: Sample Sizes for the European Scaled Average Bioequivalence Requirements in Four-Period Studies

	GMR							
CV_{WR}	0.85	0.90	0.95	1.00	1.05	1.10	1.15	1.20
80% Power								
30%	127	35	19	15	18	30	68	>201
35%	88	34	20	18	20	31	57	140
40%	64	31	20	18	20	28	47	98
CV: Coefficient of variation; GMR: Ratio of geometric means								
Reproduced with permission from [1249] Table A2								

TABLE 7.2: Sample Sizes for the European Scaled Average Bioequivalence Requirements in Four-Period Studies (continued)

	GMR							
CV_{WR}	0.85	0.90	0.95	1.00	1.05	1.10	1.15	1.20
45%	57	29	21	19	21	27	41	90
50%	54	28	22	20	21	27	38	100
55%	55	30	23	21	23	28	40	116
60%	60	32	25	23	25	31	44	124
65%	74	37	28	26	28	33	49	155
70%	78	40	31	28	31	38	55	167
75%	85	45	34	32	34	42	61	186
80%	95	50	38	35	37	46	66	>201
90% Power								
30%	180	49	25	19	24	42	95	>201
35%	123	48	27	22	27	43	80	>201
40%	93	42	26	23	26	39	66	165
45%	90	40	27	24	27	37	59	181
50%	102	39	27	25	27	36	60	>201
55%	123	41	29	26	29	38	63	>201
60%	139	45	32	29	31	41	71	>201
65%	159	51	36	32	35	46	81	>201
70%	172	55	40	36	40	52	97	>201
75%	195	62	43	39	44	58	106	>201
80%	>201	69	49	45	49	62	113	>201
CV: Coefficient of variation; GMR: Ratio of geometric means								
Reproduced with permission from [1249] Table A2								

7.3 Scaled Average Bioequivalence in the USA

Detailed summaries of the background for the FDA's approach to scaled average bioequivalence testing may be found in [242, 243]. To summarize, highly variable findings were observed in 11% of average bioequivalence studies submitted in the USA to the Office of Generic Drugs of the FDA from 2003 to 2005. For these highly variable studies, to meet the standard average bioequivalence requirements, sample sizes were increased in standard 2×2 bioequivalence designs by 15 to 23 subjects on average (depending upon whether AUC or Cmax or both were highly variable) relative to the sample sizes used for lower variability products. Most of the highly variable drugs were subject to extensive first-order metabolism (i.e., the liver modifies the drug extensively as it is absorbed through the gut wall to aid in excretion — see Chapter 1), but they are approved as safe and effective drugs by the FDA (and presumably have been marketed and followed for safety and efficacy for some time prior to patent expiration). The FDA therefore viewed it as a matter of public interest to develop a scaled average bioequivalence procedure to ensure availability of (less expensive) generic versions of highly variable drugs by decreasing the burden of proof on the sponsors of such generic versions. An FDA working group was formed to study the approaches to do so.

The FDA's working group [497, 498] considered the approach adopted in European guidance but recommended a different procedure be used which does not restrict the application of scaled average bioequivalence testing to ln-Cmax alone but allows for ln-AUC testing as well. As in the European procedure, this procedure accounts for the observed variability of σ^2_{WR}. For ln-AUC and for ln-Cmax separately, the following null hypothesis is to be tested:

$$H_0: \quad \frac{\delta^2}{\sigma^2_{WR}} \geq \theta \tag{7.13}$$

where $\delta = \mu_T - \mu_R$ is the difference in formulation means and σ^2_{WR} is the within-subject reference formulation variance. Here $\theta = \frac{(\ln(1.25))^2}{0.25^2} = 0.797$ based upon [497], and the denominator appears to be chosen based on the findings in [90].

Expression (7.13) is generally reparameterized to

$$H_0: \quad \delta^2 - \theta(\sigma^2_{WR}) \geq 0 \tag{7.14}$$

for the purposes of application of the methods developed in [616] to derive a confidence interval using the method-of-moments estimates $\hat{\delta}$ and $\hat{\sigma}^2_{WR}$. An approximate 95% upper confidence bound is derived for $\delta^2 - \theta(\sigma^2_{WR})$ [616], and if these upper bounds fall below 0 for both ln-AUC and ln-Cmax, then scaled average bioequivalence is demonstrated.

Application of the method of [616] to derive an approximate 95% upper bound may be found in the appendix to [1245]. In brief, upper 95% confidence bounds are derived for δ^2 and for $-\theta(\sigma^2_{WR})$ which are referred to here as UB_δ and UB_σ based upon the observed ln-AUC and for ln-Cmax separately. An approximate 95% confidence upper bound for the expression $\delta^2 - \theta(\sigma^2_{WR})$ is then

$$\hat{\delta}^2 - \theta(\hat{\sigma}^2_{WR}) + \sqrt{(UB_\delta - \hat{\delta}^2)^2 + (UB_\sigma - (-\theta(\hat{\sigma}^2_{WR})))^2}.$$

The FDA recommends [243] that a partial replicate design (sequences RRT, RTR, TRR) be used, but a replicate design (sequences RTRT, TRTR) may also be applied. A minimum of 24 subjects is required to meet the FDA's requirements.

It should be noted that, as with the European approach, certain caveats are applied. Those being that $0.80 < e^{\hat{\delta}} < 1.25$ must be shown for AUC and for Cmax, and if $\hat{\sigma}_{WR} < 0.294$ is observed in the study for ln-AUC or for ln-Cmax, then the standard average bioequivalence testing procedure using the mixed model specified in Chapter 5 [243, 395] is to be applied for that endpoint. Evidence of previous highly variable findings should be provided to the FDA when the protocol is submitted [395] as a basis for the use of the scaled average bioequivalence testing method, and this testing procedure must be stated in the study protocol.

SAS code for this approach in partial replicate and replicate designs may be found in [391, 395] and also is available on the website for replicate designs. We will apply the approach using the data from Example 4.4.

For ln-AUC, the estimate for $\hat{\delta}$ is 0.1046 with 90% CI of (0.0311, 0.1780) and for $-\theta(\hat{\sigma}^2_{WR})$ it is −0.0940 with 95% upper confidence bound of −0.0697. The resulting approximate 95% confidence bound for testing expression (7.14) is therefore

$$0.0109 - 0.0940 + \sqrt{(0.1780^2 - 0.0109)^2 + (-0.0697 + 0.0940)^2} = -0.0511.$$

Using the code available on the website, readers may confirm that the resulting approximate 95% confidence bound for testing expression (7.14) for ln-Cmax is 0.0827. So, using the data from Example 4.4, it was found that scaled average bioequivalence was demonstrated for AUC, but, as with the European approach, not for Cmax.

The required sample size, to achieve the FDA scaled average bioequivalence requirement for ln-AUC and/or ln-Cmax may be found in [1249] and are reproduced with the kind permission of Professor Endrenyi in Tables 7.3 and 7.4 for partial replicate (three-period) and replicate (four-period) designs, respectively.

So, to design a USA scaled average bioequivalence study, estimates of δ and of σ^2_{WR} are required for ln-AUC and ln-Cmax. We will use the estimates from Example 4.4 for illustrative purposes. These may be found in the previous section, and we will also apply the other assumptions made there for the purposes of this example (i.e., $\delta = 0$).

As Cmax has the larger estimate of variability, it will primarily determine the sample size. From Tables 7.3 and 7.4, we see that $n = 30$ subjects are required for scaled average bioequivalence testing using a three-period design (with sequences RRT, RTR, TRR) for 90% power and that $n = 22$ subjects are required for scaled average bioequivalence testing using a four-period replicate design (with sequences RTRT, TRTR) for 90% power. Note that the minimum number of subjects required by the FDA is 24.

Preliminary information on the success of this scaled average approach to testing for bioequivalence may be found in [244]. It also appears that the FDA has implemented a post-marketing surveillance system to ensure that efficacy and safety of generic products approved using this approach are monitored [1393].

We now turn to some additional observations on these testing procedures.

TABLE 7.3: Sample Sizes for the Scaled Average Bioequivalence Requirements of the FDA in Three-Period Studies

	GMR							
CV_{WR}	0.85	0.90	0.95	1.00	1.05	1.10	1.15	1.20
80% Power								
30%	145	45	24	21	24	39	82	>201
35%	74	37	24	22	25	34	54	109
40%	60	33	24	22	24	31	47	104
45%	59	31	23	22	24	29	43	116
50%	66	30	24	22	23	28	41	133
55%	80	30	24	22	24	28	44	172
60%	88	31	24	23	24	30	50	>201
65%	98	32	25	24	25	31	53	>201
70%	106	35	26	25	26	31	62	>201
75%	136	38	27	26	27	34	70	>201
80%	144	40	29	27	29	37	76	>201
90% Power								
30%	>201	65	33	26	32	55	122	>201
35%	106	51	32	28	32	47	77	186
40%	99	45	31	28	31	43	68	>201
45%	128	43	30	28	30	40	69	>201
50%	158	45	31	28	30	40	79	>201
55%	178	50	31	28	31	42	96	>201
60%	199	54	33	30	34	50	112	>201
65%	>201	61	35	32	36	53	125	>201
70%	>201	68	39	34	37	61	141	>201
75%	>201	80	43	37	41	68	161	>201
80%	>201	83	48	41	47	75	176	>201
CV: Coefficient of variation; GMR: Ratio of geometric means								
Reproduced with permission from [1249] Table A3								

TABLE 7.4: Sample Sizes for the Scaled Average Bioequivalence Requirements of the FDA in Four-Period Studies

	GMR							
CV_{WR}	0.85	0.90	0.95	1.00	1.05	1.10	1.15	1.20
80% Power								
30%	96	30	17	15	17	27	55	200
35%	54	26	18	16	18	24	39	79
40%	43	24	18	16	17	22	33	72
45%	44	23	18	16	17	21	32	82
50%	45	22	17	17	17	21	31	99
55%	52	22	18	17	17	21	31	116
60%	58	23	18	17	18	21	34	124
65%	74	24	19	18	18	22	36	155
70%	75	24	19	18	19	23	44	167
75%	81	26	20	19	20	24	47	186
80%	95	29	21	20	20	25	51	>201
90% Power								
30%	152	44	23	18	22	38	81	>201
35%	80	38	23	20	23	34	55	128
40%	70	32	22	20	22	30	48	158
45%	84	32	22	20	22	30	49	181
50%	102	32	23	20	22	30	54	>201
55%	123	34	23	21	22	31	61	>201
60%	139	38	24	22	24	33	71	>201
65%	159	44	26	23	25	35	81	>201
70%	172	46	26	24	27	43	97	>201
75%	195	53	29	26	29	48	106	>201
80%	>201	60	33	28	31	51	113	>201
CV: Coefficient of variation; GMR: Ratio of geometric means								
Reproduced with permission from [1249] Table A4								

7.4 Discussion and Cautions

Expanding the traditional average bioequivalence limits has been studied previously using simulation in the context of protection of public health. It was reported in [537] that

> It seems difficult to justify expanding the general BE limit to 70%/143% for Cmax, for either fasting or fed BE studies, in the average bioequivalence approach without an adequate scientific or clinical rationale other than intra-subject variability.

Demonstrating average bioequivalence for a highly variable drug is harder, but it is doable by using replicate and group-sequential designs [966] (see also Chapter 5). The benefit that one achieves by taking such an established approach is that average bioequivalence is internationally accepted (see Chapter 2), but in addition, very importantly, the average bioequivalence method is known to be protective of public health when multiple generic versions enter the marketplace [23]. Generally, when generic formulations are approved and given market access, the original marketer stops marketing the original formulation as the demand decreases with increasing supply. Patients may be routinely switched from a generic formulation to alternative generic formulations in an uncontrolled manner driven by marketplace availability and pricing when they routinely fill their prescription at the pharmacy.

Obviously, at the time of this publication, an international standard is not in place for scaled average bioequivalence. Generic to generic switching has not been extensively studied for the scaled average bioequivalence approaches.

We recommend that those using such scaled average bioequivalence approaches consult the regulatory bodies where application for market access is to be requested to ensure the acceptability of whatever approach is proposed, obviously prior to study initiation. We also recommend that those using such approaches ensure their sponsoring company clearly understands that an international standard is not yet available (as of the time of this publication).

Several authors have commented on the undesirable statistical properties of the European and USA scaled average bioequivalence methods (in particular the caveats and constraints associated with their application), and those interested in more information will find [675, 676, 905, 976, 1207, 1249, 1354] of interest. We will not comment further here except to note that we believe post-marketing safety and efficacy monitoring is wise for products which are approved using such scaled average bioequivalence approaches.

Part III

Clinical Pharmacology

8

Clinical Pharmacology Safety Studies

Introduction

One day, out of seemingly nowhere, I received a very strange request from a clinical scientist. We will call her Betty, and she asked if I could round off a confidence interval. My immediate response was, 'No. Why would anyone want to do that?'

In essence, we had derived an upper bound in a drug interaction trial of 1.2538 for AUC. Evaluation of this value relative to the acceptance level of 1.25 showed that it was higher than 1.25. We could not conclude the two treatments were equivalent. Pretty elementary. Betty wanted to round it off, so she could claim equivalence had been demonstrated.

I told her no, and left it at that. Such would misrepresent the data, and the statistics underlying the upper bound could not support "rounding it off." Clearly, as the value was higher than 1.25, the null hypothesis had not been rejected, and it was out of the realm of possibility. To my mind it was also a matter of professional integrity, and I was a bit surprised that anyone would ask such a thing. The less I said, the better off we would both be.

However, I was still new on the job, and did not know that some people will not take no for an answer, even if it is a matter of professional integrity. So began one of my most important "learning experiences" on the job. "Learning experiences" are a business euphemism for an experience no one in their right mind wants any part of, but you are stuck with it because you work there.

Rounding off turned out to be really, very important to Betty and the physician for whom she worked, and a major disagreement at the company developed. Peoples' egos became involved, and everyone who had even only a nebulous stake in this (or a potentially related) issue felt compelled to comment. Academic experts were paid and consulted. Opinions were sought from the FDA on the topic. Many internal meetings on the topic were held, and (despite their best efforts to avoid it) several senior vice presidents had to be consulted and in the end backed us up: "No rounding."

Years later FDA guidance [373] was issued saying the same thing, but, as is often the case, such business precedes regulatory guidance by many years.

Guess who was at the center of this argument? It was a rough experience (for what I still feel was a ridiculous request), but I learned a lot from interacting with such people on such a thing and from watching how they and many other people behaved. If I had it to do over again, I would have followed a different approach to dealing with such people. I call it the "Nurse" approach in honor of the people whom I saw do it.

We had a drug intended for the treatment of hypertension (high blood pressure) which caused migraines if given at high doses. We discovered this in the first study in man (which is designed for this purpose, see Section 8.1), and carefully worked out at which dose the problem started. These were bad migraines — the throwing-up kind. The study team wanted to stop the study, but a chief medic said to continue. The rationale was that they wanted to explore more doses before going to the next study.

There was no point in continuing. The study had defined the maximum tolerated dose, completing its objective. We were at an impasse with the medic involved. We discussed the ethical issue of continuing (i.e., not), but were told headache and emesis were not a serious enough side effect to warrant not exploring further. Egos began to become involved. Senior vice presidents were again getting phone calls.

This came to an abrupt stop, and the nurses put a stop to it. I am told that they told chief medic that, if he wanted to continue, he'd have to come down and clean up the vomit himself. The study ended the next day. That was not the official reason logged in the study file, and it is hearsay, but I think it is probably true.

The moral of the story is that, when you are asked to do something you consider inappropriate, put the person who is asking in your shoes. When they will actually have to get their own hands (or shoes) dirty to do such a thing and take personal accountability for it, you will be surprised at how the pressure to do so suddenly lets up. If not, then try "No".

When exploring safety, it is important that we get it right for the sake of each and every patient who will take the product. Everyone has a stake in this assessment. Even the people who develop and sell drugs may themselves have to take them one day! All drugs have side-effects and should be presumed to be unsafe if used incorrectly. Some side-effects can be very serious and life-threatening.

The role of clinical pharmacology safety studies is to define how the body handles the drug such that side-effects can be predicted in a rational, scientific manner. This assessment determines how the drug should be used correctly to treat the condition under study. Every decimal point matters. Do not cut any corners which would compromise patients' safety, and ensure your findings represent the data accurately, so that the people using the drug can make a fully informed decision.

8.1 Background

All other things considered, it is comparatively easy to tell when a drug is efficacious. The drug should change something about the body or its characteristics for the better, making people live longer or healthier or both. A drug that does not offer such benefit (referred to as medical utility or efficacy, see Chapter 2) would presumably not be approved for sale to a human population. The problem in drug development is to detect, observe, and ensure that the change is to the benefit of patients.

Drugs that are unsafe, producing unwanted, nonbeneficial side-effects, presumably should not be approved. This, however, constitutes a more complex issue (and one that is still evolving). The difficulty is how to deduce how and when a drug is safe. In contrast to efficacy assessment, in safety assessment the problem is to assess and ensure that no clinically relevant change in the health status of patients results from use of the drug beyond the decreased health status associated with natural factors (like aging, for example).

This problem initially seems similar to bioequivalence testing in that the desired outcome is to test for no change in the potential for hazard relative to control agent (say another drug in the same class) or placebo. The problem is different in that in bioequivalence testing, we understand and have a historical basis for the assessment of the potential for hazard using pharmacokinetics as a surrogate marker; i.e., if AUC goes down too much in a new formulation, efficacy may be lost, and if Cmax goes up too much, side-effects may appear.

In safety testing for new drugs, though, we do not know what the potential for hazard actually is in a human population! The relationship of rate and extent of exposure needs to be established relative to unknown (but presumably present) side-effects before such an assessment is valid scientifically.

Our working assumption is initially that the drug is not safe when given at any dose in any formulation under any circumstances to any human population. As a practical matter, it is also important to recognize that we will never be able to demonstrate the alternative to this assumption, i.e., that the drug is safe at any dose in any formulation under all circumstances when given to any person. All drugs are potentially toxic if used incorrectly; however, some may be used at appropriate, carefully selected, and studied doses in controlled circumstances to treat diseases in particular populations.

Following preclinical safety assessment to ensure that the new drug is not toxic at low doses (discussed in greater detail in the next section), clinical pharmacology safety assessment of a new drug product usually starts with giving the drug in very low doses and placebo to a robust, healthy population — normal healthy volunteers. The rationale for doing so is that if the new drug causes unexpected side-effects, healthy people are most likely to recover. It is relatively easy to monitor them closely, and any side-effects identified will not be confounded with disease (as normal healthy volunteers should not have any). Some patients may eventually be willing to tolerate side-effects if their underlying disease is treatable, but one cannot really assess that potential until one knows what the side-effects are! Sometimes, however, it is impossible to dose normal healthy volunteers (e.g., it is unethical to give a cytotoxic oncology agent to a normal healthy person). For such drugs, clinical pharmacology safety assessment begins in patients with the condition under study.

Dosing starts with very low doses, well under the no adverse effect level (NOAEL) seen in the most sensitive preclinical species, and slowly the dose is increased in these initial safety studies until

1. Side-effects are observed (e.g., nausea, headache, changes in laboratory values), or
2. Rate (Cmax) or extent (AUC) of exposure approach the NOAEL.

The intent of these small (generally cross-over [852, 853]), well-controlled, cautious designs is to carefully assess evidence of the potential of the drug to cause a hazard to people taking the drug. Note, however, that absence of evidence is NOT evidence of absence [647]. If side-effects are not observed and dosing is halted with exposures near the NOAEL, the potential for significant hazard still exists (even if remote). If a side-effect is observed, its relationship to exposure and dose may then be quantified. Additionally, once a potential hazard is identified, safety may be assessed relative to other agents used for treating the population for which the drug is intended.

The role of statistics in this setting is different from bioequivalence testing. Here, statistics are used to quantify the unknown relationship of unwanted side-effects to dose and exposure while dose is varied over the course of the study. A non-null relationship of dose or exposure to a safety endpoint demonstrates the *statistical* potential for hazard [621]. Note, however, that statistical potential does not necessarily imply that the drug is unsafe and should not be used or developed. Its benefits (efficacy) may outweigh the presence of these side-effects, but that is up to the clinicians, regulators, and patients who will be using the drug to determine. Statistics provide an impartial assessment in this setting to aid them in making this determination. All drugs are unsafe; some are useful under carefully controlled circumstances (to limit the risks involved).

Regulators do have requirements for formally studying (i.e., the size of the safety database) and how to look at safety for approval to market (see, for example, [396], [505]); however, that is not the topic here. Clinical pharmacology safety studies are used to study safety in preparation for subsequent studies in clinical development.

Once the relationship of dose and exposure to safety is understood, clinical pharmacology studies are then performed to assess under what circumstances it is safe to administer the drug. For example, one would study what happens when the drug is given with and without food or with and without another drug.

In this chapter, we will explore commonly used statistical methods for clinical pharmacology assessment of dose and assessments of certain circumstances to determine if and when the drug can be dosed with a reasonable expectation of safety while treating a disease. Such studies limit but do NOT eliminate the potential for hazard when using a drug. Hazards cannot be eliminated with 100% certainty, as we know from Chapter 1.

Note that "reasonable expectation" is not well defined in regulatory guidance. Safety is currently an emerging scientific topic (e.g., [626]). Whether a drug is safe (or not) is subjective. Physicians, patients, regulators, and drug-makers all have different opinions on the topic.

Operationally, and usually, statistics are derived post hoc — after the study has ended. Decisions about what dose to give in these studies and how to dose titrate are made by clinical personnel. The role of statistics is to assess and precisely quantify the relationship of dose to pharmacokinetics and dose to safety endpoints once the study is completed.

In some situations ([946, 962, 1139, 1142, 1143]), quantitative interactive models may be used to assist clinical personnel in selecting doses "on-line," and we will consider an example in the next section. This is by no means an exhaustive list of work on this topic, and readers may wish to examine recent publications on the topic (e.g., [1232], [282], and [1329, 1332]). These procedures use models to predict what effects will be observed at different doses to aid in clinical decision making. However, the final decision about what dose is used is the physician's responsibility and the subject's or patient's responsibility before taking a drug.

Safety assessment in clinical pharmacology and drug development is a rapidly evolving science. It has not always done well in the rush to get drugs to needy patient populations. Historically [1222], over-dosing is common as a result, and there have been numerous circumstances where the approved dose of drug has been reduced once the drug has been on the market for a time. It has been said [979] that in the 20th century drugs were presumed to be safe until shown otherwise. However, increasing attention from regulatory agencies is being applied to this area in light of recent safety risks [1121], and major refinements and improvements in how we test for safety in clinical studies may be expected in the coming years.

Some areas (e.g., pharmacokinetics in pregnancy) have not been well studied [718], and we encourage those engaging in what limited research there is in such areas to take advantage of modelling techniques (e.g., this chapter as a starting point) to maximize the information from such limited data sources.

8.2 First-Time-in-Humans

The administration of a drug to humans for the first time generates a great deal of excitement in the sponsoring organization and is an exciting time for everyone involved. New therapies offer potential benefit to numerous patients. Before such a drug can be administered, however, it must undergo an extensive battery of in vitro and in vivo preclinical testing. In certain nations (e.g., USA, Europe), first-time-in-humans study protocols and their supporting preclinical information must also be submitted to and approved by the relevant regulatory authorities (see [356] for an example).

Regulators will, in general, desire to review the following items prior to administration of a new drug to humans [356]:

1. The first-time-in-humans (FTiH) study protocol,
2. Information on the chemistry, manufacturing, and control/stability of the drug manufacturing process,
3. Information on preclinical pharmacology and toxicology in vitro and in vivo stud-

ies (containing, at a minimum, an integrated summary of animal toxicology study findings and the study protocols), and

4. Any human experience with the investigational drug (e.g., if studies were carried out in a different nation).

We now turn to consideration of the FTiH trial design, conduct, and analysis and will not discuss these regulatory requirements further here.

In contrast to bioequivalence trials (the objective of which is to confirm equivalence of different formulations), the objective of FTiH and other Phase I trials is to learn [1142] about the safety, pharmacokinetic, and pharmacodynamic properties of the drug being studied. The application of statistics to this topic of drug development is fundamentally different from that used in the confirmatory setting of bioequivalence, though the study designs, conduct, and models used in such studies are similar.

The approach to data analysis and interpretation is typically inductive (see Chapter 5) in that those performing FTiH and Phase 1 studies have a "rough" idea of how the drug will behave (from the preclinical testing described previously). Studies are performed and data are collected to reinforce this "rough" idea. The role of statistics in this setting is to employ the tools discussed previously (Chapter 1: randomization, replication, blinding, blocking, and modelling) to ensure the estimates provided by such studies are accurate and precise.

It would be desirable if the preclinical findings were perfectly predictive of what one would observe in humans for a new drug, but this is not always the case. There are interspecies differences which preclude such a possibility (for example, see Chapter 31 [30]). George Box stated that, "To find out what happens to a system when you interfere with it you have to interfere with it (not just observe it)" [105], and the assumption made for any new drug is that it will cause undesirable side-effects (hereafter referred to as adverse events, AEs) that are dose and exposure dependent, in that the higher the dose or exposure, the more likely such an AE will occur.

An adverse experience (AE) is any untoward medical occurrence in a patient or clinical investigation subject, temporally associated with the use of a medicinal product, whether or not considered related to the medicinal product. Such events are frequently characterized as

1. Mild: An event that is easily tolerated by the subject, causing minimal discomfort and not interfering with everyday activities.
2. Moderate: An event that is sufficiently discomforting to interfere with normal everyday activities.
3. Severe: An event that prevents normal everyday activities.

A severe AE is an AE that is noticed and alarming (e.g., severe nausea or emesis), but does not necessarily require cessation of treatment (the disease under study, like cancer, might make such an event tolerable though undesirable).

In contrast, a **serious** AE (SAE) is "an event that is fatal, life-threatening, requires in-patient hospitalization or prolongs hospitalization, results in persistent or significant disability, or results in congenital anomaly or birth defect" (Chapter 14 [95]). Observation of such an SAE in a FTiH study would generally halt dosing for all subjects being studied and must be reported quickly to relevant regulatory authorities.

In FTiH trials, dose is increased as knowledge is gained of the drug's properties until a "potential for hazard" is observed. "Potential for hazard" in this context denotes the observation of conditions where it is possible for an adverse reaction to drug treatment to occur or the actual observation of a serious or severe AE. A dose just lower than this dose is defined as the maximum tolerated dose (MTD) [621].

Statistical proof of hazard (i.e., a p-value less than 0.05 for a comparison of $H_0 : \mu_D - \mu_P \leq 0$ where μ_D denotes the mean effect at a dose and μ_P denotes the mean effect on placebo [540]) may or may not be obtained in such studies. Determination of the MTD is often driven more by clinical judgment and less by statistical analysis given the limited numbers of subjects exposed to a drug in such studies. If the drug-induced rate of an adverse experience in the population is p for a particular dose, then the chance one sees at least one such event in n subjects exposed to a dose of drug in a study is $1 - (1 - p)^n$. As FTiH trials typically involve only a small number of patients or subjects (sample sizes per dose ranging from $n = 6$ to 10), p must be relatively large in order to observe an AE in the trial. For example, if $p = 0.1$ (the proportion of subjects experiencing, for example, a headache caused by a drug at a dose) and $n = 6$ subjects are studied at this dose, the probability of observing at least one subject with a headache in the trial is only 0.47 at this dose.

For a rare side-effect (drug-induced neutropenia, for example), with a $p = 0.01$, the probability of observing such an event in a FTiH trial is only 0.06 with $n = 6$. Thus FTiH trials are geared toward detection of non-rare side-effects. If the drug causes a side-effect in less than 5% to 10% of people at a given dose, it is most unlikely that such trials will observe such an event.

Cross-over designs are generally employed for the purposes of informative dose-escalation in FTiH and Phase I studies, as such designs are known to be more informative and provide better information than alternative designs [1139] and expose only a limited number of subjects to the (potentially) harmful agent. See Table 8.1, for example. Dosing is conducted in separate cohorts, sequentially, with results from each dose being reviewed prior to the next dose being administered in the next period. Periods are separated by a washout sufficient to ensure no drug is on board when the next dose is given (generally at least one week to allow for pharmacokinetic washout and review of data).

TABLE 8.1
Schematic Plan of a First-Time-in-Humans Cross-Over Study

Subject	Period 1	Period 2	Period 3	Period 4
		Cohort 1		
1	P	D1	D2	D3
2	D1	P	D2	D3
3	D1	D2	P	D3
4	D1	D2	D3	P
		Cohort 2		
5	P	D4	D5	D6
6	D4	P	D5	D6
7	D4	D5	P	D6
8	D4	D5	D6	P
		Cohort 3		
9	P	D7	D8	D9
		......		
P=Placebo; D1=Lowest Dose D2=2nd lowest dose; etc.				

Placebo is administered to serve as a control for evaluation of any AEs observed, and subjects are randomly assigned to the period in which they receive it. Subjects are generally kept blinded as to whether they have received drug or placebo in order to ensure that safety reporting and assessment of severity are unbiased by knowledge of treatment.

Depending on the NOAEL and properties of the drug under study, shorter cross-over designs (i.e., two-period or three-period designs) may be employed. For particularly toxic drugs, oncology trials of cytotoxic agents are generally conducted using a parallel group design where cohorts of patients are randomized to increasing doses of drug (Chapter 1 [95]). We will consider an example later in this chapter but will first focus attention on how to model data from a typical trial. Such techniques also apply to the shorter cross-over designs described above.

Preclinical pharmacology and toxicology data are used to choose the FTiH starting doses. The preclinical pharmacology and toxicology studies should identify a no-effect dose and a no-adverse-effect exposure level in multiple preclinical species. Allometric scaling ([371, 1027], Chapter 8 [95]) is then applied to estimate a safe starting dose. In essence, allometric scaling uses the NOAEL and accounts for differences in weight and physiology between species to yield a range of doses expected to be safe in humans. The NOAEL in the most sensitive species (i.e., the lowest NOAEL) is defined as the upper limit of human exposure (AUC and Cmax, as previously).

Once a presumed safe range of doses is estimated, an algebraic dose escalation scheme (1x, 2x, 3x, 4x, etc.), geometric dose escalation scheme (1x, 2x, 4x, 8x, etc.), or Fibonacci scheme (Chapter 1 [95] and Chapter 31 [30]) is used to determine the next dose to administer in the next period or cohort of subjects. The choice of dose escalation scheme is pre-specified in the study protocol. The choice of next dose may be reduced (but not increased) relative to the intended, protocol-specified, scheme depending on the results from the previous dose.

Subjects or patients participating in FTiH studies are monitored very closely for the occurrence of AEs. Subjects are generally required to stay in bed for at least 4 hours following a dose, and continuous monitoring of vital signs is not unusual for a period of at least 24 hours following each dose. The population enrolled into a FTiH study is generally composed of male healthy volunteers, as females are known to be more prone to drug-induced toxicity [880]. Full discussion on inclusion and exclusion criteria for subjects enrolled in FTiH trials may be found in Chapter 1 [95] and Chapter 31 [30] and will not be discussed further here.

Operationally, each cohort of subjects is brought into a clinic on a weekly basis. Following an overnight fast, the dose chosen (or placebo) is administered at roughly 8 a.m., and safety, pharmacokinetic, and pharmacodynamic (if any) measurements are taken prior to dosing and at regular intervals thereafter. These data are then used by the study team (composed at minimum of a physician, nurse, statistician, and pharmacokineticist) to support the decision on which dose to give next (or whether to halt or delay the next administration). The key responsibility for determination of which dose to administer next (if any) is a medical purview, and the statistician and pharmacokineticist are expected to provide analyses and simulations to support this medical determination if required. The statistical and pharmacostatistical approach to data analysis in this setting is exploratory (see Chapter 14 [95]). Data are modelled periodically during the study to provide an accurate and precise description of what observations have been collected to date and are used to predict which effects may be observed at future doses ([1, 501]; Chapter 18 [30]).

We first consider pharmacokinetic data generated in a typical FTiH trial. One property of such log-normal pharmacokinetic data is that variation increases with exposure [1324]. To model this behavior, a "power" model is generally utilized [1167]. Doses are increased until average exposure (AUC and/or Cmax) is observed to approach the NOAEL or some multiple of the NOAEL's value (e.g., one-tenth). For this type of design, the power model is

$$y_{ik} = (\alpha + \xi_k) + \beta(ld) + \varepsilon_{ik},$$

where α is the overall mean pharmacokinetic response at a unit dose (logDose, $ld = 0$) known in statistics as the population intercept, ξ_k is the random-intercept accounting for each subject (k) as their own control, β is the slope parameter of interest regressed on logDose (parameter ld), and ε_{ik} denotes within-subject error, as described in Chapter 3, for each log-transformed AUC or Cmax (y_{ik}) in period i. Note that period effects are assumed to be minor relative to the magnitude of effect of logDose in this analysis and are confounded with dose. Typical data arising from such a design are listed in Table 8.2 and plotted in Figure 8.1.

TABLE 8.2: Example 8.2.1: AUC and Cmax Data from a Cross-Over First-Time-in-Humans Study Design

Subject	Period	Dose	AUC	Cmax
1	2	15	666.06	307.1
1	3	45	1701.49	524.2
1	4	100	4291.86	1684.2
2	1	5	144.63	70.1
2	3	45	956.84	390.9
2	4	100	2121.55	522.0
3	1	5	187.88	55.6
3	2	15	406.06	210.1
3	4	100	2712.69	864.6
4	1	5	111.12	53.7
4	2	15	313.21	155.8
4	3	45	1006.57	548.7
6	1	5	152.64	96.3
6	3	45	1164.88	520.7
6	4	100	3025.78	1509.1
7	2	15	641.89	233.6
7	3	45	2582.20	713.0
7	4	100	4836.58	1583.7
8	1	5	420.42	212.7
8	2	15	908.93	339.3
8	4	100	8194.40	2767.2
9	1	100	3544.28	947.0
9	2	150	5298.14	778.9
9	3	200	6936.13	1424.4
10	1	100	5051.23	1713.3
10	3	200	11881.12	3543.8
10	4	250	16409.81	4610.1
12	2	150	7460.82	2143.2
12	3	200	8995.97	3708.4
12	4	250	10479.14	2604.0
14	1	100	2134.17	1664.5
14	2	150	3294.38	932.4
14	4	250	5332.19	1276.3
15	2	150	3189.74	976.2
15	3	200	4643.52	1300.7
15	4	250	4652.96	810.1

TABLE 8.2: Example 8.2.1: AUC and Cmax Data from a Cross-Over First-Time-in-Humans Study Design (continued)

Subject	Period	Dose	AUC	Cmax
16	1	100	3357.67	1134.8
16	2	150	4305.17	856.8
16	3	200	8886.62	1914.2
17	1	5	378.75	155.1
17	2	15	915.95	307.2
17	3	45	2830.42	532.8
18	1	100	1912.93	596.3
18	2	150	2684.00	602.6
18	4	250	3971.27	1792.2
19	1	100	8446.20	2110.6
19	3	200	17004.51	2766.3
19	4	250	21097.81	7313.4

Note that variation at the 150 mg dose in Example 8.2.1 (see Figure 8.1) appears to decrease relative to the 100 mg dose. This is a feature of the cross-over nature of the design and is observed due to the fact that the subjects administered the 150 mg dose are not always the same ones administered the 100 mg dose. To account for each subject as their own control, the power model is utilized to provide a population dose to pharmacokinetic response curve. This statistical relationship provides an estimate of the magnitude of a typical individual's exposure when administered a dose. Once a subject's exposure has been measured for a given dose, this individual's dose to pharmacokinetic relationship may be quantified to provide an individual assessment of potential hazard relative to the NOAEL,

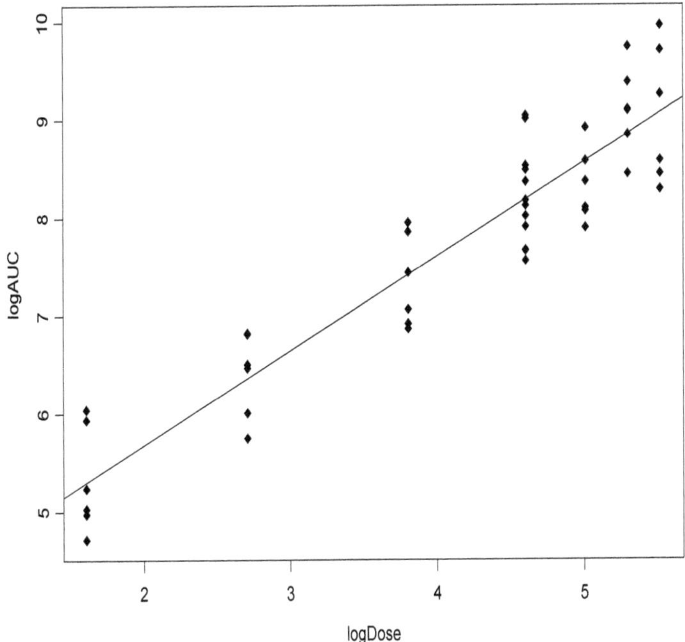

FIGURE 8.1
Estimated logDose versus logAUC Curve with Individual Data Points from Example 8.2.1

and we will consider how to do so later in this chapter. SAS code to model AUC and Cmax data from such trials is below. Doses are increased until the population dose to pharmacokinetic curve approaches the NOAEL or until a severe or serious AE is observed.

First-time-in-humans PK SAS `proc mixed` *Analysis Code Example 8.2.1 and 8.2.2*

```
proc mixed method=reml data=pk1_ftih;
    class subject;
    model lnauc=lndose/
    s ddfm=kenwardroger cl alpha=.1;
    random intercept/subject=subject;
    run;
```

SAS `proc mixed` output provides the estimates required to derive the dose to AUC or Cmax curve plotted in Figure 8.1. SAS output (not shown) estimates of parameters are given in Table 8.3.

TABLE 8.3
Parameter Estimates from Example 8.2.1

Endpoint	$\hat{\alpha}$	$\hat{\beta}$	$\hat{\sigma}_W^2$
AUC	3.75	0.96	0.01
Cmax	3.20	0.83	0.09

The parameter α in this example is the estimated logAUC (or logCmax) associated with a dose of 1 mg ($ld = 0$). The estimated population dose to pharmacokinetic response curve is calculated as

$$AUC = e^{\hat{\alpha}+\hat{\beta}(ld)}.$$

To solve for the dose expected to yield exposure at the NOAEL (the MTD), one exponentiates the above equation at $AUC = NOAEL$ after solving for ld:

$$MTD = e^{\frac{\ln(NOAEL)-\hat{\alpha}}{\hat{\beta}}}.$$

The bootstrap (see Chapter 5 and [510]) may be used to derive a confidence interval for the MTD if desired.

In our second example (Example 8.2.2, see Table 8.4) we consider a PK dataset where exposure relative to a predetermined NOAEL was of concern. Dosing was to be halted if mean AUC was in excess of 2400 ng.h/mL or Cmax exceeded 880 ng/mL (the NOAEL).

TABLE 8.4: Example 8.2.2: AUC and Cmax Data from a Cross-Over First-Time-in-Humans Study Design

Subject	Dose	AUC	Cmax
1	1	611	80.3
1	5	842	103.1
1	10	1600	167.3
2	1	1052	112.7
2	5	1584	164.7
2	10	2809	273.8
3	1	1139	98.0

TABLE 8.4: Example 8.2.2: AUC and Cmax Data from a Cross-Over First-Time-in-Humans Study Design (continued)

Subject	Dose	AUC	Cmax
3	5	1896	162.6
3	10	2531	167.9
4	1	989	89.0
4	5	1604	177.6
4	10	1817	212.8
5	1	1275	114.2
5	5	2282	173.7
6	1	947	77.7
6	5	1698	138.0
6	10	2278	240.5
7	1	603	92.3
7	5	1289	149.5
7	10	1987	225.5
8	1	867	86.4
8	5	1263	130.7
8	10	2494	276.3

Estimates of the parameters of interest may be found in Table 8.5. Here it was observed that exposure approached the NOAEL for AUC at the 10 mg dose and dosing was halted accordingly. See Figure 8.2.

Individual fitted means at each dose with 90% confidence intervals may be derived easily in SAS `proc mixed`. A statement `outp=pred` is added to the model statement after the / to output the dataset `pred` containing the relevant values. Estimated responses at other doses may be obtained by entering a missing value for the observation desired for that subject. Code to perform such analyses are provided on the website accompanying this book, and consideration is left as an exercise for interested readers.

In normal healthy volunteer studies, severe AEs are unusual, and SAEs are very unusual. Observation of an SAE should halt all dosing in a study and requires regulatory scrutiny of the event. Dose escalation is halted if severe AEs are observed. However, it is unusual for either SAEs or severe AEs to be observed in such trials. Most often dose escalation is halted when mean exposure approaches the NOAEL (as seen in the example above). Dosing for any given individual is halted if their exposure data approaches a higher than expected factor of the NOAEL.

In contrast, FTiH studies for cytotoxic agents are performed in refractory patient populations, and the goal of the study is to identify a dose causing a dose-limiting toxicity (DLT, an SAE) with X% frequency (often 30%). This is referred to as the dose expected to cause an X% response, abbreviated ED_X. The assumption is that, for such an agent to be efficacious, it must approach toxic levels. Three patients are dosed with a low dose,

TABLE 8.5
Parameter Estimates from Example 8.2.2

Endpoint	$\hat{\beta}$	$\hat{\sigma}^2_W$
AUC	0.38	0.02
Cmax	0.36	0.03

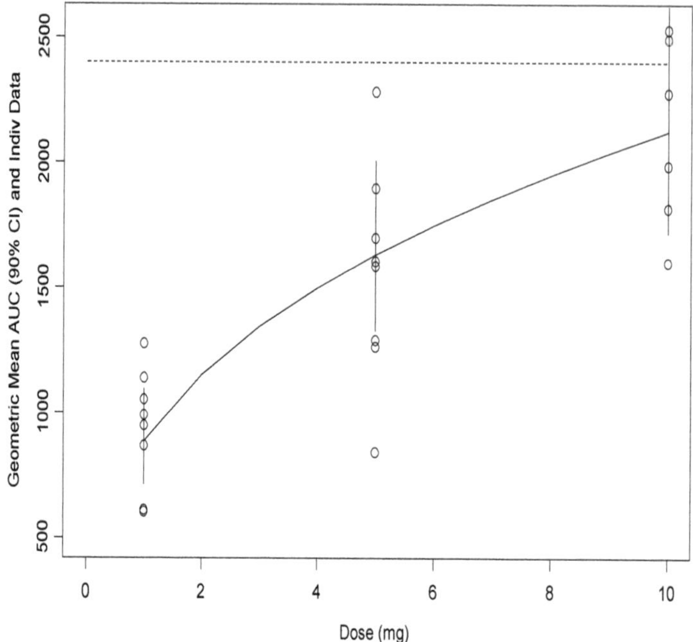

FIGURE 8.2
Estimated Dose versus AUC Curve (90% CI) with Individual Data Points from Example 8.2.2

and their responses to treatment are observed. If no DLTs are observed, another group of three patients receives the next higher dose, and their responses are observed. If one DLT is observed, another three patients are dosed at the same dose to provide reassurance that the DLT was dose related. If so, the dose is reduced is subsequent patients to refine the definition of the MTD. Once at least one DLT is observed in a group of patients and confirmed in a second cohort of three patients, the dose is reduced in subsequent patients to identify a well-tolerated dose producing DLTs in approximately the desired percentage of patients. See Table 8.6. Note that one patient did not report for dosing in the third dose group, so only two patients were dosed.

TABLE 8.6: Example 8.2.3: Dose Limiting Toxicity Data from a First-Time-in-Humans Trial

Subject	Dose(mg)	DLT
1	1	0
101	1	0
2	1	0
3	2	0
102	2	0
4	2	0
103	4	0
5	4	0
DLT=1 DLT Observed		
DLT=0 DLT not Observed		

TABLE 8.6: Example 8.2.3: Dose Limiting Toxicity Data from a First-Time-in-Humans Trial (continued)

Subject	Dose(mg)	DLT
6	6	0
104	6	0
7	6	0
8	8	0
105	8	1
106	8	0
107	8	0
9	8	0
10	8	0
108	10	0
11	10	0
12	10	0
109	12.5	0
110	12.5	0
13	12.5	0
111	16	0
112	16	0
14	16	0
15	16	0
113	21	1
114	21	1
16	21	1
17	18	0
18	18	0
19	18	0
115	18	0
20	18	0
116	18	0
21	18	1
22	18	0
23	18	1
117	18	0
118	18	0
24	18	1
25	18	1
26	18	0
119	18	0
DLT=1 DLT Observed DLT=0 DLT not Observed		

DLTs are denoted as occurring (1) or not occurring (0) for each individual patient in Table 8.6. Note that these studies are not placebo controlled and are generally conducted open-label or with only the patients blinded to treatment. Such DLT data is considered as "binomial" data (denoting a 0 or 1 response), and the proportion of DLTs as a function of dose may be modelled using a technique known as logistic regression.

To do so, the proportion (P) is defined such that

$$P = \frac{1}{1 + e^{-(\alpha+\beta(ld))}}$$

where β is the slope of a regression of $\ln(P/1 - P) = L$ (known as a logit-transformation) on logDose such that $L = \alpha + \beta(ld)$. The parameter α is the intercept at $ld = 0$.

Analysis is straightforward using `proc genmod` in SAS as follows (see code below). One calls the dataset (specifying in a `DESCENDING` statement that SAS should model the probability that DLT is 1) and instructs SAS to model the DLTs as a function of logDose. The statement `dist=b` informs SAS that DLT is a binomial endpoint, and `link=logit` specifies that a logit transformation should be used.

First-Time-in-Humans DLT SAS `proc genmod` *Analysis Code Example 8.2.3*

```
proc genmod data=dlt1 DESCENDING;
    model dlt=lndose/dist=b
    link=logit cl alpha=0.1;
    run;
```

SAS output (not listed) yielded an estimate of -10.5083 for α and 3.3846 for β for Example 8.2.3. This yields the dose-response curve for the proportion of DLTs of Figure 8.3.

We can see that the ED_X is approximately

$$e^{\frac{\ln(X/1-X)-\hat{\alpha}}{\hat{\beta}}}.$$

For example, the estimated ED_{30} is 17.4 mg in this analysis.

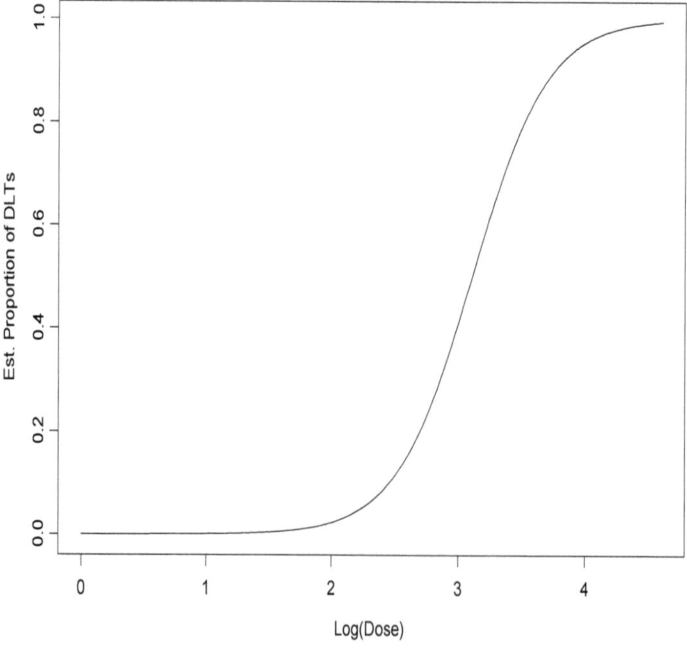

FIGURE 8.3
Estimated Proportion of DLTs versus logDose from Example 8.2.3

Note that variation is not taken into account (though it could be) in the calculation of the ED_X. A simple means to do so is to bootstrap the dataset (see Chapter 5) and derive the ED_X in each bootstrapped dataset. The 5th and 95th percentiles of the bootstrapped datasets for ED_X serve as a 90% confidence interval for our estimate of ED_X in this case the estimated confidence interval from 1000 bootstraps was 14.1 to 25.4 mg. SAS code to perform this analysis is provided on the website accompanying this book.

Similar procedures may be used to model adverse events in cross-over trials. See [652] for additional details on such techniques. However, given the relative infrequency of AEs in normal healthy volunteer FTiH studies, we do not discuss such application further here.

Intuitively, the use of interactive modelling techniques would seem to add value for such studies. Such techniques utilize data as they are collected, and the models described above, to provide clinicians with an assessment of the safety profile for their choice of future doses. Several techniques have been developed but are infrequently utilized in FTiH studies, as experience with them is limited (Chapter 1 [95]). An overview of techniques to aid in decision making in this setting may be found in [1329]. See the Technical Appendix for an example of code to perform interactive assessments of PK data in FTiH studies. Those using such interactive techniques are cautioned that "All models are wrong, but some are useful" [107] and should note that the use of such techniques supplements, **but in no way should substitute for**, clinical conduct, experience, and expertise. Choice of dose is ultimately a clinical responsibility.

At the end of the FTiH study, the single dose MTD [621] should have been defined. This MTD will possibly be based on observed nonserious AEs, but most likely will be based on observed human exposure levels relative to the NOAEL defined in preclinical studies. These studies should definitely provide data to reinforce ideas on the properties of the drug's pharmacokinetics with dose in relation to the NOAEL. In some cases, evidence of pharmacodynamic activity will also be observed, and we will consider methods for modelling of such data in a later chapter.

Note that the MTD, once defined in this study, is not a constant. As knowledge about the drug accumulates while drug development progresses, it can (and most likely will) change, as can the NOAEL. We now turn to the next study, which typically occurs in Phase I.

8.3 Sub-Chronic Dosing Studies

Following the FTiH study, a sub-chronic (sometimes referred to as a "repeat" dosing) study is performed. The main intent of this trial is to confirm that the MTD defined in the FTiH trial holds true upon repeated administration. In this study again, pharmacokinetic and safety data are most of interest, though pharmacodynamic data may be collected if appropriate. Level of blinding (open-label, single-blind, etc.) and choice of population are generally the same as in the FTiH trial. It is unusual for such trials to involve the dosing of patients with the disease for which the treatment is intended. Most often, normal healthy volunteers are dosed for this purpose as in the FTiH trial.

Eligible subjects are randomized to receive either placebo or a dose of drug up to the MTD defined in the FTiH trial. Each dose is administered to 9 to 12 subjects in a cross-over fashion. In the first period, a single dose is given, and pharmacokinetic measurements are collected out to at least five half-lives. Following this, in the second period, subjects receive the same dose at regular, repeated intervals for at least five half-lives, and pharmacokinetic measurements are taken following the last dose over the sampling interval. Following an evaluation of the data collected in the first cohort of 9 to 12 subjects (see Table 8.7), the next highest dose is administered for the next cohort up to the MTD identified in the FTiH

TABLE 8.7
Schematic Plan of a Sub-Chronic Dosing Cross-Over Study

Subject	Period 1	Period 2
Cohort 1		
1	D1	RD1
2	P	RP
3	D1	RD1
4	D1	RD1
5	P	RP
6	D1	RD1
7	D1	RD1
8	P	RP
9	D1	D1
Cohort 2		
11	MTD	RMTD
12	MTD	RMTD
13	P	RP
14	MTD	RMTD
15	P	RP
16	MTD	RMTD
17	MTD	RMTD
18	P	RP
19	MTD	RMTD

P=Single Dose of Placebo
RP=Repeated Doses of Placebo
D1=Single Dose of Well-Tolerated Dose
RD1=Repeated Doses to Steady State
MTD=Single Dose of MTD
RMTD=Repeated Doses of MTD to Steady State

trial. The placebo treatment is included to provide a control group for the purposes of safety assessment comparisons, and we will consider an example later where effects were observed in liver function.

The first order of analysis is to assess whether *clearance* is the same after the single dose and after repeated doses. The dose of drug divided by AUC defines a pharmacokinetic parameter known as Clearance (Cl). More precisely, for an orally dosed drug,

$$Cl_s = \frac{F(dose)}{AUC(0-\infty)},$$

following a single dose of drug (subscript s), denoting the volume of blood cleared of drug in a unit of time for a single dose. The parameter F is absolute bioavailability (discussed in Chapter 11). When such a drug is dosed repeatedly to steady state, the pharmacokinetic collections on the final dosing day provide an estimate for

$$Cl_{ss} = \frac{F(dose)}{AUC(0-\tau)},$$

where τ is the frequency of dosing (24 h if dosed once a day, 12 h if dosed twice a day) and the subscript ss denotes steady state. Steady state concentrations are achieved when the rate of drug being eliminated from the body equals the amount of drug dosed (e.g., dose/hour). In general, this occurs when the drug is dosed repeatedly for at least five half-lives at regular intervals (see Chapters 1 and 2 for a definition of pharmacokinetic half-life).

If $Cl_s = CL_{ss}$ or equivalently in this setting $AUC(0-\tau) = AUC(0-\infty)$ for all doses, then the drug has the property of stationarity of clearance. This property is desirable, as it makes the drug very easy to dose. All else being equal, one can be started on a dose estimated to achieve safe and effective drug concentrations, and these concentrations may be maintained by simply taking the same dose at regular intervals. In contrast, if $AUC(0-\tau)$ is larger than $AUC(0-\infty)$, then the starting dose might need to be reduced to maintain safe concentrations relative to the NOAEL over time when dosing repeatedly.

Our first example (8.3.1 in Table 8.8) consists of AUC and Cmax data from a sub-chronic dosing study where nine subjects received a dose of either 5, 10, or 20 mg in the first period (accompanying placebo treated subjects are omitted from this discussion as they did not contribute pharmacokinetic data). In the second period, these subjects received the same dose of drug once a day for seven days. On day seven, pharmacokinetic measurements were taken just prior to last the last dose and over the next 24 hours.

TABLE 8.8: Example 8.3.1: AUC and Cmax Data from a Sub-Chronic Dosing Cross-Over Study Design

Subject	Dose	$AUC(0-inf)$ S	$AUC(0-\tau)$ SS	Cmax S	Cmax SS
47	5	2.81	5.11	0.267	0.423
48	5	6.31	8.13	0.415	0.620
49	5	7.26	8.01	0.468	0.627
50	5	3.60	6.67	0.410	0.480
52	5	6.82	7.38	0.356	0.591
53	5	1.76	5.17	0.225	0.390
54	5	6.11	8.16	0.471	0.569
55	5	6.09	6.23	0.409	0.483
57	5	2.10	3.36	0.316	0.316
60	10	9.33	11.22	0.820	0.962
61	10	7.31	8.21	0.624	0.723
62	10	9.57	20.85	0.625	1.861
64	10	15.62	16.48	0.798	1.169
65	10	5.56	6.79	0.493	0.574
66	10	11.81	18.08	0.576	1.303
69	10	7.23	10.51	0.723	0.883
71	10	8.35	13.97	0.583	1.056
72	10	5.70	13.80	0.585	1.157
95	20	12.92	30.35	1.514	2.220
99	20	26.05	53.11	2.009	3.902
102	20	23.12	38.61	1.562	2.517
104	20	12.32	29.33	1.002	2.219
105	20	16.35	26.20	1.181	1.844
106	20	20.21	29.47	1.360	1.893
107	20	13.53	27.55	0.970	1.965
108	20	7.70	19.97	0.744	1.447
110	20	14.22	35.91	0.988	2.322
S=Single Dose, SS=Steady State					

For this type of design, the power model is

$$y_{jk} = (\alpha + \xi_k) + \beta_1(ld) + \phi_j + \beta_2(ld(\phi_j)) + \varepsilon_{jk},$$

where β_1 is the slope parameter of interest regressed on logDose (parameter ld), α and ξ_k are defined as in Section 8.2, ϕ_j denotes the day being studied (j denotes repeat or single dose), β_2 is the slope regressed on logDose on each study day (to account for potential heterogeneity between days within-subjects), and ε_{jk} denotes within-subject error as described in Chapter 3 for each logAUC or logCmax (y_{jk}). If repeat dosing does not impact logAUC or logCmax, then ϕ and β_2 should be zero. Under those circumstances, the model reduces to the same form used in Section 8.2.

Implementation in SAS is straightforward. `proc mixed` is called, and subject and day are specified as classifications. Each endpoint (logAUC or logCmax) is then modelled as a function of logDose, day, and the interaction between logDose and day. Subject is specified as the random intercept, as was done previously using the `random` statement, and desired estimates for the mean effect at each day are output using the `lsmeans` statement. Note that an `at` statement is included in each `lsmeans` statement to instruct SAS to derive estimates at the appropriate choices of logDose (corresponding to doses of 5, 10, and 20) and compare these between days.

Sub-Chronic Pharmacokinetic Data Analysis 8.3.1 — SAS `proc mixed` *Code:*

```
proc mixed data=pk method=reml;
    class subject day;
    model lnauc=lndose day lndose*day
    /ddfm=kenwardroger s cl alpha=0.1;
    random intercept/subject=subject;
    lsmeans day/at lndose=1.6094 diff cl alpha=0.1;
    lsmeans day/at lndose=2.3026 diff cl alpha=0.1;
    lsmeans day/at lndose=2.9957 diff cl alpha=0.1;
    run;

proc mixed data=pk method=reml;
    class subject day;
    model lncmax=lndose day lndose*day
    /ddfm=kenwardroger s cl alpha=0.1;
    random intercept/subject=subject;
    lsmeans day/at lndose=1.6094 diff cl alpha=0.1;
    lsmeans day/at lndose=2.3026 diff cl alpha=0.1;
    lsmeans day/at lndose=2.9957 diff cl alpha=0.1;
    run;
```

SAS output (not shown) estimates of parameters may be found in Table 8.9. The parameters $\hat{\alpha}$ are the common intercept (response at logDose of zero following repeated dosing), and $\hat{\phi}$ is adjustment to this response following a single dose. The sum of $\hat{\alpha} + \hat{\phi}$ should approximately coincide with the intercept obtained from the FTiH trial, all else being equal (i.e., if formulation or other factors like the pharmacokinetic assay have not changed between trials). The MTD relative to the NOAEL for repeat dosing may be derived as

$$e^{\frac{\ln NOAEL - \hat{\alpha}}{\hat{\beta}_1 + \hat{\beta}_2}}$$

in this design. Confidence intervals for the MTD may again be derived using the bootstrap.

TABLE 8.9
Parameter Estimates from Example 8.3.1

Endpoint	$\hat{\alpha}$	$\hat{\beta}_1$	$\hat{\phi}$	$\hat{\beta}_2$	$\hat{\sigma}^2_W$
AUC	-0.035	0.93	-0.035	0.23	0.04
Cmax	-2.43	0.87	-0.02	0.21	0.03

The assessment of stationarity of clearance is accomplished using the findings of the `lsmeans` statements, and relevant outputs may be found in Table 8.10 for logAUC. It was observed that clearance was clearly not stationary for this drug, as $AUC(0-\tau)$ was significantly larger than $AUC(0-\infty)$, and accumulation appears to increase with increasing dose. Results on the natural scale may be obtained by exponentiating the findings below. The assessment for Cmax is left as an exercise for interested readers.

In our second example, we turn to modelling of the properties of the pharmacokinetic concentration versus time curve. In this study, modelling of this curve generally initiates, as the data are rich compared to that collected in later patient studies (where sparse sampling schemes may be employed, see [365]). To clarify, subsequent studies in patients may not be able to employ an extensive pharmacokinetic data collection, as done in Phase I, as it is not convenient to keep patients in-clinic for the lengthy period needed to collect a full pharmacokinetic profile. The profile is modelled in the sub-chronic dosing studies so that pharmacokinetic profiles can be simulated for a patient population when sparse collections are obtained in subsequent studies.

In the sub-chronic dosing study, each subject receiving an active dose of drug (not placebo) should contribute a drug concentration in plasma versus time profile, as shown in Table 8.11 for Subject 47. Additional data from this study may be found in `conc.sas7bdat` on the website accompanying this book.

We will choose here to utilize SAS for the nonlinear mixed effect modelling of such data; however, several other statistical packages are readily available (SPLUS, NONMEM, WINNONLIN, PKBUGS, etc., [1048]) and may be used for this purpose. The models employed are nonlinear (as obviously the concentration over time is not linear) and mixed effect in that each subject has an individual profile. Readers interested in more details should see [1379] and [1271].

For this type of design, we will model the available pharmacokinetic data using what is known as a one-compartment [30] nonlinear mixed effect model for the purposes of illustration based on the SAS procedure described in [1073] for `proc nlmixed`. Interested readers may use the data in `conc.sas7bdat` on the website accompanying this book to evaluate alternative models. This model assumes that drug is absorbed into the body according to rate k_{ai} (where i denotes subject) and is eliminated from the body according to rate k_{ei}.

TABLE 8.10
Stationarity of Clearance Assessment from Example 8.3.1

Dose	logDose	logAUC(0-τ)-logAUC(0-∞)	90% CI
5	1.61	0.34	(0.19, 0.49)
10	2.30	0.50	(0.40, 0.59)
20	3.00	0.66	(0.51, 0.81)

TABLE 8.11
Pharmacokinetic Concentration Data from Subject 47 of `conc.sas7bdat` following a Single Dose of 5 mg

Subject	Dose	Time	Conc. ng/mL
47	5	0	.
47	5	0.25	0.117
47	5	0.5	0.221
47	5	0.75	0.266
47	5	1	0.267
47	5	1.5	0.232
47	5	2	0.19
47	5	4	0.178
47	5	6	0.125
47	5	8	0.138
47	5	10	0.145
47	5	12	0.126
47	5	16	0.079
47	5	24	0.051
47	5	36	.
47	5	48	.
47	5	72	.
47	5	96	.

Concentration c_{it} at time t for subject i is modelled as follows:

$$c_{it} = (e^{-k_{ei}t} - e^{-k_{ai}t})\frac{k_{ei}k_{ai}(Dose)}{Cl_i(k_{ai} - k_{ei})} + \varepsilon_{it},$$

where ε_{it} represents within-subject residual error, Cl_i is the clearance for subject i assumed to be of the form $e^{\beta_1 + b_{1i}}$, with β_1 being an unknown constant adjusted for each subject as appropriate to b_{1i}. Similarly, k_{ai} is considered to be a function of the form $e^{\beta_2 + b_{2i}}$, and k_{ei} is considered to be a function of the form $e^{\beta_3 + b_{3i}}$. The parameters b_{1i}, b_{2i}, and b_{3i} are considered to be independent random normal variables with null mean and some nonzero variance in similar fashion to the REML methods described for bioequivalence in Chapter 5.

Implementation in SAS is straightforward. First the data should be sorted by subject to accommodate SAS requirements. The SAS procedure `proc nlmixed` is then called, and, following the specification of starting values, the equation described above is specified. Note that here we have assumed concentration is normally distributed. It may be more appropriate to model concentration as log-normally distributed, and this can be accomplished by a log-transformation in a data step. Similarly, instead of modelling concentration as a function of dose, logDose may be more appropriate.

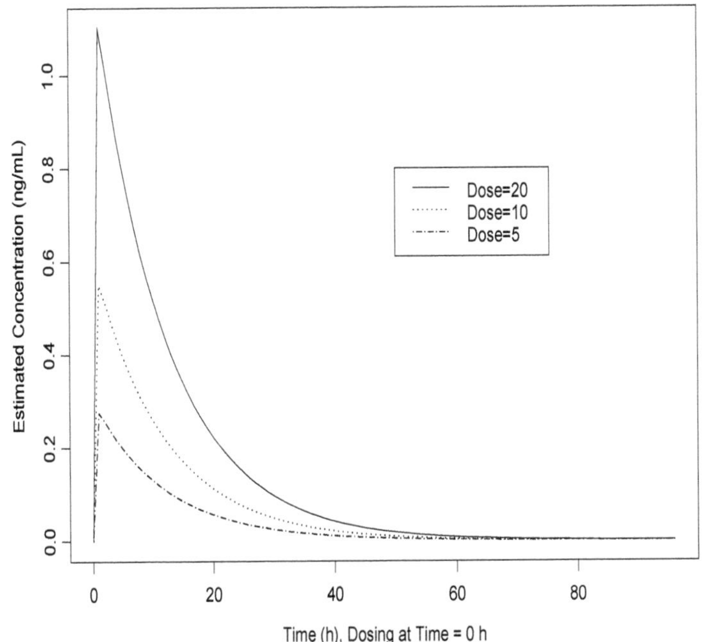

FIGURE 8.4
Estimated Concentration versus Time (h) Profile from Phase I Concentration Data in `conc.sas7bdat`

Nonlinear Mixed Effect Pharmacokinetic Data Analysis of Phase 1 Concentration Data in `conc.sas7bdat` - *SAS* `proc nlmixed` *Code:*

```
proc sort data=my.conc;
    by subject dose time;run;

proc nlmixed data=my.conc;
    parms beta1=0.4 beta2=1.5 beta3=-2 s2b1=0.04
    s2b2=0.02 s2b3=0.01 s2=0.25;
    cl = exp(beta1+b1);
    ka = exp(beta2+b2);
    ke = exp(beta3+b3);
    pred=dose*ke*ka*(exp(-ke*time)-exp(-ka*time))/
    (cl*(ka-ke));
    model conc ~ normal(pred,s2);
    random b1 b2 b3 ~ normal([0,0,0],[s2b1,0,
    s2b2,0,0,s2b3]) subject=subject;
    predict pred out=pred;
    run;
```

In this code, s2b1, s2b2, and s2b3 are the variances associated with b_{i1}, b_{i2}, and b_{i3}, respectively. The parameter s2 is the estimate of within-subject variance. Estimated parameters may be found in Table 8.12, and a plot of the estimated concentrations for each dose versus time may be found in Figure 8.4.

TABLE 8.12
Estimated PK Model Parameters from Phase I Concentration Data in `conc.sas7bdat`

Parameter	Estimate	95% CI
β_1	0.35	0.23,0.47
β_2	1.46	1.30,1.63
β_3	-2.47	-2.58,-2.36
s2b1	0.04	0.01,0.08
s2b2	0.03	-0.02,0.09
s2b3	0.01	-0.01,0.02
s2	0.011	0.009,0.013

Predicted concentrations from the model are output to a dataset `pred` using the statement `predict pred out=pred;` in the above code. These values may be used to construct residual plots for each subject and across subjects to assess model fit using the following SAS code. Some evidence of poor model fit is evident at low concentrations; however, overall, the model appears to provide an adequate description of the data.

Nonlinear PK Analysis Model Diagnostic Code:

```
proc sort data=pred;
    by subject dose time;run;
data pred;set pred;
    st_resid=(conc-Pred)/StdErrPred;
    run;
proc rank data=pred normal=blom out=nscore;
    var st_resid;
    ranks nscore;
data nscore;
  set nscore;
  label nscore="Normal Score";
  label stres="Residual";
  label pred="Predicted Value";
    run;
proc plot vpercent=50 data=nscore;
    plot st_resid*pred/vref=0;
    plot st_resid*nscore;
    run;
```

In subsequent studies, when limited concentration data are collected from patients at a given time on a given dose, these data can be used with the model findings above to simulate a population pharmacokinetic profile. This can then be used to assess the exposure levels in that patient population relative the NOAEL, and we will discuss how such assessments may be done in Chapter 11. Similar models are used to characterize the concentrations after repeat dosing. Clearance is differentiated between single and repeat dosing as appropriate to the findings of the stationarity of clearance assessment.

We now consider findings of alanine aminotransferase (ALT) elevation which were observed in a repeat dose trial. ALT elevations are potentially indicative of liver injury and were monitored each day in this study. Such elevations can occur spontaneously and unpredictably, in response to strenuous exercise, for instance. Of concern here, however, was that

TABLE 8.13
ALT Data from Subject 4 of `liver.sas7bdat`

Subject	Period	Dose	Day	ALT
4	2	50	1	13
			2	13
			3	16
			4	15
			5	18
			6	24
			7	25
			8	29
			9	34
			10	36
			11	34
			12	33
			13	45
			14	43

these elevations were presumed to be drug induced. Although the ALT returned to baseline upon cessation of treatment (data not shown), it was of interest to model the behavior of ALT with dose over time to provide clinical with a means of designing a monitoring plan in subsequent studies. For this assessment, we will treat ALT as being log-normally distributed and model it as a function of logDose.

Data from Subject 4 (who received 50 mg) may be found in Table 8.13. The data for the remaining subjects may be found in the dataset `liver.sas7bdat` on the website accompanying this book. For this subject we see little indication of a response to drug treatment until day 5, whereupon the ALT begins to increase.

For this type of design, the power model for ALT is an extension of the model used for pharmacokinetic data earlier in this section:

$$y_{jk} = \alpha + \phi_j + \beta_1(ld) + \beta_2(ld(\phi_j)) + \varepsilon_{jk},$$

where ϕ_j denotes the day being studied (j denotes days 1 to 14) for each logALT (y_{jk}). If dosing does not impact logALT, then β_1 and β_2 should be zero. We presume that ALT responses from day to day within a subject are related to each other, with the degree of correlation decreasing with increasing time between days, and will partition this aspect of variance associated with ϕ_j from the within-subject variation ε_{jk} in our model.

Here, `proc mixed` is called, and subject and day are specified as class variables. The endpoint of interest (logALT) is then modelled as a function of logDose, day, and the interaction between logDose and day. The correlation between days is partitioned from the within-subject variance using a `repeated` statement specifying that the correlation occurs within each subject. The desired estimates for the mean effect at each day are output using the `lsmeans` statement. Note that an `at` statement is again included in each `lsmeans` statement to instruct SAS to derive estimates at the appropriate choices of logDose (corresponding to doses of approximately zero to 3000).

Sub-Chronic ALT Data Analysis of `liver.sas7bdat` - *SAS* `proc mixed` *Code:*

```
proc mixed data=liver;
    class subject day;
    model lnalt=day lndose day*lndose
    /DDFM=KENWARDROGER S outp=out;
    repeated day/type=AR(1) subject=subject;
    lsmeans day/at lndose=-11.5129 CL alpha=0.01;
    lsmeans day/at lndose=3.91 CL alpha=0.01;
    lsmeans day/at lndose=4.61 CL alpha=0.01;
    lsmeans day/at lndose=5.01 CL alpha=0.01;
    lsmeans day/at lndose=5.52 CL alpha=0.01;
    lsmeans day/at lndose=6.21 CL alpha=0.01;
    lsmeans day/at lndose=6.62 CL alpha=0.01;
    lsmeans day/at lndose=6.91 CL alpha=0.01;
    lsmeans day/at lndose=7.60 CL alpha=0.01;
    lsmeans day/at lndose=8.01 CL alpha=0.01;
    ods output LSMeans=my.means1;
    run;
```

In this dataset, for this population (recall these are normal healthy volunteers), statistically significant logDose related ($p = 0.0415$) increases in ln-ALT were observed, and these changes increased with increasing dose ($p = 0.0024$). The estimates of ALT elevation for the 50 mg (logDose of 3.91) and the 3000 mg dose (logDose of 8.01) are presented in Table 8.14, exponentiated back to the original scale.

TABLE 8.14: Estimated ALT Data (based on `liver.sas7bdat`) from the Sub-Chronic Dosing Study Design

Dose	Day	Est. ALT	90% CI
50	1	15.5	12.9,18.5
50	2	14.9	12.5,17.9
50	3	15.2	12.7,18.2
50	4	17.1	14.3,20.5
50	5	20.9	17.5,25.1
50	6	25.4	21.2,30.5
50	7	28.3	23.6,33.9
50	8	29.4	24.5,35.2
50	9	30.1	25.1,36.1
50	10	31.1	26.0,37.3
50	11	31.1	26.0,37.3
50	12	29.5	24.6,35.3
50	13	30.6	25.5,36.6
50	14	31.5	26.2,37.7
3000	1	15.4	12.3,19.2
3000	2	14.9	11.9,18.6
3000	3	15.2	12.1,18.9
3000	4	17.3	13.9,21.7
3000	5	22.1	17.7,27.7
3000	6	27.9	22.3,34.8
3000	7	31.8	25.5,39.8
Upper Limit of Normal ALT=34			

TABLE 8.14: Estimated ALT Data (based on `liver.sas7bdat`) from the Sub-Chronic Dosing Study Design (continued)

Dose	Day	Est. ALT	90% CI
3000	8	33.3	26.6,41.6
3000	9	34.4	27.5,43.1
3000	10	35.4	28.3,44.2
3000	11	34.9	27.9,43.7
3000	12	32.6	26.1,40.8
3000	13	33.5	26.8,41.9
3000	14	34.5	27.5,43.2
Upper Limit of Normal ALT=34			

For the 50 mg dose, we see ALT elevations beginning on day 4 and continuing throughout the dosing interval. Potentially hazardous elevations may be expected seven days after beginning dosing (when the 90% upper bound crosses the upper limit of normal). ALT elevations were slightly greater as dose was increased to 3000 mg and potentially hazardous ALT elevations were encountered a day sooner.

Models similar to these may be used to test for proof of safety (see Chapter 9) and to model the behavior of pharmacodynamic effects (see Chapter 10). We now turn to another safety topic.

8.4 Food Effect Assessment and Drug-Drug Interactions (DDIs)

Following the studies described in the previous two sections, the maximum tolerated dose should have been identified when a single dose of drug has been given and when a dose of drug is given repeatedly. By that point, drug developers should have a good handle on what the body does to the drug in isolation.

Note that what has not been done at this point is as important as what has been learned. Drug development at this stage should have confirmed that the potential for hazard when taking the drug is low when given at certain doses over a period of limited duration. If a potential hazard with dose has been identified, it may be necessary to explicitly study the drug to provide "proof of safety" under a variety of potential clinical uses; see Chapter 9 for one such example.

Other preclinical and clinical studies later in development will be needed if the drug is to be given chronically for longer intervals. Additionally, the behavior of the drug in people with disease and different ethnicity (Chapter 11) has not yet been established.

However, no one actually takes a drug in isolation. Patients are expected to take the drug with food on occasion and may be expected to take it while taking other agents (whether or not the label precludes such [1222]). In this context, alcohol is an agent; over-the-counter vitamins and pharmaceuticals are other examples of agents, etc. How the body handles the drug when coadministered under such circumstances is the subject of this section.

As we know (Chapter 2), when a drug is taken it undergoes absorption, distribution, and metabolism and is eventually eliminated from the body (ADME). Dosing a drug with food may impact how the drug is absorbed. Dosing of a drug with other agents can impact distribution and, more frequently, metabolism. This can slow down or speed up elimination of the drug substance from the body. If elimination is decreased, exposure to drug may increase to the point where it is not well tolerated. Alternatively, if elimination is enhanced, the dose of drug may not be sufficient to cause an efficacious response.

Lack of a meaningful pharmacokinetic difference when a drug product is administered with and without food or with and without a concomitantly administered agent or medication can often be assessed using the results of small cross-over studies and applying a TOST approach [1191]. Rate of bioavailability as measured by Cmax is held, under this approach, to be a surrogate marker for safety for drugs in the marketplace. Comparable or decreased mean Cmax following administration with or without food or a concomitantly administered medication is indicative of similar safety hazards to that when dosed alone. Increases in mean Cmax are potentially suggestive of a less acceptable safety profile for the drug under study. Similarly, comparable mean AUC following administration with or without food or a concomitantly administered medication are indicative of safety and efficacy in that condition. The magnitude of decrease or increase in exposure can be used to adjust the dosing strategy for the drug product under study.

As with bioequivalence, pharmacokinetics serve as a tool for assessing safety in this context. Such a assessment limits the potential for hazard established in the first-time-in-humans and sub-chronic dosing studies, but does not eliminate it entirely.

We first consider an example of a cross-over study assessing the potential for dosing with a meal to impact exposure (food effect). This is followed by two examples of drug interaction trials.

Dosing of a drug product with a meal can change absorption of the drug substance by [370]

1. Delaying gastric emptying,
2. Stimulating bile flow,
3. Changing gastrointestinal pH,
4. Increasing splanchnic blood flow,
5. Changing luminal metabolism,
6. Causing physical or chemical interactions with the formulation or drug substance

The effect of food on absorption is typically studied using an open-label, randomized, 2×2 cross-over trial in normal healthy volunteers. See Chapter 3 and [370] for details. Subjects (normal healthy volunteers) are randomized to receive one of two sequences of treatment regimens. Subjects receive a dose of drug following an overnight fast, are washed out for five half-lives, and then receive the same dose of drug following a meal, or vice-versa.

Note the change in terminology in this section to *regimen* instead of formulation. In a food effect study, the formulation is the same; only the conditions of dosing (with or without a meal) are changed. The use of the descriptor regimen denotes that the dose of drug under study is the same, but study conditions are altered to study the ADME properties. In Example 8.4.1 (below), regimens A and B denote dosing without (regimen A) and with (regimen B) a meal. As with bioequivalence testing, absence of a food effect is concluded if the 90% confidence intervals for AUC and Cmax $\mu_B - \mu_A$ fall within the standard bioequivalence acceptance limits of $-\ln 1.25, \ln 1.25$ [370].

We now turn to an example of such testing for food effect. In this trial (Example 8.4.1), 20 normal healthy volunteers were randomly assigned to sequences AB and BA, and AUC and Cmax were measured following dosing in each period Table 8.15.

TABLE 8.15: Example 8.4.1: AUC and Cmax Data from a 2 × 2 Food Effect Cross-Over Study Design

Subject	Seq	AUC A	AUC B	Cmax A	Cmax B
1	AB	5836	8215	1953	1869
2	BA	9196	9895	1769	2446
3	AB	7809	7222	3409	1501
4	BA	6443	18864	1916	4232
5	BA	5875	5911	1884	2087
6	AB	9937	6186	2807	1743
7	BA	10275	9135	2532	2736
8	AB	4798	6211	1912	1541
9	BA	8940	9810	1939	2216
10	AB	10739	14734	1908	3645
11	AB	10549	10937	4042	2120
12	BA	8374	10853	3702	2001
13	BA	16510	13205	3411	2840
14	AB	7534	5648	2119	1684
15	AB	9473	13407	4194	3074
16	BA	5118	9399	2294	1538
17	AB	4686	7504	1487	1839
18	BA	6122	11027	1857	2063
19	AB	14059	15765	3142	3120
20	BA	6841	8104	1883	1954
A=Fasted Dose, B=Fed Dose					

Data were analyzed using the procedures of Chapter 3 based on the following `proc mixed` code.

Food Effect Example 8.4.1 — SAS `proc mixed` *Code:*

```
proc mixed data=pk_food;
    class sequence subject period regimen;
    model logauc=sequence period regimen/
    ddfm=kenwardroger;
    random subject(sequence);
    lsmeans regimen/pdiff cl alpha=0.1;
    estimate 'Food Effect for logAUC' regimen -1 1;
    run;

proc mixed data=pk_food;
    class sequence subject period regimen;
    model logcmax=sequence period regimen/
    ddfm=kenwardroger;
    random subject(sequence);
    lsmeans regimen/pdiff cl alpha=0.1;
    estimate 'Food Effect for logCmax' regimen -1 1;
    run;
```

Food Effect Example 8.4.1 — SAS `proc mixed` *Code:*

```
proc mixed data=pk_food;
    class sequence subject period regimen;
    model tmax=sequence period regimen/
    ddfm=kenwardroger;
    random subject(sequence);
    lsmeans regimen/pdiff cl alpha=0.1;
    estimate 'Food Effect for Tmax' regimen -1 1;
    run;
```

Dosing with food significantly ($p = 0.0363$) increased the extent of exposure (AUC) to this drug product by approximately 20%, with an estimate of food effect ($\mu_B - \mu_A$) of 0.1788 (90% confidence interval 0.0417, 0.3158) on the log-scale. Although rate of exposure (Cmax) was not significantly changed ($p = 0.4142$), lack of food effect could not be concluded, as the estimate of food effect was -0.0758 (90% confidence interval -0.2330, 0.0814) on the log-scale. Tmax was significantly prolonged following dosing with a meal (data may be found on the website accompanying this book), with food effect estimated to be 1.7 h (90% confidence interval 1.28 h, 2.11 h).

From these data, it is possible to conclude that dosing with food affects the absorption of this drug product, increasing the overall exposure to drug (AUC) and delaying its maximal concentration. These changes do not likely present a hazard to patients using the drug, as Cmax was not increased following a meal, and the increase in AUC was not deemed clinically relevant (requiring a change in dose to correct).

We now turn to the statistical assessment of drug interactions. Drugs can interact with each other in a number of ways involving the ADME properties [30, 95]. As with food effects, absorption may be impacted; however, the most common interaction relates to how the liver metabolizes the drug substances. Metabolic inhibition denotes that one drug prevents the metabolism of the other, usually resulting in increased exposure to the substance. Alternatively, drugs may have no effect on each other or a drug might induce the metabolism of the other, indicating that metabolism activity is enhanced in the body, likely leading to decreased exposure to drug.

Note that metabolism is only one way that drugs can interact. Other examples include protein binding interactions, transporter interaction, etc. See [95] Chapter 2 and [30] Chapter 14 for more details. In this section, we will discuss the topic of drug interactions, focusing on those introduced by the CYP450 liver enzyme system for simplicity; however, the clinical and statistical assessments used are similar to the other interaction types.

The CYP450 (cytochrome P450) enzyme family is responsible for the majority of metabolic drug interactions known to occur [364]. This type of drug metabolism is focused in the body's liver, and the liver uses multiple subfamily enzyme systems to metabolize drug products after they are ingested and as they circulate through the blood. The subfamilies include, in decreasing order of importance and frequency [95]

1. 3A4,
2. 2C9,
3. 2A6,
4. 2C8, 2E1,
5. 1A2,
6. 2B6,
7. 2D6, 2C19, etc.

Inhibition or induction of drugs metabolized by these systems may result in changed exposure levels, presumably and potentially putting the safety of patients at risk. Clinical studies are used to assess this potential.

In vitro testing [359] may preclude or enhance the need to do such a study. The predictive value of such in vitro testing for drug metabolism by the CYP450 family has become increasingly accurate and reliable in recent years, and generally, clinical drug interaction trials are only conducted when an in vitro system identifies a particular subfamily as being of potential concern. Such concern may arise if the new drug inhibits or induces the metabolism of other drugs by a certain subfamily or if the new drug is itself metabolized by a particular subfamily — the route for which may be inhibited or induced by another product.

To assess the potential changes in exposure, a steady state randomized or non-randomized cross-over design is most often used. In general, subjects are dosed to steady state with one product alone (Regimen A in the following examples), and in the alternative regimen are dosed to steady state with the potential metabolic inhibitor or inducer in tandem (Regimen B). AUC, Cmax, and other pharmacokinetic endpoints are derived at appropriate times following dosing to evaluate the potential changes in exposure [364].

Non-randomized cross-over designs (see Example 8.4.3 below) may be used if washout of the probe drug (i.e., the drug being probed for a potential interaction) is long or if an extended dosing period is necessary to achieve steady state exposure. It should be noted that it is possible to administer several probe drugs at the same time to evaluate multiple pathways of metabolism at once. These are known as "cocktail" drug interaction trials. See [1137] for an example.

Our first drug interaction example is a randomized cross-over study in 20 normal healthy volunteers where a probe drug's metabolism was inhibited when given with a new drug at steady state. The increase in exposure was studied to determine whether coadministration represented a risk to patients using the probe drug. SAS code to analyze such data is the same as that applied in Chapter 3 and may be found below Table 8.16.

TABLE 8.16: Example 8.4.2: AUC and Cmax Data from a 2 × 2 Drug Interaction Cross-Over Study Design for Metabolic Inhibition

Subject	Seq	AUC A	AUC B	Cmax A	Cmax B
1	BA	21.9	28.1	2.16	2.27
2	AB	17.9	14.8	1.63	1.39
3	BA	14.8	22.2	1.21	2.38
4	AB	19.4	17.0	1.59	1.64
6	AB	28.2	28.2	2.77	2.84
7	AB	25.3	17.1	1.98	1.84
8	BA	24.0	25.4	1.71	1.90
10	AB	27.8	33.2	2.68	2.57
11	BA	17.0	20.6	1.98	2.49
12	AB	19.3	23.6	2.37	3.29
14	AB	29.9	27.5	2.43	2.22
15	AB	20.5	22.3	1.92	2.04
16	BA	24.3	29.9	2.26	2.83
17	BA	27.5	32.5	1.92	2.27
18	AB	16.9	17.4	1.66	1.91
19	AB	33.1	39.0	3.39	2.88

A=Probe Drug
B=Probe Drug Plus a Metabolic Inhibitor

TABLE 8.16: Example 8.4.2: AUC and Cmax Data from a 2 × 2 Drug Interaction Cross-Over Study Design for Metabolic Inhibition (continued)

Subject	Seq	AUC A	AUC B	Cmax A	Cmax B
20	BA	14.7	22.1	1.63	2.66
21	BA	29.3	43.2	2.46	3.79
22	AB	23.3	31.6	3.06	2.57
23	BA	23.1	24.3	2.66	2.56
A=Probe Drug B=Probe Drug Plus a Metabolic Inhibitor					

Inhibitor Drug Interaction Example 8.4.2 — SAS `proc mixed` *Code:*

```
proc mixed data=pk_inhi;
    class sequence subject period regimen;
    model logauc=sequence period regimen/
    ddfm=kenwardroger;
    random subject(sequence);
    lsmeans regimen/pdiff cl alpha=0.1;
    estimate 'DDI Effect for logAUC' regimen -1 1;
    run;

proc mixed data=pk_inhi;
    class sequence subject period regimen;
    model logcmax=sequence period regimen/
    ddfm=kenwardroger;
    random subject(sequence);
    lsmeans regimen/pdiff cl alpha=0.1;
    estimate 'DDI Effect for logCmax' regimen -1 1;
    run;
```

Dosing with the metabolic inhibitor significantly changed AUC and Cmax of the probe drug (p = 0.0056 and 0.0094, respectively). Adminstration with the metabolic inhibitor increased the extent of exposure (AUC) to this drug product by approximately 13% with an estimate of interaction ($\mu_B - \mu_A$) of 0.1254 (90% confidence interval 0.0563, 0.1946) on the log-scale. The maximal concentration (Cmax) was also increased by 13% with an effect size of 0.1245 (90% confidence interval 0.0503, 0.1987) on the log-scale. Other data (Tmax, etc.) measured in this study may be found on the website accompanying this book. Interested readers should note that C24 (the concentration of probe drug 24 hours following dosing) and renal clearance (CLR) were significantly altered by combination dosing; however, Tmax was not.

Our second drug interaction example is a non-randomized cross-over study in 20 normal healthy volunteers where a probe drug's metabolism was induced when given with a new drug at steady state. The decrease in exposure was studied to determine whether coadministration represented a risk to patients using the probe drug. SAS code to analyze such data are similar to that applied in Chapter 3 and may be found below. Note that this was a non-randomized cross-over study, so period and sequence effects are confounded with regimen (and were not fitted in the model). This type of design is acceptable [364] when period effects can be expected to be small relative to the effect of the regimen Table 8.17.

TABLE 8.17: Example 8.4.3: AUC and Cmax Data from a Drug Interaction Cross-Over Study Design for Metabolic Induction

Subject	Seq	AUC A	AUC B	Cmax A	Cmax B
1	AB	37.73	9.38	3.84	2.75
2	AB	18.22	5.07	2.74	0.97
3	AB	10.30	5.75	1.87	1.98
4	AB	22.11	4.32	4.32	1.15
5	AB	16.31	5.83	3.24	1.15
6	AB	20.47	6.80	3.23	1.32
7	AB	16.02	3.32	1.71	0.72
8	AB	10.73	3.38	1.99	1.07
9	AB	13.93	3.72	1.92	0.97
10	AB	24.32	4.25	2.99	0.59
11	AB	31.67	6.82	3.03	1.01
12	AB	10.97	3.40	2.03	0.48
13	AB	55.49	7.72	4.90	2.20
14	AB	13.65	4.16	1.73	0.65
15	AB	23.97	6.13	3.27	1.78
16	AB	14.07	2.65	2.65	0.50
17	AB	6.51	2.59	1.32	0.91
18	AB	19.60	3.32	3.07	0.56
19	AB	18.80	2.96	2.83	0.66
20	AB	28.25	3.32	3.11	0.69

A=Probe Drug
B=Probe Drug Plus a Metabolic Inducer

Inducer Drug Interaction Example 8.4.3 — SAS `proc mixed` *Code:*

```
proc mixed data=pk_indu;
    class subject regimen;
    model logauc=regimen/ddfm=kenwardroger;
    random subject;
    lsmeans regimen/pdiff cl alpha=0.1;
    estimate 'DDI Effect for logAUC' regimen -1 1;
    run;

proc mixed data=pk_indu;
    class subject regimen;
    model logcmax=regimen/ddfm=kenwardroger;
    random subject;
    lsmeans regimen/pdiff cl alpha=0.1;
    estimate 'DDI Effect for logCmax' regimen -1 1;
    run;
```

Dosing with the metabolic inducer significantly changed AUC and Cmax of the probe drug ($p < 0.0001$ for both endpoints). Adminstration with the metabolic inducer decreased the extent of exposure (AUC) to this drug product by approximately 75%, with an estimate of interaction ($\mu_B - \mu_A$) of -1.4199 (90% confidence interval -1.5686, -1.2713) on the log-scale. The maximal concentration (Cmax) was also decreased by 63%, with an effect size of -0.9996 (90% confidence interval -1.1883, -0.8109) on the log-scale. Other data (half-life, Tmax, etc.) measured in this study may be found on the website accompanying this book. Interested readers should note that half-life was significantly altered by combination dosing; however, Tmax was not.

While a combination of dosing with these products may be presumed to be safe (as exposure was decreased), it may not be desirable. Changes in exposure of this magnitude might lead to the probe drug being inefficacious, and alternative dosing strategies might need to be employed to ensure adequate probe drug is available in the body to succeed in establishing an effective treatment.

The sample size required to have sufficient power for food effect designs and TOST assessment [370] is derived according to the procedures developed in Chapter 3. In drug interaction trials, regulatory guidance [321, 397] calls for TOST assessment relative to the traditional bioequivalence acceptance limits of $-\ln 1.25$ to $\ln 1.25$ as an option. More commonly, no-effect boundaries are predetermined by means of assessing how much change in exposure would necessitate a change in dose for the probe drug to be safe and efficacious. These limits need not be symmetric, and R code provided in previous chapters may be modified to address this situation.

Lower and upper acceptance limits are not always available from the literature, and even if they are, regulators may not agree with whatever the sponsor defines. Under such circumstances, an estimation approach [661] can be useful when the magnitude of no-effect boundaries are not known and the main study objective is to provide evidence of what the potential value, or range of values, may be, or when the sample size is in part set by feasibility, and we wish to provide an idea of the precision the trial is likely to provide for the drug interaction effect of interest.

In such cases, the intent is to provide an estimate of the expected width or precision of the plausible range of values as expressed by a confidence interval. This will help satisfy our expectation with regard to acceptability and applicability of study results in the knowledge that "The confidence interval can be thought of as the set of true but unknown differences that are statistically compatible with the observed difference" [475].

Then, as described in Chapter 3, Equation (3.8), a 90% confidence interval for $\mu_T - \mu_R$ is

$$\hat{\mu}_T - \hat{\mu}_R \pm t_{0.95}(n-2)\sqrt{\frac{2\hat{\sigma}_W^2}{n}},$$

when the sample size in each sequence is equal and n is the overall sample size. For the purposes of this discussion, we presume a standard 2×2 cross-over is used, but alteration for alternative designs is easily accomplished and is left as an exercise for the interested reader. Consider

$$w_\delta = t_{0.95}(n-2)\sqrt{\frac{2\hat{\sigma}_W^2}{n}}.$$

This function provides a precision estimate for the true mean difference. Goodman and Berlin [475] note that use of a method like that proposed above should be exercised with caution, as, in a situation where the study design is truly intended to support a test of hypothesis, the approach corresponds to a test using only 50% power when precision is equal to the difference of interest. Similarly, in situations where a TOST equivalence approach is intended, the method presented in this equation corresponds to a two one-sided hypothesis test with 50% power when precision is equal to the equivalence range of interest.

Sample Size Code for Precision in DDI Studies:

```
data a;
    * total number of subjects
    (needs to be a multiple of number
    of sequences, seq);
n=20; seq=2;
    * significance level;
a=0.05;
    * variance of difference of two observations
    on the log scale;
    * sigmaW = within-subjects standard deviation;
sigmaW=0.2; s=sqrt(2)*sigmaW;
    * error degrees of freedom for cross-over
    with n subjects in total
    assigned equally to seq sequences;
n2=n-seq;
    run;

data b; set a;
* calculate precision;
    t=tinv(1-a,n2);
    SE=s/(sqrt(n));
* precision on log-scale;
    w=t*SE;
* precision on natural-scale;
    exp_w=(exp(t*SE)-1)*100;
    run;

proc print data=b; run;
```

In this case, the precision on the natural scale would be calculated as 12%, indicating that the confidence limits will lie about that far from the point estimate for the difference in means. If greater precision is desired, the sample size may be increased, or decreased if lesser precision is needed.

Note that this expression of precision denotes that the limits of the 90% confidence interval for the ratio of geometric means will lie within 12% of that ratio. Increasing the sample size lowers this percentage, i.e., improving precision. Decreasing the sample size increases this percentage, i.e., providing poorer precision. There is no regulatory guidance on what degree of precision is required in such designs. It is the purview of the sponsor to determine this number and its expression. One could, for example, use w on the natural-logarithmic scale as the precision measurement of interest.

In some cases, such a pharmacokinetic safety assessment will not suffice, and a more rigorous assessment of safety may be called for to protect patients using the drug. Under such circumstances, often a specific biomarker is of interest. Such an example — QTc — will be considered in the next chapter.

8.5 Dose Proportionality

In developing drugs, sponsoring companies spend a great deal of time and energy mapping pharmacokinetic exposure to drug (concentration in blood, AUC, Cmax, etc.) with clinical outcomes relating to safety and efficacy. When working in a clinical setting, physicians do not often have access to pharmacokinetic data from their patients. In practice, therefore, they vary doses in their patients to cause clinical benefit, and limit dosing to ensure undesirable side-effects (e.g., nausea, emesis) do not occur. Consider a situation where one administers a dose sure to be efficacious, but observes an unacceptable side-effect (e.g., nausea). Dose proportionality, the subject of this section, helps one determine which lower dose should next be tried to improve tolerability while still attaining efficacy.

In the previous studies discussed in this chapter, an understanding of the dose to exposure to safety relationship will have been established. One of the things prescribers need to know is how much exposure changes when the dose is changed, so that in changing doses for a given patient, they can balance a change in dose with desirable outcomes and undesirable side-effects.

When one increases the dose of a drug product, this does not necessarily result in a proportional change in exposure. There are physiologic, biologic, and chemical limits to how much drug substance the body will absorb, distribute, metabolize, and excrete. However, over the therapeutic dose range (the maximum effective and tolerated dose less the minimum effective dose), it is important to know that, if one, say, doubles the dose, then double the rate and extent of exposure results — and vice versa [1167].

The assessments of rate and extent of exposure in the first-time-in-humans and sub-chronic dosing studies will yield a good practical understanding of the shape of the dose-to-exposure relationship (as described in previous sections). However, assessments of dose proportionality in the first-time-in-humans study are confounded with period effects. These effects are known to occur in pharmacokinetic studies and may impact inference [1089]. Assessments of dose proportionality in the sub-chronic dosing study are generally under-powered for robust statistical assessment as the study is parallel group. While knowledge gained from these studies, in general, is adequate for clinical development, for approval at regulatory agencies (in preparation for giving the drug to large populations), a more robust study may be done to confirm that the shape of the dose-to-exposure relationship is well understood.

In some situations, therefore, a confirmatory dose proportionality study is performed just prior to regulatory filing with the final to-be-marketed formulation. Many different models may be used to examine dose proportionality [1167]. This section will focus on the application of the power model (described in Section 8.2) for this assessment. In this setting, we will assume a randomized cross-over design is used to assess dose proportionality, with at least three doses in the therapeutic range being considered. Normal healthy volunteers receive a dose of drug after an overnight fast, with administration of each dose separated by a washout period of at least five half-lives using a Williams square design (see Chapter 4).

There is some incentive for pharmaceutical companies to perform such a confirmatory dose proportionality study. If dose proportionality is demonstrated, then regulatory agencies typically only require that bioequivalence be demonstrated at the highest dosing strength if another formulation is developed subsequently. Regulators have found that to do otherwise results in undesirable results (e.g., [1356]). If dose proportionality is not present, one may be required to demonstrate bioequivalence for a new formulation at each dosing strength if a new formulation is developed [966], and that can be challenging.

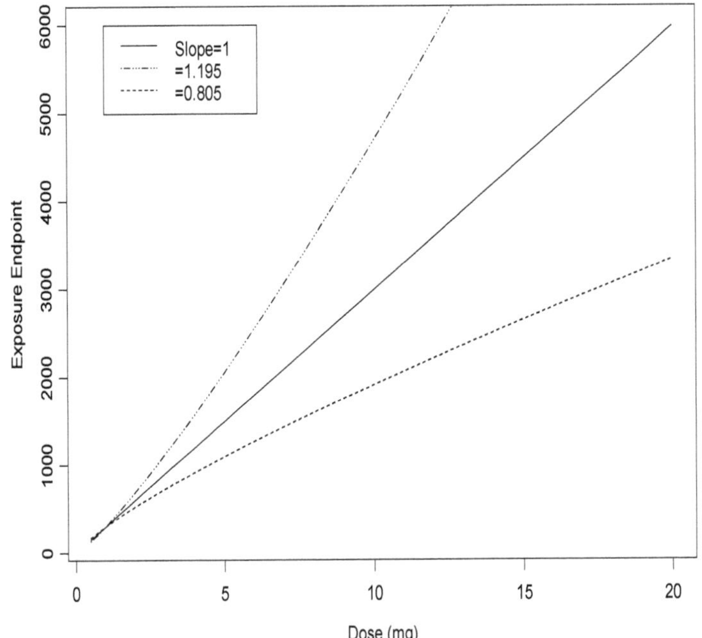

FIGURE 8.5
Dose-to-Exposure (AUC or Cmax) Relationship for β from 0.8 to 1.2

For this type of confirmatory dose proportionality design, the model is

$$y_{ijk} = \alpha + \beta(ld) + \pi_j + \gamma_i + \xi_{k(i)} + \varepsilon_{ijk},$$

where α, β, and logDose (ld) are as previously described, π_j and γ_i identify the period j of sequence i, $\xi_{k(i)}$ is the random intercept accounting for each subject within sequence as their own control, and ε_{ijk} denotes within-subject error as described in Chapter 3 for each log-transformed AUC or Cmax (y_{ijk}).

When one exponentiates both sides of this equation, AUC or $Cmax = c(d^{\beta})$ where c is a value composed of the exponentiated sum of estimates of sequence, subject, and period fixed effects, plus residual error, and d is dose. When $\beta = 1$, the drug is dose proportional as AUC or $Cmax = cd$. When one wishes to change the dose, it is easy to predict what AUC or Cmax will result. If $\beta \neq 1$, one can still predict what AUC or Cmax will result from changing the dose, but the calculation is more complex (as the relationship of dose to the exposure endpoint, AUC or Cmax, is nonlinear).

Consider the possible shape of the resulting dose-to-exposure curves in Figure 8.5.

For $\beta = 1$, a truly dose proportional relationship is observed. For any unit change in dose, a unit change in AUC results, i.e., doubling the dose results in twice the AUC. If $\beta > 1$, a greater than dose proportional response is seen (doubling the dose results in a greater than doubling in AUC), and if $\beta < 1$, a less than dose proportional response in exposure is observed (doubling the dose results in less than a doubling in AUC).

Smith et al. [1166] showed that it is obvious to think of dose proportionality as an equivalence problem. This implies that the structure for testing dose proportionality is

$$H_{01} : \beta \leq 1 - t$$

versus

$$H_{11} : \beta > 1 - t$$

or

$$H_{02} : \beta \geq 1 + t$$

versus

$$H_{12} : \beta < 1 + t,$$

similar to the TOST used in bioequivalence testing. A systematic review in [1148] also found this to be a reasonable approach.

However, there is currently no set regulatory standard for the equivalence region. Smith et al. [1166] recommend that t be defined as

$$t = \ln \theta / \ln r$$

where θ is the minimal change in exposure beyond which one may want to adjust to maintain safe exposure levels, and r is the ratio of the maximum tolerated or effective dose to be used in the study to the minimum effective dose.

In the following example, $\theta = 1.5$, as it was felt for this drug that a 50% increase in exposure might necessitate a decrease in dose. The therapeutic dose range was $1 - 8$ mg, and $r = 8$ accordingly. Therefore $t = 0.195$, and the hypotheses to be tested were

$$H_{01} : \beta \leq 0.805$$

versus

$$H_{11} : \beta > 0.805$$

or

$$H_{02} : \beta \geq 1.195$$

versus

$$H_{12} : \beta < 1.195.$$

When the parameter β lies between 0.805 and 1.195 (with sufficient confidence), this procedure judges the data adequate to support a claim of dose proportionality.

As with bioequivalence testing, a mixed model is used to assess the magnitude of β and to derive 90% confidence intervals. If the 90% confidence interval for β lies within $1 - t$ to $1 + t$, for both AUC and Cmax, dose proportionality is demonstrated.

In Example 8.5.1, a randomized cross-over study in 28 normal healthy volunteers was performed to assess dose proportionality and the effect of food. SAS code to analyze such data are similar to that applied in Chapter 3 and may be found below Table 8.18.

TABLE 8.18: Example 8.5.1: AUC and Cmax Data from a Randomized Dose Proportionality Cross-Over Study

Subject	Seq	AUC A	AUC B	AUC C	Cmax A	Cmax B	Cmax C
1	DCAB	352	746	3408	66.6	208.4	687.2
4	BACD	440	842	2560	88.9	162.6	504.0
5	CBDA	249	552	2856	66.7	124.0	601.6
6	DCAB	318	628	2560	68.9	114.4	495.2
7	ADBC	528	814	3888	98.5	177.8	826.4
8	BACD	512	1122	4680	82.8	204.8	684.8
A=1mg; B=2mg; C=8mg; D=8mg with a meal							

TABLE 8.18: Example 8.5.1: AUC and Cmax Data from a Randomized Dose Proportionality Cross-Over Study (continued)

Subject	Seq	AUC A	AUC B	AUC C	Cmax A	Cmax B	Cmax C
9	DCAB	329	750	2720	67.0	180.0	510.4
10	ADBC	374	688	2432	65.7	142.8	448.0
11	CBDA	282	994	4680	76.4	191.0	586.4
13	BACD	324	674	2584	82.1	168.8	610.4
14	CBDA	284	636	3176	61.5	108.0	532.0
15	ADBC	372	666	3200	82.8	169.4	792.0
16	DCAB	304	578	2272	67.1	123.8	440.8
17	CBDA	171	400	1696	48.0	90.2	463.2
18	DCAB	489	1054	3752	91.5	190.6	735.2
20	ADBC	267	526	1896	59.9	141.0	540.8
21	ADBC	292	620	2392	65.6	107.6	332.8
22	BACD	299	580	2488	79.2	126.8	649.6
23	DCAB	392	918	3152	64.1	291.0	615.2
24	CBDA	363	646	3448	87.3	177.2	715.2
25	ADBC	728	896	3232	75.2	130.6	571.2
27	CBDA	348	806	3360	75.5	131.0	560.8
28	DCAB	287	568	2440	69.7	146.2	578.4
29	BACD	283	620	2320	79.4	151.2	502.4
30	CBDA	246	590	2472	78.2	87.6	637.6
31	ADBC	429	786	3264	114.1	186.0	785.6
32	BACD	308	704	2616	81.0	155.2	671.2
33	BACD	462	1132	3656	85.7	174.4	656.8
A=1mg; B=2mg; C=8mg; D=8mg with a meal							

Dose Proportionality Assessment Example 8.5.1 — SAS `proc mixed` *Code:*

```
proc mixed method=reml data=pk_dp;
    class subject sequence period;
    model lnauc=sequence period lndose/
    s ddfm=kenwardroger cl alpha=.1;
    random intercept/subject=subject(sequence);
    run;

proc mixed method=reml data=pk_dp;
    class subject sequence period;
    model lncmax=sequence period lndose/
    s ddfm=kenwardroger cl alpha=.1;
    random intercept/subject=subject(sequence);
    run;
```

The estimates for β were 1.0218 and 0.9879 for logAUC and Cmax, respectively, with 90% confidence intervals contained well within 0.805 to 1.195. Therefore, dose proportionality was demonstrated. Interested readers may find data for Tmax from this study and AUC and Cmax data for the assessment of food effects (Regimen D compared to Regimen C) on the website accompanying this book. Tmax was not significantly changed by altering the dose of drug, and food did not affect the AUC and Cmax of this drug.

Determination of sample size for such a cross-over study is similar to the procedure used in bioequivalence testing [1126]. As these assessments are typically now added on to studies for multiple purposes (for example, food effect and dose proportionality may be assessed in the same study), we recommend that simulations be conducted (see Chapter 5) to study the power in such situations. Alternatively, the approach discussed in [918] may be used to approximate study power for multi-purpose designs.

8.6 Technical Appendix

This technical appendix provides an example of interactive Bayesian modelling of pharmacokinetic data in a first-time-in-humans trial. In Table 8.19, mean AUC and Cmax estimates from a preclinical species are presented.

TABLE 8.19
Exposure Estimates from a Preclinical Species

Dose	Estimated AUC	Estimated Cmax
5 mg/kg	2790	880
100 mg/kg	29,600	7600

Techniques to use these values to predict human AUC and Cmax are discussed in Chapter 30 [30] and will not be discussed further here. For the purposes of illustration, here it is assumed that only human weight needs be taken into account in predicting human exposure levels, and these estimates (assuming a 50 kg human) are provided in Table 8.20.

TABLE 8.20
Exposure Estimates for a 50 kg Human from a Preclinical Species

Dose	Estimated AUC	Estimated Cmax
5 mg	139,500	44,000
100 mg	1,480,000	380,000

We wish to use these data to derive estimates for α and β as discussed in Section 8.2; however, at this stage we have these two unknown parameters and only two data points. For pharmacokinetic data, it is possible to make the assumption that, when the dose is very small (0.0001), the resulting AUC or Cmax will be very small (0.0001). This yields three data points for two unknown parameters, and a simple regression may be performed to provide prior distributions for α and β. SAS code to perform this analysis may be found on the website accompanying this book. Other means (e.g., expert elicitation) may also be used to derive such estimates for α and β, and we refer interested readers to an excellent review in [442].

In this case, it is estimated that $\hat{\alpha} \sim N(3.43, 0.52)$ and $\hat{\beta} \sim N(1.36, 0.0081)$ where N denotes the normal distribution with (mean, variance) from a regression of logAUC on logDose. We utilize the mean estimates for these parameters in the code below, but assume that the variance associated with them is very wide (reflecting the uncertainty inherent in allometric scaling calculations).

Example 8.2.2 AUC data were analyzed in WINBUGS using the following computer code (based on the code from the RATS WINBUGS example):

Interactive Bayesian First-Time-in-Humans WINBUGS Analysis Code for Example 8.2.2

```
model
    {for( i in 1 : N )
    {
    for( j in 1 : T )
    {
    Y[i , j] ~ dnorm(mu[i , j],tau.c)
    mu[i , j] <- alpha[i] + beta[i] * x[j]
    }
    alpha[i] ~ dnorm(alpha.c,alpha.tau)
    beta[i] ~ dnorm(beta.c,beta.tau)
    }
    tau.c ~ dgamma(0.001,0.001)
    sigma <- 1 / sqrt(tau.c)
    alpha.c ~ dnorm(3.43,1.0E-6)
    alpha.tau ~ dgamma(0.001,0.001)
    beta.c ~ dnorm(1.36,1.0E-6)
    beta.tau ~ dgamma(0.001,0.001)
    lnmtd <- (7.78-alpha.c)/(beta.c)
    mtd <- exp(lnmtd)
    }
```

This model may be used interactively as data are collected to estimate individual responses (monitoring mu[i , j]) and the MTD.

As with the original analysis, attention is focused on the MTD relative to the NOAEL (2400 for illustration purposes). The MTD in this analysis is estimated as 13.8 mg (using the median posterior density of 100,000 iterations after a burn-in of 1000 iterations). A Bayesian 90% confidence interval for the MTD is 8.4 to 25.7 mg. Similar analyses may be performed for Cmax, and this is left as an exercise for the reader.

9

QTc

Introduction

No one can be expected to pay 100% attention to 100% of the issues and data encountered in clinical pharmacology 100% of the time, so one should be forgiven for not recognizing immediately that QTc is a critical endpoint in drug development.

My boss stepped in one day to alert me to the fact that I now had a new project. We were developing an anti-arrythmia drug. There were a number of ongoing clinical pharmacology trials that were delivering data, and results would be needed "Stat" to enable the company to make an investment decision.

I was used to this by this time. No one ever came by and said we had plenty of time to get a job done, with no rush, and that senior management was happy to wait as long as we needed to get the job done properly at our convenience (i.e., without interfering with all the other work we had to do). I was hopeful at that time that maybe one day I would get a project like that, but that has happened exactly one time since then.

In any event, arrythmia denotes an irregular heartbeat. Some are benign, but some are fatal, and the drug we were developing was intended to prevent its occurrence. To do so, my boss informed me that the drug would impact the ECG. I nodded sagely, and after she left I looked it up in my trusty medical dictionary. ECG denotes an electrocardiogram — a tracing of the electrical activity of the heart over time (we will see a typical one later in this chapter). What I was expecting when the data came in, therefore, was a lot of ECG tracings from which I would measure amplitude, trough to trough time intervals, and other summary measures to statistically describe the activity following dosing with our drug relative to placebo. These would obviously be related to the aortas and ventricles I remembered from 8th grade anatomy, so this should not have been too bad.

What I received, however, was a dataset of alphabet soup with numbers. There were measurements taken for PR, QRS, QT, RR, QTc, QTcB, QTcF, QTcI (to name a few) in addition to text fields describing T-wave morphology. All of these were measured in triplicate following dosing with placebo and our drug in a pretty large number of patients at many times over the course of a day. There was not an ECG to be seen, nor any ventricles. It was a completely unidentifiable mass of unbelievable gobbledygook seemingly produced by a team of junior medics with slide rules, protractors, and way too much time on their hands. I found out later it was done by senior medics and had been done this way since the 1920s.

My guess (which turned out later to be correct) was that these endpoints (PR, etc.) were measuring time relative to the voltage of the heart. But in this instance my medical dictionary let me down. QTc was not in there.

This left me with three options to try to figure out what was going on:

1. *Ask my statistical colleagues (they did not know, or said they did not, as they did not want to talk about it).*
2. *Go downstairs and talk to Denny about what this stuff was (since the report was needed yesterday), but the problem with talking to Denny was that he would want to know about the data for a couple of other projects I was working on, and I did not want to field twenty questions when all I needed was one answer.*
3. *Go to lunch.*

After lunch, I talked to Denny and got a crash course on the heart and electrocardiology. QTc turned out to be very important, not only for this drug, but also as a general issue in drug development. We will devote this chapter to QTc, as it is now an important issue in clinical pharmacology assessments of drug safety for all drug products.

9.1 Background

An electrocardiogram (ECG) measures the electrical activity of the heart over time. Usually, eight "leads" or electrical monitors are placed on a patient's upper torso and back along certain predetermined vectors out from the heart. These leads then monitor the electrical output of the heart to construct a graph of the polarization and depolarization of different parts of the heart during a beat. See Figure 9.1. This pattern is repeated over and over again while the heart beats.

The different parts of the ECG are denoted by letters and referred to as "waves" and "complexes." For instance, the first "bump" is referred to as the P-wave. The nadir of the first dip begins the QRS-complex, and the wave immediately following this complex is the T-wave. In some ECGs, there is a following wave known as the U-wave, but this is unusual in normal healthy volunteers.

On the ECG tracing, the QT interval is defined as the amount of time between the initiation of the QRS complex and the conclusion of the T-wave. QT interval duration is measured in milliseconds (msec), by computer algorithm, and measures of how long it takes the heart to repolarize and prepare for its next beat. The longer it takes to repolarize, the more time between beats, and the less oxygen gets to cells.

QT duration is dependent upon gender, age, health status, menstrual cycle, and a great number of other factors. QT changes naturally over the course of the day, and QT duration can be prolonged by food and is changed by exercise. Some drugs prolong the QT interval (i.e., delay the heart's ability to repolarize). If QT is prolonged sufficiently in humans,

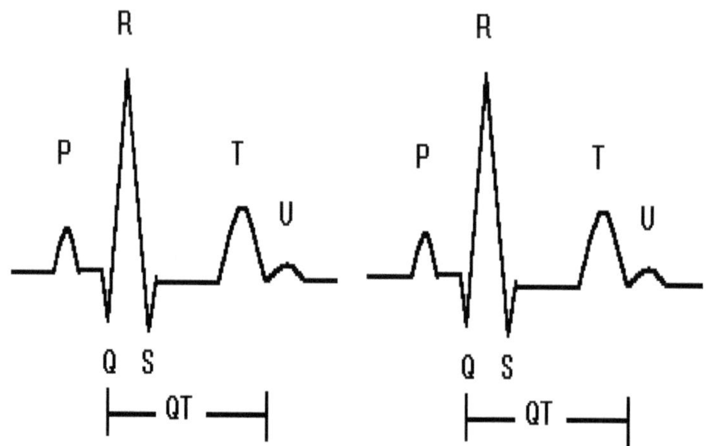

FIGURE 9.1
A Typical 12-Lead ECG Interval

potentially fatal cardiac arrhythmias can result. Torsades de pointes, most often referred to in connection with QT, as these are known to be related, is a malignant ventricular arrhythmia known to occur infrequently in individuals who are genetically predisposed to this condition and sometimes in response to drug therapy [1008].

Prolongation of the QTc interval has been observed to be related to increased risk of torsades de pointes in an exponential fashion [894]. The QT interval is highly correlated with how fast the heart is beating overall (measured by determining RR, the length of time between one R on the ECG and the next R). Therefore, in measuring QT, the interval is usually corrected to derive a QTc (QT interval corrected for heart rate). Common corrections were developed by Fridericia [432] and Bazett [54], and many authors have published on better ways to correct for heart rate in recent years, e.g., [265]. Bazett's correction has been observed to overcorrect QTc at some heart rates ([971, 1022, 1203]) and is not generally used for the purposes of safety assessment described in this chapter. We will not dwell further here on the application of correction factors in this setting, and will utilize Fridericia's correction (QT is corrected by division of the cube-root of RR such that $QTcF = \frac{QT}{RR^{1/3}}$) in subsequent discussion, as it appears unrelated to heart rate according to recent reports [1022], [1203].

QTc prolongation is a necessary but not sufficient condition for occurrence of and has a qualitative relationship to clinical arrhythmias [626]. One must, by definition, have a prolonged QTc just prior to the occurrence of torsades de pointes, but a prolonged QTc can occur without the occurrence of torsades de pointes. In general, a prolonged QTc in a patient with several other risk factors [15] may result in torsades de pointes. Prolongation from baseline (usually taken first thing in the morning) in an individual greater than 60 msec or an absolute value of QTc beyond 500 msec is deemed a clinical safety signal [626].

Drugs known to prolong the QTc interval have been responsible for killing people. This potential was observed for Terfenadine [577], [1005]-[1006], Cisapride [1359], and other examples [1222]. Terfenadine and Cisapride were approved and marketed compounds when the deaths due to the drugs occurred. The potential for this effect was identified only after the drugs were marketed to a large number of patients, and these and several other drugs were withdrawn from the market to protect patient safety [1222]. This highlighted the need for thorough assessment of the potential for QTc prolongation prior to approval.

New drugs, and potentially existing drugs seeking new indications, must study and rule out the potential for prolongation of QTc [626]. This thorough study will rule out the presence of a QT/QTc prolongation, or inform how much monitoring for QTc potential will be necessary to establish safety to market in confirmatory trials. Mean prolongation of QTc in excess of 5 to 8 msec will merit greater scrutiny in confirmatory trials. Prolongation greater than 20 msec will likely result in refusal to market unless the benefit of the drug product far outweighs the risk of QTc prolongation and clinical arrythmia (e.g., for an oncology agent).

Even if such a product were approved, it would likely have stringent warnings and requirements limiting its use to patients where benefit clearly outweighs risk. However, such labelling has been observed to be ineffective in the past at protecting patients in the marketplace [1222].

Now that the reasons behind assessment of QTc prolongation have been developed, we turn to discussion of how to model data from a thorough QTc study. This will be followed by a section on design of thorough QTc studies, and last we will consider how to interpret the results of such trials.

9.2 Modelling of QTc Data

To illustrate an approach to the modelling of QTc data, we will consider some data from a previous trial. Normal healthy volunteers are generally [626] the population dosed in such studies, as it is felt that QTc prolongation observed in that population does not pose a great risk, and findings are readily applicable to patient populations.

Fridericia's correction to the QT interval was used, and the study was a fully randomized cross-over design. The objective of the trial was to detect changes in QTc induced by the study drug over and above those introduced by a control agent, and ECGs were manually over-read by a qualified, blinded cardiologist.

In our example dataset, three single-dose regimens (C, D, E) were studied relative to placebo control (Regimen F). Regimen E was a known mild prolonger of the QTc interval (included to serve as a positive control), and regimens C and D were a therapeutic and supra-therapeutic dose of a moderate QTc prolonging agent. Forty-one subjects were included in the example dataset, and QTc was measured in triplicate at baseline (time 0) and over the course of the day at set times following dosing. Triplicate (three ECGs) measurements were averaged at each time of ECG sampling (i.e., 0, 0.5,1, 1.5, 2.4, 4, etc.) for inclusion in analysis, and samples out to four hours post dose were included in the example dataset for ease of presentation and discussion.

Consider some of the first subject's QTc data as listed in Table 9.1 of Example 9.1 below.

Unlike bioequivalence, where only one AUC or Cmax observation was of interest in each period, in this setting the pattern of QTc response within and across periods is of interest. Such repeated-measures, time-series data are inherently more complex to model. However, many methods are available to do so.

The analysis of such repeated-measures data arising in cross-over studies with baseline control is described in [691]. This analysis accounts for each subject as their own control, the correlation between measurements within-period, and accounts for baseline, period, and regimen effects. SAS code is given in [691] and may be found for application to this data on the website.

To describe the pattern of overall response to treatment, the model-adjusted means are output (along with their correlation and variance-covariance matrix) in the `mixed` procedure

TABLE 9.1
First Subject's Data in Example 9.1

Subject	Regimen	Time(h)	QTc(msec)
1	C	0.0	358
1	C	0.5	356
1	C	1.0	361
1	C	1.5	362
1	C	2.5	354
1	C	4.0	355
1	D	0.0	373
1	D	0.5	381
1	D	1.0	389
		......	

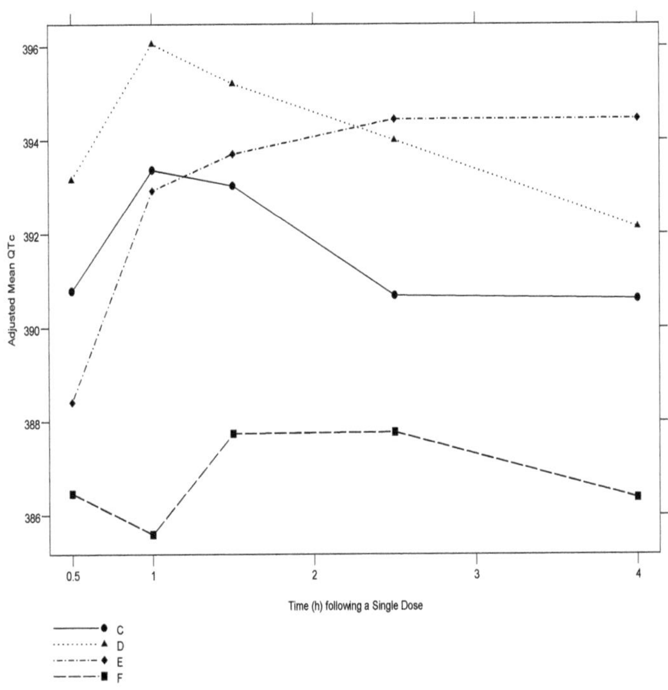

FIGURE 9.2
Mild and Moderate QTc Prolongation ($n = 41$) in Example 9.1

`lsmeans` and `ODS` statements. The `mixed` procedure accounts for effects as described above and provides adjusted mean estimates for use in describing the average effect of treatment. These are plotted for Example 9.1 in Figure 9.2.

The adjusted mean estimates derived from the mixed model are known as "BLUP" in that they are denoted as *Best Linear Unbiased Predictors.* They are asymptotically unbiased estimators for the behavior of mean QTc in the population being studied, and, as with bioequivalence, will serve to compare the properties of the different treatments.

In Figure 9.2, mild (Regimen E) and moderate degrees of prolongation (Regimen C) relative to Regimen F (placebo) are observed with slightly greater prolongation being observed at the supra-therapeutic dose of the drug being studied (Regimen D). In this context, "mild" refers to a QTc prolongation that does not begin until some time after a dose of drug is administered and which rapidly dissipates over time. "Moderate" QTc prolongation, in contrast, denotes a QTc prolongation that begins rapidly after a dose is administered and is maintained over a substantial part of the dosing interval. Both mild and moderate prolongation refer to effect sizes greater than zero but less than the ICH E14 [626] level of probable concern for causing torsades de pointes of 20 msec [1222].

As we begin considering statistical methods to compare these responses, we should consider one other important issue in the modelling of repeated-measures data. That is, that the mean responses within a regimen and across regimens are correlated given the nature of the cross-over study design and repeated-measures ECG data. As these adjusted means are derived from a cross-over trial, the adjusted means between regimens are also

TABLE 9.2
Mean Changes (90% CI) between Regimens Following a Single Dose in Example 9.1 ($n = 41$)

Comparison	Time	Difference	90%CI
C-F	0.5	4.3347	(2.0800,6.5894)
	1	7.7805	(5.0546,10.5063)
	1.5	5.2887	(2.3696,8.2077)
	2.5	2.9160	(-0.09164,5.9236)
	4	4.2413	(1.1931,7.2894)
D-F	0.5	6.7032	(4.4579,8.9485)
	1	10.4697	(7.7514,13.1880)
	1.5	7.4574	(4.5451,10.3696)
	2.5	6.2239	(3.2259,9.2219)
	4	5.7655	(2.7288,8.8023)

C = Therapeutic Dose
D = Supra-Therapeutic Dose
F = Placebo

correlated. Therefore, when we begin comparing treatments, we can account for the fact that adjusted means between treatments are correlated and that adjusted means are also correlated across time.

These comparisons account for the correlation between regimens at each individual time (i.e., that Regimen C is correlated with Regimen F at time 0.5, for example); however, they do not account for the correlation between means across the time interval of ECG sampling (that the means at time 0.5 h are correlated with the means at time 1 h, etc.). It is up to the user, however, to determine which means of controlling the Type 1 and 2 error rates should be employed, and SAS does not automatically do so. To begin the discussion on this topic, we first consider the results (not adjusted for correlation across time) as presented in Table 9.2.

In Example 9.1, it is observed that moderate and statistically significant (note lower 90% confidence bounds exceed zero) QTc prolongation is observed in Regimens C and D within a half-hour of dosing and remains prolonged out to four hours post dosing. Now that models and simple statistical procedures to compare data between regimens have been developed, we discuss statistical procedures to control the Type 1 and 2 error rates in testing for QTc prolongation.

9.3 Interpreting QTc Modelling Findings

As with bioequivalence testing, in the context of QTc testing, we are interested in confirming that a difference in treatments is **not** present. It is presumed that the drug of interest does prolong QTc until it is demonstrated not to be the case. The hypotheses of interest are therefore similar to bioequivalence testing, and the burden of proof remains on the sponsor of the study to demonstrate that QTc prolongation does not occur.

Here we are generally interested in confirming that QTc is not prolonged following dosing over an appropriate period of time when the drug could cause such an effect. The model estimates described in the last section will be used to test for an effect over the appropriate ECG sampling interval. In this setting the null hypothesis for comparison of the test drug (T, at either the therapeutic or supra-therapeutic dose) relative to placebo (P) is

$$H_0 : \mu_{Ti} - \mu_{Pi} \geq \Delta \tag{9.1}$$

for at least one i where i denotes ECG samples collected over the relevant times of sampling and Δ is a predetermined, reasonable no-effect goalpost (defined in [626]). This hypothesis is to be tested against the alternative hypothesis

$$H_1 : \mu_{Ti} - \mu_{Pi} < \Delta \tag{9.2}$$

for all i in the sampling interval. This is another application of the intersection-union test [1314].

Performing this test is simple and straightforward. One simply derives the comparisons of interest between treatments using SAS as described in the last section (Table 9.2) and evaluates the magnitude of the upper bound of the 90% confidence intervals over the relevant interval of sampling relative to the chosen Δ. The level of Δ in [626] was a subject of much debate when [626] was being developed; however, if we choose 8–10 msec for discussion purposes, we see that the null hypothesis is not rejected for the mild and moderate QTc prolongers of Example 9.1, as the upper confidence bounds fall above those levels.

This is not terribly unexpected given the nature [1314] of the testing procedure being used. As we know from bioequivalence testing, Type 1 and 2 errors can occur in testing of such situations.

		The Truth	
		Trt is NOT Safe	Trt IS Safe
Statistics from study show that	Eq. (9.1) NOT Rejected (Trt NOT Safe)	Right answer!	Wrong answer (Type 2 error)
	Eq. (9.1) IS Rejected (Trt IS Safe)	Wrong answer (Type 1 error)	Right answer!

To prove that a treatment is safe under this approach, it must be shown that it is safe over the entire sampling interval. The intersection-union test is known to protect against Type 1 errors at a very conservative level (i.e., less than or equal to the desired level of 5%). This makes the occurrence of a Type 1 error infrequent, a desirable property of such a testing procedure. The risks associated with admitting to the marketplace a drug that prolongs QTc were discussed in Section 9.1, and it is clear that regulators should be concerned (and conservative) with control of the Type 1 error rate.

The potential for a Type 2 error is best controlled in design. Techniques for doing so are

1. Increase the sample size (n),
2. Increase the number of ECGs collected at each time point (r)

Both these actions result in smaller confidence intervals about the model estimates of effect, increasing the precision of the study, yielding more confidence in the understanding of the exact properties of the treatment.

In practice, a combination of both is done as appropriate to the treatment under study. We could most likely prevent the occurrence of a Type 2 error by increasing the sample size to $n = 30$ to 40 subjects or equivalently by increasing the number of ECGs collected at each timepoint from $r = 1$ to $r = 3$ to 4 ECGs (working to reject Equation (9.1) with a $\Delta = 10$ msec). In working practice, sponsors of such trials get very depressed when a Type 2 error occurs, so they generally do both.

Note that sample sizes and ECG sampling under this approach also detect even mild and moderate degrees of QTc prolongation as shown in Example 9.1.

ICH E14 [626] goes into a great deal of complex detail on how to demonstrate that a drug does not affect QTc. To rule out that QTc prolongation occurs for a particular treatment, it must be shown that, in comparing the study drug to placebo at therapeutic and supra-therapeutic doses,

> the largest time-matched mean difference (baseline-subtracted) for the QTc interval is around 5 msec or less, with a one-sided 95% confidence interval that excludes an effect $>$ 10 msec [626].

To perform this procedure one would inspect Table 9.2 for the maximum difference in adjusted means and then use an appropriate statistical procedure to construct a confidence interval on this quantity, accounting for its correlation to all the other comparisons at other ECG sampling times. Mathematically, this procedure is quite complex. In practice, however, it turns out to be equivalent [1314] to the intersection-union test when using the SAS repeated-measures cross-over model described in [691].

The high degree of correlation in QTc data over time also suggests that the intersection-union testing procedure is not terribly conservative in terms of the type 1 error rate. The estimate of autoregressive correlation (a measure of how related data are across time for individual subjects) was 0.9 in the Placebo data of Example 9.1 (a value of 1 would indicate perfect correlation). So, although slightly conservative in its control of Type 1 errors, intersection-union testing will likely meet regulatory, sponsor, and statistical considerations for testing of safety for the issue of QTc prolongation.

Up to now, we have discussed comparisons of a given treatment with a control. However, in trials performing thorough QTc assessments, it is not unusual for multiple doses and a positive control treatment to be employed [626]. See Example 9.1 where supra-therapeutic and therapeutic doses were employed. As the number of doses increases, so too does the possibility of a Type 1 or 2 error. To control these probabilities, one should follow the principles of proof of safety testing described by Hauschke and Hothorn [540] for this setting [971]. A predefined testing procedure should be used to logically order statistical tests to mitigate the probability of a Type 1 error. One (step-up) procedure is as follows:

1. Compare the therapeutic dose to placebo. If Equation (9.1) is rejected in favor of Equation 9.2, then the therapeutic dose is acceptable (proof of safety has been demonstrated) and proceed to Step 2; otherwise, stop and conclude that safety has not been demonstrated at the therapeutic dose **and** the supra-therapeutic dose.

2. Compare the supra-therapeutic dose to placebo. If Equation (9.1) is rejected in favor of Equation (9.2) for the supra-therapeutic dose, then the supra-therapeutic dose is acceptable (proof of safety has been demonstrated); otherwise, stop and conclude that safety has not been demonstrated at the supra-therapeutic dose but was at the therapeutic dose.

Another (step-down) procedure is as follows:

1. Compare the supra-therapeutic dose to placebo. If Equation (9.1) is rejected in favor of Equation (9.2) for the supra-therapeutic dose, then the supra-therapeutic dose and the therapeutic doses are acceptable (proof of safety has been demonstrated); otherwise, conclude that safety has not been demonstrated at the supra-therapeutic dose but conduct additional testing at the therapeutic dose by proceeding to Step 2.
2. Compare the therapeutic dose to placebo. If Equation (9.1) is rejected in favor of Equation (9.2), then the therapeutic dose is acceptable (proof of safety has been demonstrated); otherwise, stop and conclude that safety has not been demonstrated at the therapeutic dose **and** the supra-therapeutic dose.

A sequentially rejecting procedure [540] is appropriate for application under the assumption that QTc prolongation increases with dose. This relationship has been observed for most drugs known to prolong the QTc interval [1222]. The role of the positive control (if any) in this context is discussed later in this section.

Alternatives to the intersection-union test are available. Such statistical testing procedures control Type 1 error at the precise level of 5% while minimizing the probability of a Type 2 error based upon correlations observed in the data. One such technique is Westfall's SimIntervals approach [1317] based upon [1127] and [219] using an SAS program available in [1318]. As the regulatory acceptance of such an approach is unknown, however, we do not discuss it further here. Note that the bootstrap may also be useful in this context [1320].

Turning now to an additional consideration, it should be noted that ICH E14 [626] also recommends that a positive control be used to confirm that the study has the potential to pick up mild to moderate QTc prolongation. Example 9.1 included such a randomized positive control (Regimen E), and we now consider how one might assess such data.

Such a test for positive control prolongation is not consistent with the intersection-union test previously described. This constitutes a union-intersection test [273] where we are interested in confirming that significant prolongation is observed at some time following the dose of positive control relative to placebo. The model estimates described in the last section will be used to test for an effect over the appropriate ECG sampling interval or, if pre-specified in the protocol, at specific times (for example, around Tmax). In this setting the null hypothesis for comparison of the positive control (PC) relative to placebo (P) is

$$H_0 : \mu_{PCi} - \mu_{Pi} \leq \phi \tag{9.3}$$

for all i where i denotes ECG samples collected over the relevant times of sampling and ϕ is a predetermined, reasonable no-effect goalpost (suggested as 5 msec in [1391]). This hypothesis is to be tested against the alternative hypothesis

$$H_1 : \mu_{PCi} - \mu_{Pi} > \phi \tag{9.4}$$

for at least one i in the sampling interval of interest.

As is well known [273], this multiple testing approach results in an inflated probability of rejecting the null hypothesis of interest, and one must adjust the Type 1 error rate for each i comparison to maintain the overall Type 1 error rate at the level desired by regulators. Considering the positive control data of Example 9.1 and adjusting the confidence intervals using the simple Bonferroni approach [273], we find that the null hypothesis is not rejected, as all lower bounds fall below 5 msec. However, several bounds fall above 0, showing that statistically significant prolongation can be detected. The choice of 5 msec in [1391] is somewhat debatable, and those designing such studies should consult with regulators to ensure they meet the local requirement for the positive control comparison (if any).

In practice, one should also consider alternative testing procedures such as [61], but there are many such procedures (see [273] for an excellent summary). One would not need to adjust the Type 1 error rate if one pre-specified in the protocol the time of testing (e.g., at or around observed Tmax).

9.4 Design of a Thorough QTc Study in the Future

The objectives of thorough QTc studies in the future will be to

1. Confirm that the new drug does not prolong QTc to a clinically relevant extent (Equation (9.1)), or
2. Measure the extent to which a drug prolongs QTc.

Given the potential risks induced when QTc is prolonged, it is expected that such compounds will likely be screened out of consideration early in drug development, and that in most cases the first objective will be the primary objective of most trials.

In either case, however, QTc will be measured at baseline and over a 24-hour sampling period following dosing with the therapeutic dose of study drug, a supra-therapeutic dose of study drug, placebo, and possibly a positive control (e.g., Moxifloxacin, an antibiotic known to prolong QTc.) As with bioequivalence testing, normal healthy volunteers will generally be used as the study population [626].

When selecting a design to assess Equation (9.1), a cross-over design will likely be the most sensitive and efficient in providing data to assess the null hypothesis. If a drug truly has no effect on QTc, then one would not expect carry-over effects to be an issue in the use of cross-over designs for the trial. If, however, there is suspicion that the drug may prolong QTc and the drug has a long-half life, then a parallel group trial may also be used to test Equation (9.1) to avoid the potential for carry-over to confound interpretation of the results.

The simulation code discussed in Chapter 5 is readily adaptable to this situation, and we recommend that those designing such studies engage in simulation experimentation based on previous data from their own protocols and labs and whatever statistics and model they choose to employ to determine sample size.

When using cross-over designs, it should be noted that period effects occur in such thorough QTc assessments, and treatments should be fully randomized throughout the study periods to ensure that period effects are not confounded with treatment effects. Period effects can be induced by small period-to-period differences when using a manual over-reader for the ECGs, and it is expected that computer algorithmic measurement is less prone to such effects.

Computer algorithmic measurement is not perfect, however. It is known to be conservative in its assessment of the end of the T-wave, erring on the side of caution to ensure that individual QTc values of potential concern (QTc $>$ 500 msec) are captured. Computer algorithmic measurement is held [626] to be biased in such individual value assessment; however, as the analyses conducted as described in Sections 9.2 to 9.3 account for baseline QTc and each subject as their own control, it would not be expected that such measurement bias introduced by using a computer algorithm would impact statistical inference for Equation (9.1).

Thorough QTc evaluations will generally be conducted in late Phase II or in parallel with the confirmatory trials for regulatory submission. Such trials cannot be conducted unless one has a good idea of the therapeutic and supra-therapeutic doses for the drug of interest, and firm knowledge of these is generally not available until one has demonstrated proof-of-concept and done some work in dose-finding in patients.

The choice of Δ has been noted as worthy of further discussion in the draft ICH E14 guidance [626] and has been defined as 8 msec for the purposes of opening the discussion. It was originally proposed as 5 msec, then changed to 7.5 in ICH discussions, before taking on the value of 8 msec. Dependence on choice of endpoint was highlighted in [971]. In the final Step 4 guidance [626], 10 msec was defined as the Δ.

Throughout this chapter we have used 90% confidence intervals to describe the QTc data. However, readers will note that Section 9.3's assessment of proof of safety is primarily driven by inspection of only the upper bound of the confidence interval. We have chosen to employ these confidence intervals to recognize that regulation [626] on this topic is imperfect. As discussed previously, the choice of Δ is ill-defined, and QTc is a necessary but not sufficient condition for the development of torsades de pointes. As discussed in Chapter 1 (Bernoulli's Principle 8), we should not attribute more weight to such a matter than its due and should view the safety assessments made from the statistics for QTc with some level of caution. ICH E14 [626] is simply a tool being used to protect the public. It is thought that, had this been done, people would not have died. The reader should recall that, as per discussion in Chapter 1, in reality, complete certainty of safety cannot be achieved by such safety testing.

In such a context, the 90% confidence intervals serve a dual purpose. They provide the basis for the QTc safety assessment (using the upper bound), but should mild or moderate prolongation be observed, the lower confidence bound and point estimate serve to place this effect size in context and to evaluate its statistical significance and probability of hazard [540].

A positive control does not add value in a thorough QTc evaluation when testing for a new treatment's safety at therapeutic and supra-therapeutic doses relative to placebo. However, its inclusion does add value if a statistically significant prolongation is observed (i.e., the lower bound of the CI is nonnegative). In drugs known to prolong QTc, the positive control's inclusion in a thorough assessment serves as a method to construct ' 'no worse than" statistical tests.

Consider the comparison of Regimen D to E in Example 9.1 as described in Table 9.3.

In Table 9.3, we see that QTc was prolonged more than the positive control after the supra-therapeutic dose early in the sampling interval, appeared similar in the middle of the sampling, and was slightly lower than the positive control at 4 hours post dose. Although we cannot conclude that the new drug poses no risk of QTc prolongation, the statistically

TABLE 9.3
Mean Changes (90% CI) between Test Drug and Positive Control Following a Single Dose in Example 9.1 ($n = 41$)

Comparison	Time	Difference	90%CI
D-E	0.5	4.7463	(2.4999,6.9926)
	1	3.1356	(0.4160,5.8552)
	1.5	1.4963	(-1.4173,4.4100)
	2.5	-0.4471	(-3.4465,2.5523)
	4	-2.3138	(-5.3519,0.7244)
D = Supra-therapeutic Dose E = Dose of Positive Control			

significant hazard introduced by dosing with the new drug at supra-therapeutic and therapeutic doses (2 to 5 msec immediately following dosing) does not appear markedly dissimilar to that produced by the positive control later in the day.

As techniques in clinical pharmacology safety assessment have now been reviewed, we turn to the assessment of efficacy and mechanism of action for drug products.

Those interested in further reading on this QTc topic may wish to consider [102, 1258], and [1259].

10

Clinical Pharmacology Efficacy Studies

Introduction

In the later years of my career in clinical pharmacology, I was transferred to a strategic job on a committee which oversaw early clinical development of drugs in humans. A big part of this job was managing the interactions of the biostatistics and data management organization with a bunch of "data-happy" clinicians. This adjective data-happy refers to medics who love to collect data and want someone to analyze it until, as they say, the data pleads for mercy. Most often it is the statistician involved who ends up pleading for an end to the analysis. Data seldom speaks for themselves; someone usually has to interpret them. It is beneficial when working with such data-happy people to train them to perform such exploratory statistical analyses themselves. Such an action tends to cure their state of "data-happiness" quite effectively.

To clarify, clinical pharmacologists are paid, and in many cases earn their higher educational degree, developing new markers of clinical activity. As with QTc (described in Chapter 9), these take on the attributes of alphabet soup, in most cases, with the addition of numbers where the pharmacologists run out of letters — for example, CRP, IL8, IL5, LDL, VLDL, VLDL1, VLDL2, etc. Unlike statisticians, in general, they do not seem to have thought to introduce Greek letters; instead they just add more letters and numbers. My personal belief is that this is because the word-processing software packages they most use make it difficult to use Greek letters....

In any event, the point of measuring such markers in humans, and describing their behavior over time and relative to dose, is to detect the clinical effect of drugs on the body. This obviously is of great potential benefit. If one can measure such activity in the body, and if such activity is predictive of clinical outcomes (like stroke or myocardial infarction), then one could, in theory, predict the efficacy of drugs early in drug development! Even if it is not directly predictive, such knowledge should, in theory, allow one to improve understanding of how a drug works. Such knowledge of method of action is hoped to be beneficial.

My data-happy clinicians were always excited about such endpoints, and often wondered why I was not. They usually put it down to, "Statisticians are just not interested in the science of such matters...." In truth, I was interested, but after many years in clinical pharmacology, I had made a conscious decision not to get excited about (or too involved in) such data-happy clinical things because:

1. *There is a lot more involved in predicting clinical outcomes than just showing that a marker is correlated to clinical outcome, and*
2. *One comes to realize that efficacy is all well and good, but safety comes first (and, as we saw in Chapter 8, is an evolving topic).*

If one cannot find a safe and well-tolerated dose range (which is what early phase development is all about), then it really does not matter how efficacious the drug is. In my experience, most drugs fail in drug development because one cannot achieve a dose that is high enough such that the drug works without untoward side-effects, not because the drug does not work.

All this said, evaluation of drug efficacy and method of action data is an important part of clinical pharmacology, and this chapter will cover some methods for modelling the behavior of such data. We first briefly review some topics related to nomenclature, assumptions, and the statistics employed for this purpose.

10.1 Background

Traditional statisticians often fail to recognize the "learning" nature of clinical pharmacology drug development. Some have suggested that this is due to the traditional techniques inherent in how statistical science is taught at many universities. Students are taught by rote to test pre-determined hypotheses using direct, confirmatory methods (like those employed in bioequivalence testing). Few assumptions about the data are made, and one in essence achieves a positive or negative outcome.

Clinical pharmacology assessments of efficacy, however, focus on learning about a compound and its properties in humans, not confirming that it has or does not have activity. In the eyes of a drug developer, a compound may be presumed to have some level of efficacy in humans. The effect may not be clinically relevant, but that is another separate issue to be determined and studied later in drug development.

First, a drug developer should learn whether the compound does roughly what one expects in humans. This approach lends itself to indirect statistical assessment (see Bayesian discussion in Chapter 5). In this chapter, we will use commonly applied traditional modelling methods and supplement them with application of a basic Bayesian program to illustrate the use of such procedures.

As described in Chapter 2, in drug development, one should first define a safe and well-tolerated dose range in normal healthy volunteers ([621, 1142]). Traditionally, ad hoc assessment of drug activity occurs in Phase I sub-chronic dosing studies. One presumes that dose and exposure have some relationship to outcome, and applies models to quantify this expectation.

Lack of a quantified relationship in markers of human activity in Phase I is not unexpected. This can occur for many reasons, such as low sample size, lack of relevant markers of pharmacodynamic activity in a normal healthy population, or lower exposures in normal healthy volunteers relative to that to be applied in patients with the disease to be treated. As described in Chapter 8, cross-over designs (randomized or non-randomized) are traditionally applied to enhance the information gained from such trials.

Once a safe and well-tolerated dose range has been defined in Phase I studies, a pilot study is usually conducted with the new drug in a small group of patients (Phase IIa). This study is sometimes referred to as providing Proof-of-Concept [1142] in that it is expected to provide drug developers with some confidence in their notion that the drug will work. Again, one presumes that dose and exposure have some relationship to pharmacologic markers of drug activity (like blood pressure, for example), and models are applied to quantify this relationship. Unless the disease state is markedly unstable over the length of dosing (usually limited to a month in Phase IIa due to the toxicology coverage), randomized or non-randomized cross-over designs are again the designs of choice in this setting, as they provide better information ([1139, 1140]) to build the models under consideration. Sample size is limited so that if the drug proves to be unsafe in the patient population, dosing and the drug's development can be halted in a timely fashion.

ICH [621] and FDA [372] guidance on the topic calls for parallel group trials to assess such information in light of concerns with carry-over effects confounding the assessment of treatment [652]. However, such a position is logically inconsistent from a drug developer's perspective. In Phase IIa, developers work on the assumption that the drug has some level of activity. Detection of a carry-over effect in a placebo-controlled cross-over trial would constitute a positive finding, as the drug would have some pharmacodynamic activity to be "carried over"!

The information desired at this stage of development is **not** confirmatory, and those seeking a yes or no solution to questions relating to developing a drug (sometimes known as a go or no-go decision in business) are likely to be disappointed. Limited scientific evidence of clinical efficacy and understanding of method of action are generated. This information serves to modify the level of confidence a sponsor has in the likely success of a compound, hopefully (but not necessarily) in a positive manner. Often, due in part to the small sample sizes in Phase IIa, many proof of concept studies are inconclusive in a traditional statistical sense [625]. Expert judgment is usually called for in interpretation of the results.

In terms of statistics, one should establish a quantitative relationship between dose or exposure with a pharmacologic effect using a model. Many assumptions are made. For example:

1. That dose and exposure are related to the marker.
2. That the relationship between dose and exposure with the marker of interest can be expressed in a mathematical model.
3. That markers of pharmacologic activity in patients substitute for assessments of longer term clinical benefit.
4. That pharmacokinetics in plasma can predict the concentrations at the site of pharmacodynamic action.

The model(s) to be explored need not be prespecified in such exploratory, learning trials. One generally would choose to dose a limited number of patients (in the interest of their safety) with a range of doses and placebo, measure the marker of pharmacodynamic activity, and apply models to the data in a systematic, parsimonious manner to quantify the relationship of dose to the marker of interest with some degree of desired precision.

As with the study of pharmacokinetics, such models are developed over the course of drug development to help with the dosing of subsequent larger numbers of patients. Of interest is maintaining the exposure levels in a safe and well-tolerated range while achieving exposure levels of drug sufficient to treat or cure the disease condition.

Clinical pharmacologists can (and some do) overestimate the value of such exploratory data. These data are **NOT** confirmatory of efficacy in a regulatory, market-access sense [621]. As discussed in Chapter 2, regulators in general presume that a drug is not efficacious until shown otherwise. Such findings as those described above are interesting and aid regulators in determining which dose is most appropriate for initiating and treating patients ([372, 466, 621]); however, a confirmatory trial is one in which the hypotheses to be tested are stated in advance and intended to provide firm, conclusive evidence of safety and efficacy [625] for a dose and dosing regimen [621]. The statistical procedures to test for success or failure of the drug to provide benefit are prespecified [625], and a determination of a positive (or negative) outcome is straightforward. Readers interested in more details about the design and analysis of confirmatory clinical trials should see [434] and [211] for excellent summaries.

The benefits of applying exploratory clinical pharmacology techniques are tangible [866, 1026], improving the information gained from drug development for drug labelling and marketing while speeding study completion and subsequently (presumably) regulatory approval. Shortfalls of these procedures result from lack of education, validation, and analytic tools and procedures for their application ([501, 980]). One key shortcoming, highlighted in [1026], pertains to lack of knowledge of the predictive value of the pharmacodynamic marker for clinical effect (in future studies), and we now turn to further discussions on the characterization of pharmacodynamic response prior to discussing the data, models, and statistics used in such techniques.

As discussed in Chapter 2, "biomarkers" or biological markers are endpoints which are "a physical sign or laboratory measurement that occurs in association with a pathological process and that has a putative diagnostic and/or prognostic utility" ([82, 758]). This essentially means that a biomarker is an endpoint we can measure in clinical pharmacology trials (like those described in Phases I and IIa) and presumably has something to do with the disease we are studying and are hoping will be impacted (for the better) by the drug being developed.

In contrast, surrogate markers ([82, 758]) are a subset of the biomarkers that can serve as a substitute [1219] for a clinically meaningful endpoint. These clinical endpoints (also sometimes called outcomes) are a measure of how a patient with the disease to be treated "feels, functions, or survives" [758]. Lesko and Atkinson [758] further subdivide the category of clinical endpoints into

1. Ultimate outcome — a clinical endpoint such as survival, survival time, onset of serious morbidity, or symptomatic response that captures the benefits and risks of therapeutic intervention.
2. Intermediate endpoints — a clinical endpoint that is not the ultimate outcome but is nonetheless of real clinical benefit.

Clinical pharmacology assessments of efficacy focus mainly on biomarker assessment with some limited assessments of surrogate markers in relation to dose and concentration in plasma. Where possible, the concentration of drug at the site of action may be probed. Measurement of clinical endpoints usually requires lengthy studies and significant investment. Therefore, such studies are generally not undertaken in modern drug development until sufficient confidence is generated by biomarker and surrogate marker data to reassure sponsors that the investment is worth the risk. Clinical pharmacology studies therefore do not provide direct assurance of safety and efficacy in clinical endpoints.

Establishing a biomarker as a surrogate marker is not a simple process. Temple [1219] describes several criteria that must be assessed, studied, and validated before such can occur:

1. Biological plausibility including (but not limited to) consistent, extensive, and quantitative epidemiologic evidence, credible animal models, well-understood disease pathogenesis, drug mechanism of action, and surrogacy relatively late on the biological path.
2. Success in clinical trials including (but not limited to) showing that the effect on the surrogate has predicted outcomes with other drugs of the same pharmacologic class and in several other classes of drug.
3. Risk benefit and public health considerations including (but not limited to) serious or life-threatening illness with no alternative therapies.

Few endpoints would be expected to fulfill such criteria for surrogacy [418], but one thing that is very clear from the above criteria is that "A correlate does not a surrogate make [418]".

Some elements of defining a biomarker as a surrogate endpoint are statistical, and we refer interested readers to Prentice's classical work on the topic [1007] and an excellent comprehensive summary [134].

For the purposes of further discussion in this chapter, we will assume that the drug of interest has been shown to impact biomarkers in animal models and that there is reason to believe dosing with drug will translate into similar pharmacodynamic effects on relevant human biomarkers. Further discussion will therefore focus on modelling of the drug, concentration, and biomarker relationship. As in previous chapters, we will focus on the application of commonly used techniques using clinical data from previous trials. We first consider data generated in Phase I sub-chronic dosing studies followed by consideration of data from patients in Phase IIa.

10.2 Sub-Chronic Dosing

The design of sub-chronic dosing studies is described in Chapter 8. In addition to the safety assessments conducted during such trials, a plethora of data on pharmacodynamic endpoints is sometime collected to elucidate the mechanism of action of the drug being studied. These data may consist of laboratory, gene expression, or protein expression endpoints, for example.

All these pharmacodynamic data are presumably correlated with each other in one way or another. Their interrelationship may be defined in a cascade manner, in that drug treatment impacts one biological mechanism, which impacts another, which impacts another, causing responses along the way. Responses may also result from parallel biological processing of drug, in that drug treatment impacts multiple mechanisms of action in parallel, e.g., one in the heart and one in the liver at roughly the same time perhaps. Several techniques are available to assess whether treatment has an effect in such large datasets ([893, 898]), and we will utilize one commonly used technique (see Ch. 31 of [881]) in this section to test for treatment effects over time in sub-chronic dosing trials using a dataset of gene expression data before and after treatment with drug or with placebo.

See Table 10.1. Here subjects were randomly assigned to a regimen (placebo or drug treatment), had their biomarker endpoints measured on day -3, and were then dosed for 14 days with the regimen to which they were assigned with another biomarker assessment occurring on the last day of dosing (day 12).

This was a very simple sub-chronic dosing study, and looked at only one dose and placebo. In general, more doses are included in such studies, allowing for more sophisticated assessment of dose-response [621]. For this dataset, a simple model may be used to describe the data:

$$Y_{ijk} = \Gamma_j + \Upsilon_k + \Omega_{jk} + \Sigma_{ijk}$$

where Y_{ijk} is the matrix (data arranged in columns by endpoint) of observations for the endpoints of interest, Γ_j is a matrix which denotes day -3 or 12, Υ_k is placebo or drug treatment, and Ω_{jk} denotes day-by-regimen interaction, with Σ_{ijk} denoting residual variability. Here we are interested in the significance of the Ω_{jk}, as this would signal that the regimens are behaving differently across time in some manner for at least one endpoint.

The element of Ω_{jk} (and the other matrices) are arranged to correspond to the endpoint to which they relate. For example, for the data in Table 10.1,

$$\Omega_{jk} =$$

$$\begin{bmatrix} \omega_{L11} & \omega_{L12} & \omega_{L21} & \omega_{L22} \\ \omega_{M11} & \omega_{M12} & \omega_{M21} & \omega_{M22} \\ \omega_{N11} & \omega_{N12} & \omega_{N21} & \omega_{N22} \\ \omega_{O11} & \omega_{O12} & \omega_{O21} & \omega_{O22} \\ \omega_{P11} & \omega_{P12} & \omega_{P21} & \omega_{P22} \end{bmatrix}$$

TABLE 10.1
Example 10.2.1: Pharmacodynamic Biomarker Data from an Exploratory Sub-Chronic Dosing Study

Subject	Day	Regimen	L	M	N	O	P
102	-3	P	7.67	7.95	9.47	10.17	4.65
102	12	P	6.77	7.50	8.89	9.60	4.47
103	-3	D	7.60	7.69	9.60	9.41	5.04
103	12	D	7.33	7.91	9.39	9.39	5.11
104	-3	D	7.61	7.58	9.60	8.93	5.32
104	12	D	7.36	8.02	9.86	9.70	5.46
201	-3	P	6.00	7.24	8.56	8.99	3.87
201	12	P	6.66	7.52	8.88	9.60	4.38
202	-3	D	8.04	8.35	9.46	9.75	5.26
202	12	D	7.32	7.74	9.36	9.10	4.85
204	-3	D	6.83	7.53	8.75	8.82	4.67
204	12	D	6.79	7.54	8.75	8.74	4.84
205	-3	P	7.33	7.81	9.27	9.52	5.15
205	12	P	7.06	7.49	8.98	8.96	4.32
208	-3	P	7.36	7.71	9.29	9.81	5.23
208	12	P	7.43	7.86	9.48	9.32	5.23
209	-3	D	7.60	7.83	9.70	9.68	5.23
209	12	D	6.70	7.64	8.90	9.07	4.44
210	-3	D	6.76	7.69	8.86	9.05	5.12
210	12	D	6.65	7.66	8.61	9.32	4.91
211	-3	P	7.15	7.91	9.73	10.22	5.26
211	12	P	7.29	7.98	9.20	10.17	5.11
213	-3	P	6.76	7.82	9.41	9.44	5.03
213	12	P	7.50	7.95	9.37	9.38	5.18
P=Placebo; D=Dose of Drug for 14 Days							

for endpoint L, M, N, O, and P in each row, respectively, where, for example, ω_{L11} denotes the mean effect of treatment with drug on day -3 and ω_{L12} denotes the mean effect of treatment with drug on day 12, and so on.

We are interested in testing the null hypothesis:

$$\omega_{L11} = \omega_{L12} = \omega_{L21} = \omega_{L22},$$

$$\omega_{M11} = \omega_{M12} = \omega_{M21} = \omega_{M22},$$

$$\omega_{N11} = \omega_{N12} = \omega_{N21} = \omega_{N22},$$

$$\omega_{O11} = \omega_{O12} = \omega_{O21} = \omega_{O22},$$

$$\omega_{P11} = \omega_{P12} = \omega_{P21} = \omega_{P22}$$

versus the alternative that at least one of the ω_{jk} differs from the others for at least one of the endpoints.

Computation of estimates for the elements of the various matrices (like Ω_{jk}) is a complex topic beyond the scope of this book. See [893] and [898] for a description. SAS automatically performs some of these calculations [1073] using a procedure similar to `proc mixed` known as `proc glm`. Code to do so for this study is as follows.

Sub-Chronic Exploratory Multivariate Data Analysis 10.2.1 — SAS `proc glm` *Code:*

```
proc glm data=my.sc1a;
    class day regimen;
    model L M N O P = day
    regimen regimen*day;
    MANOVA h=day regimen regimen*day;
    run;
```

Here `proc glm` is called and directed to assess data from the permanent dataset `my.sc1a` (available on the website accompanying this book). The `class` statement again specifies the descriptive variables of the model, and the `model` statement specifies that endpoints L, M, N, O, and P (a subset of those available, included here for simplicity) be modelled as a function of day, regimen, and day-by-regimen interaction. The `MANOVA` statement specifies that SAS should construct tests to assess whether the study days are different (pooling across regimens), whether the regimens are different (pooling across study days), and (most of interest) whether response to treatment is different between regimens over time, testing the null hypothesis described above for these endpoints simultaneously.

Selected SAS outputs appear as follows:

Sub-Chronic Exploratory Multivariate Data Analysis 10.2.1 — Selected SAS `proc glm` *Output:*

```
MANOVA Test Criteria and Exact F Statistics for
 the Hypothesis of No Overall DAY*REGIMEN Effect
  H = Type III SSCP Matrix for DAY*REGIMEN
  E = Error SSCP Matrix
Statistic          F Value    Num DF    Den DF   Pr > F
  Wilks'Lambda     0.94          5         16    0.4801
```

Based on the p-value for day-by-regimen interaction ($p = 0.4801$), there is very little evidence to suggest that treatment with drug impacts the biomarkers considered here (endpoints L, M, N, O, and P) over the course of 14 days of treatment. This is not unexpected in Phase I drug development, as described in the previous section. At worst, such data are valuable in that they provide variability estimates for use in better sizing subsequent trials. At best, one may see some evidence of treatment effects that would also aid in designing more definitive trials later in drug development.

The downside of utilization of a multivariate statistical procedure as described above is that it is known [881] to be less powerful (prone to false negatives) than univariate methods (which we will now discuss). However, such an approach serves as a handy tool for rapid assessment of whether there is value in extensive data mining of a large pharmacodynamic dataset. It should be noted that such multivariate methods have been developed for use in cross-over designs; however, they are not much utilized (e.g., [1269]).

Another way of examining such multivariate data is to use a univariate testing procedure which accounts for multiple endpoints. Pairwise comparisons are constructed between regimens (for example) for each endpoint. As is well known, Type I error becomes inflated if and when one does not take into account the number of comparisons. To protect the experiment-wise error rate, adjustment should be made.

A full discussion of this topic is beyond the scope of this book, and we advise those considering such procedures to see the excellent summary in [273]. Such approaches to adjust for multiple endpoints and comparisons are readily implemented in modern software, and in this case, the SAS procedure `proc multtest` may be used as follows.

Sub-Chronic Exploratory Multiple Testing Data Analysis 10.2.1 — SAS `proc multtest` *Code:*

```
proc multtest data=my.sc1a
bootstrap nsample=10000;
  by day;
      class regimen;
      test mean(L M N O P);
  contrast "Regimen" 1 -1;
      run;
```

Here the resampling approach of [1316] is applied by invoking **bootstrap** in the call to **proc multtest**, specifying the number of bootstrap samples in the **nsample**. Selected output is as follows.

Sub-Chronic Exploratory Multiple Testing Data Analysis 10.2.1 — Selected SAS `proc multtest` *Output from Day 12:*

```
                        p-Values

Variable    Contrast          Raw     Bootstrap

L           Regimen        0.6451        0.9551
M           Regimen        0.7793        0.9916
N           Regimen        0.9741        0.9999
O           Regimen        0.2101        0.4836
P           Regimen        0.4991        0.8584
```

We see that the multiple testing approach yields findings of non-significance between regimens similar to the multivariate approach described above. Used in tandem, these approaches are useful for data mining and understanding large datasets. Trend tests have been developed for such multivariate datasets to consider, for example, dose-response testing [523].

For single (hopefully pre-specified in the protocol) endpoints, a more powerful approach, a dose-response analysis, will now be discussed. Here, low density lipoprotein, LDL, was measured (decreasing this surrogate marker results in clinical benefit [311]), before and after sub-chronic treatment with a randomly assigned dose of drug or placebo in each normal healthy volunteer subject. The objective of modelling in this case was to assess whether there was evidence of a response to dose in this population (normal healthy volunteers).

TABLE 10.2: Example 10.2.2: Dose, Pharmacokinetic, and Low Density Lipoprotein Data from a Sub-Chronic Dosing Study

Subject	Dose	AUC	Cmax	Baseline LDL	Post-Trt LDL
56	0	0.00	0.000	2.18	2.22
63	0	0.00	0.000	3.53	4.47
67	0	0.00	0.000	2.85	3.01
73	0	0.00	0.000	1.37	1.74
74	0	0.00	0.000	2.71	2.26
AUC and Cmax assumed 0 if Dose was 0					

TABLE 10.2: Example 10.2.2: Dose, Pharmacokinetic, and Low Density Lipoprotein Data from a Sub-Chronic Dosing Study (continued)

Subject	Dose	AUC	Cmax	Baseline LDL	Post-Trt LDL
86	0	0.00	0.000	2.93	2.78
87	0	0.00	0.000	2.80	3.09
91	0	0.00	0.000	2.40	2.59
94	0	0.00	0.000	5.33	5.36
100	0	0.00	0.000	2.04	2.32
103	0	0.00	0.000	3.31	3.21
112	0	0.00	0.000	1.92	2.05
47	5	5.11	0.423	3.03	2.89
48	5	8.13	0.620	2.59	1.95
49	5	8.01	0.627	2.05	1.72
50	5	6.67	0.480	3.06	2.66
52	5	7.38	0.591	4.01	2.80
53	5	5.17	0.390	3.27	3.52
54	5	8.16	0.569	3.25	3.35
55	5	6.23	0.483	2.52	2.38
57	5	3.36	0.316	2.14	2.14
60	10	11.22	0.962	3.98	3.13
61	10	8.21	0.723	1.70	1.78
62	10	20.85	1.861	2.96	2.05
64	10	16.48	1.169	2.28	2.54
65	10	6.79	0.574	3.09	3.64
66	10	18.08	1.303	2.13	1.77
69	10	10.51	0.883	2.15	1.78
71	10	13.97	1.056	3.45	2.98
72	10	13.80	1.157	2.77	2.25
95	20	30.35	2.220	2.47	1.88
99	20	53.11	3.902	2.31	1.88
102	20	38.61	2.517	3.13	2.93
104	20	29.33	2.219	3.68	4.27
105	20	26.20	1.844	3.20	3.10
106	20	29.47	1.893	3.16	3.40
107	20	27.55	1.965	3.35	3.18
108	20	19.97	1.447	1.84	1.98
110	20	35.91	2.322	3.44	3.36
AUC and Cmax assumed 0 if Dose was 0					

Previous experience indicated that LDL was log-normally distributed in normal healthy volunteers, so, in a manner similar to pharmacokinetic analysis, this endpoint was log-transformed for analysis following correction for baseline (in this case, simply by taking the ratio of posttreatment LDL to baseline LDL). Only a limited response was expected in normal healthy volunteers, and for the purposes of this example, a power model was utilized of the form

$$y_k = \alpha + \beta(ld) + \varepsilon_k$$

where β is the slope parameter of interest regressed on logDose (parameter ld) for the log-transformed ratio of posttreatment LDL to baseline LDL for each subject k. Note that we do not have repeated measurements within a subject, so there is no term denoting each subject as their own control or denoting the repeated measures. This is often the case in Phase I designs, as such pharmacodynamic assessments are (relatively) expensive and are of limited value due to the normal healthy population being studied and the expected portfolio attrition rates.

In this case, the power model was selected for use, as normal healthy volunteers in general do not have high LDL values, and therefore may be expected to show only a limited response to treatment (if at all). To include the placebo data (null dose) in the power model, the dose needs to be set to a value greater than 0 prior to log-transform such as 0.000001 using SAS statements such as those following in a data step (see also `dose response.sas` on the website accompanying this book):

```
if dose=0 then dose=0.000001;
```

In general, one would build such a nonlinear dose-response model after first investigating the fit of a linear dose-response model ([510, 881, 907, 1104]). In this case, the fit of a linear model is poor and indicative of heterogeneous variance. We leave confirmation of this point to the reader and encourage readers interested in more details of model building to investigate the above references. SAS code for this analysis is

Sub-Chronic Dose Response Data Analysis 10.2.2 — SAS `proc mixed` *Code:*

```
title 'Log-Ratio Power Model';run;
proc mixed data=sc2a;
    class subject;
    model ldlchg=lndose/s cl ddfm=kenwardroger
    outp=out outpm=predmean;
    run;

proc print noobs data=predmean;
    where subject<10;
    var dose alpha pred lower upper;
    run;
```

Here the log-transformed ratio of posttreatment to baseline LDL is fitted versus logDose. Residuals are output to an SAS dataset `out` for use in assessing model fit (not shown), and predicted mean values are output to an SAS dataset `predmean`. To derive estimates of dose-response, one includes "dummy" subjects (in this case, subjects 1 to 9 corresponding to doses of 0 to 80 mg, see `dose response.sas`) with dosing information in the analysis data, set but with no data on LDL response. As no LDL data are available for these "dummy" subjects, they are not included in model fitting, but SAS provides estimates of effect for these subjects in the `predmean` dataset. Selected SAS output is as follows.

Sub-Chronic Dose Response Data Analysis 10.2.2 — Selected SAS `proc mixed` *Output:*

```
The Mixed Procedure
Solution for Fixed Effects

 Effect       Estimate    Pr > |t|
 Intercept    -0.06567    0.0104
 lndose       -0.00854    0.0086

       Type 3 Tests of Fixed Effects
                 Num      Den
Effect           DF       DF     F Value     Pr > F
lndose            1       37        7.71     0.0086

DOSE      Alpha        Pred         Lower         Upper
 0        0.05       0.05226     -0.03131       0.13584
 5        0.05      -0.07941     -0.13290      -0.02592
10        0.05      -0.08533     -0.14109      -0.02957
20        0.05      -0.09125     -0.14951      -0.03299
30        0.05      -0.09471     -0.15453      -0.03489
40        0.05      -0.09716     -0.15813      -0.03620
60        0.05      -0.10062     -0.16326      -0.03799
80        0.05      -0.10308     -0.16693      -0.03923
```

In this case, we observed that LDL (adjusted for baseline) decreases with increasing logDose (estimate of -0.00854 for β with $p = 0.0086$). The values `Pred`, `Lower`, and `Upper` may be exponentiated to estimate dose-response in LDL (adjusted for baseline) on the original scale, resulting in the findings of Table 10.3.

Here we observe that dosing in normal healthy volunteers resulted in decreases of 8 to 10% in LDL (adjusted for baseline). This is promising data (in terms of effect on a surrogate marker in Phase I). However, overinterpretation of such data is not recommended. Data from normal healthy volunteers can only predict clinical outcomes under carefully controlled circumstances.

Here, these findings should increase confidence in the drug's potential to be useful in the clinic, but such data are not definitive (as patients with disease have not yet been assessed). Pairwise testing between mean responses (for example, direct comparison of 5, 10, and 20 mg to placebo), as is often done in Phase II–III dose-response testing [712], is

TABLE 10.3
LDL Dose-Response (Ratio Relative to Baseline LDL) with 95% Confidence Intervals in Sub-Chronic Dosing Study Example 10.2.2

Dose	Estimated Effect	95% CI
0	1.05	0.97 – 1.15
5	0.92	0.88 – 0.97
10	0.92	0.87 – 0.97
20	0.91	0.86 – 0.97
40	0.91	0.85 – 0.96
60	0.90	0.85 – 0.96
80	0.90	0.85 – 0.96

not recommended here, as such analyses are typically misleading in trials of such limited sample size.

Note that sample size selection is driven by safety considerations in such designs (see Chapter 8).

Models such as the above may also be useful to provide a preliminary check for association between pharmacokinetic and pharmacodynamic responses. In this case, steady state AUC and Cmax did not appear to be related to baseline-adjusted LDL changes ($p = 0.8026$ and $p = 0.6549$ for logAUC and logCmax, respectively). Absence of a significant relationship may not preclude that such an association exists [647]. As described previously, such an observation may occur due to low sample size and may be related to not having a model accounting for all relevant biologic information. In this particular case, for example, it was thought that the drug worked in the liver such that plasma pharmacokinetics were not predictive of concentrations at the site of action. Plasma concentrations in the liver may be modelled by extending the findings of Chapter 11 to allow for another compartment. As shown in Chapter 8, dose and AUC are to some extent confounded and their use in a model simultaneously is therefore of questionable validity [1024], potentially leading to model overspecification [907].

We now turn to modelling and interpretation of data in clinical pharmacology studies of patient populations.

10.3 Phase IIa and the Proof of Concept

For purposes of illustration, assume that a proof-of-concept trial was desired to test whether the LDL response in normal healthy volunteers described in the last section would result in clinical benefit when given to patients. LDL was again to be used as a surrogate marker of clinical benefit for the purposes of this trial.

Recall that about a 10% decrease in LDL was observed in normal healthy volunteers. When dosing in patients, it might be expected that approximately twice this magnitude would be observed, as

1. Patients with disease would be recruited with higher LDL (than the subjects in Phase I), allowing more of an effect of drug to be observed,
2. Dosing in patients was planned to be of at least twice the duration of Phase I, and
3. Animal efficacy data indicated that drug would be more effective than observed in the Phase I sub-chronic dosing study.

The proof-of-concept Phase IIa trial was designed in a standard [625] pessimistic fashion under the assumption (null hypothesis) that the drug would have no effect on LDL. The alternative to be tested was that treatment with drug would result in a 20% decrease (accounting for baseline) relative to placebo.

Patients with high LDL (who are not already taking some form of medication) are not easy to find. This resulted in a lengthy trial duration to recruit only 15 patients in a 2×2 cross-over design. LDL data from this trial may be found in Table 10.4. After a baseline LDL assessment in each session, patients were dosed with a drug expected to lower LDL level (or placebo) for 6 weeks.

TABLE 10.4: Example 10.3.1: Low-Density Lipoprotein Data from a Proof-of-Concept Study

Subject	Sequence	Per	Reg	Post-Trt LDL	Baseline LDL	Analysis Endpoint
2472	PA	1	P	101	98	0.031
2472	PA	2	A	89	110	-0.212
2530	AP	1	A	140	159	-0.132
2530	AP	2	P	146	151	-0.034
2535	PA	1	P	100	86	0.150
2535	PA	2	A	106	82	0.257
2540	PA	1	P	163	135	0.182
2540	PA	2	A	139	143	-0.027
2544	PA	1	P	160	147	0.086
2544	PA	2	A	99	123	-0.220
2546	AP	1	A	85	103	-0.186
2546	AP	2	P	81	92	-0.126
2548	AP	1	A	106	115	-0.077
2548	AP	2	P	96	111	-0.139
2549	PA	1	P	125	142	-0.128
2549	PA	2	A	116	126	-0.083
2560	PA	1	P	155	178	-0.140
2560	PA	2	A	108	151	-0.331
2562	PA	1	P	104	124	-0.170
2562	PA	2	A	97	104	-0.077
2650	AP	1	A	128	139	-0.087
2650	AP	2	P	132	124	0.061
2659	PA	1	P	120	108	0.102
2659	PA	2	A	101	116	-0.143
2668	PA	1	P	151	128	0.167
2668	PA	2	A	128	163	-0.241
2712	AP	1	A	120	124	-0.032
2712	AP	2	P	108	139	-0.251
2755	PA	1	P	132	147	-0.111
2755	PA	2	A	132	151	-0.137
A=Drug Treatment; P=Placebo Endpoint=Natural-log of Post-Trt LDL to Baseline LDL						

The SAS code used to analyze the analysis endpoint of Table 10.4 is the same as that used to analyze 2×2 cross-over studies in Chapter 3 and is not reproduced here. Readers interested in the code may find it on the website accompanying this book.

The findings ($n = 15$) indicated that treatment with the drug lowered LDL by only approximately 7% relative to placebo (the effect size on the log-scale was -0.07177 with a 90% confidence interval of -0.1544 to 0.01090). As the upper bound of the 90% confidence interval exceeded zero, the null hypothesis (that the drug does not significantly change LDL relative to placebo) was not rejected. This would therefore be regarded as a "failed" study.

However, the findings provide some useful information ([526, 697]):

1. The bulk of the confidence interval falls to the left of null; therefore, while we cannot conclude that this dose of drug is effective, it suggests the potential for increased doses of drug to provide significant benefit.
2. The maximum expected mean effect of this dose of drug is a 14% decrease in LDL (corresponding to the exponentiated lower confidence limit) with the effect size most likely falling around 7%. Such a small decrease might be desirable (and clinically relevant) in some patient population.

Thus, while failing to reject the null hypotheses, the study has provided some degree of useful information.

The above approach is a traditional one, and, should it be successful (as this example was not), it clearly increases confidence that the drug will be efficacious even against a pessimistic level of opinion concerning the drug's merits. Such studies need not be designed to provide such a yes-or-no answer, however. Moreover, planning a traditional hypothesis testing approach, like that described here, requires a long time. One would probably wait to analyze the data until the full ($n = 15$) complement of patients complete the study.

A Bayesian analysis (described in Chapter 5) provides a ready alternative to the traditional analysis described above. Here, we may take explicit account that an effect size of approximately 10% is our expectation and express it as a prior distribution for `delta` (the effect size of treatment with drug relative to placebo). WINBUGS code to perform a Bayesian analysis is the same as that utilized for bioequivalence testing in Chapter 5.

With data from only eight patients, such a Bayesian analysis (see Table 10.5) provides the following expectations regarding the effect size on the log-transformed scale and original scale.

From this Bayesian analysis (based on the 90th percentile), we can conclude (with only $n = 8$) that the drug has approximately a 90% probability of reducing LDL relative to placebo. Conversely, there is a lesser chance (approximately 10%) that the drug treatment is the same or worse than placebo. The effect size with this dose of drug is unlikely (less than a 5% chance, based on the 5th percentile) to be greater than a 17% decrease and is most unlikely (less than a 2.5% chance, based on the 2.5th percentile) to reach the desired decrease level of 20% in posttreatment LDL relative to placebo.

If one looks closely, this is about the same amount of information one could glean from the traditional analysis and design described above, except that this Bayesian analysis approach, if used, only takes half as many patients and half the time as the original study. Bayesian design and analysis plans such as these can be very useful tools to increase a sponsor's confidence in the properties of a compound without requiring long resource-intensive

TABLE 10.5
LDL Effect Size (Ratio Relative to Baseline LDL) from a Bayesian Statistical Analysis of a Proof-of-Concept Study Example 10.3.1 ($n = 8$)

Trt:Pbo Baseline Adj Effect Size	2.5 PTL	5 PTL	Median	90 PTL	97.5 PTL
ln-Scale	-0.2141	-0.1878	-0.07697	0.006284	0.05994
Original-Scale	0.8073	0.8288	0.9259	1.006	1.062
PTL=Percentile of the Bayesian Posterior Distribution					

studies. Such an approach is useful for internal decision making; however, use in a regulatory setting when wishing to make a claim about the properties of a drug (for the reasons discussed in Chapter 2) is of questionable validity.

An unstated reason why one often does not utilize such an approach to design and analysis is the wish to publish data from such studies. Akin to the approach to data interpretation taken by regulators, most scientific journals would question the application of such a Bayesian approach closely, as such techniques are only now becoming widely used and have been the matter of some historical debate. A group-sequential approach (described in Chapter 5) may be used if a journal-acceptable approach is desired. Here, interested readers will observe that such a group-sequential approach provides approximately the same information as the Bayesian analysis.

We now turn to consideration of extensions of dose-response modelling involving pharmacokinetic-pharmacodynamic modelling [1143]. With the publication of [621] and [372], applications of such techniques are becoming more frequent in drug development. Typically, what is done is to develop a nonlinear mixed effect models [790] for pharmacokinetics in an effect compartment ([1143], a hypothesized part of the body where pharmacodynamic effect is thought to be induced by drug treatment) and then relate that to a model of pharmacodynamic activity using a statistical model [828].

Specialized software is generally needed for such an activity. Several packages are described in [1170]. See also [1048] for a review of some data comparisons between available software packages. For the purposes of illustrating the principles involved, we will make use of a dataset involving dose, pharmacokinetics, and some data on QTc using SAS from a longitudinal, repeated-measures proof-of-concept study. Other software programs may also be used to model this data (e.g., SPLUS, PKBUGS, NONMEM, NONLINMIX), and we invite interested readers to make use of the data available on the website accompanying this book to do so.

The data used in the following examples for PK-PD modelling are quite extensive. Measurement of QTc was taken over a period of eight days to assess the properties of the compound under study (utilizing doses up to 120 mg) with pharmacokinetic assessment to measure plasma concentration taken at regular intervals. See Tables 10.6 and 10.7. The full data sets may be found on the website accompanying this book.

TABLE 10.6: Example 10.3.2: QTc Data from One Subject in a Proof-of-Concept Study

Subject	Dose(mg)	Day	Time(h)	QTc(msec)
1	80	1	0	393
1	80	1	0.5	394
1	80	1	1	399
1	80	1	1.5	400
1	80	1	2	416
1	80	1	3	418
1	80	1	4	396
1	80	1	6	402
1	80	1	8	405
1	80	1	10	393
1	80	1	12	390
1	80	1	18	388
1	80	2	0	406
1	80	2	3	413
1	80	2	12	386

TABLE 10.6: Example 10.3.2: QTc Data from One Subject in a Proof-of-Concept Study (continued)

Subject	Dose(mg)	Day	Time(h)	QTc(msec)
1	80	2	15	421
1	80	3	0	421
1	80	3	3	425
1	80	3	12	394
1	80	3	15	420
1	80	4	0	427
1	80	4	3	430
1	80	4	12	384
1	80	4	15	417
1	80	5	0	425
1	80	5	3	435
1	80	5	12	398
1	80	5	15	415
1	80	6	0	409
1	80	6	3	434
1	80	6	12	388
1	80	6	15	418
1	80	7	0	420
1	80	7	3	409
1	80	7	12	398
1	80	7	15	410
1	80	8	0	407
1	80	8	0.5	411
1	80	8	1	432
1	80	8	1.5	443
1	80	8	2	455
1	80	8	3	460
1	80	8	4	428
1	80	8	6	419
1	80	8	8	382
1	80	8	10	404
1	80	8	12	388
1	80	8	18	384
1	80	8	24	409
1	80	8	36	384
1	80	8	48	388

TABLE 10.7: Example 10.3.2: Plasma Pharmacokinetic-Pharmacodynamic Data from One Subject in a Proof-of-Concept Study

Subject	Day	Time(h)	QTc(msec)	Conc.(ng/mL)
1	1	0	393	.
1	1	0.5	394	.
1	1	1	399	8.15
1	1	1.5	400	7.89

TABLE 10.7: Example 10.3.2: Plasma Pharmacokinetic-Pharmacodynamic Data from One Subject in a Proof-of-Concept Study (continued)

Subject	Day	Time(h)	QTc(msec)	Conc.(ng/mL)
1	1	2	416	7.56
1	1	3	418	5.43
1	1	4	396	3.58
1	1	6	402	.
1	1	8	405	.
1	1	10	393	.
1	1	12	390	.
1	1	18	388	.
1	1	24	.	.
1	8	0	407	2.53
1	8	0.5	411	5.26
1	8	1	432	13.9
1	8	1.5	443	14.72
1	8	2	455	17.12
1	8	3	460	12.81
1	8	4	428	9.39
1	8	6	419	5.83
1	8	8	382	3.09
1	8	10	404	.
1	8	12	388	.
1	8	18	384	.
1	8	24	409	.
1	8	36	384	.
1	8	48	388	.

We will first build a dose-response model for these data and then will supplement it with a discussion of how to build a PK-PD model for the data to illustrate the concepts involved.

The data in Table 10.6 are consistent with repeated-measures data. As such, it can be modelled simply using a model of the form

$$y_{ijk} = \alpha + \phi_j + \tau_k + (interactions) + \beta_1(dose) + \varepsilon_{ijk},$$

where α is the common intercept, ϕ_j adjusts for study day j, τ_k adjusts for each time k, β_1 denotes the slope of dose-response. The terms of the error term ε_{ijk} are constructed recognizing that QTc responses (y_{ijk}) are correlated across time within each day for each subject (i). The interactions (not described here) are combinations of the dose, day, and time information to study whether response to a dose of the drug is dependent on the day and time of sampling. In SAS such a model can be implemented in `proc mixed` as

Dose-Response Repeated Measures Data Analysis of Example 10.3.2 — SAS `proc mixed` *Code:*

```
proc mixed data=my.poc2 method=reml;
    class subject day time;
    model qtc=dose day time
    day*time dose*day dose*time
    /DDFM=KENWARDROGER outp=out;
    repeated time/type=AR(1) subject=subject*day;
    lsmeans day*time/at dose=0 CL ALPHA=0.1;
    lsmeans day*time/at dose=25 CL ALPHA=0.1;
    lsmeans day*time/at dose=80 CL ALPHA=0.1;
    lsmeans day*time/at dose=120 CL ALPHA=0.1;
    lsmeans day*time/at dose=200 CL ALPHA=0.1;
    ods output LSMeans=my.lsmeans;
    run;
```

This model indicates (outputs not shown) that a significant, linear dose-response relationship was observed for QTc ($p < 0.0001$) and that the response changed over the course of eight days ($p < 0.0001$) and over times of ECG sampling ($p < 0.0001$). The `lsmeans` statements output the expected responses at various doses to a dataset called `my.lsmeans` for further assessment, and the dataset `out` may be used to assess model fit, as described in previous chapters. Here the model fit as assessed by residuals appeared adequate, and Table 10.8 gives the expected responses on placebo (dose of 0 mg) on day 1 and day 8, for example.

TABLE 10.8: QTc Response on Placebo on Days 1 and 8 in a Proof-of-Concept Study from Modelling of Dose-QTc Data in Example 10.3.2

Day	Time(h)	Dose	Mean QTc	95% CI
1	0	0	398	(390,405)
1	0.5	0	396	(388,405)
1	1	0	392	(384,400)
1	1.5	0	398	(390,406)
1	2	0	397	(389,405)
1	3	0	400	(392,407)
1	4	0	398	(390,406)
1	6	0	395	(387,403)
1	8	0	399	(391,407)
1	10	0	398	(390,407)
1	12	0	401	(394,409)
1	18	0	409	(401,418)
8	0	0	394	(386,402)
8	0.5	0	391	(382,399)
8	1	0	398	(389,406)
8	1.5	0	398	(390,406)
8	2	0	396	(388,405)
8	3	0	395	(388,403)
8	4	0	394	(386,402)
8	6	0	392	(383,400)
8	8	0	386	(378,395)
8	10	0	390	(381,398)

TABLE 10.8: QTc Response on Placebo on Days 1 and 8 in a Proof-of-Concept Study from Modelling of Dose-QTc Data in Example 10.3.2 (continued)

Day	Time(h)	Dose	Mean QTc	95% CI
8	12	0	392	(384,400)
8	18	0	394	(385,402)
8	24	0	391	(382,400)
8	36	0	389	(380,398)
8	48	0	393	(384,403)

In addition to confirming that a dose-response is evident, providing overall positive evidence of efficacy for the compound [621] (though we do not yet know which dose is best in terms of safety), the model's findings in terms of response on placebo are very important. These will figure prominently as we develop models for concentration to QTc response relationships. For the purposes of this example, we neglect the development of a pharmacokinetic compartment model. Readers interested in doing so should see Chapter 11 for more details. In this example, plasma concentration is therefore assumed to be the effect compartment where pharmacodynamic effect is caused by drug action.

The first step taken in modelling such data (see Chapter 4 of [108]) is to assess whether a linear relationship exists between concentration and response. This can easily be accommodated using the above SAS code (replacing dose with concentration). Eliminating nonsignificant terms, we use the following SAS model to examine the relationship of concentration to QTc where the term `pt_` denotes subject and the term `pkp_c` is concentration.

Concentration Response Repeated Measures Data Analysis — SAS `proc mixed` *Code:*

```
proc mixed data=poc2pkpd method=reml;
    class pt_ day time;
    model qtc=pkp_c time
    /DDFM=KENWARDROGER outp=out S;
    repeated time/type=AR(1) subject=pt_*day;
    run;
```

Model fit may again be examined using the dataset `out` and was observed to be adequate (not shown). Concentration was a significant ($p < 0.0001$) linear predictor of QTc with a slope of 0.38. This indicates that, as drug concentration in blood increases, so too does QTc.

If the fit was not adequate, any number of other potential nonlinear models may be fitted [907]. However, by far the favorite model used in PK-PD research is the Emax model (named for one of the parameters used in the model). Boxtel et al. [108] described these models in great detail, and we shall dwell only on simple examination of Day 8 QTc and concentration data using such a model. Interested readers may apply other models using the data on the website and may find Chapter 15 of [108] helpful for additional background materials on PK-PD modelling in cardiac repolarization.

The Emax model is described as [108]

$$E = \frac{Emax(C)}{EC50 + C} + E_0,$$

where E is the effect being modelled, E_0 is the effect observed without any drug present, C is the concentration of drug in the effect compartment, $EC50$ is the concentration needed to cause a 50% response, and $Emax$ is the maximum effect that can occur with drug treatment. This is a nonlinear (in concentration) additive model. If concentration is not related to effect, Emax and EC50 would be zero.

Here, we are interested in assessing the following model:

$$QTc_{ij}(Effect) = \frac{Emax_i * C}{EC50_i + C} + E_0 + \varepsilon_{ij}$$

on Day 8, where the subscript i denotes subject, j denotes time, and ε_{ij} is the usual term for residual error. Such a model is easily implemented in `proc nlmixed` in SAS as

Emax Concentration Response Data Analysis Example 10.3.2 — SAS `proc nlmixed` *Code:*

```
proc nlmixed data=pkpd2;
    parms beta1=4.6 beta2=5.57 s2b1=1
    s2b2=1 s2=400;
    emax = exp(beta1+b1);
    ec50 = exp(beta2+b2);
    pred=((emax*pkp_c)/(pkp_c+ec50))+e0;
    model qtc ~ normal(pred,s2);
    random b1 b2 ~ normal([0,0],[s2b1,0,
    s2b2]) subject=pt_;
    predict pred out=pred;
    run;

*Model fit assessment;
data pred;set pred;
    st_resid=(qtc-Pred)/StdErrPred;
    run;
proc rank data=pred normal=blom out=nscore;
    var st_resid;
    ranks nscore;
data nscore;
  set nscore;
  label nscore="Normal Score";
  label stres="Residual";
  label pred="Predicted Value";
    run;
proc plot vpercent=50 data=nscore;
    plot st_resid*pred/vref=0;
    plot st_resid*nscore;
    run;
```

Here `proc nlmixed` is called and applied to a dataset denoted as `pkpd2` where the placebo modelling results of the dose-response model (Table 10.8) have been used to describe E_0. In general, it is more desirable for each subject to provide such an assessment so that more informative models may be fitted [1139], but that is obviously not possible with this data as subjects were not crossed over to Placebo. Starting values must be specified for the parameters of interest (`beta1` and `beta2`, their variances, and the residual variance). As both Emax and EC50 must be positive, the exponential function is used to allow their estimated values to be such and to accommodate subject-specific adjustment, as appropriate to the data, for each parameter. The predicted values `pred` are output for assessment of model fit using residual plots using the above code (results not shown), which appeared adequate.

The model indicated that both Emax ($p < 0.0001$) and EC50 ($p < 0.0001$) were important in describing the QTc response. The estimates of Emax and EC50 were 86.8 msec (95% CI of 74.7–101) and 26.7 ng/mL (95% CI of 12.6–56.2), respectively.

One should be careful with the interpretation of such a model in early phase trials. If we assume a basal QTc of approximately 400 msec in keeping with Table 10.8, one might be tempted to interpret this model as indicative that the maximum prolongation in QTc possible with this drug would be approximately 500 msec by looking at the magnitude of the upper bound of Emax. However, Emax is in this case design dependent. Dosing was terminated at the 120 mg dose in this study, as prolongation was approaching a QTc of 500 msec (known, see Chapter 9, to be a level associated with a potentially fatal cardiac arrythmia). Note that the linear model predicts no such plateau in effect. Models such as these should be interpreted in tandem and developed further as drug development progresses from Phase II to file and beyond.

Proof-of-concept, in spite of deficiencies in application in a business setting, is a "living" topic, and new approaches become available regularly. Those interest in more information may find [826] and [122] of interest for further research.

11

Population Pharmacokinetics

Introduction

I was sitting in my office one day minding my own business (i.e., staring out the window) when I received a call from one of our clinical research scientists. I refer to it as resting one's eyes — staring out the window, that is. After staring at statistical outputs of a computer screen all day, it is good to dwell on distance for just a moment or two — if for no other reason than to keep your eyes from going bad.

If anyone gives you a hard time about it, hand them a stack of statistical outputs needing sorting out, review, and interpretation, and ask them to come back to you in two to three hours if they still really have a problem with it. They will not likely come back, and it is possible you will never see them again.

The scientist had received a message from one of our company's offices in the Far East (South Korea), requesting assistance with a statistical issue. It related to one of our key drug projects and was, to paraphrase, "How does one go about statistically analyzing pharmacokinetic data? We just did a study and do not know what to do with the data."

I was tempted to tell her I did not know either (and to call someone else), but I knew I could not get away with that.... It was my drug project; I did know how to analyze pharmacokinetic data, and even if I referred her to someone else in the company, eventually the question would make its way back to me. I was the one with the Western pharmacokinetic data to which they would wish (even though they did not know it yet) to compare these new data. I must admit I was tempted, though.

What started off as a seeming annoyance turned into a very interesting project as we began looking at the data that had been generated in South Korea, and we will discuss the statistical assessment of population pharmacokinetics at some length in this chapter. This information is generally used on the label of new drug products to ensure they are used safely and effectively in different populations. Some aspects also may impact regulatory approval of drugs.

11.1 Population and Pharmacokinetics

Beginning in the latter half of the 20th century (as computational tools became available to support its development), the study of extent and rate of exposure began and has since become the norm in drug development. This study is targeted toward achieving an understanding of the differences in the way disease-bearing patients' bodies handle a drug once a dose is taken. It is hoped that this understanding will aid in the determination and control of safe and effective dosage regimens. Most pharmacokinetic methods applied in pharmaceutical development are non-compartmental (see Chapter 2) in that the concentration of drug in plasma or blood over time is expressed as a summary measure (e.g., AUC or Cmax).

The model-based study of population pharmacokinetics is, however, a relatively recent innovation in drug development and is more of an art than a science at this time. Such techniques apply models to describe the population-specific behavior of concentration in plasma or blood as a function of dose over time. The relationship of concentration to population-specific factors is observational.

Dose is varied among populations, and the resulting pharmacokinetic measurements are quantified using models. Except in selected studies (discussed later in this chapter for the purposes of model validation), control of population-specific factors is not all that robust. Such studies are designed for other purposes (e.g., safety evaluation), and pharmacokinetic data are collected in case this can help explain any findings of concern (or benefit). While the dose is controlled, and can therefore be considered to affect or cause study outcomes, population and demographic factors are not as robustly controlled and can be termed to be **associated** with or **related to** study outcomes, not a direct cause. The purpose of this chapter is to describe procedures used to study this association between population and pharmacokinetics.

We will not review this topic in great detail and refer interested readers to summaries of this topic in [30], [95], [365], and [828]. Instead we will utilize the pharmacokinetic concentration data from Section 8.3 to review concepts in population pharmacokinetic modelling to enable an understanding of the statistical issues involved in this topic of drug development. We will continue to use the first-order compartmental model introduced in Section 8.3, as its properties lend themselves to transparent interpretation. More complex models, however, are likely to improve model fit, and we encourage interested readers to examine `conc.sas7bdat` (found on the website accompanying this book) to do so.

Statistically, the study of population pharmacokinetics may be viewed as a modelling exercise. Pharmacostatistical modelling follows several stages in this setting:

1. Model **building** based on the rich concentration data obtained from limited numbers of subjects in Phase I,
2. Statistical and practical model **assessment**,
3. Model **application** as sparse concentration data are obtained in large numbers of patients in Phases II and III,
4. **Utilization** of model estimates for labelling purposes.

We will briefly review the building and statistical assessment of an example model as illustrated in Section 8.3. Recall the concentration data for Subject 47 presented in Table 8.11 (Section 8.3). These data (and data from the other 26 subjects in `conc.sas7bdat`) were used to develop a pharmacostatistical model to describe the concentration versus time profile (see Figure 8.4 and Table 8.12). Readers will recall that model diagnostics revealed that concentrations appeared to be underestimated at low and high concentrations in this model. We now examine the practical implications of this in more detail.

From the first-order model, it is easy to derive model-based estimates for Tmax, Cmax, and AUC with accompanying confidence intervals and to compare them to the non-compartmental estimates derived using the standard techniques described in Chapter 2. SAS code for doing so in this model may be found below. Details of the derivations may be found in the Technical Appendix to this chapter. For the purposes of this example, we will examine how the model-estimated AUC differs from the non-compartmental-derived AUC. Similar procedures may be used to examine Cmax, and we encourage interested readers to use the code found on the website accompanying this book to do so. Intuitively, if the model is accurate, the estimates of AUC and Cmax from the model should approximate those found using non-compartmental methods of derivation.

The SAS code below utilizes the model of Section 8.3 to derive estimates of AUC. The code then outputs these AUC values (with confidence intervals) and compares them to the non-compartmental-derived AUCs (see Table 11.1). It was found that the estimated AUCs from the model were approximately 20% lower than those derived using the non-compartmental analysis (based on the findings for the ratio of non-compartmental AUC to model-based AUC).

Derivation of Tmax, Cmax, and AUC from Nonlinear Mixed Effect Pharmacokinetic Data Analysis of `conc.sas7bdat` *— SAS* `proc nlmixed` *Code:*

```
proc nlmixed data=my.conc;
    parms beta1=0.4 beta2=1.5 beta3=-2 s2b1=0.04
    s2b2=0.02 s2b3=0.01 s2=0.25;
    cl = exp(beta1+b1);
    ka = exp(beta2+b2);
    ke = exp(beta3+b3);
    auc=dose/cl;
    tmax=(log(ka)-log(ke))/(ka-ke);
    pred=dose*ke*ka*(exp(-ke*time)-exp(-ka*time))/
    (cl*(ka-ke));
    cmax=dose*ke*ka*(exp(-ke*tmax)-exp(-ka*tmax))/
    (cl*(ka-ke));
    model conc ~ normal(pred,s2);
    random b1 b2 b3 ~ normal([0,0,0],[s2b1,0,
    s2b2,0,0,s2b3]) subject=subject;
    predict auc out=auc;
    predict cmax out=cmax;
    predict tmax out=tmax;
    run;
```

The explanation for this discrepancy in estimates, in this manufactured example, is as follows. Interested readers will recall that in theory (see Section 8.3)

$$AUC = \frac{F(Dose)}{Cl},$$

where F denotes the ratio of absolute bioavailability. No basis for the derivation of this F is present in this dataset (as no intravenous route of administration was included in the study). In science, such "fudge factors" are often employed while learning about the science to account for differences in model estimates to actual observations (e.g., Einstein's cosmological constant [133]), and we will utilize this procedure here for the purposes of illustration. In practice, input from a pharmacokineticist should be sought to determine what procedure for adjustment should be used or if another model should be built and assessed. For the purpose of illustration, we adjust the model-estimated AUC by a factor of 1.2 using the following SAS code accordingly:

```
auc=1.2*dose/cl;.
```

Based on the model parameters and our rough estimate for F, we now have a model-based means of constructing accurate AUC estimates from concentration data (for illustration purposes). Subsequent Phase I studies collect more concentration data to enhance the understanding of the model, and at the end of Phase I, a more robust model should have been developed relating clearance (etc.) and dose to AUC and Cmax. It should be expected that the building of a model and statistical and practical assessment of its properties is an iterative and collegial process. Such models are built by statisticians and pharmacokineticists in consultation with disease area experts and their medical colleagues. Those building and assessing such models should bear in mind George Box's statement "All models are wrong, but some are useful" [107]. The idea is to build and assess a parsimonious model describing the data adequately. Adequacy of model fit and performance is to some extent subjective.

TABLE 11.1
Estimated AUC Parameters from `conc.sas7bdat`

Subject	Dose	Model AUC	Model Low B.	Non-Comp AUC	Model Upper B.	Diff.	Ratio
47	5	3.24	2.29	2.81	4.18	0.43	0.87
48	5	4.36	3.24	6.31	5.48	-1.95	1.45
49	5	4.80	3.59	7.26	6.00	-2.46	1.51
50	5	3.51	2.54	3.60	4.48	-0.09	1.03
52	5	4.23	3.10	6.82	5.37	-2.59	1.61
53	5	2.85	1.96	1.76	3.75	1.09	0.62
54	5	4.83	3.62	6.11	6.05	-1.28	1.26
55	5	3.93	2.87	6.09	5.00	-2.16	1.55
57	5	3.24	2.30	2.10	4.18	1.14	0.65
60	10	7.63	6.16	9.33	9.11	-1.70	1.22
61	10	6.45	5.12	7.31	7.78	-0.86	1.13
62	10	7.16	5.71	9.57	8.60	-2.41	1.34
64	10	8.45	6.83	15.62	10.07	-7.17	1.85
65	10	5.58	4.25	5.56	6.91	0.02	1.00
66	10	6.34	4.90	11.81	7.78	-5.47	1.86
69	10	7.36	5.93	7.23	8.80	0.13	0.98
71	10	6.68	5.30	8.35	8.07	-1.67	1.25
72	10	6.02	4.74	5.70	7.31	0.32	0.95
95	20	13.65	11.44	12.92	15.86	0.73	0.95
99	20	19.56	16.45	26.05	22.67	-6.49	1.33
102	20	18.32	15.60	23.12	21.05	-4.80	1.26
104	20	11.91	9.94	12.32	13.87	-0.41	1.03
105	20	13.16	11.05	16.35	15.27	-3.19	1.24
106	20	15.43	13.03	20.21	17.83	-4.78	1.31
107	20	11.12	9.19	13.53	13.05	-2.41	1.22
108	20	9.53	7.64	7.70	11.42	1.83	0.81
110	20	12.22	10.19	14.22	14.25	-2.00	1.16

Turning now from these topics, we consider the application of a model to emerging clinical pharmacokinetic data obtained in Phase II and III patient studies. Such data are generally more sparse than Phase I data (in that a full pharmacokinetic profile sufficient for estimation of AUC and Cmax is not obtained); however, these sparse collections are generally obtained in a far larger number of patients than were exposed to the drug in Phase I. Selected data for three subjects may be found in Table 11.2. The full simulated dataset may be found in `simulate.sas7bdat` on the website accompanying this book.

These data are concentrations from 3 of 100 simulated patients. Note that the number of concentrations obtained is limited relative to the normal healthy volunteer data (Table 8.11). Using the model developed in Phase I, we use the above SAS code to derive parameter and AUC estimates for each subject. The same code as above is used except that the starting values are based on the findings from the Phase I model in Table 8.12 using a PARMS statement of: `parms beta1=0.35 beta2=1.46 beta3=-2.47 s2b1=0.04 s2b2=0.03 s2b3=0.007 s2=0.01;`

Code for this purpose may be found in `poppk.sas` on the website accompanying this book. Model diagnostics may be applied (although not done for the purposes of this ex-

TABLE 11.2
Selected Sparse Concentration Data from Patient Studies

Subject	Dose	Time	Concentration
1	5	1	0.21
1	5	3	0.18
1	5	6	0.13
1	5	14	0.05
40	10	1	1.10
40	10	3	0.95
40	10	6	0.74
40	10	14	0.38
90	20	2	0.79
90	20	5	0.62
90	20	8	0.48
90	20	18	0.20

ample), and if model fit is poor, alternative models may be built and assessed. Parameter estimates may be found in Table 11.3 (note slight differences from the Phase I estimated parameters in Table 8.12), and resulting AUC estimates for selected patients may be found in Table 11.4.

As shown in Table 11.4, the estimates of AUC (and the other parameters) have uncertainty (error) associated with their estimation. In SAS, a Bayesian algorithm [1073] is applied to characterize this uncertainty. In theory, the bootstrap may also be applied (in addition to its use as a model diagnostic to assess model performance) to provide an estimate for the uncertainty of the estimate.

We turn now to the utilization of these estimates from the model. The first goal is to use the estimated AUCs to confirm their position relative to the NOAEL in this population. The estimated AUCs are plotted against dose in Figure 11.1 and are well below the NOAEL (not plotted).

Similar procedures may be done for the estimated Cmax, and we leave this as an exercise for interested readers.

The second goal of population pharmacokinetic analysis is to assess the estimated parameters (in this case we will use clearance) relative to factors which may influence their

TABLE 11.3
Estimated Population PK Parameters from Sparse Population Data

Parameter	Estimate	95% CI
β_1	0.45	0.39,0.52
β_2	1.47	1.11,1.83
β_3	-2.44	-2.48,-2.39
s2b1	0.10	0.08,0.11
s2b2	0	...
s2b3	0.03	0.02,0.04
s2	0.0003	0.0002,0.0004

TABLE 11.4
Selected Estimates for AUC from Sparse Concentration Data Obtained in Patient Studies

Subject	Dose	AUC	95% CI
1	5	3.00	2.37,3.63
40	10	17.10	16.03,18.17
90	20	13.09	12.17,14.01

magnitude. Examples include dose and demographic factors such as age, gender, weight, body mass index, ethnicity, and creatinine clearance (a measure of renal function). Basic statistical tools are often used to enable assessment of whether changes in these factors influence the magnitude of the estimated population pharmacokinetic parameters; see Figure 11.2.

Figure 11.2 is a plot of the estimated clearance (from the model) versus dose expressed using a standard descriptive statistical procedure known as a *boxplot*. The box encloses the 75th and 25th percentiles of the observed data, and the line in the box is the median of the observed data. The upper and lower lines extend to the 90th and 10th percentiles, respectively, with data outside these indicated using points so their status as outliers can be assessed.

In Figure 11.2, we observe that clearance appears related to dose. This relationship may be further quantified by regressing the estimated clearance on dose to assess whether the relationship is linear or nonlinear. Multiple linear regression may be performed to assess

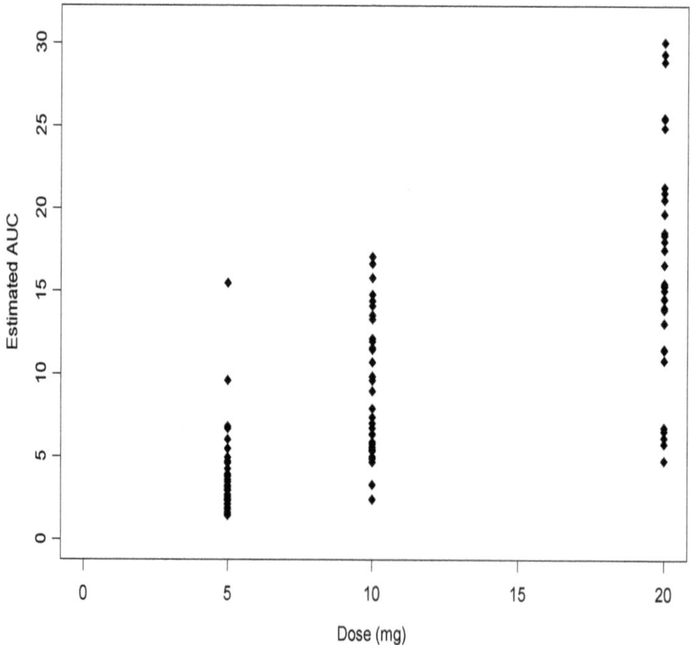

FIGURE 11.1
Estimated AUCs versus Dose from a Simulated Population Pharmacokinetic Study

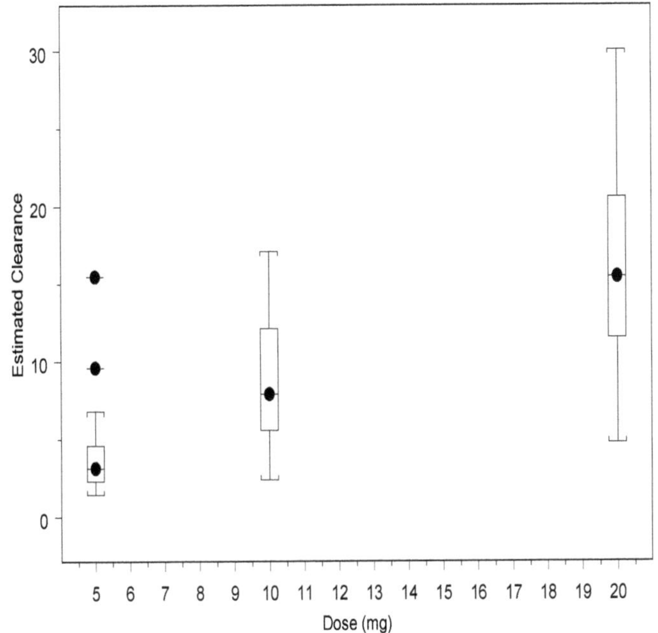

FIGURE 11.2
Boxplot of Estimated Clearance versus Dose from a Simulated Population Pharmacokinetic Study

the simultaneous relationship of other (i.e., demographic) factors [907]. We will not dwell further on such assessments here and refer interested readers to discussion in Chapter 11 of [95] for more details.

Such model-based population pharmacokinetic assessments are used to guide dosing in patients where well-controlled clinical designs are not possible (e.g., [378]) due to ethical or practical constraints. Additionally, this information will be used in labelling for the drug product [365] to ensure dosing of patients in the marketplace is appropriate to their demography and concurrent-disease states.

Exposure levels above the NOAEL or exposure levels related to a demographic factor which may be impacted by a concurrent-disease state may be the subject of specific clinical pharmacology studies to assess the relationship of exposure to disease or demography. Following a brief discussion of the determination and estimation of absolute bioavailability, we turn to several examples of such studies.

11.2 Absolute and Relative Bioavailability

As described in Chapter 1, when a drug is taken orally, it is absorbed and distributed into the body, metabolized at various sites within the body, and eventually eliminated from systemic circulation. This process is termed ADME, and the availability of drug at the site of action within the body is presumably mediated by the rates at which the various facets of ADME are performed by the body.

Consider, however, a drug that is injected or administered intravenously. Once administered, the drug is distributed to the systemic circulation from the site of entry and does not undergo first-pass metabolism. As the injected drug product circulates throughout the body, it is metabolized and eliminated. Equation (11.1) in the Technical Appendix is appropriate for such a product. This is termed 100% bioavailable, as an injected product by definition reaches the circulation intact at the time of dosing. Most oral products have different levels of bioavailability, as some drugs pass straight through the intestinal tract and are eliminated, and some drugs (like the example of the previous section) can be very rapidly absorbed in the intestinal tract. To account for this in equations like (11.1), parameters such as F can be introduced to account for the differential mode of administration (Chapter 8, [95]).

Description of absorption pharmacokinetics is a lengthy topic, and we will not discuss all aspects of its assessment. Instead, we will discuss a commonly used method to assess absolute bioavailability F using data from a cross-over clinical pharmacology trial. Such a trial need not always be performed in drug development. In certain circumstances, F can be determined by other means (see Chapter 8, [95]).

Absolute bioavailability F is a measure of the percentage of drug absorbed after oral administration relative to that in the body after administration by an intravenous route (hereafter denoted IV). This parameter F can be estimated by giving an IV dose and an oral dose of drug in a cross-over study to normal healthy volunteers and comparing their resulting AUCs.

The same approach to study design is used as in the typical bioequivalence study; however, here we do not desire to demonstrate equivalence in AUC but only to estimate F to a given degree of precision. Usually, the dose of drug administered IV and orally in such trials will differ depending on the properties of the compound to ensure that exposure levels remain safe. For example, a drug poorly absorbed after oral adminstration might have a reduced dose when administered IV to ensure concentrations remain below the NOAEL. Therefore, the AUCs are dose normalized (i.e., divided by dose) prior to analysis to ensure that an appropriate basis for comparison is obtained.

Table 11.5 contains data from a typical cross-over trial to estimate absolute bioavailability. In this case, 2 mg of drug was administered intravenously over an hour or 4 mg of drug was administered orally in a cross-over trial in $n = 12$ normal healthy subjects, and dose-normalized AUC values were derived following each administration.

The dose-normalized data of Table 11.5 were analyzed according to the methods of Chapter 3 (SAS code may be found on the website accompanying this book), and an estimate of $\mu_O - \mu_{IV}$ with a 90% confidence interval was constructed (where μ_O and μ_{IV} denote the adjusted mean logAUC following oral and IV administration, respectively). As with bioequivalence, these are exponentiated to provide an estimate of F. In this case $\hat{F}$ was 0.99 with 90% confidence bounds of 0.91 to 1.07.

Information provided by the models of this and the previous section and Chapter 8 are necessary but not always sufficient for complete understanding of the ADME properties of a drug. To complete the scientific understanding of ADME properties, a single dose, cross-over mass-balance (see Chapter 5, [95]) study is often performed in an extremely small number of normal healthy volunteers ($n = 2$ to 4 total). In such trials, subjects are administered a radio-labelled dose of drug, and blood and other bodily excretions (urine, feces) are collected and assessed for the presence of a radio-labelled substance. In another session, a standard dose of drug is given to serve as a control for the amount of drug (and radio-label) found in blood in the other session. Pharmacokinetic data from such a trial are generally not analyzed statistically (given the low sample size) but are used qualitatively

TABLE 11.5
Dose-Normalized (DN) AUC from an Absolute Bioavailability Cross-Over Trial

Subject	DN-AUC *IV*	DN-AUC Oral
1	751	818
2	897	694
3	900	954
4	537	469
5	656	665
6	665	681
7	772	578
8	930	869
9	884	1055
10	556	506
11	1029	1078
12	727	946

to confirm the scientific understanding of the ADME properties of drug products. As such, we do not consider their statistical properties here.

During the early stages of drug development, many changes are made to formulation. These may be minor (changing the color) but can be major (e.g., changing from a capsule to a tablet). Guidance [373] does not require that a bioequivalence trial be performed, but sponsoring companies will wish to confirm that AUC is similar in the new formulation to ensure that the understanding of absolute bioavailability gained in previous experimentation is robust to the change in formulation.

As with absolute bioavailability studies, bioequivalence need not be demonstrated, and such relative bioavailability trials are performed to provide the desired level of precision in the ratio of AUC in the new formulation to the old. Study design and data analysis follow the same principles of those used in bioequivalence testing as described in Chapter 3 and will not be discussed further here.

11.3 Age and Gender Pharmacokinetic Studies

As described in Section 11.1, population pharmacokinetic models will be used to relate clearance and other pharmacokinetic parameters relative to age and gender. Such models, however, are handicapped with decreasing confidence as findings are extrapolated beyond the observed data [907].

For example, clinical trials of a new drug product may only be done in adults (ages 18 years to 50 years, perhaps). The models of Section 11.1 will allow for extrapolation to lower and higher ages (down to zero and up to, say, 100+ years perhaps); however, the confidence in the model predictions decreases as distance from the observed age range increases. Of interest, then, would be how exposure will actually behave in very young people or perhaps very old people. Age pharmacokinetic studies are designed to go and check. As noted, estimates will be available from the population pharmacokinetic model, and often a limited

TABLE 11.6
AUC and Cmax Data from a Pediatric (PED) and Adult (ADT) Bioavailability Trial

Subject	Age	AUC	Cmax
201	PED	1510	88.6
202	PED	883	52.5
203	PED	1650	92.0
204	PED	1015	56.0
205	PED	1556	84.0
206	PED	1412	84.8
207	PED	1353	83.0
208	PED	1443	96.4
209	PED	1299	68.1
210	PED	560	33.5
101	ADT	1284	70.3
102	ADT	1391	73.5
103	ADT	873	50.2
104	ADT	1211	62.2
105	ADT	1233	74.1
106	ADT	1172	60.4
108	ADT	1172	60.4
109	ADT	1336	75.3
110	ADT	1348	76.8
112	ADT	1419	82.9

pharmacokinetic study is performed to assess whether these model estimates are dependable. These small age (and gender) studies are, in essence, model-validation tools.

Consider the data in Table 11.6 from a study where pediatric patient pharmacokinetics were assessed for such a purpose. Ten pediatric and ten adult subjects received a single dose of drug, and their plasma concentrations were measured in the usual fashion over time.

Note that age, weight, and height were expected to differ between the two age groups, but these were not related to clearance and concentration in the population pharmacokinetic models (data not shown). Weight, height, and kidney and liver function all differ also (hopefully for the better in the younger people).

The study was performed to assess whether exposure in juveniles was consistent with this finding. The resulting findings are observational. Demographic characteristics will differ between groups, and the adult subjects are included, not for purposes of direct comparison, but to serve as a control back to the model used in the population pharmacokinetic modelling population. Their inclusion serves as a control if unexpected findings are observed to determine if the model or some facet of the study (e.g., assay) explains the observed difference.

The objective of statistical analysis in such a setting is to estimate exposure levels with a desired level of precision and compare to the NOAEL, calibrating back to estimates from the population pharmacokinetic models. SAS code commonly used to do so follows.

Age AUC Assessment Example — SAS `proc mixed` *Code:*

```
proc mixed method=reml data=age;
    class subject age;
    model lnauc=age/
    s ddfm=kenwardroger cl alpha=.1;
    lsmeans age/cl alpha=0.1;
    repeated /group=age subject=subject;
    ods output LSMeans=auc;
    run;
```

As previously, a REML model is used to characterize the mean AUC and Cmax of such data. As this is a parallel group trial, the model simply calls for characterization of logAUC relative to age, with mean effect in each age group output in the `lsmeans` and `ods` statements. The `repeated` statement specifies that a variance estimate should be provided for each age group separately, as it may be unrealistic to expect variation to be the same in the pediatric population relative to the adult population.

Exponentiating the estimated means and 90% confidence intervals back to the natural scale, it was found that mean AUC in the adult subjects was 1234 (1138–1338) and in the pediatric subjects 1214 (1000–1474). These estimates were as expected from the population pharmacokinetic modelling and served to reassure those using the drug that the choice of dose in this population was safe relative to the NOAEL.

Similar to pediatric subjects, for elderly people, it will often be of interest to assess the findings of population pharmacokinetic models in this manner. As before, weight, height, and kidney and liver function all differ too (probably for the worse in the older people). We omit further discussion on this topic here, as the principles and analyses are similar to those used in the pediatric population.

A particularly important facet of the application of population pharmacokinetic data pertains to assessment of the relationship of gender to exposure levels. In population pharmacokinetic models, interpretation of gender's relationship to exposure is often not straightforward. Confounding with other demographic factors is significant — i.e., weight and height. In general, to obtain a good handle on whether exposure is gender related, a single-dose study of exposure levels relative to NOAEL is done early in drug development (usually just after the sub-chronic dosing study is completed, see Section 8.3) in Phase I. Inclusion of females of child-bearing potential in drug development studies is contingent on genotoxicology findings, as fetal development can be impaired or terminated by such products. Effort is made to weight match male and female volunteers from the different populations where possible.

Consider the AUC and Cmax data from a gender trial in Table 11.3. Here 18 males (M) and females (F) were given a single dose of drug, and their pharmacokinetics were measured in the usual fashion.

TABLE 11.7: AUC and Cmax Data from a Gender Bioavailability Trial

Subject	Dose	Gender	AUC	Cmax
1	1	M	354	68.4
2	1	M	219	50.5
3	1	M	228	36.5
4	1	M	216	55.6
5	1	M	405	74.6
6	1	M	306	55.5

TABLE 11.7: AUC and Cmax Data from a Gender Bioavailability Trial (continued)

Subject	Dose	Gender	AUC	Cmax
13	1	F	704	90.0
14	1	F	375	52.3
15	1	F	534	83.7
16	1	F	434	59.2
17	1	F	565	59.8
18	1	F	484	84.0
25	2	M	602	151.5
26	2	M	762	165.6
27	2	M	728	134.6
28	2	M	934	116.6
29	2	M	560	121.2
30	2	M	408	86.9
38	2	F	871	196.3
39	2	F	1104	216.0
40	2	F	777	80.1
41	2	F	592	109.7
42	2	F	728	122.5
49	5	M	2295	553.5
50	5	M	1743	307.8
51	5	M	1646	483.4
52	5	M	1523	281.4
53	5	M	1782	534.4
54	5	M	1906	375.0
61	5	F	1676	211.8
62	5	F	1493	266.7
63	5	F	2597	328.1
64	5	F	2396	242.3
65	5	F	1656	455.4
66	5	F	1355	288.8

As with the pediatric trial described above, statistical analysis of the pharmacokinetic data is geared toward providing estimates which may be used to calibrate the population pharmacokinetic findings. SAS code for this purpose follows.

Gender AUC Assessment Example — SAS `proc mixed` *Code:*

```
proc mixed method=reml data=gender;
    class subject dose gender;
    model lnauc=dose gender dose*gender/
    s ddfm=kenwardroger cl alpha=.1;
    lsmeans dose*gender/cl alpha=0.1;
    repeated /group=gender subject=subject;
    ods output LSMeans=auc;
    run;
```

Again, variability is allowed to differ between genders using a **repeated** statement, and mean logAUC is output from the **lsmeans** and **ods** statements. Exponentiating these findings back to the normal-scale, the estimates given in Table 11.8 were found.

TABLE 11.8
Mean AUC Findings from a Gender Bioavailability Trial

Dose	Gender	Mean AUC	90% CI
1	Female	506	426 – 600
2	Female	797	661 – 962
5	Female	1808	1523 – 2146
1	Male	279	235 – 332
2	Male	644	541 – 766
5	Male	1800	1514 – 2142

Relative to the population pharmacokinetic model findings (based up to this time on data from male subjects only), we see in Table 11.8 that, while mean AUC in females still falls below the NOAEL (greater than 2000 ng.h/mL for this drug at this time), average exposure in females was dramatically greater in this dataset at lower doses than would be expected from the models of male data.

Findings such as these would prompt the sponsor to reinterrogate the population pharmacokinetic model building and assessment procedures, and the concentration data of the gender trial would be utilized for this purpose. Using such techniques, it was determined that, unexpectedly, clearance was related to weight (data not shown). This enabled the team to adapt their population pharmacokinetic model to take this into account. For example, in the SAS code of Section 11.1, `beta1` might be defined as a function of weight where relevant parameters are determined from model-based regression of weight on estimated clearance.

Assessment of Cmax in age and gender trials is left as an exercise for interested readers, and SAS code to perform such analysis may be found on the website accompanying this book.

11.4 Ethnicity

Consideration of ethnicity's impact upon pharmacokinetics has long been a topic of discussion and was recently commented on in international regulatory guidance [624]. This ICH-E5 guidance [624] was intended to provide a framework for evaluating ethnic factors on a drug's efficacy and safety profile in drug development. However, the guidance has not been implemented in the local ICH regions (USA, Europe, and Japan), and there is still a great deal of question about how to interpret the guidance (e.g., [379], [909], [24], [1260]).

In most cases, the reality is that, if one wants to obtain local market approval and access, then a local randomized, blinded, well-controlled clinical trial is required. Whether one needs to perform an outcome study or a "bridging" study (using a surrogate marker) then becomes the question of concern.

ICH-E5 [624] makes the implicit assumption that registration of a drug in a new region involves new registration for a new ethnic population, and we will follow this convention in this section. As described in ICH-E5, the first of two primary requirements for a submission package is that the data requirements for registration in the new region be met — i.e., that clinical trial methodology, recordkeeping, protocol compliance and drug accountability, and informed patient consent must be acceptable in the new region [624]. The minimal data package, consisting of either data from the original region and/or data from the new region, should include an adequate characterization of the pharmacokinetics (PK), pharmacodynamics (PD), dose response, efficacy, and safety of the drug (see Chapter 1 for more details). At least pharmacokinetics [914], and preferably pharmacodynamics and dose response, should also be characterized in an ethnic population that is relevant to the new region [624] but not necessarily resident in the new region [915] (i.e., if one wants to market a drug in Japan, one has to study its properties in Japanese patients or in patients of Japanese descent).

The second requirement is the demonstration of the ability to extrapolate findings from any data from the original region to the population of the new region. It is easier to extrapolate from one region to another if the new medication is "ethnically insensitive," i.e., unlikely to behave differently in different populations. Ethnic sensitivity can be categorized into two components, intrinsic (genetic) and extrinsic (environmental), either or both of which may impact bioavailability and hence the appropriate dose and response relationship [624].

A "bridging" study, as its name implies, is designed to allow one to bridge from the original region's data in the original population to the new region with its new population. It is a [624]

> ....supplemental study performed in the new region to provide pharmacodynamic or clinical data on efficacy, safety, dosage, and dose regimen in the new region that will allow extrapolation of the foreign clinical data to the new region...

The degree of ethnic sensitivity will determine whether a study is necessary and the design of such a study (e.g., PK only, PK/PD only, in what population, etc.). ICH-E5 [624] describes several characteristics of drug products which would make such a product "ethnically insensitive." These are [624]

1. Linear pharmacokinetics
2. A flat response curve for both efficacy and safety in the range of the recommended dosage and dose regimen (this may mean the medicine is well tolerated)
3. A wide therapeutic dose range (again an indicator of good tolerability)
4. Minimal metabolism or metabolism distributed among multiple pathways
5. High bioavailability, thus less susceptibility to dietary absorption effects
6. Low potential for protein binding
7. Little potential for drug-drug, drug-diet, and drug-disease interactions
8. Nonsystemic mode of action
9. Little potential for inappropriate use

It is rare for a drug to meet all nine conditions which would make it ethnically insensitive and result in only minimal data requirements to enter new regions and markets (e.g., such as Asia). In any event, ethical and cultural considerations regarding drug use in Asia are slightly different than other international regions, and consideration should first be given to such matters (regardless of the outcome of this checklist) when designing a bridging program [1215].

Statistical approaches to bridging are in early stages of development, and no international consensus is yet available on how ethnicity bridging programs should be designed and the data analyzed. See [682], [1151], [1072], [803], [199], [804], [969], and [805] for a description of some methods which are publicly available. We will not discuss these approaches further here, as they are, in general, intended for application to bridging study data to confirm these are sufficient to permit market access. We turn to practical pharmacology-based ethnicity assessment in population pharmacokinetics and the statistics involved. These pharmacology assessments are usually carried out in drug development prior to the initiation of a bridging program and should constitute the major basis for the approach to its design.

We assume as in previous sections of this chapter that a population pharmacokinetic model has been developed (as in Section 11.1) describing concentration as a function of time and physiologic parameters (e.g., clearance, absorption constant(s), elimination constant(s), etc.) As described in Section 11.1, some of these physiologic parameters may be related to demography (e.g., weight, height, gender, etc).

When dosing a new population, it is to be expected that demographic factors may be different. As with the population pharmacokinetic assessment of gender, significant confounding with ethnicity can often be expected. For example, in the dataset which follows, Western subjects were on average heavier than South Korean subjects. The working assumption, in the absence of information, made in the early stages of model development is that the functional form of the model is the same for both populations; however, in reality the magnitude of parameters (e.g., clearance) may be dependent upon ethnicity in some, as yet unknown, way.

Once a population pharmacokinetic model is proposed and estimates are available for differences in pharmacokinetics between populations related to demographic factors, the logical next step is to conduct a validation exercise via a small focused pharmacokinetic study. Selected data from such a study in South Korean subjects are presented along with corresponding data (at the same doses) observed in Western subjects. The full data in Table 11.9 set may be found on the website accompanying this book.

TABLE 11.9: AUC and Cmax Data from a Population Pharmacokinetic Assessment of South Korean and Western Subjects

Dose (mg)	Ethnicity	Subject	AUC (ng.h/mL)	Cmax (ng/mL)	Weight (kg)	Height (cm)	Age (yrs.)
2	K	A01	1228	195.2	65.0	170	20
2	K	A02	1003	193.9	65.0	172	20
2	K	A03	1063	165.8	75.0	175	27
2	K	A04	906	215.2	64.0	172	22
2	K	A07	811	215.6	76.0	177	21
2	K	A08	928	167.5	82.0	187	21
2	K	A09	1401	136.4	65.0	178	29
2	K	A11	1099	206.1	59.0	168	26
2	W	1	746	208.4	73.7	177	28
2	W	1	734	137.7	71.7	175	28
2	W	11	994	190.9	58.7	180	20
2	W	12	552	125.7	87.6	179	38
2	W	13	675	168.7	59.5	163	36
2	W	13	566	104.9	63.6	175	26
2	W	14	637	108.0	91.7	180	28
2	W	15	666	169.4	70.7	162	30
2	W	15	728	167.2	78.0	176	32
2	W	16	578	123.8	76.2	173	36
			....				
4	K	B01	1763	345.6	64.0	174	21
4	K	B02	1638	302.4	68.0	178	25
K= South Korean; W = Western							

TABLE 11.9: AUC and Cmax Data from a Population Pharmacokinetic Assessment of South Korean and Western Subjects (continued)

Dose (mg)	Ethnicity	Subject	AUC (ng.h/mL)	Cmax (ng/mL)	Weight (kg)	Height (cm)	Age (yrs.)
4	K	B03	1894	345.8	66.0	171	25
4	K	B06	2125	373.2	69.0	182	26
4	K	B07	2289	466.4	63.0	170	26
4	K	B08	1380	336.9	68.0	181	25
4	K	B10	1557	257.2	80.0	180	23
4	K	B11	3035	335.2	57.0	169	24
4	W	1	1637	362.0	76.3	180	27
4	W	10	2109	371.0	71.3	181	30
4	W	104	1468	308.0	76.1	185	51
4	W	109	999	249.0	85.0	178	56
4	W	11	1012	174.0	109.0	200	25
4	W	115	1273	275.0	69.4	175	31
4	W	116	1322	302.0	74.6	168	22
4	W	2	1388	319.0	68.3	175	26
4	W	391	989	174.1	91.1	176	27
			....				
8	K	C01	4890	709.2	64.0	176	19
8	K	C02	3641	737.7	65.0	167	28
8	K	C04	7211	981.7	63.0	175	22
8	K	C06	3382	421.4	68.0	182	21
8	K	C07	5459	1009.0	59.0	171	28
8	K	C08	3077	769.6	71.0	179	28
8	K	C11	4144	820.0	73.0	177	24
8	K	C12	4263	673.0	61.0	180	21
8	W	1	3404	687.1	73.7	177	28
8	W	1	2942	563.6	80.5	184	26
8	W	10	3596	550.4	79.5	173	26
8	W	10	2148	462.0	76.3	182	32
8	W	100	2572	718.0	73.2	175	54
8	W	106	1997	428.0	96.8	186	43
8	W	11	4677	586.1	58.7	180	20
8	W	11	1278	320.0	96.1	178	29
8	W	112	3023	467.0	80.9	173	49
8	W	113	2959	575.0	69.8	170	53
			....				

K= South Korean; W = Western

The code used to analyze such data is similar to that used in the previous section. In this setting, it may be desirable to conduct a model-building assessment (see Chapter 2 of [907] and Chapters 2 and 4 of [510]) to determine which factors are significantly related to the endpoint under study. Accordingly, in the example that follows, weight (`wt`) was included as a covariate.

Ethnicity AUC Assessment Example — SAS `proc mixed` *Code:*

```
proc mixed data=pk method=reml maxiter=200 scoring=50;
    class subject race;
    model lnauc=race lndose wt
    /s ddfm=kenwardroger cl alpha=.1 outp=out;
    lsmeans race/CL ALPHA=0.1 DIFF=CONTROL("W");
    repeated /group=race subject=subject;
    ods output LSMeans=auc;
run;
```

For logAUC, the resulting model estimates are presented in Table 11.10. AUC was observed to be significantly related to ethnicity and weight, and was linearly related to dose. In terms of the impact of ethnicity, we can conclude from these data that weight, by itself, does not explain all of the differences in pharmacokinetics between Koreans and Westerners. The concentration data supporting this assessment would be used to rebuild the population pharmacokinetic model, allowing for other parameters to be related to ethnicity.

TABLE 11.10
Estimated Population Parameters from Evaluation of logAUC as a Function of Ethnicity, logDose, and Weight

Parameter	Estimate	95% CI
Ethnicity	0.28	0.19, 0.36
logDose	1.00	0.94, 1.05
Weight	-0.01	-0.02, -0.00

In this case, it was determined that South Koreans metabolized the drug slightly differently than Westerners (via a different CYP450 pathway, see Chapter 8). Alteration of the elimination rate constant to account for this ethnicity-related difference resulted in adequate model fit (data not shown).

Cmax was also observed to be higher in South Koreans than in the Western population. The analysis of these data is left as an exercise for interested readers and may be done using code on the website accompanying this book.

In combination with the full data package from the original region, data such as the above can serve as the basis for approval in some nations. However, several nations also require that the concentration to effect relationship (see Chapter 10) be studied and be shown to be unrelated to ethnicity. In theory, the model-based approach used should be similar.

11.5 Liver Disease

Liver disease or hepatic impairment can be caused by a number of factors. Diseases like hepatitis can cause injury to the liver and impair its function. Injury may also be chemically induced (cirrhosis via alcohol) and drug induced. In this section, we consider the pharmacokinetics of a drug in the body when patients have liver disease.

Severity of liver disease is typically measured by the Child–Pugh score [374], and subsequently categorized as healthy, mild, moderate, or severe liver function impairment, depending on the extent of damage to the liver and impairment of its function. If a drug is eliminated (in the ADME sense) by metabolism or excretion (into bile) in the liver, the drug would be expected to accumulate in the plasma. Decreased clearance of drug by the liver [30] implies increased AUC and Cmax, and, as these increase the likelihood of adverse events associated with exposure (relative to the NOAEL), would also be expected to increase. Therefore, it is important to understand the magnitude of increased exposure in patients with impaired hepatic function to determine [30] if it is necessary to reduce the dose in such patients or potentially to contraindicate the use of the drug.

We again assume that a population pharmacokinetic model has been developed from Phase I data. In tandem with this, a mass-balance radio-label ADME trial will generate information on the role of the liver in excretion and metabolism of the drug in plasma. If the liver plays only a minor role in elimination of the drug from the body ([30, 374]), then regulatory guidance suggests that study in patients with hepatic impairment is not required. However, if the role of the liver cannot be precisely determined, then a small pharmacokinetic study is generally performed to confirm the validity of the model's findings. In practice, the radio-label ADME study is expensive and takes a long time, so it is general practice to perform a small pharmacokinetic trial as described in the following.

Patients with hepatic impairment are enrolled and administered a single dose of drug in the standard clinical pharmacology sampling paradigm, and their plasma concentrations are summarized as AUC, Cmax, etc. [374]. In tandem, depending on the results of population pharmacokinetic assessment for the demographic factors involved, race, age, and weight range-matched volunteers are enrolled as a control group, administered the same single dose, and pharmacokinetics are measured. As with previous population pharmacokinetic modelling exercises, the objective of the trial is to estimate the pharmacokinetics in each group to assess the performance of the population pharmacokinetic model, not to compare the groups ("normal" and "hepatic impaired").

AUC and Cmax data from such a trial may be found in Table 11.11. In this case, population pharmacokinetic modelling of the impact of reduced clearance due to hepatic impairment led the team working on this drug to be confident that increased extent of exposure would occur in hepatic impaired patients. The model, however, was imprecise in terms of the extent to which exposure would be increased, with estimates ranging from little effect to approximately eight to ten times the exposure in normal healthy volunteers. The study was performed using a low dose to enhance the understanding of the impact of moderate hepatic impairment. The lower dose was used to ensure exposure levels would remain well below the NOAEL.

TABLE 11.11: Pharmacokinetic Data from a Clinical Pharmacology Hepatic Impairment Trial

Subject	Group	AUC (ng.h/mL)	Cmax (ng/mL)
100	HEALTHY	2572	718
101	HEPATIC	2862	374
102	HEPATIC	5225	302
103	HEPATIC	3709	441
HEALTHY (No Liver Disease)			
HEPATIC (Moderate Liver Disease)			

TABLE 11.11: Pharmacokinetic Data from a Clinical Pharmacology Hepatic Impairment Trial (continued)

Subject	Group	AUC (ng.h/mL)	Cmax (ng/mL)
104	HEPATIC	3866	258
105	HEPATIC	2675	382
106	HEALTHY	2911	504
107	HEPATIC	4321	439
108	HEPATIC	5801	434
109	HEALTHY	2701	466
110	HEALTHY	2374	606
111	HEPATIC	3023	409
112	HEALTHY	3023	467
113	HEALTHY	2344	449
114	HEALTHY	2544	386
115	HEPATIC	3352	343
116	HEALTHY	2802	422
117	HEPATIC	2768	422
118	HEPATIC	2489	554
119	HEALTHY	3715	385
120	HEPATIC	3740	488
121	HEALTHY	2088	487
122	HEALTHY	2038	474
123	HEALTHY	1703	592
124	HEPATIC	2711	301
201	HEPATIC	3164	349
202	HEPATIC	1998	303
203	HEPATIC	4270	316
204	HEPATIC	5501	773
205	HEALTHY	1983	553
206	HEALTHY	3494	728
207	HEALTHY	3962	478
208	HEALTHY	3106	493
209	HEPATIC	2897	432
210	HEALTHY	1598	392
HEALTHY (No Liver Disease) HEPATIC (Moderate Liver Disease)			

Code to analyze such data is provided below and is very similar to that used in previous model validity exercises. In cases where data are collected from mild and severe liver impairment patients, the groupings may be changed to accommodate this, or the Child–Pugh scores themselves can be used to examine the correlation between scores and the pharmacokinetics. We will consider such an approach in the next section, using renal impairment data.

Hepatic Impairment AUC Assessment Example — SAS `proc mixed` *Code:*

```
proc mixed method=reml data=liver;
    class subject group;
    model lnauc=group/s
    ddfm=kenwardroger cl alpha=.1;
    lsmeans group/cl alpha=0.1;
    repeated /group=group subject=subject;
    ods output LSMeans=auc;
    run;
```

For logAUC, the resulting back-transformed model estimates are presented in Table 11.12. AUC was increased (as expected) in the hepatic impaired patients. Assessment of Cmax is left as an exercise for interested readers, and may be performed using code on the website accompanying this book.

TABLE 11.12
Estimated Population Parameters from Evaluation of logAUC as a Function of Group

Group	Estimated Mean AUC	90% CI
HEALTHY	2653	2296, 2861
HEPATIC	3433	3045, 3869
HEALTHY (No Liver Disease) HEPATIC (Moderate Liver Disease)		

According to the suggestion in regulatory guidance [374], if a doubling in extent of exposure is observed relative to the levels used to achieve efficacy while maintaining safety in the normal patient population, the dose in hepatic-impaired patients should be adjusted downward. If exposures cannot be kept clear of the NOAEL, one would presumably not wish to expose patients to such a risk and might contraindicate. If desired, a no-effect claim may be established if a two one-sided test (similar to that used for average bioequivalence) with a clinically relevant threshold is set up a priori in the protocol [374], but we omit discussion of such an approach here, as inference and labelling based on such trials most often utilize expert clinical assessment of estimated model parameters without such formal statistical testing.

11.6 Kidney Disease

Most drugs are eliminated unchanged by the kidney or by metabolism in the liver [360]. As with hepatic impairment, renal impairment can be caused by a variety of factors, and we will not discuss these further here. As age increases, this also results in impaired functioning of the kidney.

For drugs which are eliminated from circulation by the kidney, impaired function is expected to result in decreased clearance [30]. Decreased clearance would be expected to result in increased exposure, and, as with hepatic impairment, this may result in increased likelihood of adverse experiences.

Creatinine clearance (CLcr) is a parameter often used to describe renal function [360]. This endpoint may be derived as [360]

$$CLcr = \frac{(140 - age(yrs))weight(kg)}{72(serum - creatinine(mg/dL))}.$$

This formula is multiplied by 0.85 for female subjects and represents steady-state renal function. Severity of impairment is typically characterized using these values [360]:

1. Healthy (CLcr > 80 mL/min),
2. Mild (CLcr from 50–80 mL/min),
3. Moderate (CLcr from 30–50 mL/min),
4. Severe (CLcr < 30 mL/min), and
5. ESRD (requiring dialysis).

While building a population pharmacokinetic model (see Section 11.1), the impact of renal function (assessed using creatinine clearance) on estimated parameters for plasma clearance will generally be assessed. As with hepatic impairment, if there is good scientific evidence to support this being minor (i.e., renal clearance plays only a small role in elimination and metabolism of the drug), then one need not study the issue further in drug development [360]. Note that this involves some degree of subjectivity; hence, in practice, a study is generally done to validate the understanding from the population pharmacokinetic model.

Design of such a trial is similar to the other validation exercises discussed in this chapter. Roughly equal numbers of subjects in each renal impairment severity class are recruited and given a single dose of drug with a typical clinical pharmacology pharmacokinetic sampling scheme performed. One may also study the ends of the impairment spectrum (severe versus healthy) before enrolling mild and moderates [360].

Often mentioned in the context of renal impairment is the importance of protein binding and consideration of (and derivation of) unbound concentrations and estimates of rate and extent of exposure. Drug molecules bound to protein in plasma are not active and are often removed from circulation by the kidney. Drug not bound to protein is typically the active component which, reaching the site of action, is presumed to elicit a pharmacodynamic response in the body (see Chapters 1 and 2). As protein binding may be impacted by kidney function, typically one blood sample is collected in such studies for each subject to estimate the degree of drug protein binding. If the degree of binding is pronounced (greater than 80%), the unbound concentration is used to derive an estimate of unbound AUC (AUCu) and unbound Cmax (Cmaxu) by straightforward multiplication. An example dataset may be found in Table 11.13. Note that, in this experiment, 60 mL/min was used as the cut-off between mild and moderate renal impairment as it pre-dated the [360] guidance.

TABLE 11.13: Pharmacokinetic Data from a Clinical Pharmacology Renal Impairment Trial

Group	Subject	CLcr	AUC (ng.h/mL)	Cmax (ng/mL)	AUCu (ng.h/mL)	Cmaxu (ng/mL)
HEALTHY	107	105	1523	407	1.68	0.448
HEALTHY	116	87	2426	409	3.40	0.573
HEALTHY	117	92	3919	341	.	.
HEALTHY	126	105	3351	606	.	.
HEALTHY	127	90	1851	474	2.78	0.711
HEALTHY	128	101	3487	444	5.23	0.666
HEALTHY	130	84	3719	592	7.44	1.184
HEALTHY	131	82	3046	400	4.87	0.640
HEALTHY	138	96	3282	474	4.59	0.664
HEALTHY	215	94	2823	424	4.80	0.721
HEALTHY	218	81	2765	584	3.59	0.759
HEALTHY	219	100	1860	377	3.91	0.792
MILD	102	67	2635	392	4.48	0.666
MILD	110	72	2321	320	.	.
MILD	113	68	4498	440	7.65	0.748
MILD	115	68	2727	460	4.09	0.690
MILD	118	67	3226	681	4.52	0.953
MILD	121	66	2653	401	4.51	0.682
MILD	122	73	6710	458	11.41	0.779
MILD	123	69	3991	507	6.39	0.811
MILD	124	65	2304	347	3.23	0.486
MILD	207	64	3254	455	4.88	0.683
MILD	208	71	3364	670	4.37	0.871
MILD	210	61	2271	476	3.18	0.666
MILD	212	74	3137	500	6.59	1.050
MILD	216	64	1560	323	2.18	0.452
MILD	217	71	2235	374	3.80	0.636
MODERATE	105	33	2375	495	3.80	0.792
MODERATE	106	49	3658	389	5.85	0.622
MODERATE	108	44	6638	710	13.28	1.420
MODERATE	111	53	2167	427	3.03	0.598
MODERATE	112	48	3445	517	4.82	0.724
MODERATE	114	46	3670	565	6.61	1.017
MODERATE	120	57	3108	440	5.59	0.792
MODERATE	125	58	3959	599	6.33	0.958
MODERATE	132	55	2211	286	3.76	0.486
MODERATE	133	53	3138	442	5.02	0.707
MODERATE	134	54	3003	572	3.90	0.744
MODERATE	135	53	4187	469	.	.
MODERATE	202	51	2627	337	3.68	0.472
MODERATE	203	54	2718	474	3.81	0.664

HEALTHY (No Renal Disease; CLcr> 80)
MILD (Mild Renal Disease; 60 <CLcr≤ 80)
MODERATE (Moderate Renal Disease; 30 <CLcr≤ 60)
SEVERE (Severe Renal Disease; CLcr≤ 30)

TABLE 11.13: Pharmacokinetic Data from a Clinical Pharmacology Renal Impairment Trial (continued)

Group	Subject	CLcr	AUC (ng.h/mL)	Cmax (ng/mL)	AUCu (ng.h/mL)	Cmaxu (ng/mL)
MODERATE	204	55	3410	558	5.12	0.837
MODERATE	205	55	3314	405	4.97	0.608
MODERATE	209	58	2105	352	2.53	0.422
MODERATE	213	43	2520	504	3.53	0.706
SEVERE	101	15	2290	230	.	.
SEVERE	103	22	2825	262	.	.
SEVERE	104	17	2427	370	4.13	0.629
SEVERE	109	22	2704	527	4.06	0.791
SEVERE	119	23	2237	395	6.04	1.067
SEVERE	129	18	1490	233	2.53	0.396
SEVERE	136	27	1407	329	2.67	0.625
SEVERE	137	21	3415	447	6.83	0.894
SEVERE	201	24	2325	404	.	.
SEVERE	206	6	1675	259	5.36	0.829
SEVERE	211	19	1974	329	4.15	0.691
SEVERE	214	22	2705	526	7.03	1.368
HEALTHY (No Renal Disease; CLcr> 80) MILD (Mild Renal Disease; 60 <CLcr≤ 80) MODERATE (Moderate Renal Disease; 30 <CLcr≤ 60) SEVERE (Severe Renal Disease; CLcr≤ 30)						

Code to analyze such data is provided below and is very similar to that used in previous model validity exercises. Variability is allowed to change with group using the `repeated` statement, and the relationship of the pharmacokinetic endpoint of interest (in this example, AUC) is modelled on the logscale as a function of creatinine clearance. The `estimate` statements are used to output estimates of mean AUC at various levels of creatinine clearance.

Renal Impairment AUC Assessment Example — SAS `proc mixed` *Code:*

```
proc mixed method=reml data=renal;
    class subject group;
    model lnauc=clcr/s
    ddfm=kenwardroger cl alpha=.1 outp=out;
    estimate '80' intercept 1 clcr 80/cl alpha=0.1;
    estimate '70' intercept 1 clcr 70/cl alpha=0.1;
    estimate '60' intercept 1 clcr 60/cl alpha=0.1;
    estimate '50' intercept 1 clcr 50/cl alpha=0.1;
    estimate '40' intercept 1 clcr 40/cl alpha=0.1;
    estimate '30' intercept 1 clcr 30/cl alpha=0.1;
    estimate '20' intercept 1 clcr 20/cl alpha=0.1;
    estimate '10' intercept 1 clcr 10/cl alpha=0.1;
    repeated /group=group subject=subject;
    ods output Estimates=outest;
    run;
```

TABLE 11.14
Estimated Population Parameters from Evaluation of logAUC as a function of Creatinine Clearance

Creatinine Clearance	Estimated Mean AUC	90% CI
80	2953	2651,3289
70	2869	2625,3136
60	2787	2580,3011
50	2708	2506,2926
40	2631	2406,2878
30	2557	2293,2851
20	2484	2177,2835
10	2413	2062,2825

For AUC, the resulting back-transformed model estimates are presented in Table 11.14. No relationship between creatinine clearance and AUC was observed in the renally impaired patients. Analysis of Cmax and unbound AUC and Cmax are left as an exercise for interested readers and may be performed using code on the website accompanying this book.

Generally, a log-linear relationship of total and unbound AUC and Cmax with creatinine clearance is observed. If not, transformation of creatinine clearance using a power model generally suffices to adequately describe the data. As such a model has already been described in the context of dose proportionality (see Chapter 8), this is not discussed further here.

As with hepatic impairment, based on these findings, the population pharmacokinetic model may be rebuilt, if appropriate. Dose is typically adjusted in renally impaired patients to achieve concentrations that are expected to be safe and effective. Labelling statements based on data like those described above provide the basis for the selection of dose adjustment or contraindication. [360].

11.7 Technical Appendix

Models such as

$$c_{it} = (e^{-k_{ei}t} - e^{-k_{ai}t})\frac{k_{ei}k_{ai}(Dose)}{Cl_i(k_{ai} - k_{ei})} + \varepsilon_{it} \tag{11.1}$$

may be used to easily derive estimates for Tmax, Cmax, and AUC. We provide one such example here based on the estimated parameters from the fitted model.

To derive Tmax, take the first derivative of $\hat{c}_{it}$ (the fitted model) with respect to t. The resulting equation is

$$\frac{d\hat{c}_{it}}{dt} = \frac{\hat{k}_{ai}\hat{k}_{ei}(Dose)}{\hat{C}l_i(\hat{k}_{ai} - \hat{k}_{ei})}(-\hat{k}_{ei}e^{-\hat{k}_{ei}t} + \hat{k}_{ai}e^{-\hat{k}_{ai}t}).$$

Setting this equal to zero and solving for t yields an estimate for Tmax of

$$Tmax = \frac{\ln \hat{k}_{ai} - \ln \hat{k}_{ei}}{\hat{k}_{ai} - \hat{k}_{ei}}.$$

An estimate for Cmax may be derived by taking the predicted concentration at this time point:

$$Cmax = (e^{-\hat{k}_{ei}Tmax} - e^{-\hat{k}_{ai}Tmax})\frac{\hat{k}_{ei}\hat{k}_{ai}(Dose)}{\hat{Cl}_i(\hat{k}_{ai} - \hat{k}_{ei})}.$$

To derive $AUC(0-\infty)$, take the integral from zero to infinity of $\hat{c}_{it}$ with respect to time (t):

$$\int_0^\infty \hat{c}_{it}dt = \frac{\hat{k}_{ai}\hat{k}_{ei}(Dose)}{\hat{Cl}_i(\hat{k}_{ai} - \hat{k}_{ei})}\int_0^\infty (e^{-\hat{k}_{ei}t} - e^{-\hat{k}_{ai}t})dt.$$

Integration yields

$$\frac{\hat{k}_{ai}\hat{k}_{ei}(Dose)}{\hat{Cl}_i(\hat{k}_{ai} - \hat{k}_{ei})}(\frac{1}{\hat{k}_{ei}} - \frac{1}{\hat{k}_{ai}}) = \frac{Dose}{\hat{Cl}_i}.$$

As stated in Chapter 8, we chose here to utilize SAS for the nonlinear mixed effect modelling of data; however, several other statistical packages are readily available (SPLUS, NONMEM, WINNONLIN, PKBUGS, etc., [1048]) and may be used for this purpose. Readers interested in more details of these software packages should see [1379] and [1271].

Part IV

Vaccines and Epilogue

12

Vaccine Trials

Introduction

One of my senior supervisors asked a very good question one March. He asked, "Why are you still doing this?" The question was not directed solely at me. It was asked in the context of an introduction before a team building exercise (to develop a culture to promote entrepreneurial spirit, collegiality, and a good work ethic, etc.). The question from my senior supervisor stumped me — why was I still doing this?

That got me thinking. I did the math and figured out that I had been doing clinical trial statistics for 20 years! That was sort of surprising, as I had only intended to do this for a while until something more interesting came along. It occurred to me that maybe to find something more interesting, I had better go look for it.

So while thinking and praying and talking to my wife (not necessarily in that order), I figured I'd best have a talk with my mentor later that same March at a conference we were both attending in Brazil. Bob was in his 60s and had retired from the clinical trials business after 30 years. He and I had a lot of time to talk as we shuttled back and forth from the conference, as the hotel where we were staying was some way from the conference site. He told me the happiest he'd ever been on the job was in giving his time to his old alma mater and seeing the bright enthusiastic students that came out of the school. The students and professors (or some of them) were deeply appreciative of his efforts, but he confided in me that he got a lot more out of it than they did. It was rewarding and made him feel good about all he had done in his career and was doing. Bob reassured me that a successful career in industry is a balance between putting up with petty annoyances while accomplishing objectives that serve the common good and one's own objectives.

Bob had never touched the savings from his 30 years in industry, as he still consulted during his retirement not only for companies making vaccines but also folks like the World Health Organization. He and I were working together on some new analyses for a paper that we were planning. At the close of conference dinner, he saved a seat for me, and while we watched the show, I told him that I now "got" why FDA's vaccines reviewing division was so insistent on randomized studies with pre-specified hypothesis tests (as the many, many clinical trials reported at the conference with the exception of four, one of which Bob and I worked on, were non-randomized). He laughed uproariously and said good and that the whole thing was worth it.

I departed Thursday morning to return to the USA after we rode the bus back to the conference hotel from the dinner Wednesday night, fully expecting we would be in touch back in the USA on Monday morning to wrap up the analyses being planned for our paper, but Bob never came back from the conference. He was found in his room on Friday morning by the hotel staff after attending the remainder of the conference on Thursday. He had a heart condition and had previously survived several heart attacks.

I miss Bob. He answered my senior supervisor's question among many others, while including me in his life and work, out of his own kindness. If one is lucky, one comes across at least one person like that at least once in a lifetime. They are gifts from God. If you do encounter such a treasure, I encourage you to pay attention, listen, and to pass it on.

12.1 Brief Introduction to Vaccine Research and Development

The following section is a brief overview of vaccine development and associated data of interest needed to discuss vaccine studies relating to clinical pharmacology. Readers interested in a more general discussion of statistics in vaccine development may wish to see [156] and [733].

Developing a vaccine for the market is similar in many respects to developing a drug. As with drugs, a vaccine is developed by showing regulators that it is safe (when used as recommended), that it works (when used as recommended), and that it is manufactured to high quality standards. Where development differs from drugs originates with the approach to disease management. A vaccine is a biological construct that improves the body's natural immunity to a disease — see, for example, [1136] — thereby enhancing the body's natural ability to prevent infection and disease. Diseases are, in general, caused by viruses and bacteria infecting the body, and for simplicity, these are referred to as disease vectors in the following discussion and sections.

To begin, it should be recognized that, historically, disease has killed far more people than wars have. For example, prior to its eradication via vaccination, smallpox caused approximately 300,000,000 deaths [936] in the 20th century alone. The disease vectors we are concerned with in making a vaccine are not typically killed by antibiotics, or if they are, it takes a long time and a lot of doses.

On its own, a disease vector does nothing but sit there waiting for a susceptible person to happen by, become exposed, and infect. When introduced into a susceptible organism for example, a viral disease vector infects cells, and then uses these infected cells to multiply [936].

A virus contacts a cell and attaches to its surface at a receptor (for example, measles attaches at a receptor known as CD46). The virus infects the cell by passing through the cell's plasma membrane (phagocytosis) and entering the cell's interior. Then the virus' nucleic acid expresses its genes, replicates its genome, and produces replicas which, when mature, exit the cell and begin to infect more cells.

Viral disease then results and may happen in many ways [936]. The virus itself may be toxic to cells, resulting in cell death. The virus may alter the cell's function — for example, the cell may be inhibited from making a hormone the body needs to grow or function. The immune system of the body (tasked with destroying such viruses) may need to do so by destroying the infected cells, thereby damaging tissues, organs (etc.) that are critical to the body's function.

Most disease vectors result in acute infections [936]. The incubation period for many viruses varies from 2 days to 3 weeks — e.g., the virus infects the body, spreads via the blood or nervous system, and causes damage. It is thereafter destroyed by the immune system (resulting in subsequent immunity) or causes the destruction of the organism (death). Chronic infection, by contrast, is when the immune system does not completely remove the virus (e.g., human immunodeficiency virus) and subsequent recrudescence occurs, followed by death of the organism.

Avoidance of exposure to a disease vector, hand-washing (with soap and in clean water), along with the immune system are the chief means of defense against disease vectors. The immune system recognizes antigens (proteins produced in cells when disease vectors replicate), and upon recognition, responds with specific and nonspecific factors to kill the disease vector. Nonspecific factors are produced all the time by the body — e.g., lymphoid cells, macrophages, complement factors. These float around in the blood, and "eat" or disable any disease vector they recognize. Specific factors are also introduced to the body by prior

infection/recovery or by vaccination. These result in antibodies which the body creates automatically in the immune system and/or in cell-mediated immunity when exposed to a disease vector [936].

Vaccines have been produced historically in a few ways. Attentuation is performed by taking a disease vector and passing it through an animal and tissue culture or tissue culture alone which removes or reduces the ability of the vector to cause disease. The vaccine then results in the body's immune system being primed to produce a response (e.g., antibodies) but not in disease. These are known as "live" vaccines. Measles vaccines were produced using this method.

Vaccines are also produced by chemically killing the disease vector. Administration of vaccines made this way obviously cannot cause disease (as a dead disease vector cannot replicate) but primes the body's immune system to recognize and respond to it. The Salk polio vaccine is an example of this.

Traditionally, vaccines have been used to prevent disease, e.g., smallpox. Lately, vaccines are being developed to treat existing diseases, e.g., cancer, Alzheimer's, even addiction to nicotine. Most of the remainder of this chapter will be in reference to preventative vaccines, but the concepts may be readily extended to treatment vaccines.

Turning now to discussion of endpoints, the body generates antibodies (among other things) in response to infection. Immunoglobulin is a protein of interest and has several classes: IgG, IgM, IgA, etc. Of these, IgG (immunoglobulin protein type G) is the protein most of interest in vaccination.

Antibody concentration denotes how much antibody is present in a serum sample of given size. For example IgG may be expressed in units such as μg/mL. Antibody titers are a more complex way of expressing the amount of antibody: "measure of the antibody amount in a serum sample, expressed as the reciprocal of the highest dilution of the sample" that "results a certain assay read-out" [918]. That is, a serum sample is diluted 1:8 (8 parts water or other neutral substance is added to the sample). Dilution continues 1:16, 1:32, 1:64, 1:128, etc., and an antigen (antibody-producing substance) is added. Each dilution is then assayed to see if a reaction occurs.

Let us suppose that we are interested in the titer which results in 50% killing of a given disease vector. We take serum samples from subjects after vaccination in a study, produce the dilutions for each subject's serum sample, add a precise amount of disease vector to each and every dilution, and see how much each titer of the sample kills. For example, consider the following results for a given subject's sample: 1:8 kills 100%, 1:16 kills 75%, 1:32 kills 50%, 1:64 kills 25%, 1:128 kills 0%. The titer we'd be interested in is 1:32. Titers obviously have no units — they are divided out by dilution, and the titer is typically referred to by the inverse dilution. That is 1:32 is analyzed as a data point with value 32.

Concentrations and titers are log-normally distributed [732] and are analyzed in very similar fashion to pharmacokinetic data [72]. A caution of particular note to vaccines — concentrations and titers are produced using biologic assays, and such assays have specifications. These are the lower limit of quantification (LLOQ, we can trust numbers above this point), the lower limit of detection (LLOD, below here one does not get a finding consistently), and the upper limit of quantification (ULOQ, beyond which the assay cannot generate a consistent finding). Thus such data are not really normally distributed after natural-log transformation, but the central limit theorem protects us (within reason). When it does not, there are approaches to dealing with missing data; those interested may wish to review [766, 942, 1095, 1383].

As with drugs, safety data collected in vaccine studies are generally binary, repeated measures; i.e., one has (1) or does not have (0) a safety reaction of given type at a given visit or time interval of reporting. Statistically of interest is $100(\hat{p})$ where $\hat{p} = r/n$ where r is the number of events designated 1 and n is the number of subjects. We can use a variety of analysis techniques [280] on these data, ranging from application of the binomial distribution to Fisher's exact test to more sophisticated methods as described in Chapter 8. We will consider common methods used for analysis in vaccine development in the next section.

There are a few types of adverse events which are of particular interest following vaccination. Local reactions are events that are sometimes known as reactogenicity. Vaccines are typically given by injection, and local reactions relate to safety observations at the site of injection (or in the immediate vicinity). These events include things like

1) Tenderness (None, Mild, Significant, Any),

2) Induration=Swelling (None, Mild, Moderate, Severe, Any),

3) Erythema=Reddening (None, Mild, Moderate, Severe, Any).

Systemic events are adverse events typically related to the immune response to vaccine, such as

1) Fever (None, 38–39°C, 39–40°C, >40°C, Any),

2) Decreased appetite,

3) Irritability,

4) Increased/decreased sleep,

5) Hives,

6) Use of medication to treat or prevent symptoms (i.e., fever), etc.

Local reactions and systemic events are binary, repeated measures data, and the percentage of the observed number of events amongst the subjects potentially experiencingat a given time interval (and maybe duration) are the data of most interest. These are typically presented as percentagesin reporting.

There are other types of vaccine data. Carriage data and outcome data are two examples. Carriage studies assess whether a subject is carrying the disease vector (i.e., infected) at a given visit. See, for example, [32, 235, 236, 299]. Vaccine efficacy studies assess whether disease itself is observed at a given visit. Both types of data are generally treated as binary, repeated measures data. These types of event data will involve comprehensive algorithms for endpoint definition (typically in the study protocol and statistical analysis plan). Measurement will involve microbiology measurement (e.g., cultures) and results will involve categories (e.g., serogroups [71]). Those interested in more information on carriage and efficacy studies for vaccines should review [503, 504, 918]. The analysis of such data is beyond the scope of this chapter, and we will confine our attention to immunogenicity and to safety data in the following sections, as these are the most pertinent to clinical pharmacology trials in vaccines.

Studies in Phase I through IV vaccine development follow the same paradigm of development as discussed for drugs in Chapter 1. As our emphasis is upon clinical pharmacology vaccine trials, we first discuss Phase I vaccine studies before turning to vaccine proof-of-concept studies. We will then discuss concomitant vaccination studies and lot consistency studies, ending with a brief discussion of cross-over study designs in vaccine development.

12.2 Phase I Vaccine Studies

As discussed in Chapter 1, clinical development of a product, with the exception of only the most toxic products targeted for the treatment of cancer, initiates with the study of the product in normal healthy adult male volunteers in what is known as Phase I. These studies are typically small, well controlled, data intensive, dose escalating, and placebo controlled. The primary objective of these studies for vaccines is to determine a safe dose and dosing regimen (e.g., once a month for three months) for later dosing in studies involving subjects who may be exposed to the disease vector of concern.

Dose and dosing regimen for the vaccine are examined with respect to their impact on immunogenicity and on safety, in particular with regard to local reactions and systemic events. The goal is to identify a dose and dosing regimen resulting in desired antibody levels without the occurrence of unacceptable side-effects. Side-effects like local reactions or systemic events may be tolerable even if significantly higher than placebo, depending upon the disease vector of concern — for example, the Measles-Mumps-Rubella vaccine is well known to result in fever in some recipients following vaccination; however, the benefit in terms of preventing disease outweighs the risk. Dosing in adult volunteers is generally followed by studies in children or the elderly, depending upon the disease vector being considered.

Like drugs, by the end of such studies in Phase I, dose-finding studies in normal healthy volunteers should provide a safe (and potentially efficacious) dose and dosing regimen for further studies in subjects at risk, an initial description of immunogenicity and safety to support the choice of dose and regimen, and provide seed data for the powering of Phase II and III studies.

Also considered during Phase I is the use of an adjuvant. These are substances included in the vaccine which are used to enhance the body's immune response to a given dose of vaccine and are often associated with increased reactions compared to un-adjuvanted vaccines. At this stage in Phase 1, there will be some preclinical knowledge of whether the adjuvant enhanced immunogenicity in preclinical (non-human) species, but the dose of the adjuvant must also be studied in parallel with studying the dose and dosing regimen of vaccine. The use of factorial study designs [561] is readily applicable in this context, as multiple doses of vaccine, adjuvant, and schedule are potential factors.

However, study designs for vaccines in Phase I are constrained in that dose escalation procedures must be followed, as discussed in Chapter 8. That is, for example, consider a vaccine with two potential doses ($D_1 =$ Low, $D_2 =$ High), two potential doses of adjuvant ($A_1 =$ Low, $A_2 =$ High), and two potential schedules ($S_1 =$ once per month for three months, $S_2 =$ once a week for three weeks). The $D_1 : A_1 : S_1$ combination would need to be studied to ensure subject safety (relative to placebo) before initiating combinations like $D_2 : A_1 : S_1$, $D_1 : A_1 : S_2$, etc. At each stage, eligible subjects are randomly assigned to either the desired combination or to placebo.

Ignoring schedule for a moment, and assuming there is only one dose of an adjuvant to consider (denoted A1 if administered), then an example of the design of a Phase I study could appear as given in Table 12.1. That is, in the first stage, 12 subjects would be randomly assigned to receive a low dose of vaccine ($n = 9$) or placebo ($n = 3$). If acceptable safety data are observed, then an additional 12 subjects would be randomly assigned to receive a low dose of vaccine with adjuvant ($n = 9$) or placebo ($n = 3$) in parallel with another 12 subjects who would be randomly assigned to receive a middle dose of vaccine ($n = 9$) or placebo ($n = 3$), and so forth, depending upon the observed safety findings.

Such studies are difficult to double blind, but this obstacle may be overcome by use

TABLE 12.1
Schematic Plan of a Phase I Study

Stage	Dose	Adjuvant	N (Vaccinated)	N (Placebo)
1	Low		9	3
2	Low	A1	9	3
2	Middle		9	3
3	Middle	A1	9	3
3	High		9	3
4	High	A1	9	3

of an unblinded pharmacy with the use of double dummy administrations (e.g., saline injections) where warranted. It is recommended that at least single blinding be applied, as local reactions and systemic events are self-reported by the subject, typically in modern studies using an electronic diary which is filled out by each subject each day for a period of time following vaccination. Of particular concern, at each stage, is that care should be taken to ensure that protocol-specified subject inclusion and exclusion criteria are rigorously applied. If these are allowed to change over time, then the analysis of vaccine dose, adjuvant, and schedule may be confounded by changes in population factors, potentially biasing the results. For example, if younger subjects are enrolled at higher doses relative to lower doses, dose would be confounded with age in the data analysis.

Generally, at this stage of vaccine development, only small batches of vaccine and adjuvant are made. This limits the potential sample size of such studies (in addition to the ethical requirements of Phase I to expose only small numbers of subjects to potential risk). Once dose, adjuvant, and schedule are identified in Phase I, larger batches of clinical grade material are developed to enable powered studies.

Sample size may be varied at each stage during the trial as specified in protocol. For example, it may be thought (based upon pre-clinical data) that the lower doses will not result in desired immunogenicity. Once studied, then the higher doses may be studied using larger numbers of subjects to more precisely define the safety and immunogenicity profile. In the example given in Table 12.1, one would do so by, for example, randomizing 12:4 vaccine:placebo in the middle dose groups, and perhaps 18:6 in the high dose groups. This sort of approach is not unusual [473] and is increasingly becoming the norm in Phase I development.

Consider a three-dose, one-adjuvant, placebo-controlled Phase I design with fevers observed, as shown in Table 12.2. Note that there are 18 subjects receiving placebo in this design, and it is not unusual to pool their data in practice for analysis.

For a given dose group, the observed frequency of an event is defined as $\hat{p} = r/n$ where r is the number of events, and n is the sample size in that group. The Clopper–Pearson lower and upper confidence bounds [213] are $\frac{r(f_l)}{r(f_l)+(n-r+1)}$ and $\frac{(r+1)(f_u)}{(n-r)+(r+1)f_u}$, respectively, where f_l is the 2.5th percentile of the F-distribution with $2r$ and $2(n-r+1)$ degrees of freedom and f_u is the 97.5th percentile of the f-distribution with $2(r+1)$ and $2(n-r)$ degrees of freedom.

One can apply SAS code as given below to derive 95% confidence bounds for the proportion of fevers in each dose group.

TABLE 12.2
Number of Fevers Observed in Each Dose Group in a Phase I Study

Dose	Adjuvant	Fever	N
1	1	0	9
1	0	1	9
10	1	4	9
10	0	3	9
100	1	3	9
100	0	9	9
0	0	0	18
Adjv=1 denotes present, 0 absent			

```
data prev_ct;set mock;
prev=r/n;
prev_pct=100*prev;
df1=2*r;df2=2*(n-r+1);df3=2*(r+1);df4=2*(n-r);
f_l=finv(0.025,df1,df2);f_u=finv(0.975,df3,df4);
run;

data prev_ct;set prev_ct;
if r=0 then f_l=1;if r=n then f_u=1;
prev_l=100*(r*f_l)/((r*f_l)+(n-r+1));
prev_u=100*((r+1)*f_u)/((n-r)+((r+1)*f_u));
run;
```

Clopper–Pearson confidence intervals are termed *exact* intervals, as they are based directly on the binomial distribution. "Exact" is a misnomer and denotes that the coverage probability of the confidence interval is at least 95% — it may well be higher. Thus such an exact interval may be overly wide. By contrast, the classical normal approximation may be too narrow (i.e., less than 95% coverage rate). As the normal approximation is held to be too narrow, we will only discuss exact approaches here.

Consider the findings of Table 12.3. Note the overlap of confidence intervals with the exception of the highest dose (no adjuvant) and placebo. Note the counterintuitive result — the fever rate is higher at the high dose with no adjuvant than with adjuvant. Such observations are not unusual when the n is low.

A few useful asides. The "rule of 3" is a simple way of stating an approximate 95% confidence interval for p in the special case that no events have been observed. The rule of 3 interval is approximately $(0, 3/n)$. Also, keeping in mind that overlap of half the length of one arm corresponds approximately to statistical significance at $p = 0.05$ can be helpful for a quick appreciation of tables and figures that display confidence intervals by group, when p-values are not reported [232]. The key (understated) assumption in the use of this rule of thumb is independence. This can only be assumed for each randomized dose group relative to placebo in Phase I vaccine studies, as such studies are dose escalating (i.e., from low to high doses). Strictly speaking, therefore, statistical inference in such studies focusses upon the effect of each dose relative to placebo.

TABLE 12.3
Findings from a Phase I Study

Dose	Adjuvant	Fevers %	95% LB	95% UB
1	1	0.0	0.0	33.6
1	0	11.1	0.3	48.2
10	1	44.4	13.7	78.8
10	0	33.3	7.5	70.1
100	1	33.3	7.5	70.1
100	0	100.0	66.4	100.0
0	0	0.0	0.0	18.5
Adjv=1 denotes present				

We can also easily formally compare the proportions between dose groups and placebo using a variety of procedures such as Fisher's exact test. To compare the observed proportion of fevers at the middle dose to placebo, SAS code to do so is

```
Title 'Middle Dose:Pbo';run;
data middle;input group $ category $ Count @@;
cards;
A yes 7 A no 11 B yes 0 B no 18
;
proc freq data=middle order=data;weight count;
tables category*group/chisq;run;
```

This results in a Fisher's exact p-value of 0.0076, indicating that the two dose groups differ significantly in their rate of observed fevers, with the middle dose being significantly higher than placebo. The low dose does not result in a significant difference, but the high dose group clearly is even more significant relative to placebo. These analyses are left as an exercise for interested readers.

To determine whether the difference is clinically important, one may wish to examine confidence intervals for the difference in the observed proportions. A large number of statistical approaches are available to do so — see [1071]. The Chan and Zhang approach [154] is often used and may be implemented in StatXact using SAS code as follows:

```
Title 'Middle Dose:Pbo';run;
proc binomial data = middle
max_time=30 gamma = 0.000001
out = ex_diff;
riskdiff / ex one;
po group;
ou category;
weight count;
run;
```

This results in a point estimate and 95% confidence interval comparing the proportion of fevers observed for the middle dose of 0.3889 (0.1545, 0.6425), again indicating that the two dose groups differ significantly in their rate of observed fevers, with the middle dose being significantly higher than placebo but also providing a plausible range of values for the true

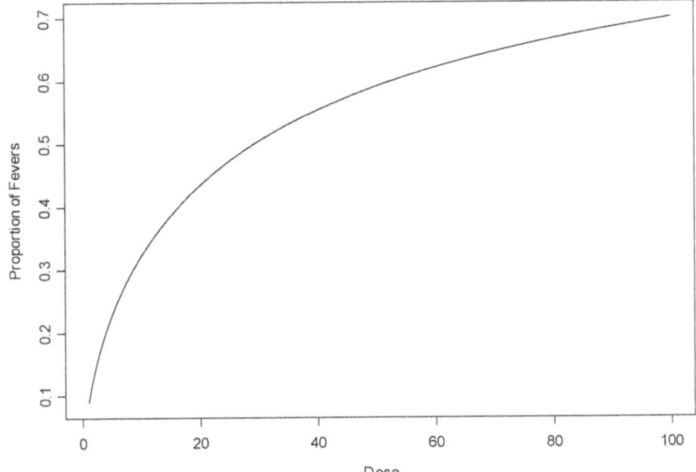

FIGURE 12.1
Model Estimates for Proportion of Events (Fevers) versus Dose in a Phase I Study

effect size. Interested readers may find that the low dose compared to placebo results in a point estimate and 95% confidence interval of 0.0556 (-0.1328, 0.2736) and 0.6667 (0.4074, 0.8666) for the high dose.

As discussed in Chapter 8, the proportion (p) can be defined such that

$$p = \frac{1}{1 + e^{-(\alpha+\beta(ld))}}$$

where β is the slope of a regression of $\ln(p/1-p) = L$ (known as a logit-transformation) on logDose such that $L = \alpha + \beta(ld)$. Using `proc genmod` in SAS as was done in Chapter 8, SAS output (not listed) yielded an estimate (95% CI) of -2.33 (-3.64, -1.02) for $\hat{\alpha}$ and 0.69 (0.29, 1.08) for β for the above example, yielding estimated proportions of fevers with dose as given in Figure 12.1.

Data are sparse in Phase I, so it is likely that adjuvant and placebo must be neglected in such a model to get the model to fit. More formal testing approaches among the doses [273] may be employed but are not frequently needed in Phase I, as the usual assumptions around independence among the doses does not apply. One is not testing confirmatory hypotheses in Phase I as one is learning. As data accumulates across Phase I studies, it is desirable to use the principles of meta-analysis [1326] to study differences between doses, and such is becoming the norm in later phases of development during submission (e.g., [1233]). However, such meta-analysis is beyond the scope of this chapter.

In the next section, we discuss analyses pertaining to proof-of-concept concerning immunogenicity data. We therefore will not discuss this data here.

At the end of Phase I, it is to be expected that the dose, adjuvant, and schedule for the vaccine have been identified, and in particular that administration meets the desired target profile for safety (so far). The next step is to move to Phase II studies in the target population and establish proof-of-concept (PoC). Historically, the transition probability of success from Phase I to Phase II is approximately 64% [264]. Acceptable safety with some evidence of immunogenicity is all that needs to be seen, so the bar to progression into Phase II is not very high.

12.3 Proof-of-Concept and Phase II

As dose, adjuvant, and schedule have been identified in Phase I, vaccine development in terms of manufacturing scales up to allow for larger studies. Hence, between Phase I and II, there is usually a formulation change. Phase II studies, and in particular the proof-of-concept study or studies, have a triple purpose — first to assess whether the safety and immunogenicity results of the dose, adjuvant, and schedule identified in Phase I still hold true, but also to generate sufficient data in the target population to support investment decisions, and also to allow for the design of Phase III confirmatory studies.

The design of Phase II studies in vaccines is almost always a randomized, parallel group, double blinded, longitudinal study. Safety data is collected after each vaccine administration, and immunogenicity data is collected approximately 1 month after the primary series of vaccination. Some vaccines are given in only one dose, but for most vaccines (e.g., polio vaccines, for example), multiple doses are given over time, and immunogenicity is assessed following the last dose. Subjects from the target population (for example, infants or the elderly or an at-risk population) are randomized to receive the vaccine (according to the dose, adjuvant, and schedule identified in Phase I) or placebo (or a positive control vaccine if one is available).

The proof-of-concept study should be designed to meet a pre-identified immunogenicity target as follows:

		The Truth	
		Vaccine does NOT meet target	Vaccine does meet target
Stats from	Vaccine does NOT meet target	Right answer!	Wrong answer (Type 2 error)
the study show that	Vaccine does meet target	Wrong answer (Type 1 error)	Right answer!

In this case, both the Type 1 (false positive, α) and 2 (false negative, β — note that power equals $1 - \beta$) errors are risks the **sponsor** carries in making an investment decision. As the data generated in Phase II will form the basis of power calculations for Phase III, regulators will be involved in review of the findings, and, additionally under modern legislation, sponsors are required to publish their data. Therefore, while more latitude is given at this stage of development in terms of the choice of α and β, sponsors do not have full freedom to choose any level desired. It is most usual in practice to set $\alpha = 0.05$, but it is common for the sponsor to carry increased risk of a false negative at this stage of development ($0.2 < \beta < 0.3$ are not uncommon.)

For the purposes of this section, we will assume that one primary immunogenicity endpoint has been chosen for the purposes of powering the proof-of-concept study. Multistrain and disease vaccines are becoming common with emerging technology, and we will discuss powering for such multiple vaccine endpoints later in this chapter.

As discussed earlier, for immunogenicity data, antibody and titer data are held to be log-normally distributed. For the purpose of this example, it is assumed that it was desired that the 4-fold response rate for vaccine for Strain 1 significantly exceeds that of placebo (three other strains were also assessed as secondary endpoints). In practice, additional criteria may be desired; for example, the lower bound of the estimate for the difference in response rate between vaccine and placebo might need to exceed 20% to achieve the desired target.

SAS code like the following may be used to power such a study:

```
proc power;
    twosamplefreq test=fisher
   alpha      =   0.05
       PROPORTIONDIFF = 0.5, 0.6, 0.7, 0.8
       REFPROPORTION= 0.05
       power          = 0.8
       npergroup         = .;
 run;
```

A low 5% placebo response rate was assumed along with vaccine increasing response rates from 50 to 80%. Type 1 error was set at 5%, and the desired Type 2 error rate was defined as 20%. Readers may verify using the above code that, to meet the immunogenicity objective, only $n = 8 - 16$ subjects per group were required. However, as will be seen in the following example, a larger sample size was selected to mitigate the risk of a Type 2 error in addition to providing a safety database sufficient for regulators to endorse progression to larger Phase III confirmatory studies.

Anonymous baseline and post-vaccination titer data from a randomized, double blinded, placebo controlled proof-of-concept trial may be found on the website accompanying the book and are shown in Table 12.4. We will study the Strain 1 titer data as the primary endpoint for the proof-of-concept assessment.

SAS code is available on the website accompanying this book to calculate geometric mean titers and to compare Vaccine to Placebo, accounting for baseline. As shown in Table 12.4, while comparable at baseline, following vaccination, higher geometric titers were observed in the vaccine group relative to placebo. Inspection of the raw data shows that, in both groups, titers above the assay lower limit of quantification were observed for some subjects at baseline. This is consistent with the disease vector under study in that in this population some subjects will have been exposed to infection that did not cause disease. The geometric mean ratio for Vaccine to Placebo following vaccination was 20.4 with a 95% confidence interval (10.1, 41.1) accounting for baseline titer in the mixed model. Clearly a statistically significant increase in geometric mean titers was observed following vaccination.

Geometric mean fold rises [918] may be easily calculated from the summary statistics; however, it should be noted that their use in interpretation of data (for example, post- as compared to pre-vaccination) is not favored by regulatory agencies in part due to findings of [72]. When examining post-vaccination to pre-vaccination data, it is more usual to dichotomize the data into a binary endpoints, typically by use of a 4-fold rise indicator endpoint (e.g., those subjects experiencing a 4 times or greater antibody level or titer post-vaccination relative to their pre-vaccination level are denoted as a 1, otherwise 0). Those subjects with pre-vaccination data less than the assay lower limit of quantification (LLOQ) should show 4 times the LLOQ level or greater following vaccination to be denoted

TABLE 12.4
Strain 1 Pre-vaccination and Post-vaccination Geometric Mean Titres (GMT) from Proof-of-Concept Vaccine Trial

Strain	Treatment	Pre-Vax GMT	Post-Vax GMT
1	Vaccine	2.73	50.57
1	Control	2.13	2.53

responders. This is common practice, but those using such approaches are well advised to be aware of the decrease in study power resulting from dichotomization of continuous data [402].

After dichotomization, the same approaches to analyzing binary safety data as described in the previous section may then be applied to the resulting binary immunogenicity data. SAS code is available on the website accompanying this book to allow interested readers to do so. For Strain 1, there was one 4-fold responder who received placebo ($n = 36$), and for vaccinated subjects, there were 54 4-fold responders ($n = 71$). The observed difference in the proportion of 4-fold responders between vaccinated and placebo subjects was therefore 73.3% (Fisher's exact $p < 0.0001$) with a 95% confidence interval of (58.2%, 83.7%) derived using [154].

Along with understanding of the geometric means by group, these types of responder data are generally sufficient to achieve proof-of-concept (i.e., support investment decisions) by defining the normal level of response and how many subjects' immune systems clearly demonstrated that the vaccine causes an immunogenic reaction. This assumes that the safety profile remains the same as Phase I, but as that aspect was discussed in the previous section, we will not revisit it here.

Increasingly, where multiple disease strain vectors are involved in a single vaccine, dichotomization to 0 (did not respond to any or did not respond to all strains) or 1 (responded to all strains) is also being considered as a regulatory endpoint. Additional data for three strains are available in the dataset used as an example in this section (available on the website) for those readers interested in exploring this type of analysis.

Following the proof-of-concept study (or studies), confidence will have been generated that the vaccine will meet the sponsor's desired target profile. This will then lead to a decision on whether or not to invest further in large Phase III confirmatory studies to reach the marketplace. Even if a vaccine has demonstrated proof-of-concept, a decision to invest may not be made for reasons such as competing projects (with higher priority), insufficient expectation of return on investment, competitive landscape (e.g., another sponsor has a vaccine that will precede the sponsor's vaccine to market), among other reasons.

The data will also inform end of Phase II meetings with regulators in the USA (known as Scientific Advice meetings in the European Union). Findings will also define to some extent the confirmatory studies and data required for approval to market. These meetings occur after completion of Phase II (assuming a positive investment decision) and when all relevant data are available for regulatory review. More or less, this is where the major Western regulatory bodies give the go-ahead (or their views) on Phase III protocols. Similar procedures are used in Japan. Specific questions are asked of the regulators to seek their opinions on key issues for Phase III. Their opinion is informed based on a summary of findings from Phases I and II.

Topics discussed at these meetings cover everything from study design, to adequacy of the safety database, to particulars of the immunogenicity and efficacy assessments, to how the lab will run the assays, how randomization will be performed, etc. Essentially, this is the last chance to ask for regulatory input prior to the the implementation of Phase III and the resulting pre-submission meetings (which occur after Phase III findings are available for review but prior to actual submission of all the relevant clinical study reports).

The chance of success decreases in this phase of development. Going from Phase II to III is harder — there are more hurdles to surmount. The transition probability is historically about 39% [264]. One needs to see the right dose, acceptable safety, acceptable regimen (i.e., scheduling) with clear evidence of immunogenicity (and potentially some demonstration of efficacy), a positive decision to invest by the sponsor, plus regulatorys' views, so the bar to progression is higher.

The data generated in Phase II is from the desired target population. For the powering of Phase III studies, we therefore recommend that simulations be performed to understand the various implications of regulatory feedback relative to Phase III study design and analysis planning. We now turn to consideration of lot consistency studies.

12.4 Lot Consistency

Lot consistency is the demonstration by the vaccine's manufacturer that the vaccine can be manufactured over and over again. Vaccines are more "grown" than "made," and, similar to the genesis of clinical bioequivalence testing for drugs, experience has led regulators to believe that consistency based on technical specifications need not ensure consistent clinical responses.

Lots of vaccine are made in sequential basis at various sites. Manufacturers must take three large (generally manufacturing scale) sequentially made lots and compare their immunogenicity properties in a clinical trial. The interest is in confirming that the lots are essentially the same to prove that the manufacturer has the production under control. This makes the approach to design and analysis an equivalence problem [734], very similar to bioequivalence testing.

The null hypothesis is that the lots are not the same, and sufficient clinical data are to be collected to reject this hypothesis.

		The Truth	
		Lots are NOT equivalent	Lots ARE equivalent
Stats from	Lots are NOT equivalent	Right answer!	Wrong answer (Type 2 error)
the study show that	Lots ARE equivalent	Wrong answer (Type 1 error)	Right answer!

Type 1 error is again termed regulatory risk (i.e., risk for regulators that lots are deemed equivalent and approved for marketing when in fact they are not). Type 2 error in this study is also called sponsor's risk (i.e., risk for the sponsor that they cannot conclude equivalence when in fact the lots are equivalent).

Assume (for now) that the vaccine gives one antibody response, and we derive a geometric mean (μ_L) for each lot to describe its properties. Under this approach to inference, the usual null hypothesis to find differences was reformulated to correspond to the structure of testing the question of lot equivalence:

$$H_{01}: \quad \mu_L - \mu_{L'} \leq -\Delta \tag{12.1}$$

versus the alternative

$$H_{11}: \quad \mu_L - \mu_{L'} > -\Delta$$

OR

$$H_{02}: \quad \mu_L - \mu_{L'} \geq \Delta \tag{12.2}$$

versus the alternative

$$H_{12}: \quad \mu_L - \mu_{L'} < \Delta$$

for all combinations across lots $L = 1$–3 where $L \neq L'$.

So the situation is a bit more complex than that usually encountered in bioequivalence testing in that all three two one-sided null hypotheses (Lot 1–2, 1–3, and 2–3 for Equations 12.1 and 12.2) must be rejected in order to conclude that the lots 1, 2, and 3 are equivalent.

If three manufacturing lots are shown to be equivalent (i.e., not too large and not to small for all responses of interest), then the manufacturing process is confirmed as stable at that point in time. Periodic manufacturing inspections are carried out by regulatory agencies subsequently to ensure that this state of control is not allowed to deteriorate. Major changes in site of manufacture are not really encouraged by regulators, and may trigger additional such studies following approval.

The primary objective of such a trial is "To demonstrate that the immune responses induced by 3 lots of vaccine are equivalent when measured 1 month after the vaccination regimen." There are often a plethora of secondary objectives — e.g., concomitant vaccination, safety relative to a control, etc.

The study design itself is parallel group (to lot), randomized (to lot), and double blind. A randomized control group may also be included for the purpose of confirmatory immunogenicity or for safety comparisons (see the previous sections of this chapter). Inclusion and exclusion criteria are standardized, and, following the required number of vaccinations, blood samples for immunogenicity assay are collected 14–42 days (usually a month) following the last vaccination.

Randomization and dosing are matters to monitor closely. Eligible subjects will be randomly assigned to one of the lots (or control if included), and these regimens are designated L1, L2, L3, or C for lot 1, lot 2, lot 3, or control, respectively, in the following materials. If a sequence of vaccinations is being applied (i.e., 2–3 doses separated by a period of time), it is important to ensure that the subject receives the right lot at each individual vaccination. Most interactive randomization systems are not designed with this in mind, and statisticians should take steps in the protocol to ensure it is done correctly, as it is obviously undesirable that a subject who is randomized to, say, L1 to get L2 at one dose (as that comparison would then be biased toward the alternative). Obviously if a subject receives more than 1 lot in such a circumstance, they are not strictly evaluable as randomized and can be excluded from the inferential population, if designated in the protocol and statistical analysis plan.

The model to be used is very simple for only one endpoint. The response to each lot is viewed as $\ln(y_{Li}) = \alpha + \tau_L + \varepsilon_i$ where $\ln(y_{Li})$ is the natural-log of the response variable (IgG, etc.) for lot $L = 1 - 3$ subject $i = 1 - n_L$, $\alpha + \tau_L = \mu_L$ denotes the mean response across subjects $i = 1 - n_L$ of lot L =1–3, and ε_i is the residual variance where $Var(\varepsilon_i) = \sigma^2$. Note that this model assumes a common between-subject variance across lots. While this is frequently done, we can be more specific such that $\ln(y_{Li}) = \alpha + \tau_L + \varepsilon_{Li}$ with $Var(\varepsilon_{Li}) = \sigma_L^2$. There may be reason to do this, as we will consider in the following example.

In reality as a practical matter, there is usually more than one endpoint. The response to each lot is then viewed as $\ln(y_{Lji}) = \alpha_j + \tau_{Lj} + \varepsilon_{ji}$ where $\ln(y_{Lji})$ is the natural-log of the response variable (IgG, etc.) for lot L subject $i = 1 - n_L$ for response variable j, $\alpha_j + \tau_{Lj} = \mu_{Lj}$ denotes the mean response across subjects $i = 1 - n_L$ in lot L, and ε_{ji} is the residual variance where $Var(\varepsilon_{ji}) = \sigma_j^2$ for response variable j.

This model describes the mean response for each variable j in each lot. The interest is then to test for equivalence using the two one-sided tests as follows.

$$H_{01}: \quad \mu_{Lj} - \mu_{L'j} \leq -\Delta \tag{12.3}$$

versus the alternative

$$H_{11}: \quad \mu_{Lj} - \mu_{L'j} > -\Delta$$

OR

$$H_{02}: \quad \mu_{Lj} - \mu_{L'j} \geq \Delta \tag{12.4}$$

versus the alternative

$$H_{12}: \quad \mu_{Lj} - \mu_{L'j} < \Delta$$

for all combinations across lots $L = 1–3$ for each response variable j where $L \neq L'$.

Each of the two one-sided testing procedures must be successfully rejected across all j endpoints and all three lots for equivalence to be demonstrated.

The two one-sided testing approach for lot consistency (as with bioequivalence) is an intersection-union test (IUT). There are $L \times (j)$ two one-sided tests, and the global null hypothesis is

$$H_0 : \bigcup_j TOST_j$$

versus alternative

$$H_1 : \bigcap_j TOST_j$$

As such, the experimentwise true Type 1 error rate is conservatively controlled, as described in Section 4.7.

In lot consistency, unlike bioequivalence, regulators require that $\alpha = \frac{0.05}{2} = 0.025$ for each one-sided test, and 95% confidence intervals will be used for inference. The acceptance criteria, Δ, is also in part a criteria determined by regulators. In theory, one would look at how much antibody must change in order for protection of the vaccine to wane and take some percentage of that to set this criterion [743]. However, at this point in vaccine development, confirmatory trials will not have been done, nor in general will longitudinal studies to look at antibody over time have been done. We fall back on precedent in such situations, and in general $\Delta = \ln(2) = 0.6931$ has historically been used. Where one wants to be extra sure, a requirement of $\Delta = \ln(1.5) = 0.4055$ may be applied. This criterion should be included in the lot consistency protocol and reviewed by regulators before initiating the clinical trial.

In practice, as with bioequivalence, most sponsors do not actually construct the t-tests for the TOST and derive p-values. Most sponsors construct 95% confidence intervals for this purpose. If all the lower and upper bounds of the lot to lot confidence intervals fall within $-\Delta, \Delta$ for all j endpoints, then the two null hypotheses are successfully rejected each time, and equivalence is demonstrated.

A dataset based on a lot consistency study containing $n = 200$ randomized, double-blinded subjects per lot (overall $n = 600$) with IgG measured 1 month following vaccination for four serotypes (A–D) may be found on the website accompanying this book. The lot consistency acceptance criteria is $\Delta = 0.6931$. For one subject in each of lot groups 1, 2, and 3, for example, the ln-IgG data were

subject	group	serotype	lnigg
1	1	A	0.47990
1	1	B	-0.48936
1	1	C	0.75303
1	1	D	1.28451
201	2	A	0.38591
201	2	B	-0.82267
201	2	C	0.95563
201	2	D	1.23691
401	3	A	-0.34689
401	3	B	-0.39631
401	3	C	0.22147
401	3	D	0.39233

We first will assume that between-subject variance is homogeneous across lots and perform analysis using the following SAS code:

```
proc mixed data=trialf method=reml
ITDETAILS maxiter=200;
by serotype;
class group;
model lnigg=group;
estimate '1-2' group 1 -1 0/cl alpha=0.05;
estimate '1-3' group 1 0 -1/cl alpha=0.05;
estimate '2-3' group 0 1 -1/cl alpha=0.05;
ods output Estimates=test;
run;
```

For serotype A, we observe that our estimate for $\sigma_A^2 = 0.7794$:

```
Covariance Parameter
      Estimates

Cov Parm       Estimate

Residual          0.7794
```

The test for a group effect finds that at least one of the lots significantly differs from the others ($p = 0.0266$):

```
        Type 3 Tests of Fixed Effects

                  Num       Den
Effect             DF        DF     F Value     Pr > F

group               2       597        3.65     0.0266
```

However, lot consistency was demonstrated for serotype A as the confidence intervals fall within the acceptance limits:

```
Estimates
Label         Lower           Upper

L1-L2      -0.2965         0.05024
L1-L3      -0.05814         0.2886
L2-L3        0.06501        0.4118
```

Recall that $(-\Delta, \Delta) = (-0.6931, 0.6931)$ is the acceptance region.

Note that the standard error for all lot comparisons is the same and is $\sqrt{\frac{2(\sigma^2)}{n}} = \sqrt{\frac{2(0.7794)}{200}} = 0.08828$.

```
Estimates


                          Standard
Label      Estimate          Error        DF

L1-L2       -0.1231        0.08828       597
L1-L3        0.1152        0.08828       597
L2-L3        0.2384        0.08828       597
```

There is not clear guidance on whether to allow for heterogeneous variance between-lots, but as a statistical matter as far back as Satterthwaite [1074, 1075], there has been capability to do this.

We now allow for differing between-subject variance across lots (`repeated/group=group`), but importantly must use Satterthwaite's formulae (`DDFM=SATTERTH`) to derive the appropriate degrees of freedom using the following SAS code:

```
proc mixed data=trialf method=reml
ITDETAILS maxiter=200;
by serotype;
class group;
model lnigg=group/DDFM=SATTERTH;
repeated /group=group;
estimate 'L1-L2' group 1 -1 0/cl alpha=0.05;
estimate 'L1-L3' group 1 0 -1/cl alpha=0.05;
estimate 'L2-L3' group 0 1 -1/cl alpha=0.05;
ods output Estimates=test;
run;
```

The between-subject variance is is allowed to differ across lots. For serotype A, we observe that our estimates are

Covariance Parameter Estimates

Cov Parm	Group	Estimate
Residual	group 1	0.7835
Residual	group 2	0.7453
Residual	group 3	0.8094

Note that the average of these is 0.7794.

The test for a group effect still finds that at least one of the lots significantly differs from the others ($p = 0.0266$):

Type 3 Tests of Fixed Effects

Effect	Num DF	Den DF	F Value	Pr > F
group	2	393	3.66	0.0266

Note that the denominator degrees of freedom is changed.

Lot consistency was still demonstrated for serotype A, as the confidence intervals fall within the acceptance limits

Estimates

Label	Lower	Upper
L1-L2	-0.2950	0.04873
L1-L3	-0.06020	0.2907
L2-L3	0.06506	0.4117

The standard error differs between lot comparisons, as does the degrees of freedom:

```
 Estimates


                              Standard
Label      Estimate             Error        DF

L1-L2       -0.1231           0.08743       398
L1-L3        0.1152           0.08925       398
L2-L3        0.2384           0.08817       397
```

Interested readers may perform these analyses for serotypes B–D using the data and code on the website. Overall, from this analysis, we can conclude that these lots are consistent.

Alternative approaches to inference do exist. Wiens' [1335] approach to analysis is slightly different in that it tries to reduce the data across lots by the use of an order statistic. One derives the minimum of

$$\frac{\Delta - |\hat{\mu}_{Lj} - \hat{\mu}_{L'j}|}{SE_{Lj-L'j}}$$

across all lot $L \neq L'$ combinations and for all j endpoints and compares it to the $100(1-\frac{\alpha}{2})$ percentile of the normal distribution [918, Ch. 6.5.2].

However, the findings of [1314, Ch. 7] showed that such an order statistic turns out to be equivalent to the intersection-union test. Plus, as a practical matter, if one fails, one wants to know which lot and endpoint was at fault, so a global test isn't really useful, and one ends up doing the intersection-union test as a practical matter anyway.

The above example uses all available immunogenicity data. However, it is not unusual for protocol violations to occur in practice — for example, a subject might receive a prohibited vaccine in error during the study. Such subjects would be excluded from the per-protocol (sometimes known as evaluable) immunogenicity data prior to unblinding. For vaccines, usually, regulatory agencies require that the per-protocol data be the primary basis for inference [581]; however, they also in general want an all-available analysis done and any discrepancies (if any) brought to light. In contrast, for safety assessment, it is desired to err on the side of caution. This dataset would include anyone who receives at least one dose of a vaccine.

An additional caution is that the staff doing the assays for immunogenicity and safety assessments should be blinded to lot as a matter of good clinical practice. Documentation of any protocol violations and exclusions from per-protocol datasets should be in place prior to unblinding the trial. This applies as a general rule to all Phase II and III studies.

A reasonable question remains: how does one sample size a study for multiple comparisons across endpoints and across different lots? Under the IUT, an equation-based approach is available and will be illustrated using an example. For sample sizing, first assume there is one antibody ($j = 1$) to consider. For this one endpoint, where $\mu_L - \mu_{L'}$ can vary up to 0.3, we apply code as follows:

```
title "One Endpoint";run;
proc power;
twosamplemeans test=equiv_diff
alpha=0.025
lower=-0.6931 upper=0.6931
stddev=1.17
meandiff=0,0.3
power=0.8,0.9
npergroup=.
;run;
```

Here $\Delta = \ln(2)$, $\alpha = 0.05$ (so 95% confidence intervals are to constructed in analysis corresponding to each test of the TOST at 2.5%, $\sigma^2 = 1.38$ so $\sigma = \sqrt{1.38} = 1.17$ is the between-subject standard deviation assumed to be homogeneous across lots, and 80–90% power is desired.

Selected outputs look like

```
         Computed N Per Group

Mean      Nominal      Actual     N Per
Diff        Power       Power     Group

 0.0          0.8       0.801        61
 0.0          0.9       0.905        76
 0.3          0.8       0.803       141
 0.3          0.9       0.901       188
```

Lot $\mu_L - \mu_{L'}$ does not have to be precisely 0 to be equivalent, so it is safer to assume some sort of random differences in response will be observed when determining sample size, and 0.3 will be utilized in the following derivations. In this case, $n = 188$ per lot would be needed for the study to have at least 90% power for one of the lot-to-lot comparisons.

Using the formula from [918, p. 45], and noting that there are three lot-to-lot comparisons of interest,

$$Power \geq \sum_{L=1}^{3} P_j - (3-1) = 3(0.901) - 2 = 0.703$$

where P_j is the estimate of power for endpoint $j = 1$ in each of the three (correlated) lot-to-lot comparisons. Obviously, the overall power of the study should not be this low, so the individual comparisons' power must be adjusted upwards to compensate as follows:

```
title "One Endpoint";run;
proc power;
twosamplemeans test=equiv_diff
alpha=0.025
lower=-0.6931 upper=0.6931
stddev=1.17
meandiff=0.3
power=0.965
npergroup=.
;run;
```

Then, when increasing the desired power by $(0.90^{1/3} = 0.965$, SAS output (not shown) derives the estimated power as 0.966 with $n = 254$ per lot, and, accounting for the three lot-to-lot comparisons, the overall study power would be

$$Power \geq \sum_{L=1}^{3} P_j - (3-1) = 3(0.966) - 2 = 0.898.$$

Turning now to a more realistic situation, for six endpoints j = 1-6 where $\mu_L - \mu_{L'}$ can vary up to 0.3 and $\sigma^2_{j=1-6} = 0.74, 0.58, 0.56, 0.74, 0.73, 1.38$, we apply code as follows. The desired power 0.983 again is derived by taking the minimum desired overall power and dividing by the reciprocal of the number of endpoints (i.e., $0.9^{1/6} = 0.9826$).

```
title "J=6 Endpoints";run;
proc power;
twosamplemeans test=equiv_diff
alpha=0.025
lower=-0.6931 upper=0.6931
stddev=0.86,0.76,0.75,0.86,0.85,1.17
meandiff=0.3
power=0.9826
npergroup=.
;run;
```

First, we need to get in the right vicinity of the desired sample size for an individual lot-to-lot across these $j = 1$-6 multiple endpoints, and then we will account for the additional impact of additional lot-to-lot comparisons. It is seen that in the selected output below that $n = 295$ per lot are required for the most variable endpoint $j = 6$:

```
        Computed N Per Group


                Std      Actual     N Per
Index           Dev       Power     Group
    1          0.86       0.983       160
    2          0.76       0.983       125
    3          0.75       0.983       122
    4          0.86       0.983       160
    5          0.85       0.983       156
    6          1.17       0.983       295
```

The expected powers for all $j = 1$-6 endpoints at $n = 295$ per group are needed to perform an accurate overall power derivation for the study as follows:

```
title "J=6 Endpoints";run;
proc power;
twosamplemeans test=equiv_diff
alpha=0.025
lower=-0.6931 upper=0.6931
stddev=0.86,0.76,0.75,0.86,0.85,1.17
meandiff=0.3
power=.
npergroup=295
;run;
```

The estimates for power arising for each endpoint $j = 1$-6 are as follows.

```
   Computed Power
       Std
Index  Dev     Power
1      0.86    >.999
2      0.76    >.999
3      0.75    >.999
4      0.86    >.999
5      0.85    >.999
6      1.17    0.983
```

So, using the [918] approach above to derive overall power based upon $n = 295$ per lot, we find that, for an individual lot-to-lot comparison,

$$Power_L \geq \sum_{j=1}^{6} P_j - (6-1) = 5(0.999) + 0.983 - 5 = 0.978,$$

and as we have three lot-to-lot comparisons of interest to account for,

$$Power \geq \sum_{L=1}^{3} Power_L - (3-1) = 3(0.978) - 2 = 0.934.$$

As with bioequivalence studies, power should be constrained to be greater than 90% in lot consistency studies, as it is a show stopper (i.e., major review issue) if control of manufacturing is not demonstrated. Simulation (see Section 5.3) may easily be used to verify such power and sample size estimates, and we encourage interested readers to make use of the SAS code available on the website to do so. An example may be found in [770].

We now turn to a topic very much akin to drug-drug interaction studies (see Section 8.4). These are concomitant vaccination studies used to study whether vaccines can be administered at the same time.

12.5 Concomitant Vaccination

Vaccines are usually administered via injection, and going to a physician's office or a vaccine clinic requires time and resources. Generally, when one is vaccinated, one may receive more than one vaccine at a time to ensure protection as soon as possible for vulnerable populations. Recommended scheduling from the CDC (Centers for Disease Control and Prevention, USA) may be found in [16]. Other nations adapt such schedules to their own specific populations' needs.

For example, around the age of 1 year the CDC recommends that toddlers receive vaccinations for hepatitis B, haemophilus influenza type b, pneumococcal influenza, measles, mumps, rubella, varicella, hepatitis A, and meningitis! Obviously, one cannot and should not give all these vaccinations at once, and in practice, the schedule is staggered to ensure that the required number of vaccines and doses are administered over time. Before reasonable recommendations can be made, regulators must be shown data to give them confidence that giving vaccines together (for example, hepatitis A, pneumococcal, and varicella vaccines at age 1) do not interfere with each other in terms of priming the body's immune system to respond to a disease vector.

Registration and regulation of vaccines are done "locally." By local, we mean that a dossier is submitted to a particular regulatory agency for a particular nation (or set of nations, e.g., Europe). The local regulatory agency reviews and approves (or modifies or refuses) the application for access to market with respect to their specific population. As local regulators are involved, local requirements will come into play. For example, some regulatory agencies (e.g., Japan) require that vaccinations be given at separate visits unless a clinical trial has been done *in their population* to confirm "lack of interference." Others will accept foreign data.

Generally, regulators assume their population is not the same as others studied elsewhere, unless epidemiology has confirmed that the population response to disease and/or vaccine is similar enough to neglect. As this is rarely the case, clinical trials to confirm lack of interference when vaccines are given together (concomitantly) must be done locally. For example, if Japan's PMDA wants to confirm that a given new vaccine does not impact MMR (measles, mumps, and rubella) antibody generation, then the study must be done in Japanese toddlers.

In such studies, it is desired to confirm that giving vaccines together results in antibody levels for each vaccine that are the same as if each vaccine was given alone. Moreover, vaccines do have local and systemic side-effects, and it is desired to confirm that these are the same when given together versus separately. The same thing applies to the adverse event profile. Essentially, lack of interference corresponds to showing regulators that, in their population, the vaccines are safe and effective when used together.

These studies can be done in Phase II or Phase III. They may be done in Phase II to enable a pivotal study in Phase III in a particular region's population (by reducing the requirement that dosing of the new vaccine be done independently of any others in that region). If used in Phase III, they are used in tandem with pivotal studies to allow for local market access following approval, and in support of recommending bodies.

To be more specific, objectives for a concomitant vaccination study may be

1) To demonstrate that the immune responses induced by the influenza vaccine (or whatever the concomitant vaccine of interest) when administered concomitantly with the test vaccine (influenza+test) are equivalent to the immune responses induced by influenza vaccine alone.

2) To demonstrate that the immune responses induced by the test vaccine when administered concomitantly with the influenza vaccine (influenza+test) are equivalent to the immune responses induced by test vaccine alone.

Comparisons of interest are therefore influenza+test:influenza alone for influenza immune responses, and influenza+test:test alone for test vaccine immune responses. We use influenza vaccine here for the purpose of this example, but in principle, any of the many vaccines that are recommended could be used here.

Although not explicitly stated as a primary objective, as a practical matter it is the case that safety comparisons of interest are of important magnitude. Vaccines are generally given to healthy populations, and an unacceptable side-effect profile (e.g., fever, soreness) could result in practitioners not administering the vaccines together even if warranted by lack of interference. We have studied safety previously, however, and here will therefore confine our attention to the immune responses.

For the concomitant vaccine (e.g., influenza), there will generally be guidance on what level of continuous response is required for efficacy (either in the product's label or in regulatory guidance). For example, for influenza, one must look at the proportion of subjects achieving at least a 4-fold increase in the post-vaccination hemagglutination inhibition assay (HAI) titer (i.e., seroconversion) for each influenza virus subtype. As such levels are not generally defined at this stage for the test vaccine, one generally will use the geometric mean concentration (or titer as the case may be) to establish equivalence, as was done in the previous section to assess lot consistency.

The test and concomitant vaccines will not look alike. Therefore, there will be a need for a double dummy for both vaccines (i.e., a placebo). This makes the desired randomized arms of the study look like

Group 1: influenza vaccine + test vaccine.

Group 2: influenza vaccine (+ test placebo).

Group 3: (influenza placebo +) test vaccine.

TABLE 12.5
Schematic Plan of a Concomitant Vaccination Study

Group	Period 1	Period 2
1	F+T	FP+TP
2	F+TP	FP+T
3	FP+T	F+TP
F: influenza vaccine; FP: placebo for influenza T: test vaccine; TP: placebo for test		

Note that group 3 will need to have an influenza catch-up when the subjects come in to get their post-vaccination blood samples (one can't leave people unprotected from the influenza). See Table 12.5. This means for the purpose of blinding one must give an influenza "shot" and a "test" shot in each period.

Periods 1 and 2 are generally separated by one month to allow for immunogenicity blood sampling just prior to the period 2 vaccinations to study the responses to the vaccines given in period 1. The time between is not a wash-out period in the traditional sense as discussed previously but is intended to be sufficient time to ensure the body mounts the desired immune response to vaccination. A blood sample is collected prior to vaccination in each study period to define baseline response (period 1) and post-vaccination 1 response (e.g., for 4-fold endpoints) prior to vaccination in period 2. A blood sample is not taken following vaccinations in period 2, as within-subject comparisons are not of interest.

This is referred to as a randomized, double blind, double dummy cross-over design. Note that period 2 for group 2 is the same as period 1 for group 3. One may be tempted to economize and measure the test immune response in group 2 following vaccination in period 2, but it is important to beware of carry-over effects (and period effects and direct by carry-over interaction). Use of such a reduced design is only appropriate if period and carry-over effects can be assumed to be negligible.

Sample size need not be equal between groups 1, 2, and 3 as we will see later. Indeed, given what we know about dichotomizing data, it will not come as surprise that group 1 and 2 need to be larger than group 3 in general. However, inclusion and exclusion criteria must be uniformly applied, and personnel doing the assays for the influenza and the test vaccine immune responses should be blinded to group to ensure no bias is introduced.

In general, immune responses to test placebo (TP) and to influenza placebo (FP) are not of interest (as both will generally be below the limit of quantification for the assays involved). Equivalence is of interest in both settings, and we return to the TOST for inference.

We will refer to the acceptance region for the concomitant vaccine as $\mp\Theta$. Recall that the data for the concomitant vaccine will in general be dichotomized $(0,1)$ where 0 denotes a non-response (in the context of influenza, a less than 4-fold increase in titer from baseline) and 1 denotes a response (e.g., for influenza, a 4-fold increase in titer from baseline). The number of responses in a given group i are binomial distributed, with p_i being the unknown parameter of interest (estimated as r_i/n_i in each group where r_i is the number of responding subjects and n_i is the number of subjects from group $i = 1 - 2$).

The interest is then to test for equivalence in the proportion of responders.

$$H_{01}: \quad p_{1j} - p_{2j} \leq -\Theta_j \tag{12.5}$$

versus the alternative

$$H_{11}: \quad p_{1j} - p_{2j} > -\Theta_j$$

OR

$$H_{02}: \quad p_{1j} - p_{2j} \geq \Theta_j \tag{12.6}$$

versus the alternative

$$H_{12}: \quad p_{1j} - p_{2j} < \Theta_j$$

for each response variable j in groups 1 and 2. Θ may be made specific to endpoint j (e.g., different criteria for different vaccine responses to combination vaccines like Tdap or MMR). In our case, for influenza, regulators require $\Theta_j = 0.1$ for each of the 4-fold HAI responses (j = 1-3). As equivalence must be shown for all j responses, Type 1 error is controlled conservatively by the intersection-union testing procedure as discussed in Section 4.7.

A formula for deriving the sample size per group for independent proportions is given in Formula 12.12 of [666]. Input parameters are α, β, Θ, and expected values of p_1 and p_2. Here we desire $\alpha = 0.05$, $\beta = 0.03$, $\Theta = 0.1$, and expected values of $p_1 = 0.5$ and $p_2 = 0.5$. Resulting sample size is n = 853 per group (in groups 1 and 2) using the following SAS code. Note that power $1 - \beta = 1 - 0.03 = 0.97$ is adjusted upwards as the influenza vaccine generates three (or more) types of antibodies to provide overall study-wise power of at least 90% (i.e., $0.97^3 > 0.90$).

```
data julious_2009;
*formula 12.12 for 3 independent antibodies;
power=0.97;beta=1-power;b_2=1-(beta/2);
alpha=0.05;a_2=1-(alpha/2);
z_a=quantile('NORMAL',a_2);
z_b=quantile('NORMAL',b_2);
p_1=0.5;p_2=0.5;p_avg=(p_1+p_2)/2;
s_1=(p_1*(1-p_1))+(p_2*(1-p_2));
part1=z_a*(sqrt(s_1));
s_2=2*p_avg*(1-p_avg);
part2=z_b*(sqrt(s_2));
num=(part1+part2)**2;
theta=0.1;den=theta**2;npergroup=num/den;
run;
```

Recall that we needed n = 251 per group for the test vaccine (see the previous section), so group 3 need only have that number of subjects. However, as shown, for influenza we need n = 853 per group, and groups 1 and 2 need to be larger. It is fine to use unequal sample sizes in study design, e.g., a 3:3:1 ratio for groups 1:2:3, respectively. This should be specified in the protocol, and if lab procedures for assay are adapted accordingly (not recommended), special care must be taken to ensure the blind is maintained.

Using the data of this design, 4-fold responder and non-responder influenza data in groups 1 and 2 are given in Table 12.6.

An exact procedure to derive a confidence interval $p_1 - p_2$ should be specified in the protocol in practice; here we will apply the Chan and Zhang approach [154] discussed previously in this chapter. Interested readers may use the code given earlier in this chapter to verify that equivalence may be concluded for HAI1, HAI2, and HAI3, as the 95% confidence intervals for $\hat{p}_1 - \hat{p}_2$ for all endpoints fall within the interval -0.10, 0.10. Note that a statistically significant decrease was observed for HAI2, but this is not unexpected given the sample size involved. As in bioequivalence testing, equivalence may be demonstrated even if a statistically significant difference is observed provided the confidence limits fall within the acceptance interval.

TABLE 12.6
Data from a Concomitant Influenza Vaccination Study

Group	Type	Responder	Non-Responder	N
1	HAI1	436	417	853
2	HAI1	428	425	853
1	HAI2	504	349	853
2	HAI2	549	304	853
1	HAI3	685	168	853
2	HAI3	687	166	853
1: influenza vax + test vax 2: influenza vax + test placebo				

Comparisons of geometric means were described in the previous section. Here we will simply note the findings from comparison of groups 1 to 3 on the ln-transformed scale for each of four serotypes (A–D). The estimates, and lower and upper findings denote the difference between groups 1 and 3 on the ln-scale and the corresponding lower and upper 95% confidence bounds, respectively. Equivalence may not be concluded for serotype C based upon an acceptance range of $\Delta = \mp 0.6931$. The point estimate and lower confidence bound for serotype C fell below the acceptance boundary.

serotype	Estimate	Lower	Upper	Probt
A	-0.2404	-0.4073	-0.0736	0.0048
B	0.1244	-0.0307	0.2795	0.1157
C	-0.7321	-0.8838	-0.5804	<.0001
D	-0.0030	-0.1744	0.1685	0.9729

While equivalence was demonstrated for the test vaccine when given concomitantly with influenza vaccine for the influenza vaccine responses, it appears administration of influenza vaccine decreases the test vaccine antibody response to serotype C when given concomitantly. Depending on how important serotype C is, the label for the test product may designate that these vaccines should not be given together. If this was an enabling study for Phase III, in all likelihood they would not be given together, as the sponsor will not be interested in diminishing the effect of the test vaccine in the pivotal trials needed for registration. That approach would likely carry into the label if the vaccine is approved thereafter for marketing.

12.6 Cross-Over Trials in Vaccines

As discussed in earlier chapters, in a cross-over study, subjects are randomized to a sequence of treatments over time, with repeated measurements being taken after each treatment. The benefits of within-subject estimation of treatment effects are well known [652, 1113] but may be underutilized in some settings due to the presence of carry-over effects. That is, the effect of a prior treatment remains with the subject while evaluating the effect of a subsequent treatment.

TABLE 12.7
Schematic Plan of a Balaam Design Cross-Over Study

Sequence Group	Period			Number of Subjects
	1	Washout	2	
1(AA)	A	—	A	n_1
2(AB)	A	—	B	n_2
3(BA)	B	—	A	n_3
4(BB)	B	—	B	n_4
A=Regimen 1, B=Regimen 2				

These carry-over effects are typically regarded as nuisances (see Chapter 5), and cross-over designs have been developed to ensure treatment effects are not confounded with carry-over effects [652] among other parameters. However, the potential for differential carry-over effects complicates design, and in some instances has led to recommendations to use simpler (parallel group) designs in biopharmaceutical development (see, for example, [621], [735]) when a washout period [1102] cannot be used to confirm the assumption that carry-over effects are negligible relative to treatment effects.

A Balaam design [652] is one example of a design developed to ensure carry-over effects are not confounded with treatment and period effects. In such a design subjects are randomized to one of four sequences of treatment administration. We will denote these sequences as AA, AB, BA, and BB (see Table 12.7) where A denotes one treatment and B the other. The administration of each treatment is separated by a wash-out period appropriate to the products under study. While within-subject estimates of treatment effect are only possible in the AB and BA sequences, the application of the AA and BB sequences serve to allow for the estimation of carry-over effects in combination with treatment and period effects.

The value of Balaam's design rests on the assumption that there is no carry-over-by-treatment interaction, i.e., that carry-over from the first administration of A and from B in the AA and BB sequences is the same as in the change-over sequences [652].

For vaccines, such cross-over studies may be done to identify the potential for "boosting" immune response, identifying opportune time of re-vaccination, and/or for the identification of potential alternative dosing regimens (when multiple vaccines of differing mechanism and/or coverage are available) among other reasons. Carry-over for vaccines (and in such designs) is obviously not only assumed but is also desired. As such, application of cross-over designs is infrequent but not unknown (e.g., [125]).

An in-depth discussion of the mechanisms of vaccine carry-over effects is beyond the scope of this section. We recommend the reader consult [686] and [918] for an introduction to these topics. For our purposes here, it should be recognized that carry-over from a vaccine can result from multiple mechanisms — e.g., antibody may remain in the body for an extended period of time and/or elements within the body's immune system may be primed to recognize and mount an immune response to antigens even if limited or no circulating antibody remains present, or both.

Mean natural-logarithm (ln) transformed antibody titer data from such a Balaam design are plotted for six antibody types in Figure 12.2. Pre-vaccination and post-vaccination blood samples were obtained in this design in both study periods. Antibody titer data were combined across two randomized, double blind, clinical studies in the same nation with identical inclusion and exclusion criteria (healthy subjects aged 60–64 years at time of first

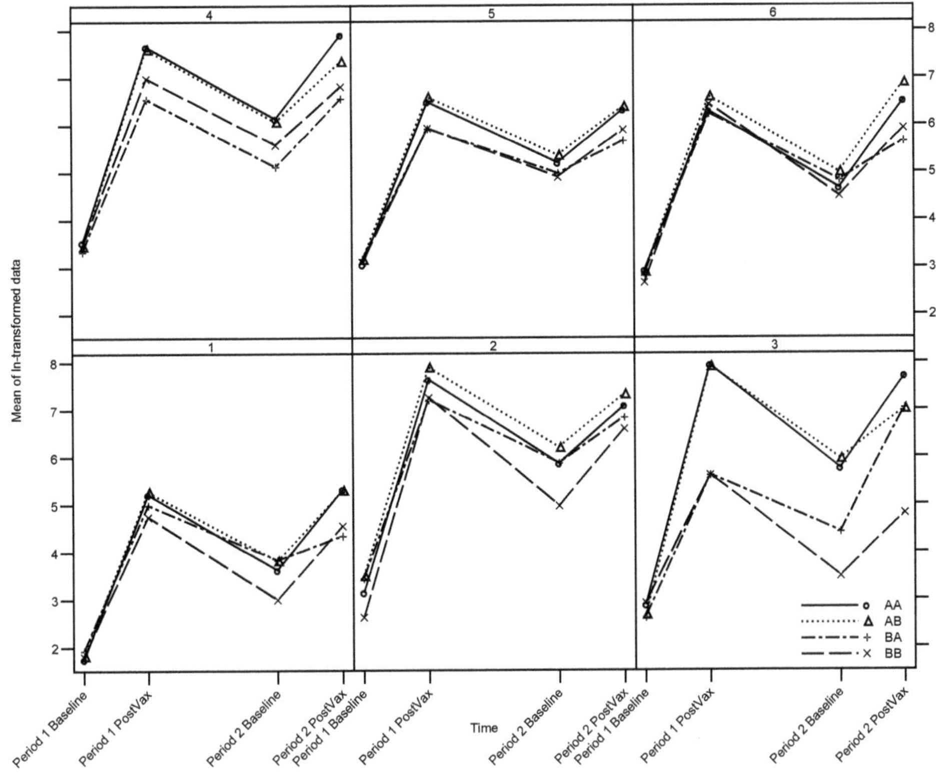

FIGURE 12.2
Mean ln-Transformed Titer Data by Vaccine Sequence versus Time Matrix Plot for Antibody Types 1–6 for Periods 1 and 2, prior to and 1 Month following Vaccination

vaccination), controls (e.g., allowance for concomitant vaccination, assays), and vaccination/sampling schedules and materials. Time between vaccinations varied by a minimum of one to a maximum of four years across the studies. The total sample size was $n = 1113$ subjects ($n = 284$ for sequence AA, $n = 404$ for sequence AB, $n = 236$ for sequence BA, $n = 189$ for sequence BB). The time between vaccinations is referred to as a wash-out, and, as a practical matter, a lengthy time period is generally used between such vaccinations to ensure an appropriate immune response is provoked by the body and can be provoked in subsequent vaccinations. Also, as a practical matter, vaccinations in adults typically can occur at roughly one year intervals as a maximum (i.e., when undertaking an annual physical exam).

In practice, estimates and confidence intervals from analysis on the ln-transformed scale are typically exponentiated (back-transformed) to describe the data (or to test for non-inferiority, super-efficacy, etc.) We focus on the statistics here and neglect such alternative presentations without loss of generality. All results in this section are presented on the ln-scale.

A traditional vaccine statistical analysis of such continuous repeated measures, cross-over data is described in [918]. In brief, comparisons are first constructed between regimens by period to compare vaccine response following each vaccination. See Table 12.8. The vaccines (A and B) are compared directly in the first period (A-B) following vaccination and thereafter between sequences following repeated vaccinations.

TABLE 12.8
Example: Traditional Analysis of Differences in Mean ln-Titer between Vaccine Groups and Following Sequences of Dosing from a Cross-Over Vaccine Trial

Type	A-B Period 1 (p-value)	AA-BA Period 2 (p-value)	AA-BB Period 2 (p-value)
1	0.37(0.0006)	0.98(<0.0001)	0.77(<0.0001)
2	0.56(<0.0001)	0.25(0.0997)	0.49(0.0014)
3	2.31(<0.0001)	0.67(0.0005)	2.90(<0.0001)
4	0.88(<0.0001)	1.34(<0.0001)	1.08(<0.0001)
5	0.62(<0.0001)	0.65(<0.0001)	0.42(0.0015)
6	0.15(0.2367)	0.85(<0.0001)	0.58(0.0004)
A: New Vaccine; B: Original Vaccine			
H_0: Mean Difference between Groups (or Sequence) = 0			
Period 2 Comps. AA-AB, BA-BB, etc. on File			

Two of the potential comparisons of interest in period 2 between sequences are given in Table 12.8 to conserve space. In the period 2 assessments, carry-over is assumed to exist, but it is not estimated. The comparisons by period are not confounded with period effects (as analysis is within period); however, the analysis of period 2 data is confounded in that treatment and carry-over are both involved in the resulting estimates across sequences.

The traditional analysis becomes more complex thereafter. In general practice [918], period 2 data are compared to period 1 data, and comparisons of interest are constructed between sequences. Period effects [652] are assumed to be null (by default) in such an analysis. This is a strong assumption, and, as we will see, it is problematic when period effects are directly estimated later in this report. See Table 12.9. Carry-over and treatment remain confounded when comparing sequences of vaccine administration in this assessment.

Finally, in part to attempt to account for carry-over, pre-vaccination titers may be taken into account. See Table 12.10. Pre-vaccination ln-titers were subtracted from post-vaccination in each study period and then compared across periods between sequences.

TABLE 12.9
Example: Traditional Analysis of Period 2-1 ln-Titer Following Sequences of Dosing from a Cross-Over Vaccine Trial

Type	AA-BA Period 2-1 (p-value)	AA-BB Period 2-1 (p-value)
1	0.87(<0.0001)	0.31(0.0257)
2	-0.06(0.6658)	0.20(0.1721)
3	-1.31(<0.0001)	0.62(0.0005)
4	0.29(0.0574)	0.43(0.0053)
5	0.26(0.0186)	-0.03(0.8036)
6	0.85(<0.0001)	0.66(<0.0001)
A: New Vaccine; B: Original Vaccine		
H_0: Mean Difference between Sequences = 0		
Period 2-1 Comps. AA-AB, BA-BB, etc. on File		

TABLE 12.10
Example: Traditional Analysis of Pre-Vaccination Adjusted Differences in Period 2-1 for ln-Titer between Sequences of Dosing from a Cross-Over Vaccine Trial

Type	AA-BA (p-value)	AA-BB (p-value)
1	0.81(0.0008)	-0.36(0.1410)
2	-0.38(0.2891)	-0.41(0.2852)
3	-2.74(<0.0001)	-1.66(<0.0001)
4	-0.68(0.0516)	-0.38(0.2872)
5	-0.16(0.5039)	-0.47(0.0490)
6	1.27(0.0001)	0.66(0.0492)
A: New Vaccine; B: Original Vaccine		
H_0: Mean Difference between Ratios across Periods between Sequences = 0		
Period 2-1 Comps. AA-AB, BA-BB, etc. on File		

Beyond the overly complex nature of interpretation of such multiple data analyses, these approaches highlight the need for analysis of such data accounting properly for period and carry-over effects for a quantitative understanding of the characteristics of each vaccine and repeated administration. A modelling approach based on [652] will now be described for this purpose.

The model chosen for application here for each type of ln-titer y_{ijk}, separately, is derived from [652] and is

$$y_{ijk} = \mu_{d[i,j]} + \pi_j + \lambda_{d[i,1]} + \xi_{k(i)} + \varepsilon_{ijk}, \tag{12.7}$$

where $d[i,j] = R$ or T and identifies the vaccine in period (π_j, $j = 1-2$) with potential carry-over $\lambda_{d,1} = \lambda_A$ or λ_B from period 1. We assume that $\xi_{k(i)}$ and ε_{ijk} are independent random variables such that $\mathrm{E}(\xi_{k(i)}) = 0$, $Var(\xi_{k(i)}) = \sigma_B^2$, $\mathrm{E}(\varepsilon_{ijk}) = 0$ and $Var(\varepsilon_{ijk}) = \sigma_W^2$, where σ_B^2 is the between-subject variance and σ_W^2 is the within-subject variance. E denotes the expected value (i.e., population mean) for a given parameter, and Var denotes its variance. We also assume that the $\xi_{k(i)}$ are independent among themselves and that the ε_{ijk} are independent among themselves. SAS code is given in [652] and is not reproduced here.

The p-values in Table 12.11 denote the tests of model parameters for treatment effects $\mu_A = \mu_B$, carry-over effects $\lambda_A = \lambda_B$, and period effects $\pi_1 = \pi_2$ in columns 2 through 4, respectively. The estimates of effect correspond to $\mu_A - \mu_B$, $\lambda_A - \lambda_B$, $\pi_1 - \pi_2$ in columns 2 through 4, respectively.

Additional models may be easily explored. For example, baseline may be added as a period-specific covariate following the principles described in [691, Section 4.2] with SAS code given in the appendix to said paper, and we discuss the application of such a model later in this section.

At best, the traditional analysis findings of Tables 12.8–12.10 should be regarded as a supplement to Figure 12.2 and permits additional qualitative assessments. One could conclude from the plot (and Tables 12.8 and 12.9) that vaccine A provides a similar or greater response relative to vaccine B for some of these endpoints (types 1–6). Administration of vaccine A prior to vaccine B results in a higher response whether one gives vaccine A or B in the second period. Finally, administration of sequence AA results in higher average ln-titer relative to BB for all types. The magnitude of treatment effects relative to carry-over effects

TABLE 12.11
Example: Model-Based Cross-Over and Carry-Over Analysis of ln-Titer from a Cross-Over Vaccine Trial

Type	Vaccine A-B (*p*-value)	Carry-over A-B (*p*-value)	Period 1-2 (*p*-value)
1	-0.08(0.2182)	0.69(<0.0001)	-0.12(0.0599)
2	0.24(0.0003)	0.39(0.0001)	0.34(<0.0001)
3	1.70(<0.0001)	1.19(<0.0001)	-0.45(<0.0001)
4	0.51(<0.0001)	0.72(<0.0001)	-0.27(0.0002)
5	0.17(0.0016)	0.33(<0.0001)	0.00(0.9841)
6	-0.05(0.4724)	0.83(<0.0001)	-0.30(<0.0001)
A: New Vaccine; B: Original Vaccine			

is unclear, and no potential for other confounders is taken into direct account (unless an observer is very astute).

Inspection of pre-vaccination average ln-titers in Figure 12.2 is sufficient to suggest that a carry-over effect is present and differentiable between vaccines (as is indeed desired).

The findings of Table 12.9 are very challenging to interpret in this context. Reference to Figure 12.2 aids somewhat in interpretation. When vaccine B is administered in period 1, average ln-titers return closer to basal levels prior to vaccination in period 2. This results in a larger baseline subtracted value in period 2 if vaccine B was given first in period 1. As a generalization, then, once one is vaccinated with vaccine A, ln-titers are maintained higher, and there is therefore less "boosting" with a subsequent dose of either vaccine due to greater carry-over.

Assessments of significance in Tables 12.8–12.10 may therefore be misleading, as the *p*-values are confounded between multiple effects (treatment, period, and carry-over.) They serve to indicate that something statistically significant is happening, but an accurate and precise analysis is needed to pick out which are the key contributing factors for a given comparison of interest.

The traditional approach is admittedly quite complex. However, more importantly, it is non-quantitative with respect to the effects of interest in such a design space. That is, treatment, period, sequence, and carry-over effects are in part confounded in these analyses unless strong assumptions are made regarding period effects in particular. The assumption of null period effects is quite unsafe — if for no other reason than findings from other therapy areas [1089].

Period effects should be expected in such vaccine trials due to the duration of wash-out, in combination with other factors, making an assumption of null unlikely. This is not surprising if considered carefully. As is well known, immunity among populations varies over time naturally and in response to outbreaks of disease. Moreover, when a significant part of a population is vaccinated, herd immunity may develop. Additionally, changes will likely be made to an assay over the course of years (e.g., reagents must be changed upon expiration or when amounts run out). It would also be surprising if clinical conditions could be maintained with an exactness necessary to nullify period effects (e.g., staff changes are to be expected over the years of such vaccine trials). If nothing else, the shipping company taking blood samples to the lab may change between period 1 and 2 (with potentially different storage conditions). All such potential factors may of themselves contribute to a period effect. Therefore, vaccine cross-over designs should expect and protect against their occurrence by design.

The need for a model-based approach such as [652] seems justified given the complex, confounded findings of traditional analysis. In this example, it is found that a single model can supply all of the information required by multiple analyses of the same dataset. This is true, however, if and only if one is willing to set up the experimental conditions to permit it. If one were not permitted to administer the BB sequence, for example, due to ethical concerns with re-administration of the B vaccine, then a proper quantitative understanding of such data is not possible.

Conclusions with regard to the effect of vaccination with A-B are altered when accounting for period effects and carry-over. Type 1 changes from statistically significant to non-significant for comparison of treatment effects of vaccine A to B. This is probably real given the more accurate and precise nature of the within-subject comparison. This finding is not of concern, as the effect is still non-inferior relative to vaccine B (data on file).

Notably, period effects were significant for all types except for 1 and 5. The magnitude relative to traditional estimates of A-B from period 1 are interesting. With the exception of type 5, the absolute effect appears to be quite a percentage of the traditional estimate of the treatment effect (see Table 12.8).

Carry-over is significant across all types 1–6 and supports that dosing with Vaccine A results in benefit in terms of higher maintenance of ln-titers over time for these endpoints.

Baseline-adjusted model-based assessment (as described in [691]) improves the precision of the model but does not change any of the fundamental conclusions as regards treatment, period, and carry-over effects (data on file).

In summary, the purpose of this section was to give an example of a model-based approach to see whether it resulted in findings which represented an improvement over the traditional method(s). A "simple" [1102] approach to carry-over was adopted to assess whether this was possible and, if so, whether value was added by taking such an approach. More precise methods are available [1106]. While such carry-over models have been the subject of debate in the study of drugs, we are not aware of previous quantitative comparative reports in the area of vaccines using a Balaam design. Especially in a therapy area like vaccines, where wash-out may not be physiologically possible given priming of the body's immune system, we deem it important to account where possible for an effect like carry-over, even if the approach taken is not precisely consistent with the body's processes and mechanisms involved in generating immune responses.

As a practical matter, therefore, period effects should be expected in vaccine cross-over trials and estimated in analysis. Carry-over effects also should be accounted for in design and in modelling of vaccine cross-over data by default, in some manner, as they are desired and expected. It should be noted that the simple model applied in this section should not be regarded as adequate in all such situations. It is a starting point to understanding such data, in combination with the pre-vaccination titers, and should be viewed as useful for developing a quantitative understanding of the data.

13

Epilogue

Final Words

Many people in business and medicine regard statistics as at best a nuisance, or as a challenging (frequently incomprehensible) and therefore best ignored subject (whenever possible), or at worst as an hinderance to science. Even Einstein liked to say that "God doesn't gamble." [133].

In the short term while making biopharmaceuticals, we cannot operate with complete certainty and have to depend upon statistics as a guide to making safe, effective, quality products. In clinical biopharmaceutical development, statistics are used to quantify and manage the uncertainties associated with human use of biopharmaceuticals — not to eliminate uncertainty. If statistics are not used well, the trend toward increased length and cost in biopharmaceutical development [377] will continue.

Clinical pharmacology and many aspects of biopharmaceutical development are evolving, and will continue to do so. These changes are good, as they would be expected to improve the biopharmaceuticals that are produced for the people who need them. Changes in medicine and science such as these represent new challenges for statisticians, but the raw materials to meet the needs of the science are available. Change is not so bad once one gets used to it. The same can be said of statistics.

We hope that our readers have found this second edition useful as a starting point for making some of the concepts associated with statistics in clinical pharmacology more transparent. To conclude this work, we wish all our past, present, and future readers good luck with their research.

Part V

Bibliography

Bibliography

[1] Aarons, L., Karlsson, M., Mentre, F., Rombout, F., Steimer, J.-L., van Peer, A., and Invited COST B15 Experts (2001) The role of modelling and simulation in phase I drug development. *European Journal of Pharmaceutical Sciences*, **13**, 115–122.

[2] Abdel-Rahman, S., Reed, M., Wells, T., Kearns, G. (2007) Considerations in the rationale design and conduct of Phase 1-2 pediatric clinical trials: Avoiding the problems and pitfalls. *Clinical Pharmacology and Therapeutics*, **81**, 483–494.

[3] Agnelli, G., Prandoni, P., Becattini, C., Silingardi, M., Taliani, M., Miccio, M., Imberti, D., Poggio, R., Ageno, W., Pogliani, E., Porro, F., Zonzin, P. for the Warfarin Optimal Duration Italian Trial Investigators (WODIT-PE) (2003) Extended oral anti-coagulant therapy after a first episode of pulmonary embolism. *Annals of Internal Medicine*, **139**, 19–26.

[4] Ahr, G., Voith, B., Kuhlmann, J. (2000) Guidances related to bioavailability and bioequivalence: European perspective. *European Journal of Drug Metabolism and Pharmacokinetics*, **25**, 25–27.

[5] Akaike, H. (1973) Information theory and an extension of the maximum likelihood principle. *Second International Symposium on Information Theory*, 267–281.

[6] Akritas, M., Bershady, M. (1996) Linear regression for astronomical data with measurement errors and intrinsic scatter. *The Astrophysical Journal*, **470**, 706–714.

[7] Albert J., Ioannidid, J., Reichelderfer, P., Conway, B., Coombs, R., Crane, L., DeMasi, R., Dixon, D., Flandre, P., Hughes, M., Kalish, L., Larntz, K., Lin, D., Marschner, I., Munoz, A., Murray, J., Neaton, J., Pettinelli, C., Rida, W., Taylor, J., Welles, S. (1998) Statistical issues for HIV surrogate endpoints: point/counterpoint. *Statistics in Medicine*, **17**, 2435–2462.

[8] Alberti, K., Zimmet, P., Shaw, J. for the IDF Epidemiology Task Force Consensus Group (2005) The metabolic syndrome — A new worldwide definition. *The Lancet*, **366**, 1059–1062.

[9] Ali, M., Talukder, E. (2005) Analysis of longitudinal binary data with missing data due to dropouts. *Journal of Biopharmaceutical Statistics*, **15**, 993–1007.

[10] Al-Marzouki, S., Roberts, I., Marshall, T., Evans, S. (2005). The effect of scientific misconduct on the results of clinical trials: A Delphi survey. *Contemporary Clinical Trials*, **26**, 331–337.

[11] Alonso, A., Molenberghs, G. (2007) Surrogate marker evaluation from an information theory perspective. *Biometrics*, **63**, 180–186.

[12] Al-Sallami, H.S., Kumar, V.V.P., Landersdorfer, C.B., Bulitta, J.B., Duffull, S.B. (2009) The time course of drug effects. *Pharmaceutical Statistics*, **8**, 176–185.

[13] Altman, D.G., Bland, J.M. (1983) Measurement in medicine: The analysis of method comparison studies. *The Statistician*, **32**, 307–317.

[14] Altman, D.G., Bland, J.M. (1995) Absence of evidence is not evidence of absence. *British Medical Journal*, **311**, 485.

[15] Amankwa, A., Krishnan, S., Tisdale, J. (2004) Torsades de pointes associated with fluoroquinilones: Importance of concommitant risk factors. *Clinical Pharmacology and Therapeutics*, **75(3)**, 242–247.

[16] American College of Immunization Practice. (2012) http://www.cdc.gov/vaccines/recs/acip.

[17] Amoros, J. (2014) Recapturing Laplace. *Significance*, **July 2014**, 38–39.

[18] Anderson, K.C., Pazdur, R., Farrell, A.T. (2005) Development of effective new treatments for multiple myeloma. *Journal of Clinical Oncology*, **23, No. 28**, 1–5.

[19] Anderson, S. (1993) Individual bioequivalence: A problem of switchability [with discussion]. *Biopharmaceutical Reports*, **2**, 1–11.

[20] Anderson, S. (1995) Current issues in individual bioequivalence. *Drug Information Journal*, **29**, 961–964.

[21] Anderson, S., Hauck W.W. (1983) A new procedure for testing equivalence in comparative bioavailability and other clinical trials. *Communications in Statistical Theory and Methods*, **12**, 2663–2692.

[22] Anderson, S., Hauck W.W. (1990) Consideration of individual bioequivalence. *Journal of Pharmacokinetics and Biopharmaceutics*, **18**, 259–273.

[23] Anderson, S., Hauck W.W. (1996) The transitivity of bioequivalence testing: Potential for drift. *International Journal of Clinical Pharmacology and Therapeutics*, **34**, 369–374.

[24] Ando, Y., Uyama, Y. (2012) Multiregional clinical trials: Japanese perspective on drug development strategy and sample size for Japanese subjects. *Journal of Biopharmaceutical Sciences*, **22**, 977–987.

[25] Ansbacher, R. (1990) Interchangeability of low dose oral contraceptives. *Contraception*, **43**, 139–147.

[26] Antithrombotic Trialists' Collaboration (2002) Collaborative meta-analysis of randomised trials of anti-platelet therapy for prevention of death, myocardial infarction, and stroke in high risk patients. *British Medical Journal*, **324**, 71–86.

[27] Antman, E. (2001) Clinical trials in cardiovascular medicine. *Circulation*, **103**, e101–e104.

[28] Aoyagi, N. (2000) Japanese guidance on bioavailability and bioequivalence. *European Journal of Drug Metabolism and Pharmacokinetics*, **25, No. 1**, 28–31.

[29] Aregay, M., Shkedy, Z., Molenberghs, G., David, M.-P., Tibaldi, F. (2013) Model-based estimates of long-term persistence of induced HPV antibodies: A flexible subject-specific approach. *Journal of Biopharmaceutical Statistics*, **23**, 1228–1248.

[30] Atkinson, A., Daniels, C., Dedrick, R., Grudzinskas, C., Markey, S., eds. (2001) *Principles of Clinical Pharmacology.* Academic Press, San Diego.

[31] Atkinson, A., Lalonde, R. (2007) Introduction to quantitative methods in pharmacology and clinical pharmacology: An historical perspective. *Clinical Pharmacology and Therapeutics*, **82**, 3–6.

[32] Aurenen, K., Arjas, E., Leino, T., Takala, A. (2000) Transmission of pneumococcal carriage in families: A latent Markov process model for binary longitudinal data. *Journal of the American Statistical Association*, **95**, 1044–1053.

[33] Australia Therapeutic Goods Administration, Australian Regulatory Guidelines for Prescription Medicines (2002) Appendix 15, Biopharmaceutical Studies.

[34] Awad, A. (2012) Application of information theory to bio-equivalence problem. *Journal of Bioequivalence and Bioavailability*, **4**, 10–13.

[35] Baker, S. (2006) A simple meta-analytic approach for using a binary surrogate endpoint to predict the effect of intervention on a true endpoint. *Biostatistics*, **7**, 58–70.

[36] Balakrishnan, N., Ma, C.W. (1990) A comparative study of various tests for the equality of two population variances. *Journal of Statistical Computing and Simulation*, **35**, 41–89.

[37] Balthasar, J.P. (1999) Bioequivalence and bioequivalency testing. *American Journal of Pharmaceutical Education*, **63**, 194–198.

[38] Bang, H., Jung, S., George, S. (2005) Sample size calculation for simulation-based multiple testing procedures. *Journal of Biopharmaceutical Statistics*, **15**, 957–967.

[39] Barbieri, M.M., Liseo, B., Petrella, L. (2000) Bayes factors for Fieller's problem. *Biometrika*, **87**, 717–723.

[40] Barrett, J.S., Batra, V., Chow, A., Cook, J., Gould, A.L., Heller, A., Lo, M.-W., Patterson, S.D., Smith, B.P., Stritar, J.A., Vega, J.M., Zariffa, N. (2000) PhRMA perspective on population and individual bioequivalence and update to the PhRMA perspective on population and individual bioequivalence. *Journal of Clinical Pharmacology*, **40**, 561–572.

[41] Barthel, F., Babiker, A., Royston, P., Parmar, M. (2006) Evaluation of sample size and power for multi-arm survival trials allowing for non-uniform accrual, non-proportional hazards, loss to follow-up, and cross-over. *Statistics in Medicine*, **25**, 2521–2542.

[42] Bartlett, M.S. (1936) Properties of sufficiency and statistical tests. *Proceedings of the Royal Statistical Society, Series A*, **154**, 124–137.

[43] Basson, R.P., Ghosh, A., Cerimele, B.J., DeSante, K.A., Howey, D.C. (1998) Why rate of absorption inferences in single dose bioequivalence studies are often inappropriate. *Pharmaceutical Research*, **15**, 276–279.

[44] Bate, S., Jones, B. (2002) The construction of universally optimal uniform cross-over designs. *GSK BDS Technical Report*, **2002-06**, 1–42.

[45] Bauchner, H. (2013) Editorial changes for clinical trials and the continued changes in medical journalism. *Journal of the American Medical Association*, E1–E2.

[46] Bauer, P. (1989) Multistage testing with adaptive designs. *Biometric und Informatik in Medizin und Biologie*, **20**, 130–148.

[47] Bauer, P. (1991) Multiple testing in clinical trials. *Statistics in Medicine*, **10**, 871–890.

[48] Bauer, P., Bauer, M.M. (1994) Testing equivalence simultaneously for location and dispersion of two normally distributed populations. *Biometrical Journal*, **6**, 643–660.

[49] Bauer, P., Kieser, M. (1996) A unifying approach for confidence intervals and testing of equivalence and difference. *Biometrika*, **83**, 934–937.

[50] Bauer, P., Rohmel, J., Maurer, W., Hothorn, L. (1998) Testing strategies in multi-dose experiments including active control. *Statistics in Medicine*, **17**, 2133–2146.

[51] Bauer, P., Koenig, F. (2006) The reassessment of trial perspectives from interim data — A critical view. *Statistics in Medicine*, **25**, 23–36.

[52] Bauer, R., Guzy, S., Ng, C. (2007) A survey of population analysis methods and software for complex pharmacokinetic and pharmacodynamic models with examples. *The AAPS Journal*, **9**, E60–E83.

[53] Bayes de Lunda, A., Guindo, J., Borja, J., Roman, M., Madoery, C. (1990) Recasting the approach to the treatment of potentially malignant ventricular arrythmias after the CAST study. *Cardiovascular Drugs and Therapy*, **4**, 651–656.

[54] Bazett, H. (1920) An analysis of time relations of electrocardiograms. *Hcart*, **7**, 353–367.

[55] Bekersky, I., Dressler, D., Colburn, W., Mekki, Q. (1999) Bioequivalence of 1 and 5 mg Tacrolimus capsules using a replicate study design. *Journal of Clinical Pharmacology*, **39**, 1032–1037.

[56] Bell, C.B., Smith Haller, H. Smith (1969) Bivariate symmetry tests: Parametric and nonparametric. *The Annals of Mathematical Statistics*, **40, No. 1**, 259–269.

[57] Bellavance, F., Tardif, S. (1995) A nonparametric approach to the analysis of three-treatment three-period cross-over data. *Biometrika*, **82**, 865–875.

[58] Benet, L.Z., Goyan, J.E. (1995) Bioequivalence and narrow therapeutic index drugs. *Pharmacotherapy*, **15**, 433–440.

[59] Benet, L.Z. (1999) Understanding bioequivalence testing. *Transplantation Proceedings*, **31, Suppl A**, 7S–9S.

[60] Benet, L.Z. (2000) Permeability, metabolism, transporters and systemic exposure. *European Journal of Drug Metabolism and Pharmacokinetics*, **1**, 68–68.

[61] Benjamini, Y., Hochberg, Y. (1995) Controlling the false discovery rate: A practical and powerful approach to multiple testing. *Journal of the Royal Statistical Society, Series B*, **57**, 289–300.

[62] Berger, R.L. (1992) Multiparametric hypothesis testing and acceptance sampling. *Technometrics*, **24**, 295–300.

[63] Berger, R.L., Hsu, J.C. (1996) Bioequivalence trials, intersection–union tests, and equivalence confidence sets. *Statistical Science*, **11**, 283–319.

[64] Berger, E., Patel, K., Anwar, S., Davies, W., Sheridan, D.J. (2005) Investigation of the effects of physiological and vasodilation-induced autonomic activation on the QTc interval in healthy male subjects. *British Journal of Clinical Pharmacology*, **60**, 17–23.

[65] Bergstrand, M., Karlsson, M.O. (2009) Handling data below the limit of quantification in mixed effect models. *The AAPS Journal*, **11**, 371–380.

[66] Berman, B. (2013) It's random. *Astronomy*, **41**, 11.

[67] Berry, D.A. (1997) Teaching elementary Bayesian statistics with real applications in science. *The American Statistician*, **51, No. 3**, 241–261.

[68] Berry, S., Berry, D. (2004) Accounting for multiplicities in assessing drug safety: A three-level hierarchical model. *Biometrics*, **60**, 418–426.

[69] Berry, D., Ayers, G. (2006) Symmetrized percent change for treatment comparisons. *The American Statistician*, **60**, 27–31.

[70] Best, N.G., Tan, K.K.C., Gilks, W.R., Spiegelhalter, D.J. (1995) Estimation of population pharmacokinetics using the Gibbs sampler. *Journal of Pharmacokinetics and Biopharmaceutics*, **23, No. 4**, 407–435.

[71] Bewick, T., Sheppard, C., Greenwood, S., Slack, M., Trotter, C., George, R., Lim, W. (2012) Serotype prevalence in adults hospitalised with pneumococcal non-invasive community-acquired pneumonia. *Thorax*, **67**, 540–545.

[72] Beyer, W., Palache, A., Luchters, G., Nauta, J., Osterhaus, A. (2004) Seroprotection rate, mean fold increase, seroconversion rate: Which parameter adequately expresses seroresponse to influenza vaccination? *Virus Research*, **103**, 125–132.

[73] Bhatt, D., Fox, K., Hacke, W., Berger, P., Black, H., Boden, W., Cacoub, P., Cohen, E., Creager, M., Easton, J., Flather, M., Haffner, S., Hamm, C., Hankey, G., Johnston, S., Mak, K., Mas, J., Montalescot, G., Pearson, T., Steg, G., Steinbuhl, S., Weber, M., Brennan, D., Fabry-Ribaudo, L., Booth, J., Topol, E. for the CHARISMA Investigators (2006) Clopidogrel and aspririn versus aspirin alone for the prevention of atherothrombotic events. *New England Journal of Medicine*, **354**, 1706–1717.

[74] Bhatt, D., Steg, P., Ohman, E., Hirsch, A., Ikeda, Y., Mas, J.-L., Goto, S., Liau, C.-S., Richard, A., Rother, J., Wilson, P. for the REACH Registry Investigators (2007) International prevalence, recognition, and treatment of cardiovascular risk factors in outpatients with atherothrombosis. *Journal of the American Medical Association*, **295**, 180–189.

[75] Bhattaram, V., Booth, B., Ramchandani, R., Beasley, B., Wang, Y., Tandon, V., Duan, J., Baweja, R., Marroum, P., Uppoor, R., Rahman, N., Sahajwalla, C., Powell, J., Mehta, M., Gobburu, J. (2005) Impact of pharmacometrics on drug approval and labelling decisions: A survey of 42 new drug applications. *The AAPS Journal*, **7**, E503–E512.

[76] Bhattycharyya, L., Dabbah, R., Hauck, W., Sheinin, E., Yeoman, L., Williams, R. (2005) Equivalence studies for complex active ingredients and dosage forms. *The AAPS Journal*, **7**, E786–E812.

[77] Bhaumick, D., Amatya, A., Normand, S., Greenhouse, J., Kaizar, E., Neelon, B., Gibbons, R. (2012) Meta-analysis of rare binary adverse event data. *Journal of the American Statistical Association*, **107**, 555–567.

[78] Bhoj, D.S. (1979) Testing equality of variances of correlated variates with incomplete data on both responses. *Biometrika*, **66**, 681–683.

[79] Bickel, P.J., Doksum, K.A. (1977) *Mathematical Statistics*. Holden Day, San Francisco.

[80] Biedermann, S., Dette, H., Zhu, W. (2006) Optimal designs for dose-response models with restricted design spaces. *Journal of the American Statistical Association*, **101**, 747–759.

[81] Bigger, J. (1990) Clinical aspects of trial design: What can we expect from the Cardiac Arrythmia Suppression Trial (CAST)? *Cardiovascular Drugs and Therapy*, **4**, 657–664.

[82] Biomarker Definition Working Group (2001) Biomarkers and surrogate endpoints: Preferred definitions and conceptual framework. *Clinical Pharmacology and Therapeutics*, **69**, 89–95.

[83] Bjornsson, E. (2006) Drug-induced liver injury: Hy's rule revisited. *Clinical Pharmacology and Therapeutics*, **79**, 521–528.

[84] Blackwelder, W.C. (1982) Proving the null hypothesis in clinical trials. *Controlled Clinical Trials*, **3**, 345–353.

[85] Blakesley, V. (2005) Current methodology to assess bioequivalence of levothyroxine sodium products is inadequate. *The AAPS Journal*, **7**, E42–E46.

[86] Bloomfield, D.M., Kost, J.T., Ghosh, K., Hreniuk, D., Hickey, L.A., Guitierrez, M.J., Gottesdiener, K., Wagner, J.A. (2008) The effect of moxifloxacin on QTc and implications for the design of thorough QTc studies. *Clinical Pharmacology and Therapeutics*, **84**, 475–480.

[87] Blume, H.H., Midha, K.K., eds. (1993) Conference Report. In: Bio-International: Bioavailability, Bioequivalence, and Pharmacokinetics. *Medpharm Stuttgart*, 13–23.

[88] Blume, H.H., Schug, B.S. (2000) Biopharmaceutical characterization of herbal medicinal products: Are in vivo studies necessary? *European Journal of Drug Metabolism and Pharmacokinetics*, **25, No. 1**, 41–48.

[89] Blumenthal, R., Kapur, N. (2006) Can a potent statin actually regress coronary atherosclerosis? *Journal of the American Medical Association*, **295**, E1–E3.

[90] Boddy, A.W., Snikeris, F.C., Kringle, R.O., Wi, G.C.-G., Oppermann, J.A., Midha, K.K. (1995) An approach for widening the bioequivalence acceptance limits in the case of highly variable drugs. *Pharmaceutical Research*, **12**, 1865–1868.

[91] Bois, F.Y., Tozer, T.N., Hauck, W.W., Chen, M.L., Patnaik, R., Williams, R. (1994) Bioequivalence: Performance of several measures of extent of absorption. *Pharmaceutical Research*, **11**, 715–722.

[92] Boisclair, C., Casais, M., Foote, M., Lepin, J., Peters, J., Peterson, D. (2007) Continuous marketing applications: Experiences of three biotechnology companies. *Drug Information Journal*, **41**, 101–109.

[93] Bolton, S. (2005) Bioequivalence studies for levothyroxine. *The AAPS Journal*, **7**, E47–E53.

[94] Bolton, S., Bon, C. (2008) Statistical considerations: Alternative designs and approaches for bioequivalence assessments. *Clinical Research and Regulatory Affairs*, **25**, 119–137.

[95] Bonate, P., Howard, D., eds. (2004) *Pharmacokinetics in Drug Development: Clinical Study Design and Analysis.* AAPS Press, Arlington, VA.

[96] Bonate, P. (2005) Recommended reading in population pharmacokinetic pharmacodynamics. *The AAPS Journal*, **7**, E363–E373.

[97] Bonate, P. (2006) *Pharmacokinetic-Pharmacodynamic Modeling and Simulation.* Springer, New York.

[98] Bonetti, P., Lerman, L., Lerman, A. (2003) Endothelial dysfunction: A marker of atherosclerotic risk. *Arteriosclerosis Thrombosis and Vascular Biology*, **23**, 168–175.

[99] Bonham, G.H. (1995) Health and environment: Public health decisions based on evidence, psychology and politics. *Environmetrics*, **6**, 311–318.

[100] Boos, D., Hoffman, D., Kringle, R., Zhang, J. (2007) New confidence bounds for QT studies. *Statistics in Medicine*, **26**, 3801–3817.

[101] Boudes, P. (2006) The challenges of new drugs benefits and risk analysis: Lessons from the ximelagatran FDA cardiovascular advisory committee. *Contemporary Clinical Trials*, **27**, 432–440.

[102] Bouvy, J., Koopmanschap, M., Shah, R., Schellekens, H. (2012) The cost-effectiveness of drug regulation: The example of thorough QT/QTc studies. *Clinical Pharmacology and Therapeutics*, **91**, 281–288.

[103] Bowman, F. (2005) Spatio-temporal modelling of localised brain activity. *Biostatistics*, **6**, 558–575.

[104] Box, G.E., Cox, D.R. (1964) An analysis of transformations. *Journal of the Royal Statistical Society, Series B*, **26**, 211–243.

[105] Box, G.E. (1966) Use and abuse of regression. *Technometrics*, **8**, 625–629.

[106] Box, G., Tiao, G. (1972) *Bayesian Inference in Statistical Analysis, 1992 Wiley Classics Library Edition.* John Wiley & Sons, New York.

[107] Box, G.E. (1979) Robustness in the strategy of scientific model building. In *Robustness in Statistics*, Launer, R.L., Wilkinson, G.N., eds., 201–236. Academic Press, New York.

[108] Boxtel, C., Holford, N., Danhof, M., eds. (1992) *The In Vivo Study of Drug Action.* Elsevier, New York.

[109] Bradburn, M., Deeks, J., Berlin, J., Localio, A. (2007) Much ado about nothing: A comparison of the performance of meta-analytical methods with rare events. *Statistics in Medicine*, **26**, 53–77.

[110] Breslow, N. (1990) Biostatistics and Bayes [with discussion]. *Statistical Science*, **5**, 269–298.

[111] Bretz, F. (2006) An extension to the William's trend test to general unbalanced linear models. *Computational Statistics and Data Analysis*, **50**, 1735–1748.

[112] Bretz, F., Hsu, J., Pinheiro, J., Liu, Y. (2008) Dose findings — A challenge in statistics. *Biometrical Journal*, **50**, 480–504.

[113] Bristol, D.R. (1991a) Testing equality of treatment variances in a 2×2 cross-over study. *Journal of Biopharmaceutical Statistics*, **1**, 185–192.

[114] Bristol, D.R. (1991b) A confidence interval for the ratio of treatment variances in a 2×2 cross-over study. *Journal of Biopharmaceutical Statistics*, **1**, 237–245.

[115] Bristol, D. (2007) The choice of two baselines. *Drug Information Journal*, **41**, 55–61.

[116] Brown, B.W. (1980) The cross-over experiment for clinical trials. *Biometrics*, **36**, 69–79.

[117] Brown, E.B., Iyer, H.K., Wang, C.M. (1997) Tolerance intervals for assessing individual bioequivalence. *Statistics in Medicine*, **16**, 803–820.

[118] Brown, H.K., Kempton, R.A. (1994) The application of REML in clinical trials. *Statistics in Medicine*, **13**, 1601–1617.

[119] Brown, L.D., Hwang, J.T.G., Munk, A. (1997) An unbiased test for the bioequivalence problem. *Annals of Statistics*, **25**, 2345–2367.

[120] Brown, L.B., Casella, G., Hwang, G. (1995) Optimal confidence sets, bioequivalence, and the limacon of Pascal. *Journal of the American Statistical Association*, **90**, 880–889.

[121] Brown, M.B., Forsythe, A.B. (1974) Robust tests for the equality of variances. *Journal of the American Statistical Association*, **69**, 364–367.

[122] Brown, M., Chuang-Stein, C., Kirby, S. (2012) Designing studies to find early signals of efficacy. *Journal of Biopharmaceutical Statistics*, **22**, 1097–1108.

[123] Brumback, B., Berg, A. (2008) On effect-measure modification: Relationships among changes in the relative risk, odds ratio, and risk difference. *Statistics in Medicine*, **27**, 3453–3465.

[124] Brunk, H.D. (1958) On the estimation of parameters restricted by inequalities. *Annals of Mathematical Statistics*, **29**, 437–455.

[125] Bryan, J., Henry, C., Hoffman, A., South-Paul, J., Smith, J., Cruess, D., Spieker, J., de Medina, M. (2001) Randomized, cross-over, controlled comparison of two inactivated hepatitis A vaccines. *Vaccine*, **19**, 743–750.

[126] Budescu, D.V. (1982) The power of the F test in normal populations with heterogeneous variances. *Educational and Psychological Measurement*, **42**, 409–416.

[127] Buice, R.G., Subramanian, V.S., Duchin, K.L., Uko-Nne, S. (1996) Bioequivalence of a highly variable drug: An experience with Nadolol. *Pharmaceutical Research*, **13**, 1109–1115.

[128] Bultz, B.D., Carlson, L.E. (2005) Emotional distress: The sixth vital sign in cancer care. *Journal of Clinical Oncology*, **23**, 6440–6441.

[129] Bungay, S., Gentry, P., Gentry, R. (2003) A mathematical model of lipid-mediated thrombin generation. *Mathematical Medicine and Biology*, **20**, 105–129.

[130] Buoen, C., Bjerrum, O., Thomsen, M. (2005) How first-time-in-humans studies are being performed: A survey of phase I dose-escalation trials in healthy volunteers published between 1995 and 2004. *Journal of Clinical Pharmacology*, **45**, 1123–1136.

[131] Burdick, R.K., Graybill, F.A. (1992) *Confidence Intervals on Variance Components.* Marcel Dekker, New York.

[132] Burdick, R.K., Sielken, R.L. (1978) Exact confidence intervals for linear combinations of variance components in nested classifications. *Journal of the American Statistical Association*, **73**, 632–635.

[133] Burnham, R. (2005) The man who remade the universe. *Astronomy*, **33**, 39–41.

[134] Burzykowski, T., Molenberghs, G., Buyse, M., eds. (2005) *The Evaluation of Surrogate Endpoints.* Springer, New York.

[135] Burzykowski, T., Buyse, M. (2006) Surrogate threshold effect: An alternative measure for meta-analytic surrogate endpoint validation. *Pharmaceutical Statistics*, **5**, 173–186.

[136] Cai, T., Pepe, M., Zheng, Y., Lumley, T., Jenny, N. (2006) The sensitivity and specificity of markers for event times. *Biostatistics*, **7**, 182–197.

[137] Califf, R.M., Kramer, J.M. (2008) The balance of benefit and safety of rosiglitazone: Important lessons for our system of drug development and postmarketing assessment. *Pharmacoepidemiology and Drug Safety*, **17**, 782–786.

[138] Calvert, R.T. (1996) Bioequivalence and generic prescribing: A pharmacy view. *Journal of Pharmacy and Pharmacology*, **48**, 9–10.

[139] Campbell, G. (2006) The role of statistics in medical devices — The contrast with pharmaceuticals. *Biopharmceutical Reports*, **14**, 1–8.

[140] Canadian Guidance for Industry (1992) Conduct and Analysis of Bioequivalence Studies — Part A.

[141] Canadian Guidance for Industry (1996) Conduct and Analysis of Bioequivalence Studies — Part B.

[142] Canafax, D.M., Irish, W.D., Moran, H.B., Squiers, E., Levy, R., Pouletty, P., First, M.R., Christians, U. (1999) An individual bioequivalence approach to compare the intra-subject variability of two Ciclosporin formulations, SangCya and Neoral. *Pharmacology*, **59**, 78–88.

[143] Cannon, C., Braunwald, E., McCabe, C., Radner, D., Rouleau, J., Belder, R., Joyal, S., Hill, K., Pfeffer, M., Skene, A. for the Pravastatin or Aotorvastatin evaluation and infection therapy - thrombolysis in myocardial infarction 22 Investigators. (2004) Intensive versus moderate lipid lowering with statins after acute coronary syndromes. *New England Journal of Medicine*, **350**, 1495–1504.

[144] Cantilena, L., Koerner, J., Temple, R., Throckmorton, D. (2006) FDA evaluation of cardiac repolarisation data for 19 drugs and drug candidates. *Clinical Pharmacology and Therapeutics*, **79**, P29.

[145] Carpenter, J., Bithell, J. (2000) Bootstrap confidence intervals: When, which, what? A practical guide for medical statisticians. *Statistics in Medicine*, **19**, 1141–1164.

[146] Carrasco, J., Jover, L. (2005) The structural error-in-equation model to evaluate individual bioequivalence. *Biometrical Journal*, **5**, 623–634.

[147] Carter, B.L., Noyes, M.A., Demmler, R.W. (1993) Differences in serum concentrations of and responses to generic verapamil in the elderly. *Pharmacotherapy*, **13**, 359–368.

[148] Cartwright, A.C. (1991) International harmonisation and consensus DIA meeting on bioavailability and bioequivalence requirements and standards. *Drug Information Journal*, **25**, 471–482.

[149] Cartwright, M., Cohen, S., Fleishaker, J., Madani, S., McLeod, J., Musser, B., Williams, S. (2010) Proof of concept: A PhRMA position paper with recommendations for best practice. *Clinical Pharacology and Therapeutics*, **87**, 278–285.

[150] Casella, G., George, E.J. (1992) Explaining the Gibbs sampler. *The American Statistician*, **46**, 167–174.

[151] Cerutti, R., Rivolta, G., Cavalieri, L., Di Giulio, C., Grossi, E., Vago, T., Baldi, G., Righini, V., Marzo, A. (1999) Bioequivalence of Levothyroxine tablets administered to a target population in steady state. *Pharmacological Research*, **39**, 193–201.

[152] Cesana, M., Cerutti, R., Grossi, E., Fagiuoli, E., Stabilini, M., Stella, F., Luciani, D. (2007) Bayesian data mining techniques: The evidence provided by signals detected in single-company spontaneous reports databases. *Drug Information Journal*, **41**, 11–21.

[153] Chan, I. (1998) Exact tests of equivalence and efficacy with a non-zero lower bound for comparative studies. *Statistics in Medicine*, **17**, 1403–1413.

[154] Chan, I.S.F., Zhang, Z. (1999) Test-based exact confidence intervals for the difference of two binomial proportions. *Biometrics*, **55**, 1202–1209.

[155] Chan, I.S.F., Li, S., Matthews, H., Chan, C., Vessey, R., Sadoff, J., Heyse, J. (2002) Use of statistical models for evaluating antibody response as a correlate of protection against varicella. *Statistics in Medicine*, **21**, 3411–3430.

[156] Chan, I., Wang, W., Heyse, J. (2003) Vaccine Clinical Trials. *Encyclopedia of Biopharmaceutical Statistics.* Marcel Dekker, New York.

[157] Chan, K., Lee, S.-Y., Cheng, C., Shih, P.-L. (1998) Assessing the potential bioequivalence requirement for oral immediate release dosage form: Post approval changes for cardiovascular drugs. *Journal of Food and Drug Analysis*, **6, No. 3**, 537–552.

[158] Chang, W., Chuang-Stein, C. (2004) Type I error and power in trials with one interim futility analysis. *Pharmaceutical Statistics*, **3**, 51–59.

[159] Charbonnel, B., Dormandy, J., Erdmann, E., Massi-Benedetti, M., Skene, A., on behalf of the PROactive study investigators (2004) The prospective pioglitazone clinical trial in macrovascular events (PROactive). *Diabetes Care*, **27**, 1647–1653.

[160] Chaturvedi, A., Bhatti, M.I., Kumar, K. (2000) Bayesian analysis of disturbances variance in the linear regression model under assymetric loss assumptions. *Applied Mathematics and Computation*, **114**, 149–153.

[161] Charvat, B., Brookmeyer, R., Herson, J. (2009) The effects of herd immunity on the power of vaccine trials. *Statistics in Biopharmaceutical Research*, **1**, 108–117.

[162] Chen, C., Wang, H., Snapinn, S.M. (2003) Proportion of treatment effect (PTE) explained by a surrogate marker. *Statistics in Medicine*, **22**, 3449–3459.

[163] Chen, K.-W., Li, G., Sun, Y. (1996) A confidence region approach for assessing equivalence in variability of bioavailability. *Biometrical Journal*, **4**, 475–487.

[164] Chen, M.-L., Lee, S.-C., Ng, M.-J., Schuirmann, D. (1998) Gender analysis of bioequivalence trials. *Clinical Pharmacology and Therapeutics*, **63, No. 2**, 145–145.

[165] Chen, M.-L. (1997) Individual bioequivalence — A regulatory update. *Journal of Biopharmaceutical Statistics*, **7**, 5–11.

[166] Chen, M.-L., Patnaik, R., Hauck, W.H., Schuirmann, D.J., Hyslop, T., Williams, R. (2000a) An individual bioequivalence criterion: Regulatory considerations. *Statistics in Medicine*, **19**, 2821–2842.

[167] Chen, M.-L., Lee, S.-C., Ng, M.-J., Schuirmann, D., Lesko, L.J., Williams, R.L. (2000b) Pharmacokinetic analysis of bioequivalence trials: Implications for sex-related issues in clinical pharmacology and biopharmaceutics. *Clinical Pharmacology and Therapeutics*, **68**, 510–521.

[168] Chen, M.-L., Lesko, L.J. (2001a) Individual bioequivalence revisited. *Clin Pharmacokinet*, **40, No. 10**, 701–706.

[169] Chen, M.-L., Shah, V., Patnaik, R., Adams, W., Hussain, A., Conner, D., Mehta, M., Malinowski, H., Lazor, J., Huang, S.-M., Hare, D., Lesko, L., Sporn, D., Williams, R. (2001b) Bioavailability and bioequivalence: An FDA regulatory overview. *Pharmaceutical Research*, **18, No. 12**, 1645–1650.

[170] Chen, M.-L. (2005) Confounding factors for sex differences in pharmacokinetics and pharmacodynamics: Focus on dosing regimen, dosage form, and formulation. *Clinical Pharmacology and Therapeutics*, **78**, 322-329.

[171] Chen, M.-L., Lee, V.H.L. (2008) Equivalence-by-design: Targeting *in vivo* drug delivery profile. *Pharmaceutical Research*, **25**, 2723–2730.

[172] Chen, M.-L., Davit, B., Lionberger, R., Wahba, Z., Ahn, H., Yu, L. (2011) Using partial area for evaluation of bioavailability and bioequivalence. *Pharmaceutical Research*, **28**, 1939–1947.

[173] Chen, M.-L., Straughn, A., Sadrieh, N., Faustino, P., Ciavarella, A., Meibohm, B., Yates, C., Hussain, A. (2007) A modern view of excipient effects on bioequivalence: Case study of sorbitol. *Pharmaceutical Research*, **24**, 73–80.

[174] Chen, Y., Chang, Y. (2007) Identification of the minimum effective dose for right-censored survival data. *Computational Statistics and Data Analysis*, **51**, 3213–3222.

[175] Cheng, Y., Shen, Y. (2005) Bayesian adaptive designs for clinical trials. *Biometrika*, **92, No. 3**, 633–646.

[176] Chervoneva, I., Hyslop, T., Hauck, W. (2007) A multivariate test for population bioequivalence. *Statistics in Medicine*, **26**, 1208–1223.

[177] Chevret, S., ed. (2006) *Statistical Methods for Dose Finding Experiments.* Wiley, West Sussex, England.

[178] Cheung, Y. (2005) Coherence principles in dose-finding studies. *Biometrika*, **92**, 863–873.

[179] Chi, E.M. (1994) M-estimation in cross-over trials. *Biometrics*, **50**, 486–493.

[180] Chiacchierini, R., Seidman, M. (1997) Perspectives on clinical studies for medical device submissions. www.fda.gov/cdrh/guidance.html.

[181] Chick, S., Barth-Jones, D., Koopman, J. (2001) Bias reduction for risk ratio and vaccine effect estimators. *Statistics in Medicine*, **20**, 1609–1624.

[182] Chien, J., Friedrich, S., Heathman, M., de Alwis, D., Sinha, V. (2005) Pharmacokinetic-pharmacodynamics and the stages of drug development: Role of modelling and simulation. *The AAPS Journal*, **7**, E544–E559.

[183] China State Drug Administration (2003) Drug Registration Regulation.

[184] Chinchilli, V.M. (1996) The assessment of individual and population bioequivalence. *Journal of Biopharmaceutical Statistics*, **6**, 1–14.

[185] Chinchilli, V.M., Elswick, R.K. (1997) The multivariate assessment of bioequivalence. *Journal of Biopharmaceutical Statistics*, **7**, 113–123.

[186] Chinchilli, V.M., Esinhart, J.D. (1996) Design and analysis of intra-subject variability in cross-over experiments. *Statistics in Medicine*, **15**, 1619–1634.

[187] Chinchilli, V., Phillips, B., Mauger, D., Szefler, S. (2005) A general class of correlation coefficients for the 2×2 cross-over design. *Biometrical Journal*, **47**, 644–653.

[188] Choi, L., Caffo, B., Rohde, C. (2008) A survey of the likelihood approach to bioequivalence trials. *Statistics in Medicine*, **27**, 4874–4894.

[189] Choudhary, P.K., Nagaraja, H.N. (2005) Assessment of agreement using intersection-union principle. *Biometrical Journal*, **47**, 1–8.

[190] Choudhury, R., Fuster, V., Badimon, J., Fisher, E., Fayad, Z. (2002) MRI and the characterisation of atherosclerotic plaque. *Arteriosclerosis Thrombosis and Vascular Biology*, **22**, 1065–1074.

[191] Chow, S.C. (1990) Alternative approaches for assessing bioequivalence regarding normality assumptions. *Drug Information Journal*, **24**, 753–762.

[192] Chow, S.C. (1988) A new procedure for the estimation of variance components. *Statistics and Probability Letters*, **6**, 349–355.

[193] Chow, S.C. (1997a) Guest editor's note: Recent issues in bioequivalence trials. *Journal of Biopharmaceutical Statistics*, **7, No. 1**, 1–3.

[194] Chow, S.C., Liu, J. (1997b) Meta-analysis for bioequivalence review. *Journal of Biopharmaceutical Statistics*, **7, No. 1**, 97–111.

[195] Chow, S.C., Liu, J., eds. (1998) *Design and Analysis of Animal Studies in Pharmaceutical Development.* Marcel Dekker, New York.

[196] Chow, S.C., Liu, J. (2000) *Design and Analysis of Bioavailability and Bioequivalence Studies, 2nd ed.* Marcel Dekker, New York.

[197] Chow, S.C., Shao, J. (1988) A new procedure for the estimation of variance components. *Statistics and Probability Letters*, **6**, 349–355.

[198] Chow, S.C., Shao, J., Wang, H. (2002a) Individual bioequivalence testing under 2×3 designs. *Statistics in Medicine*, **21**, 629–648.

[199] Chow, S.C., Shao, J., Hu, O. (2002b) Assessing sensitivity and similarity in bridging studies. *Journal of Biopharmaceutical Statistics*, **12**, 385–400.

[200] Chow, S.C., Shao, J., Wang, H. (2003) In vitro bioequivalence testing. *Statistics in Medicine*, **22**, 55–68.

[201] Chow, S.C., Shao, J., Wang, H. (2003b) *Sample Size Calculations in Clinical Research.* Marcel Dekker, New York.

[202] Christopher, D., Adams, W., Amann, A., Bertha, C., Byron, P., Doub, W., Dunbar, C., Hauck, W., Lyapustina, S., Mitchell, J., Morgan, B., Nichols, S., Pan, Z., Singh, G., Tougas, T., Tsong, Y., Wolff, R., Wyka, B. (2007) Product quality research institute evaluation of cascade impactor profiles of pharmaceutical aerosols. Part 3: Final report on a statistical procedure for determining equivalence. *AAPS Pharmaceutical Science and Technology*, **8, Article 90**, E1–E10.

[203] Chuang-Stein, C., Shih, W. (1991) A note on the analysis of titration studies. *Statistics in Medicine*, **10**, 323–328.

[204] Chuang-Stein, C., Le, V., Chen, W. (2001) Recent advancements in the analysis and presentation of safety data. *Drug Information Journal*, **35**, 377–397.

[205] Chuang-Stein, C., Anderson, K., Gallo, P., Collins, S. (2006a) Sample size reestimation: A review and recommendations. *Drug Information Journal*, **40**, 475–484.

[206] Chuang-Stein, C. (2006b) Sample size and the probability of a successful trial. *Pharmaceutical Statistics*, **5**, 305–309.

[207] Chuang-Stein, C. (2006c) A cautionary note on design implications when the primary endpoint is a stratified analysis of a binary endpoint. *Biometrical Journal*, **48**, 978–993.

[208] Chuang-Stein, C., Stryszak, P., Dmitrienko, A., Offen, W. (2007) Challenge of multiple co-primary endpoints: A new approach. *Statistics in Medicine*, **26**, 1181–1192.

[209] Chuang-Stein, C., Entsuah, R., Pritchett, Y. (2008) Measures for conducting comparative benefit:risk assessment. *Drug Information Journal*, **42**, 223–233.

[210] Chuang-Stein, C., Kirby, S., French, J., Marshall, S. (2009) An enhanced approach to quantitative decision making in drug development. *Presentation to Collegeville Stats Forum.*

[211] Chuang-Stein, C., Kirby, S. (2014) The shrinking or disappearing observed treatment effect. *Pharmaceutical Statistics*, **13**, 277–280.

[212] Clinical Pharmacology and Therapeutics Editorial Team. (2010) Statistical guide for *Clinical Pharmacology and Therapeutics. Clinical Pharmacology and Therapeutics*, **88**, 150–152.

[213] Clopper, C., Pearson, E. (1934) The use of confidence or fiducial limits illustrated in the case of the binomial. *Biometrika*, **26**, 403–414.

[214] Cohen, M. H., Moses, M.L., Pazdur, R. (2002) Gleevec for the treatment of chronic myelogenous leukemia: U.S. food and drug administration regulatory mechanisms, accelerated approval, and orphan drug status. *The Oncologist*, **7**, 390–392.

[215] Cohen, M.H., Johnson, J.R., Chen, Y.-F., Sridhara, R., Pazdur, R. (2005) FDA drug approval summary: Erlotinib (Tarceva) tablets. *The Oncologist*, **10**, 461–466.

[216] Colaizzi, J.L., Lowenthal, D.T. (1986) Critical therapeutic categories: A contraindication to generic substitution? *Clinical Therapeutics*, **8**, 370–379.

[217] Colburn, W.A., Keefe, D.L. (2000) Bioavailability and bioequivalence: Average, population, and/or individual. *Journal of Clinical Pharmacology*, **40**, 559–600.

[218] COMMIT: Clopidogrel and Metropolol in Myocardial Infarction Trial collaborative group. (2005) Addition of clopidogrel to aspirin in 45,852 patients with acute myocardial infarction: Randomised placebo-controlled trial. *The Lancet*, **366**, 1607–1621.

[219] Conforti, M., Hochberg, Y. (1987) Sequentially rejective pairwise testing procedures. *Journal of Statistical Planning and Inference*, **17**, 193–208.

[220] Cook, T., Benner, R., Fisher, M. (2006) The WIZARD trial as a case study of flexible clinical trial design. *Drug Information Journal*, **40**, 345–353.

[221] Cook, J., Davit, B., Polli, J. (2010) Impact of biopharmaceutics classification system-based biowavers. *Molecular Pharmaceutics*, **7**, 1539–1544.

[222] Cornell, R.G. (1980) Evaluation of bioavailability data using non-parametric statistics. *In Drug Absorption and Disposition: Statistical Considerations*; Albert, K., ed., 51–57, American Pharmaceutical Association.

[223] Cornell, R.G. (1991) Nonparametric tests of dispersion for the two period cross-over design. *Commumications in Statistical Theory and Methodology*, **20**, 1099–1106.

[224] Corpet, D.E., Pierre, F. (2005) How good are rodent models of carcinogenesis in predicting efficacy in humans? A systematic review and meta-analysis of colon chemoprevention in rats, mice and men. *European Journal of Cancer*, **41**, 1911–1922.

[225] Corsini, A. (2003) The safety of HMG-CoA reductase inhibitors in special populations at high cardiovascular risk. *Cardiovascular Drugs and Therapy*, **17**, 265–285.

[226] Cortese, G., Andersen, P. (2009) Competing risks and time-dependent covariates. *Biometrical Journal*, **51**, 138–158.

[227] Cox, D.R. (1967) Fieller's theorem and a generalization. *Biometrika*, **54**, 567–572.

[228] Crowder, M.J., Kimber, A.C., Smith, R.L., Sweeting, T.J. (1991) *Statistical Analysis of Reliability Data.* Chapman and Hall, London.

[229] Crow, E.L., Shimizu, K. (1988) *Lognormal Distributions.* Marcel Dekker, New York.

[230] Crowe, B., Xia, H., Berlin, J., Watson, D., Shi, H., Lin, S., Kuebler, J., Schriver, R., Santanello, N., Rochester, G., Porter, J., Oster, M., Mehrotra, D., Li, Z., King, E., Harpur, E., Hall, D. (2009) Recommendations for safety planning, data collection, evaluation and reporting, during drug, biologic, and vaccine development: A report of the safety planning, evaluation, and reporting team. *Clinical Trials*, **6**, 430–440.

[231] Cui, L., Hung, J., Wang, S.-J. (1999) Modification of sample size in group sequential clinical trials. *Biometrics*, **55**, 853–857.

[232] Cumming, G. (2009) Inference by eye: Reading the overlap of independent confidence intervals. *Statistics in Medicine*, **28**, 205–220.

[233] CURE: Clopidogrel in unstable angina to prevent recurrent events trial investigators (2001) Effects of clopidogrel in addition to aspirin in patients with acute coronary syndromes without ST-segment elevation. *New England Journal of Medicine*, **345**, 494–502.

[234] Cytel (1995) *StatXact 3 for Windows: Statistical Software for Exact Nonparametric Inference (User Manual).* Cytel Software Corporation, Cambridge, MA.

[235] Dagan, R., Givon-Lavi, N., Fraser, D., Lipsitch, M., Siber, G., Kohberger, R. (2005) Serum serotype-sepcific pneumococcal anticapsular immunoglobulin G concentrations after immunization with 9-valent conjugate pneumococcal vaccine correlate with nasopharyngeal acquisition of pneumococcus. *Journal of Infectious Disease*, **192**, 367–376.

[236] Dagan, R., Patterson, S., Juergens, C., Greenberg, D., Givon-Lavi, N., Porat, N., Gurtman, A., Gruber, W., Scott, D. (2013) Comparative immunogenicity and efficacy of 13-valent and 7-valent pneumococcal conjugate vaccine in reducing nasopharyngeal colonization: A randomized double-blind trial. *Clinical Infectious Diseases*, **57**, 952–962.

[237] D'Angelo, G., Potvin, D., Turgeon, J. (2001) Carry-over effects in bioequivalence studies. *Journal of Biopharmaceutical Statistics*, **11**, 27–36.

[238] Daniels, M.J., Kass, R.E. (2001) Shrinkage estimators for covariance matrices. *Biometrics*, **57**, 1173-1184.

[239] Dann, R.S., Koch, G.G. (2008) Methods for one-sided testing of the difference between proportions and sample size considerations related to non-inferiority clinical trials. *Pharmaceutical Statistics*, **7**, 130–141.

[240] Dannenberg, O., Dette, H., Munk, A. (1994) An extension of Welch's approximate t-solution to comparative bioequivalence trials. *Biometrika*, **81, No. 1**, 91–101.

[241] Davidian, M., Giltinan, D.M. (1995) *Nonlinear Models for Repeated Measurement Data.* Chapman and Hall, London.

[242] Davit, B.M., Conner, D.P., Fabian-Fritsch, B., Haidar, S.H., Jiang, X., Patel, D.T., Seo, P.R.H., Suh, K., Thompson, C.L., Yu, L.X. (2008) Highly variable drugs: Observations from bioequivalence data submitted to the FDA for generic new drug applications. *The AAPS Journal*, **10**, 148–156.

[243] Davit, B., Conner, D. (2010) USA Chapter, in *Generic Drug Development*, Kanfer, I, Shargel, S., eds., pp 254–281. Informa Healthcare, New York.

[244] Davit, B., Chen, M., Conner, D., Haidar, S., Kim, S., Lee, C., Lionberger, R., Makhlouf, F., Nwakama, P., Patel, D., Schuirmann, D., Yu, L. (2012) Implementation of a reference-scaled average bioequivalence approach for highly variable generic drug products by the US Food and Drug Administration. *The AAPS Journal*, **14**, 915–924.

[245] Davit, B., Braddy, A., Conner, D., Yu, L. (2013) International guidelines for bioequivalence of systemically available orally administered generic drug products: A survey of similarities and differences. *The AAPS Journal*, **15**, 974–990.

[246] Dawid, A.P. (1988) Symmetry models and hypotheses for structured data layouts. *Journal of the Royal Statistical Society, Series B*, **50, No. 1**, 1–34.

[247] Dawson, J.D. (1998) Sample size calculations based on slopes and other summary statistics. *Biometrics*, **54**, 323–330.

[248] Day, S., Altman, D. (2000) Blinding in clinical trials and other studies. *British Medical Journal*, **321**, 504.

[249] Day, S. (2002) Changing times in pharmaceutical statistics: 2000-2020. *Pharmaceutical Statistics*, **1**, 75–82.

[250] DeAngelis, C., Fontanarosa, P. (2010) Ensuring integrity in industry-sponsored research. *Journal of the American Medical Association*, **303**, 1196–1198.

[251] De Santis, F. (2006) Power priors and their use in clinical trials. *The American Statistician*, **60**, 122–129.

[252] Dean, B.D., Borenstein, J.E., Henning, J.M., Knight, K., Merz, C.N.B. (2004) Can change in high-density lipoprotein cholesterol levels reduce cardiovascular risk? *American Heart Journal*, **147, No. 6**, 966–976.

[253] DeBruin, M., Langendijk, P., Koopmans, R., Wilde, A., Leufkens, H., Hoes, A. (2006) In-hospital cardiac arrest is associated with use of non-antiarrythmic QTc-prolonging drugs. *British Journal of Clinical Pharmacology*, **63**, 216–223.

[254] DeCook, R., Nettleton, D., Foster, C., Wurtele, E. (2006) Identifying differentially expressed genes in unreplicated multiple-treatment microarray timecourse experiments. *Computational Statistics and Data Analysis*, **50**, 518–532.

[255] Dempster, A.P., Selwyn, M. R. (1984) Statistical and computational aspects of mixed model analysis. *Applied Statistics*, **33, No. 2**, 203–214.

[256] Desfrere, L., Zohar, S., Morville, P., Brunhes, A., Chevret, S., Pons, G., Moriette, G., Reyes, E., Treluyers, J.M. (2005) Dose-finding study of ibuprofen in patent ductus arteriosus using the continual reassessment method. *Journal of Clinical Pharmacy and Therapeutics*, **30**, 121–132.

[257] Dette, H., Bretz, F., Pepelyshev, A., Pinhiero, J. (2008) Optimal designs for dose-findings studies. *Journal of the American Statistical Association*, **103**, 1225–1237.

[258] Diaz, F., Berg, M., Krebill, R., Welty, T., Gidal, B., Alloway, R., Privitera, M. (2013) Random-effects linear modelling and sample size tables for two special cross-over designs of average bioequivalence studies: The four-period, two-sequence, two-formulation and six-period, three-sequence, three-formulation designs. *Clinical Pharmacokinetics*, **52**, 1033–1043.

[259] Diener, H., Bogousslavsky, J., Brass, L., Cimminiello, C., Csiba, L., Kaste, M., Leys, D., Matias-Guiu, J., Rupprecht, H. on behalf of the MATCH Investigators. (2004) Aspirin and clopidogrel compared to clopidogrel alone after recent ischaemic stroke or transient ischaemic attack in high-risk patients (MATCH): Randomised, double-blind, placebo controlled trial. *The Lancet*, **364**, 331–337.

[260] Diletti, E., Hauschke, D., Steinijans, V.W. (1991) Sample size determination for bioequivalence assessment by means of confidence intervals. *International Journal of Clinical Pharmacology, Therapeutics, and Toxicology*, **29**, 1–8.

[261] DiMasi, J. (2001) New drug development in the USA from 1963 to 1999; Risks in new drug development — Approval success rates for investigational drugs. *Clinical Pharmacology and Therapeutics*, **69**, 286–307.

[262] Dimasi, J., Hansen, R., Grabowski, H. (2003) The price of innovation: New estimates of drug development costs. *Journal of Health Economics*, **22**, 151–185.

[263] DiMasi, J.A., Faden, L. (2009) Factors associated with multiple FDA review cycles and approval phase times. *Drug Information Journal*, **43**, 201–225.

[264] DiMasi, J., Feldman, L., Seckler, A., Wilson, A. (2010) Trends in risks associated with new drug development: Success rates for investigational drugs. *Clinical Pharmacology and Therapeutics*, **87**, 272–277.

[265] Dmitrienko, A., Smith, B. (2003) Repeated-measures models in the analysis of QT-interval data. *Pharmaceutical Statistics*, **2**, 175–190.

[266] Dmitrienko, A., Sides, G., Winters, K., Kovacs, R., Rebhun, D., Bloom, J., Groh, W., Eisenberg, P. (2005) Electrocardiogram reference ranges derived from a standardised clinical trial population. *Drug Information Journal*, **39**, 395–405.

[267] Dmitrienko, A., Offen, W., Wang, O., Xiao, D. (2006a) Gatekeeping procedures in dose-response clinical trials based on the Dunnett test. *Pharmaceutical Statistics*, **5**, 19–28.

[268] Dmitrienko, A., Wang, M.-D. (2006b) Bayesian predictive approach to interim monitoring in clinical trials. *Statistics in Medicine*, **25**, 2178–2195.

[269] Dmitrienko, A., Wiens, B., Westfall, P. (2006c) Fallback tests in dose-response clinical trials. *Journal of Biopharmaceutical Statistics*, **16**, 745–755.

[270] Dmitrienko, A., Tamhane, A., Wang, X., Chen, X. (2006d) Stepwise gatekeeping procedures in clinical trial applications. *Biometrical Journal*, **48**, 984–991.

[271] Dmitrienko, A., Tamhane, A. (2007) Gatekeeping procedures with clinical trial applications. *Pharmaceutical Statistics*, **6**, 171–180.

[272] Dmitrienko, A., Beasley, C., Mitchell, M. (2008) Design and analysis of thorough QTc studies. *Biopharmaceutical Network Report 2008-04-29*, www.biopharmnet.com.

[273] Dmitrienko, A., Tamhane, A., Bretz, F., eds. (2009) *Multiple Testing Problems in Pharmaceutical Statistics.* Chapman and Hall/CRC Press, London.

[274] Doctor, R.N., Newton, D.P., Pearson, A. (2001) Managing uncertainty in research and development. *Technovation*, **21**, 79–90.

[275] Donner, A., Hauck, W.W., Zou, G. (2005) The impact of missing values in the concentration-time curve on the assessment of bioequivalence. *Pharmaceutical Statistics*, **4**, 91–99.

[276] Dormandy, J., Charbonnel, B., Eckland, D., Erdmann, E. et al. on behalf of the PROactive investigators (2005) Secondary prevention of macrovascular events in patients with type 2 diabetes in the PROactive study (prospective pioglitazone clinical trial in macrovascular events): A randomised clinical trial. *The Lancet*, **366**, 1279–1289.

[277] Doyle, Sir A. C. (1890) Chapter 1 *The Sign of Four*, appearing in *The Complete Sherlock Holmes.* Doubleday, New York.

[278] Dragalin, V., Fedorov, V. (1999a) Kullback–Liebler distance for evaluating bioequivalence. *SB BDS Technical Report 1999-03.*

[279] Dragalin, V., Fedorov, V. (1999b) The total least squares method in individual bioequivalence evaluation. *SB BDS Technical Report 1999-04.*

[280] Dragalin, V., Fedorov, V., Cheuvart, B. (2002) Statistical approaches to establishing vaccine safety. *Statistics in Medicine*, **21**, 877–893.

[281] Dragalin, V., Fedorov, V., Patterson, S., Jones, B. (2003) Kullback-Leibler divergence for evaluating bioequivalence. *Statistics in Medicine*, **22**, 913–930.

[282] Dragalin, V., Fedorov, V. (2004) Adaptive model-based designs for dose-finding studies. *GSK BDS Technical Report 2004-02.*

[283] Dragalin, V., Fedorov, V., Wu, Y. (2006) Optimal designs for bivariate probit models. *GSK BDS Technical Report 2006-01.*

[284] Dragalin, V., Fedorov, V., Wu, Y. (2008) Two-stage design for dose-finding that accounts for both safety and efficacy. *Statistics in Medicine*, **27**, 5156–5176.

[285] Dubois, A., Lavielle, M., Gsteiger, S., Pigeolet, E., Mentre, F. (2011) Model-based analyses of bioequivalence cross-over trials using the stochastic approximation expectation maximisation algorithm. *Statistics in Medicine*, **30**, 2582–2600.

[286] Duffull, S. B. (2001) Design of clinical pharmacology trials. *Clinical and Experimental Pharmacology and Physiology*, **28**, 905–912.

[287] Duffull, S.B., Kirkpatrick, C.M.J., Green, B., Holford, N.H.G. (2005) Analysis of population pharmacokinetic data using nonmem and winbugs. *Journal of Biopharmaceutical Statistics*, **15**, 53–73.

[288] Dumville, J., Hahn, S., Miles, J., Torgerson, D. (2006) The use of unequal randomisation ratios in clinical trials: A review. *Contemporary Clinical Trials*, **27**, 1–12.

[289] Dunger-Baldouf, C., Racine, A., Koch, G. (2006) Re-treatment studies: Design and analysis. *Drug Information Journal*, **40**, 209–217.

[290] Dunnett, C.W., Gent, M. (1977) Significance testing to establish equivalence between treatments, with special reference to data in the form of 2×2 tables. *Biometrics*, **33**, 593–602.

[291] Eaton, M., Muirhead, R., Mancuso, J., Kolluri, S. (2006) A confidence interval for the maximum mean QT interval change caused by drug effect. *Drug Information Journal*, **40**, 267–271.

[292] Ebbutt, A.F. (1984) Three-period crossover designs for two treatments. *Biometrics*, **40**, 219–224.

[293] Efron, B. (1987) Better bootstrap confidence intervals. *Journal of the American Statistical Association*, **82, No. 397**, 171–185.

[294] Efron, B., Tibshirani, R.J. (1993) *An Introduction to the Bootstrap.* Chapman and Hall, New York.

[295] Efron, B. (2007) Size, power, and false discovery rates. *The Annals of Statistics*, **35**, 1351–1377.

[296] Eisenhauer, E., Twelves, C., Buyse, M. (2006) *Phase I Cancer Clinical Trials.* Oxford University Press, Oxford.

[297] Ekbohm, E. (1981) A test for the equality of variances in the paired case with incomplete data. *Biometrical Journal*, **3**, 261–265.

[298] Ekbohm, G., Melander, H. (1989) The subject-by-formulation interaction as a criterion of interchangeability of drugs. *Biometrics*, **45**, 1249–1254.

[299] Ekholm, A., Jokinen, J., Kilpi, T. (2002) Combining regression and association modelling for longitudinal data on bacterial carriage. *Statistics in Medicine*, **21**, 773–791.

[300] El-Tahtawy, A.A., Tozer, T.N., Harrison, F., Lesko, L., Williams, R. (1998) Evaluation of bioequivalence of highly variable drug using clinical trial simulations. II: Comparison of single and multiple-dose trials using AUC and Cmax. *Pharmaceutical Research*, **15**, 98–104.

[301] El-Tahtawy, A., Harrison, F., Zirkelbach, J., Jackson, A. (2011) Bioequivalence of long half-life drugs — Informative sampling determination — Parallel designed studies. *Bioequivalence and Bioavailability*, **3**, 56–61.

[302] El-Tahtawy, A., Harrison, F., Zirkelbach, J., Jackson, A. (2012) Bioequivalence of long half-life drugs — Informative sampling determination — Using truncated area in parallel-designed studies for slow sustained-release formulations. *Journal of Pharmaceutical Sciences*, **101**, 4337–4346.

[303] Ellenberg, J.H. (1973) The joint distribution of the standardized least squares residuals from a general linear regression. *Journal of the American Statistical Association*, **68**, 941–943.

[304] Ellenberg, S., Fleming, T., DeMets, D. (2002) *Data Monitoring Committees in Clinical Trials: A Practical Perspective.* Wiley, West Sussex, England.

[305] Ellenburg, S. (2004) Analytical, practical, and regulatory issues in prevention studies. *Statistics in Medicine*, **23**, 297–303.

[306] EMEA, European Agency for the Evaluation of Medicinal Products, Committee for Proprietary Medicinal Products (1999) Note for guidance on the clinical evaluation of new vaccines. http://www.emea.eu.int/index/

[307] EMEA, European Agency for the Evaluation of Medicinal Products, Committee for Proprietary Medicinal Products (2000) Points to consider on switching between superiority and non-inferiority. http://www.emea.eu.int/index/

[308] EMEA, European Agency for the Evaluation of Medicinal Products, Committee for Proprietary Medicinal Products (2001) Guidance on the investigation of bioavailability and bioequivalence. http://www.emea.eu.int/index/

[309] EMEA, European Agency for the Evaluation of Medicinal Products, Committee for Proprietary Medicinal Products (2002a) Note for guidance on clinical investigation of medicinal products in the treatment of diabetes mellitus. http://www.emea.eu.int/index/

[310] EMEA, European Agency for the Evaluation of Medicinal Products, Committee for Proprietary Medicinal Products (2002b) Points to consider on multiplicity issues in clinical trials. http://www.emea.eu.int/index/

[311] EMEA, European Agency for the Evaluation of Medicinal Products, Committee for Proprietary Medicinal Products (2004) Note for guidance on clinical investigation of medicinal products in the treatment of lipid disorders. http://www.emea.eu.int/index/

[312] EMEA, European Agency for the Evaluation of Medicinal Products, Committee for Proprietary Medicinal Products (2006a) Concept paper for an addendum to the note for guidance on the investigation of bioavailability and bioequivalence: Evaluation of bioequivalence of highly variable drugs and drug products. http://www.emea.eu.int/index/

[313] EMEA, European Agency for the Evaluation of Medicinal Products, Committee for Proprietary Medicinal Products (2006b) Guideline on clinical investigation of medicinal products for prophylaxis of high intra- and post-operative venous thromboembolic risk. http://www.emea.eu.int/index/

[314] EMEA, European Agency for the Evaluation of Medicinal Products, Committee for Proprietary Medicinal Products (2006c) Guideline on similar biological medicinal products containing biotechnology-derived proteins as active substance: Non-clinical and clinical issues. http://www.emea.eu.int/index/

[315] EMEA, European Agency for the Evaluation of Medicinal Products, Committee for Proprietary Medicinal Products (2006d) Guideline on the choice of the non-inferiority margin. http://www.emea.eu.int/index/

[316] EMEA, European Agency for the Evaluation of Medicinal Products, Committee for Proprietary Medicinal Products. (2007a) Draft guideline on the evaluation of medicinal products for cardiovascular disease prevention. http://www.emea.eu.int/index/

[317] EMEA, European Agency for the Evaluation of Medicinal Products, Committee for Proprietary Medicinal Products. (2007b) Guideline on clinical evaluation of new vaccines. http://www.emea.eu.int/index/

[318] EMEA, European Agency for the Evaluation of Medicinal Products, Committee for Proprietary Medicinal Products (2009) Guideline on the requirements for clinical documentation of orally inhaled products including the requirements for demonstration of therapeutic equivalence between two inhaled products for use in the treatment of asthma and chronic obstructive pulmonary disease in adults and for use in the treatment of asthma in children and adolescents. http://www.emea.eu.int/index/

[319] EMEA, European Agency for the Evaluation of Medicinal Products, Committee for Proprietary Medicinal Products (2010a) Guideline on the investigation of bioequivalence. http://www.emea.eu.int/index/

[320] EMEA, European Agency for the Evaluation of Medicinal Products, Committee for Proprietary Medicinal Products (2010b) Guideline on missing data in confirmatory clinical trials. http://www.emea.eu.int/index/

[321] EMEA, European Agency for the Evaluation of Medicinal Products, Committee for Proprietary Medicinal Products (2012) Guideline on the investigation of drug interactions. http://www.emea.eu.int/index/

[322] EMEA, European Agency for the Evaluation of Medicinal Products, Committee for Proprietary Medicinal Products (2013) Questions and answers: Positions on specific questions addressed to the pharmacokinetics working party, Rev. 7. http://www.emea.eu.int/index/

[323] Emerson, S., Kittelson, J., Gillen, D. (2007) Frequentist evaluation of group sequential clinical trial designs. *Statistics in Medicine*, **26**, 5047–5080.

[324] Enas, G.G., Andersen, J.S. (2001) Enhancing the value delivered by the statistician throughout drug discovery and development: Putting statistical science into regulated pharmaceutical innovation. *Statistics in Medicine*, **20**, 2697–2708.

[325] Endrenyi, L., Fritsch, S., Yan, W. (1991) Cmax/AUC is a clearer measure than Cmax for absorption rates in investigations of bioequivalence. *International Journal of Clinical Pharmacology, Therapy, and Toxicology*, **29**, 394–399.

[326] Endrenyi, L., Schulz, M. (1993) Individual variation and the acceptance of average bioequivalence. *Drug Information Journal*, **27**, 195–201.

[327] Endrenyi, L. (1994) A method for the evaluation of individual bioequivalence. *International Journal of Clinical Pharmacology and Therapeutics*, **32**, 497–508.

[328] Endrenyi, L. (1995) A simple approach for the evaluation of individual bioequivalence. *Drug Information Journal*, **29**, 847–855.

[329] Endrenyi, L. (1997) Some issues for the consideration of individual bioequivalence. *Journal of Biopharmaceutical Statistics*, **7, No. 1**, 35–39.

[330] Endrenyi, L., Czimadia, F., Tothfalusi, L, Chen, M.L. (1998a) Metrics comparing simulated early concentration profiles for the determination of bioequivalence. *Pharmaceutical Research*, **15**, 1292–1299.

[331] Endrenyi, L., Amidon, G.L., Midha, K.K., Skelly, J.P. (1998b) Individual bioequivalence: Attractive in principle, difficult in practice. *Pharmaceutical Research*, **15**, 1321–1325.

[332] Endrenyi, L., Hao, Y. (1998c) Assymetry of the mean-variability tradeoff raises questions about the model in investigations of individual bioequivalence. *International Journal of Clinical Pharmacology, Therapy, and Toxicology*, **36**, 1–8.

[333] Endrenyi, L., Midha, K.K. (1998d) Individual bioequivalence—Has its time come? *European Journal of Pharmaceutical Sciences*, **6**, 271–277.

[334] Endrenyi, L., Tothfalusi, L. (1999) Subject-by-formulation interaction in determination of individual bioequivalence: Bias and prevalence. *Pharmaceutical Research*, **16**, 186–190.

[335] Endrenyi, L., Taback, N., Tothfalusi, L. (2000) Properties of the estimated variance component for subject-by-formulation interaction in studies of individual bioequivalence. *Statistics in Medicine*, **19**, 2867–2878.

[336] Endrenyi, L., Tothfalusi, L. (2008) Evaluation of bioequivalence for highly variable drugs. *Clinical Research and Regulatory Affairs*, **25**, 93–117.

[337] Endrenyi, L., Tothfalusi, L. (2009) Regulatory conditions for the determination of bioequivalence of highly variable drugs. *Journal of Pharmacy and Pharmaceutical Science*, **12**, 138–149.

[338] Endrenyi, L., Tothfalusi, L. (2012) Metrics for the evaluation of bioequivalence for modified-release formulations. *The AAPS Journal*, **14**, 813–819.

[339] Endrenyi, L., Tothfalusi, L. (2013) Determination of bioequivalence for drugs with narrow therapeutic index: Reduction of the regulatory burden. *Journal of Pharmacy and Pharmaceutical Science*, **16**, 676–682.

[340] Engel, B. (1990) The analysis of unbalanced linear models with variance components. *Statistica Neerlandica*, **44**, 195–219.

[341] Erdman, E, Morelock, M. (2007) A study of kinetics: The estimation and simulation of systems of first-order differential equations. *SAS User Group Proceedings*, 1–8.

[342] Erdmann, E., Dormandy, J., Charbonnel, B., Massi-Benedetti, M., Koules, I. et al. on behalf of the PROactive investigators. (2007) The effect of pioglitazone on recurrent myocardial infarction in 2,445 patients with type 2 diabetes and previous myocardial infarction. *Journal of the American College of Cardiology*, **49**, 1772–1780.

[343] Ereshefsky, L., Meyer, M. (2001) Comparison of the bioequivalence of generic versus branded Clozapine. *Journal of Clinical Psychiatry*, **62(Suppl 5)**, 3–27.

[344] Esinhart, J.D., Chinchilli, V.M. (1994a) Extensions to the use of tolerance intervals for the assessment of individual bioequivalence. *Journal of Biopharmaceutical Statistics*, 4, 39–52.

[345] Esinhart, J.D., Chinchilli, V.M. (1994b) Sample size considerations for assessing individual bioequivalence based on the method of tolerance intervals. *International Journal of Clinical Pharmacology and Therapeutics*, **32**, 26–32.

[346] Everson-Stewart, S., Emerson, S. (2010) Bio-creep in non-inferiority clinical trials. *Statistics in Medicine*, **29**, 2769–2780.

[347] Fan, X., DeMets, D. (2006) Conditional and unconditional confidence intervals following a group sequential test. *Journal of Biopharmaceutical Statistics*, **16**, 107–122.

[348] Fay, M., Halloran, E., Follmann, D. (2007) Accounting for variability in sample size estimation with applications to non-adherence and estimation of variation and effect size. *Biometrics*, **63**, 465–474.

[349] Fay, M. (2010) Confidence intervals that match Fisher's exact or Blaker's exact tests. *Biostatistics*, **11**, 373–374.

[350] FDA Guidance (1987) Guidance for in-vivo bioequivalence study for slow release potassium-chloride tablets and capsules. http://www.fda.gov/cder/guidance/

[351] FDA Guidance (1989) Guidance for the in-vitro portion of bioequivalence requirements for metaproterenol sulfate and albuterol inhalation aerosols (metered dose inhalers). http://www.fda.gov/cder/guidance/

[352] FDA Guidance (1992) Statistical procedures for bioequivalence studies using a standard two treatment cross-over design.

[353] FDA Guidance (1993) Interim guidance — Cholestyramine powder in-vitro bioequivalence. http://www.fda.gov/cder/guidance/

[354] FDA Guidance (1994) Phenytoin sodium capsules, tablets, and suspension in vivo bioequivalence and in-vitro dissolution testing. http://www.fda.gov/cder/guidance/

[355] FDA Guidance (1995a) Topical dermatologic corticosteroids: In-vivo bioequivalence. http://www.fda.gov/cder/guidance/

[356] FDA Guidance (1995b) Content and format of investigational new drug applications (INDs) for Phase 1 studies of drugs, including well-characterized, therapeutic, biotechnology-derived products. http://www.fda.gov/cder/guidance/

[357] FDA Guidance (1996) Clozapine tablets in-vivo bioequivalence and in-vitro dissolution testing. http://www.fda.gov/cder/guidance/

[358] FDA Preliminary Draft Guidance (1997a) In vivo bioequivalence studies based on population and individual bioequivalence approaches.

[359] FDA Guidance (1997b) Drug metabolism, drug interaction studies in the drug development process: Studies in-vitro. http://www.fda.gov/cder/guidance/

[360] FDA Guidance (1998a) Pharmacokinetics in patients with impaired renal function — Study design, data analysis, and recommendations for dosing and labeling. http://www.fda.gov/cder/guidance/

[361] FDA Letter regarding IND 51,171 (March 17, 1998) Private communication on Bayesian analysis of Study 539 for Paxil-CR.

[362] FDA Draft Guidance (1999a) BA and BE studies for orally administered drug products: General considerations.

[363] FDA Draft Guidance (1999b) Average, population, and individual approaches to establishing bioequivalence.

[364] FDA Guidance (1999c) In-vivo drug metabolism, drug-interaction studies — Study design, data analysis, and recommendations for dosing and labeling. http://www.fda.gov/cder/guidance/

[365] FDA Guidance (1999d) Population Pharmacokinetics. http://www.fda.gov/cder/guidance/

[366] FDA Guidance (2000a) Waiver of in vivo bioavailability and bioequivalence studies for immediate-release solid oral dosage forms based on a biopharmaceutics classification system. http://www.fda.gov/cder/guidance/

[367] FDA Guidance (2000b) Bioavailability and bioequivalence studies for orally administered drug products: General considerations.

[368] FDA Guidance (2000c) Levothyroxine sodium tablets — In vivo pharmacokinetic and bioavailability studies and in vitro dissolution testing. http://www.fda.gov/cder/guidance/

[369] FDA Guidance (2001) Statistical approaches to establishing bioequivalence. http://www.fda.gov/cder/guidance/

[370] FDA Guidance (2002a) Food-effect bioavailability and fed bioequivalence studies. http://www.fda.gov/cder/guidance/

[371] FDA Draft Guidance (2002b) Estimating the safe starting dose in clinical trials for therapeutics in adult healthy volunteers. http://www.fda.gov/cder/guidance/

[372] FDA Guidance (2003a) Exposure-response relationships – Study design, data analysis, and regulatory applications. http://www.fda.gov/cder/guidance/

[373] FDA Guidance (2003b) Bioavailability and bioequivalence studies for orally administered drug products: General considerations. http://www.fda.gov/cder/guidance/

[374] FDA Guidance (2003c) Pharmacokinetics in patients with impaired hepatic function: Study design, data analysis, and impact on dosing and labeling. http://www.fda.gov/cder/guidance/

[375] FDA Draft Guidance (2003d) Bioavailability and bioequivalence studies for nasal aerosols and nasal sprays for local action. Appended with statistical information (1999). http://www.fda.gov/cder/guidance/

[376] FDA Draft Guidance (2003e) Statistical guidance on reporting results from studies evaluating diagnostic tests. www.fda.gov/cdrh/guidance.html.

[377] FDA Position Paper (2004a) Challenge and opportunity on the critical path to new medical products.

[378] FDA Draft Guidance (2004b) Pharmacokinetics in pregnancy — Study design, data analysis, and impact on dosing and labeling. http://www.fda.gov/cder/guidance/

[379] FDA Guidance for Industry (2004c) E5 — Ethnic factors in the acceptability of foreign clinical data: Questions and answers. http://www.fda.gov/cder/guidance/

[380] FDA Guidance (2005a) Clinical trial endpoints for the approval of cancer drugs and biologics. http://www.fda.gov/cder/guidance/

[381] FDA Draft Guidance (2005b) Drug-diagnostic co-development concept paper. www.fda.gov/cdrh/guidance.html.

[382] FDA Guidance (2006a) Exploratory IND studies. http://www.fda.gov/cder/guidance/

[383] FDA Guidance (2006b) Guidance for industry — Providing regulatory submissions in electronic format — Human pharmaceutical product applications and related submissions using the eCTD specifications. http://www.fda.gov/cder/guidance/

[384] FDA Draft Guidance (2006c) Draft guidance for the use of Bayesian statistics in medical device clinical trials. http://www.fda.gov/cdrh/guidance.html

[385] FDA Guidance (2007a) Guidance for industry — Drug-induced liver injury: Premarketing clinical evaluation. http://www.fda.gov/cder/guidance/

[386] FDA Guidance (2007b) Guidance for industry — Clinical data needed to support the licensure of seasonal inactivated influenza vaccines. http://www.fda.gov/cder/guidance/

[387] FDA Guidance (2008a) Draft guidance for industry — End-of-phase 2A meetings. http://www.fda.gov/cder/guidance/

[388] FDA Guidance (2008b) Guidance for industry — General principles for the development of vaccines to protect against global infectious diseases. http://www.fda.gov/cber/guidlines.htm

[389] FDA Guidance (2009a) Guidance for industry — Requirements for submission of bioequivalence data; Final rule. http://www.fda.gov/cder/guidance/

[390] FDA Guidance (2009b) Draft guidance for industry — Postmarketing studies and clinical trials. http://www.fda.gov/cder/guidance/

[391] FDA Guidance (2010a) Draft guidance on progesterone. http://www.fda.gov/cder/guidance/

[392] FDA Guidance (2010b) Draft guidance for industry — Non-inferiority clinical trials. http://www.fda.gov/cder/guidance/

[393] FDA Guidance (2010c) Draft guidance for industry — Qualification process for drug development tools. http://www.fda.gov/cder/guidance/

[394] FDA Guidance (2010d) Draft guidance for industry — Adaptive design clinical trials for drugs and biologics. http://www.fda.gov/cder/guidance/

[395] FDA Guidance (2011a) Updated draft guidance on progesterone. http://www.fda.gov/cder/guidance/

[396] FDA Guidance (2012) Draft guidance for industry — Determining the extent of safety data collection needed in late stage premarket and postapproval clinical investigations. http://www.fda.gov/cder/guidance/

[397] FDA Guidance (2012b) Draft guidance for industry — Drug interaction studies - Study design, data analysis, implications for dosing, and labeling recommendations. http://www.fda.gov/cder/guidance/

[398] Federer, W.T., Raghavarao, D. (1975) On augmented designs. *Biometrics*, **31**, 29–35.

[399] Fedorov, V., Hackl, P. (1997) *Model-Oriented Design of Experiments.* Springer, New York.

[400] Fedorov, V., Jones, B., Jones, M., Zhigljavsky, A. (2004) Estimation of the treatment difference in multicenter trials. *Journal of Biopharmaceutical Statistics*, **14, No. 4**, 1037–1063.

[401] Fedorov, V., Liu, T. (2005) *Randomized Discontinuation Trials: Design and Efficiency.* GSK BDS Technical Report 2005-03.

[402] Fedorov, V., Mannino, F., Zhang, R. (2009) Consequences of dichotomization. *Pharmaceutical Statistics*, **8**, 50–61.

[403] Feingold, M., Gillespie, B.W. (1996) Cross-over trials with censored data. *Statistics in Medicine*, **15**, 953–967.

[404] Fenech, A., Harville, D. (1991) Exact confidence sets for variance components in unbalanced mixed linear models. *The Annals of Statistics*, **19**, 1771–1785.

[405] Fieller, E. (1954) Some problems in interval estimation. *Journal of the Royal Statistical Society, Series B*, **16**, 175–185.

[406] Fiessinger, J., Huisman, M., Davidson, B., Bounameaux, H., Francis, C., Eriksson, H., Lundstrom, T., Berkowitz, S., Nystrom, P., Thorsen, M., Ginsberg, J for the THRIVE Treatment Study Investigators. (2006) Ximelagatran vs. low-molecular-weight heparin and warfarin for the treatment of deep vein thrombosis: A randomized trial. *Journal of the American Medical Association*, **293**, 681–689.

[407] Filloon, T.G. (1995) Estimating the minimum therapeutically effective dose of a compound via regression modeling and percentile estimation. *Statistics in Medicine*, **14**, 925–932.

[408] Fine, G. (2007) Consequences of delayed treatment effects on analysis of time-to-event endpoints. *Drug Information Journal*, **41**, 535–539.

[409] Fireman, B., Lee, J., Lewis, N., Bembom, O., van der Laan, M., Baxter, R. (2009) Influenza vaccination and mortality: Differentiating vaccine effects from bias. *American Journal of Epidemiology*, **170**, 650–656.

[410] Cornish, E.A., Fisher, R.A. (1937) Moments and cumulants in the specification of distributions. *Extrait de la Revue de l'Institut International de Statistique*, **4**, 1–14.

[411] Fisher, L.D., van Belle, G. (1993) *Biostatistics, A Methodology for the Health Sciences.* John Wiley and Sons, New York.

[412] Fisher, L.D. (1999) Carvedilol and the Food and Drug Administration (FDA) approval process: The FDA paradigm and reflections on hypothesis testing. *Controlled Clinical Trials*, **20**, 16–39.

[413] Flather, M., Farkouh, M., Pogue, J., Yusuf, S. (1997) Strengths and limitations of meta-analysis: Larger studies may be more reliable. *Controlled Clinical Trials*, **18**, 568–579.

[414] Fletcher, D.J., Lewis, S.M, Matthews, J.N.S. (1990) Factorial designs for cross-over clinical trials. *Statistics in Medicine*, **9**, 1121–1129.

[415] Fleiss, J.L. (1971) On the distribution of a linear combination of independent chi squares. *Journal of the American Statistical Association*, **66**, 142–144.

[416] Fleiss, J.L. (1986) Letter to the editor: On multiperiod cross-over studies. *Biometrics*, 449–450.

[417] Fleiss, J.L. (1989) A critique of recent research on the two treatment cross-over design. *Controlled Clinical Trials*, **10**, 237–243.

[418] Fleming, T., DeMets, D. (1996) Surrogate endpoints in clinical trials: Are we being misled? *Annals of Internal Medicine*, **125**, 605–613.

[419] Fleming, T. (2005) Surrogate endpoints and FDA's accelerated approval process. *Health Affairs*, **24**, 67–78.

[420] Fleming, T., Koch, G., Powers, J. (2008) Current issues in non-inferiority trials. *Statistics in Medicine*, **27**, 317–352.

[421] Floyd, J., Nguyen, D., Lobins, R., Bashir, Q., Doll, D., Perry, M. (2005) Cardiotoxicity of cancer therapy. *Journal of Clinical Oncology*, **23**, 7685–7696.

[422] Fluehler, H., Hirtz, J., Moser, H.A. (1981) An aid to decision making in bioequivalence assessment. *Journal of Pharmacokinetics and Biopharmaceutics*, **9**, 235–243.

[423] Fosser, C., Duczynski, G., Agin, M., Wicker, P., Darpo, B. (2009) Comparison of manual and automated measurements of the QT interval in healthy volunteers: An analysis of five thorough QT studies. *Clinical Pharmacology and Therapeutics*, **86**, 503–506.

[424] Fox, A. (2010) Biosimilar medicines — New challenges for a new class of medicine. *Journal of Biopharmaceutical Statistics*, **20**, 3–9.

[425] Frangakis, C.E., Rubin, D.B. (2002) Principal stratification in causal inference. *Biometrics*, **58**, 21–29.

[426] Freedman, L., Spiegelhalter, D., Parmar, M. (1994) The what, why, and how of Bayesian clinical trials monitoring. *Statistics in Medicine*, **13**, 1371–1383.

[427] Freeman, P. (1989) The performance of the two-stage analysis of two treatment, two period cross-over trials. *Statistics in Medicine*, **8**, 1421–1432.

[428] Freidlin, B., Simon, R. (2005) Evaluation of randomized discontinuation design. *Journal of Clinical Oncology*, **23**, 5094–5098.

[429] Freidlin, B., Korn, E. (2007) Release of data from an ongoing randomised clinical trial for sample size adjustment or planning. *Statistics in Medicine*, **26**, 4074–4082.

[430] French, N., Gordon, S., Mwalukomo, T., White, S., Mwafulirwa, G., Longwe, H., Mwaiponya, M., Zijlstra, E., Molyneux, M., Gilks, C. (2010) A trial of 7-valent pneumococcal conjugate vaccine in HIV-infected adults. *New England Journal of Medicine*, **362**, 812–822.

[431] Friberg, L., Isbister, G., Duffull, S. (2005) Pharmacokinetic-pharmacodynamic modelling of QT interval prolongation following citalopram overdoses. *British Journal of Clinical Pharmacology*, **61**, 177–190.

[432] Fridericia, L. (1920) Die systolendauer im elecktrokardiogramm bei normalen menschen und bei herzkranken. *Acta Medica Scandinavia*, **53**, 469–486.

[433] Friede, T., Kieser, M. (2006) Sample size recalculation in internal pilot study designs: A review. *Biometrical Journal*, **48**, 537–555.

[434] Friedman, L., Furberg, C., DeMets, D. (1998) *Fundamentals of Clinical Trials, 3 ed.* Springer, New York.

[435] Friesen, M.H., Walker, S.E. (1999) Are the current bioequivalence standards sufficient for the acceptance of narrow therapeutic index drugs? Utilization of a computer simulated warfarin bioequivalence model. *Journal of Pharmacy and Pharmaceutical Sciences*, **2**, 15–22.

[436] Frison, L., Pocock, S. (1992) Repeated measures in clinical trials: Analysis using mean summary statistics and its implications for design. *Statistics in Medicine*, **11**, 1685–1704.

[437] Gaffney, M. (1992) Variance components in comparative bioavailability studies. *Journal of Pharmaceutical Sciences*, **81**, 315–317.

[438] Gallo, P., Chuang-Stein, C., Dragalin, V., Gaydos, B., Krams, M., Pinheiro, J. (2006) Adaptive designs in clinical drug development — An executive summary of the PhRMA working group with comments and rejoinder. *Journal of Biopharmaceutical Statistics*, **16**, 275–312.

[439] Ganju, J., Izu, A., Anemona, A. (2008) Sample size for equivalence trials: A case study from a vaccine lot consistency trial. *Statistics in Medicine*, **27**, 3743–3754.

[440] Garcia-Arieta, A., Gordon, J. (2012) Bioequivalence requirements in the European Union: Critical discussion. *The AAPS Journal*, **14**, 738–748.

[441] Gardner, W., Lidz, C.W., Hartwig, K.C. (2005) Authors' reports about research integrity problems in clinical trials. *Contemporary Clinical Trials*, **26**, 244–251.

[442] Garthwaite, P., Kadane, J., O'Hagan, A. (2005) Statistical methods for eliciting probability distributions. *Journal of the American Statistical Association*, **100**, 680–700.

[443] Gaudreault, J., Potvin, D., Lavigne, J., Lalonde, R.L. (1998) Truncated area under the curve as a measure of relative extent of bioavailability: Evaluation using experimental data and Monte Carlo simulations. *Pharmaceutical Research*, **15, No. 10**, 1621–1629.

[444] Geischke, R., Steimer, J.-L. (2000) Pharmacometrics: Modeling and simulation tools to improve decision making in clinical drug development. *European Journal of Drug Metabolism and Pharmacokinetics*, **25**, 49–58.

[445] Geisser, S. (1982) Aspects of the predictive and estimative approaches in the determination of probabilities. *Biometrics Supplement: Current Topics in Biostatistics and Epidemiology*, 75–85.

[446] Gelfland, A.E., Hills, S.E., Racine-Poon, A., Smith, A.F.-M. (1990a) Illustration of Bayesian inference in normal data models using Gibbs sampling. *Journal of the American Statistical Association*, **85**, 972–985.

[447] Gelfand, A.E., Smith, A.F.-M. (1990b) Sampling-based approaches to calculating marginal densities. *Journal of the American Statistical Association*, **85**, 398–409.

[448] Gelman, A., Carlin, J., Stern, H., Rubin, D. (2004) *Bayesian Data Analysis, 2nd ed.* Chapman and Hall, CRC Press, London.

[449] Geman, S., Geman, D. (1984) Stochastic relaxation, Gibbs distributions, and the Bayesian restoration of images. *IEEE Transactions on Pattern Analysis and Machine Intelligence*, **6**, 721–741.

[450] Generali, J.A., Danish, M.A., Rosenbaum, S.E. (1995) Knowledge of and attitudes about adverse drug reaction reporting among Rhode Island pharmacists. *The Annals of Pharmacotherapy*, **29**, 365–369.

[451] George, E.I., McCulloch, R.E. (1993) Variable selection via Gibbs sampling. *Journal of the American Statistical Association*, **88, No. 423**, 881–889.

[452] Genz, A., Miwa, T., T, X. M., and Hothorn. (2015) R package mvtnorm: Multivariate normal and t distributions.

[453] Ghosh, K., Hesney, M., Sarkar, S., Thiyagarajan, B. (1996) Comprehensive criteria for population and individual bioequivalence. *Proceedings of the American Statistical Association, Biopharmaceutics Chapter*, 77-81.

[454] Ghosh, P., Khattree, R. (2003) Bayesian approach to average bioequivalence using Bayes' factor. *Journal of Biopharmaceutical Statistics*, **13**, 719–734.

[455] Ghosh, P., Rosner, G. (2007) A semi-parametric Bayesian approach to average bioequivalence. *Statistics in Medicine*, **26**, 1224–1236.

[456] Ghosh, S., Majumder, P.P. (1999) Mapping a quantitative trait locus via the EM algorithm and Bayesian classification. *Genetic Epidemiology*, **19**, 97–126.

[457] Giesbrecht, F., Burns, J. (1985) Two-stage analysis based on a mixed model: Large sample asymptotic theory and small-sample simulation results. *Biometrics*, **41**, 477–486.

[458] Gilbert, P., Qin, L., Self, S. (2008) Evaluating a surrogate endpoint at three levels, with application to vaccine development. *Statistics in Medicine*, **27**, 4758–4778.

[459] Gilbert, P. (2012) Assessing immune correlates of protection via estimation of the vaccine efficacy curve. *International Society for Clinical Biostatistics, Vaccines Subcommittee Web Seminar Series, November 2012.*

[460] Gilbertson, R.J. (2005) ERBB2 in pediatric cancer: Innocent until proven guilty. *The Oncologist*, **10**, 508–517.

[461] Gilks, W.R., Richardson, S., Spiegelhalter, D. (1996) *Markov Chain Monte Carlo in Practice*, Chapman and Hall, New York.

[462] Gilmour, A.R., Thompson, R., Cullis, B.R. (1995) Average information REML: An efficient algorithm for variance parameter estimation in linear mixed models. *Biometrics*, **51**, 1440–1450.

[463] Glickman, M.E., Kao, M.-F. (2005) Apo-E genotypes and cardiovascular diseases: A sensitivity study using cross-validatory criteria. *Biometrical Journal 47*, **4**, 541–553.

[464] Glimm, E., Maurer, W., Bretz, F. (2009) Heirarchical testing of multiple endpoints in group-sequential trials. *Statistics in Medicine*, **29**, 219–228.

[465] Glueck, D.H., Muller, K.E. (2003) Adjusting power for a baseline covariate in linear models. *Statistics in Medicine*, **22**, 2535–2551.

[466] Gobburu, J., Marroum, P. (2001) Utilisation of pharmacokinetic-pharmacodynamic modelling and simulation in regulatory decision making. *Clinical Pharmacokinetics*, **40**, 883–892.

[467] Godbillon, J., Cardot, J.B., LeCaillon, G., Sioufi, A. (1996) Bioequivalence assessment: A pharmaceutical industry perspective. *European Journal of Drug Metabolism and Pharmacokinetics*, **21**, 153–158.

[468] Godwin, H.J. (1955) On generalizations of Tchebychef's inequality. *American Statistical Association Journal*, 923–945.

[469] Goldberg-Alberts, R., Page, S. (2006) Multivariate analysis of adverse events. *Drug Information Journal*, **40**, 99–110.

[470] Goldblatt, D., Southern, J., Andrews, N., Ashton, L., Burbidge, P., Woodgate, S., Pebody, R., Miller, E. (2009) The immunogenicity of 7-valent pneumococcal conjugate vaccine versus 23-valent polysaccharide vaccine in adults aged 50-80 years. *Clinical Infectious Diseases*, **49**, 1318–1325.

[471] Goldblatt, D., Ashton, L., Zhang, Y., Antonello, J., Marchese, R. (2011) Comparison of a new multiplex binding assay versus the enzyme-linked immunosorbent assay for measurement of serotype-specific pneumococcal capsular polysaccharide IgG. *Clinical Vaccine and Immunology*, **18**, 1744–1751.

[472] Golkowski, D., Friede, T., Kieser, M. (2014) Blinded sample size re-estimation in cross-over bioequivalence trials. *Pharmaceutical Statistics*, **13**, 157–162.

[473] Gonen, M. (2005) A Bayesian evaluation of enrolling additional patients at the maximum tolerated dose in phase I trials. *Contemporary Clinical Trials*, **26**, 131–140.

[474] Good, I.J. (1993) Comments, conjectures, and conclusions. *Journal of Statistical Computation and Simulation*, **47**, 89–90.

[475] Goodman, S., Berlin, J. (1994) The use of predictive confidence intervals when planning experiments and the misuse of power when interpreting results. *Annals of Internal Medicine*, **121**, 200–206.

[476] Goodsaid, F., Frueh, F. (2007) Biomarker qualification pilot process at the US Food and Drug Administration. *The AAPS Journal*, **9**, E105–E108.

[477] Gorst-Rasmussen, A., Spiegelhalter, D., Bull, C. (2007) Monitoring the introduction of a surgical intervention with long term consequences. *Statistics in Medicine*, **26**, 512–531.

[478] Gossger, N., Snape, M., Yu, L.-M., Finn, A., Bona, G., Esposito, S., Principi, N., Diez-Domingo, J., Sokal, E., Becker, B., Kieninger, D., Prymula, R., Dull, P., Ypma, E., Toneatto, D., Kimura, A., Pollard, A., for the European MenB Vaccine Study Group (2012) Immunogenicity and tolerability of recombinant serogroup B meningococcal vaccine administered with or without routine infant vaccinations

according to different immunization schedules. *Journal of the American Medical Association*, **307**, 573–582.

[479] Gott, J. (1982) Creation of open universes from de Sitter space. *Nature*, **295**, 304–307.

[480] Gotzsche, P. (2006) Lessons from and cautions about non-inferiority and equivalence randomized trials. *Journal of the American Medical Association*, **295**, 1172–1174.

[481] Gould, A.L. (1993) Sample sizes for event rate equivalence trials using prior information. *Statistics in Medicine*, **12**, 2009–2023.

[482] Gould, A.L. (1995) Group sequential extensions of a standard bioequivalence testing procedure. *Journal of Pharmacokinetics and Biopharmaceutics*, **23**, 57–86.

[483] Gould, A.L. (1997) Discussion of individual bioequivalence by M.L. Chen. *Journal of Biopharmaceutical Statistics*, **7**, 23–29.

[484] Gould, A.L. (2000) A practical approach for evaluating population and individual bioequivalence. *Statistics in Medicine*, **19**, 2721–2740.

[485] Gould, A.L. (2005) timing of futility analyses for 'proof of concept' trials. *Statistics in Medicine*, **24**, 1815–1835.

[486] Gould, A. (2007) Accounting for multiplicity in the evaluation of 'signals' obtained by data mining from spontaneous report adverse event databases. *Biometrical Journal*, **49**, 151–165.

[487] Grahnan, A., Hammarlund, M., Lundqvist, T. (1984) Implications of intra individual variability in bioavailability studies of furosemide. *European Journal of Clinical Pharmacology*, **27**, 595–602.

[488] Graybill, F.A., Wang, C.H. (1980) Confidence intervals on nonnegative linear combinations of variances. *Journal of the American Statistical Association*, **75**, 869–873.

[489] Green, W. (2005) New questions regarding bioequivalence of levothyroxine preparations: A clinician's response. *The AAPS Journal*, **7**, E54–E58.

[490] Grieve, A.P. (1985) A Bayesian analysis of the two-period cross-over design for clinical trials. *Biometrics*, **21**, 467–480.

[491] Grieve, A.P. (1990) Cross-over vs. parallel designs. In *Statistical Methodology in the Pharmaceutical Sciences*, Berry, D., ed., 239–270, Marcel Dekker, New York.

[492] Grieve, A.P. (2007) 25 years of Bayesian methods in the pharmaceutical industry: A personal, statistical bummel. *Pharmaceutical Statistics*, **6**, 261–281.

[493] Grizzle, J.E. (1965) The two-period changeover design and its use in clinical trials. *Biometrics*, **21**, 467–480.

[494] Guilbaud, O. (1993) Exact inference about the within-subject variability in 2×2 cross-over studies. *Journal of the American Statistical Association*, **88**, 939–946.

[495] Guilbaud, O. (1999) Exact comparisons of means and variances in 2×2 cross-over trials. *Drug Information Journal*, **33**, 455–469.

[496] Gwaza, L., Gordon, J., Welink, J., Potthast, H., Hansson, H., Stahl, M., Garcia-Arieta, A. (2012) Statistical approaches to indirectly compare bioequivalence between generics: A comparison of methodologies employing artemether/lumefrantine 20/120 mg tablets as prequalified by WHO. *European Journal of Clinical Pharmacology*, **68**, 1611–1618.

[497] Haidar, S., Davit, B., Chen, M.-L., Conner, D., Lee, L., Li, Q., Lionberger, R., Makhlouf, F., Patel, D., Schuirmann, D., Yu, L. (2007) Bioequivalence approaches for highly variable drugs and drug products. *Pharmaceutical Research*, **25**, 237–241.

[498] Haidar, S., Makhlouf, F., Schuirmann, D., Hyslop, T., Davit, B., Conner, D., Yu, L. (2008) Evaluation of a scaling approach for the bioequivalence of highly variable drugs. *AAPS Journal*, **10**, 450–454.

[499] Hald, A. (1990) *A History of Probability and Statistics and Their Applications before 1750.* John Wiley and Sons, New York.

[500] Hald, A. (1998) *A History of Mathematical Statistics from 1750 to 1930.* John Wiley and Sons, New York.

[501] Hale, M., Gillespie, W.R., Gupta, S.K., Tuk, B., Holford, N. (1996) Clinical trial simulation. *Applied Clinical Trials*, 6, 35–40.

[502] Halloran, M., Struchiner, C., Longini, I. (1997) Study designs for evaluating different efficacy and effectiveness aspects of vaccines. *American Journal of Epidemiology*, **146**, 789–803.

[503] Halloran, M. (2006) Overview of vaccine field studies: Types of effects and designs. *Journal of Biopharmaceutical Statistics*, **16**, 415–427.

[504] Halloran, M., Longini, I., Struchiner, C. (2010) *Design and Analysis of Vaccine Studies.* Springer, New York.

[505] Hammad, T., Pinhiero, S., Neyarapally, G. (2011) Secondary use of randomized controlled trials to evaluate drug safety: A review of methodological considerations. *Clinical Trials*, **8**, 559–570.

[506] Hanauske, A.-R., Chen, V., Paoletti, P., Niyikiza, C. (2001) Pemetrexed disodium: A novel antifolate clinically active against multiple solid tumors. *The Oncologist*, **6**, 363–373.

[507] Hanna, N., Shepherd, F.A., Fossella, F.V., Pereira, J.R., DeMarinis, F., von Pawel, J., Gatzemeier, U., Tsao, T.C.Y., Pless, M., Muller, T., Lim, H.-L., Desch, C., Szondy, K., Gervais, R., Shaharyar, Manegold, C., Paul, S., Paoletti, P., Einhorn, L., Bunn, P.A. (2004) Randomized phase III trial of pemetrexed versus docetaxel in patients with non-small-cell lung cancer previously treated with chemotherapy. *Journal of Clinical Oncology*, **22, No. 9**, 1589–1597.

[508] Hare, D., Foster, T. (1990) The Orange Book: The FDA's advice on therapeutic equivalence. *American Pharmacy*, **NS30**, 35–37.

[509] Harel, O., Zhou, X.-H. (2007) Multiple imputation: Review of theory, implementation, and software. *Statistics in Medicine*, **26**, 3057–3077.

[510] Harrell, F. (2001) *Regression Modelling Strategies.* Springer, New York.

[511] Harrison, L.I. (2000) Commentary on the FDA draft guidance for bioequivalence studies for nasal aerosols and nasal sprays for local action: An industry view. *Journal of Clinical Pharmacology*, **40**, 701–707.

[512] Harville, D.A. (1969) Expression of variance-component estimators as linear combinations of independent noncentral chi-square variates. *The Annals of Mathematical Statistics*, **40, No. 6**, 2189–2194.

[513] Harville, D.A. (1976) Confidence intervals and sets for linear combinations of fixed and random effects. *Biometrics*, **32**, 403–407.

[514] Harville, D.A. (1977) Maximum likelihood approaches to variance component estimation and to related problems. *Journal of the American Statistical Association*, **72**, 320–340.

[515] Harville, D.A. (1978) Alternative formulations and procedures for the two-way mixed model. *Biometrics*, **34**, 441–453.

[516] Harville, D.A. (1979) Some useful representations for constrained mixed-model estimation. *American Statistical Association*, **74, No. 365**, 200–206.

[517] Harville, D.A. (1981) Unbiased and minimum-variance unbiased estimation of estimable functions for fixed linear models with arbitrary covariance structure. *The Annals of Statistics*, **9, No. 3**, 633–637.

[518] Harville, D.A. (1985) Decomposition of prediction error. *Journal of the American Statistical Association*, **80**, 132–138.

[519] Harville, D.A. (1990) BLUP (best linear unbiased prediction) and beyond. *AdStMetGen*, 239–276.

[520] Harville, D.A., Carriquiry, A.L. (1992) Classical and Bayesian prediction as applied to an unbalanced mixed linear model. *Biometrics*, **48**, 987–1003.

[521] Harville, D.A., Jeske, D.R. (1992) Mean squared error of estimation or prediction under a general linear model. *Journal of the American Statistical Association*, **87**, 724–731.

[522] Harville, D.A., Zimmermann, A.G. (1996) The posterior distribution of the fixed and random effects in a mixed-effects linear model. *Journal of Statistical Computing and Simulation*, **54**, 211–229.

[523] Hasler, M., Hothorn, L. (2012) A multivariate Williams-type trend procedure. *Statistics in Biopharmaceutical Research*, **4**, 57–65.

[524] Hasselblad, V., Kong, D. (2001) Statistical methods for comparison to placebo in active-control trials. Drug Information Journal, 35, 435–449.

[525] Hauck, W.W., Anderson S. (1984) A new statistical procedure for testing equivalence in two-group comparative bioavailability trials. *Journal of Pharmacokinetics and Biopharmaceutics*, **12**, 83–91.

[526] Hauck, W.W., Anderson S. (1986) A proposal for interpreting and reporting negative studies. *Statistics in Medicine*, **5**, 203–209.

[527] Hauck, W.W., Anderson, S. (1991) Individual bioequivalence: What matters to the patient. *Statistics in Medicine*, **10**, 959–960.

[528] Hauck, W.W., Anderson S. (1992) Types of bioequivalence and related statistical considerations. *International Journal of Clinical Pharmacology, Therapy, and Toxicology*, **30**, 181–187.

[529] Hauck, W.W., Anderson S. (1994) Measuring switchability and presciptability: When is average bioequivalence sufficient? *Journal of Pharmacokinetics and Biopharmaceutics*, **22**, 551–564.

[530] Hauck, W.W., Anderson, S. (1999) Some issues in the design and analysis of equivalence trials. *Drug Information Journal*, **33**, 109–118.

[531] Hauck, W.W., Hyslop, T., Anderson, S., Bois, F.Y., Tozer, T.N. (1995) Statistical and regulatory considerations for multiple measures in bioequivalence testing. *Clinical Research and Regulatory Affairs*, **12**, 249–265.

[532] Hauck, W.W, Chen, M.L., Hyslop, T., Patnaik, P., Shuirmann, D., Williams, R., for the FDA Individual Bioequivalence Working Group (1996) Mean differences versus variability reduction: Tradeoff in aggregate measures for individual bioequivalence. *International Journal of Clinical Pharmacology, Therapy, and Toxicology*, **34**, 535–541.

[533] Hauck, W.W., Hauschke, D., Diletti, E., Bois, F.Y., Steinijans, V.W., Anderson, S. (1997a) Choice of Student's t or Wilcoxon based confidence intervals for assessment of bioequivalence. *Journal of Biopharmaceutical Statistics*, **7**, 179–189.

[534] Hauck, W.W, Bois, F.Y., Hyslop, T., Gee, L., Anderson, S. (1997b) A parametric approach to population bioequivalence. *Statistics in Medicine*, **16**, 441–454.

[535] Hauck, W.W., Preston, P.E., Bois, F.Y. (1997c) A group sequential approach to cross-over trials for average bioequivalence. *Journal of Biopharmaceutical Statistics*, **7**, 87–96.

[536] Hauck, W.W., Hyslop, T., Chen, M.L., Patnaik, R., Williams, R.L., and the FDA Population/Individual Bioequivalence Working Group (2000) Subject-by-formulation interaction in bioequivalence: Conceptual and statistical issues. *Pharmaceutical Research*, **17**, 375–380.

[537] Hauck, W.W., Parekh, A., Lesko, L., Chen, M.-L., Williams, R. (2001) Limits of 80%-125% for AUC and 70%-143% for Cmax — What is the impact on bioequivalence studies? *International Journal of Clinical Pharmacology and Therapeutics*, **39**, 350–355.

[538] Hauschke, D., Steinijans, V.W., Diletti, E. (1990) A distribution free procedure for the statistical analysis of bioequivalence studies. *International Journal of Clinical Pharmacology, Therapy, and Toxicology*, **28**, 72–78.

[539] Hauschke, D., Steinijans, V.W., Hothorn, L.A. (1996) A note on Welch's approximate t-solution to bioequivalence assessment. *Biometrika*, **83, No. 1**, 236–237.

[540] Hauschke, D., Hothorn, L. (1998) Safety assessment in toxicological studies: Proof of safety versus proof of hazard. In *Design and Analysis of Animal Studies in Pharmaceutical Development,* Chow, S., and Liu, J., eds., 197–226, Marcel Dekker, New York.

[541] Hauschke, D., Kieser, M., Diletti, E., Burke, M. (1999) Sample size determination for proving equivalence based on the ratio of two means for normally distributed data. *Statistics in Medicine*, **18**, 93–105.

[542] Hauschke, D., Steinijans, V.W. (2000) The US draft guidance regarding population and individual bioequivalence approaches: Comments by a research-based pharmaceutical company. *Statistics in Medicine*, **19**, 2769–2774.

[543] Hauschke, D. (2002) Letter to the Editor and Correspondence on "A Note on Sample Size Calculation in Bioequivalence Trials" by Chow and Wang (2001;28:155-169). *Journal of Pharmacokinetics and Pharmacodynamics*, **29**, 89–102.

[544] Hauschke, D., Slacik-Erben, R., Hensen, S., Kaufmann, R. (2005a) Biostatistical assessment of mutagenicity studies by including the positive control. *Biometrical Journal*, **47**, 82–87.

[545] Hauschke, D., Pigeot, I. (2005b) Establishing efficacy of a new experimental treatment in the "gold standard" design with correspondance and rejoinder. *Biometrical*, **47**, 782–798.

[546] Hauschke, D., Knoerzer, D. (2006) Letter to the editor commenting upon "Comparison of sample size formulae for 2×2 cross-over designs applied to bioequivalence trials" by Siqueira, A. et al. and reply. *Pharmaceutical Statistics*, **5**, 231–233.

[547] Hauschke, D., Steinijans, V., Pigeot, I. (2007a) *Bioequivalence Studies in Drug Development*. John Wiley & Sons, West Sussex

[548] Hauschke, D. (2007b) Letter to the editor on "An introductory note to the CHMP guideline: Choice of the non-inferiority margin and data monitoring committees" with Rejoinder by Brown, D., Volkers, P., and Day, S. *Statistics in Medicine* 2006;25:1623-1627. *Statistics in Medicine*, **26**, 230–236.

[549] Haynes, J.D. (1981) Statistical simulation study of new proposed uniformity requirement for bioequivalency studies. *Journal of Pharmaceutical Sciences*, **70**, 673–675.

[550] Hazarika, M., White, R.M., Johnson, J.R., Pazdur, R. (2004) FDA drug approval summaries: Pemetrexed (Alimta). *The Oncologist*, **9**, 482–488.

[551] Hedayat, A., Stufken, J., Yang, M. (2006) Optimal and efficient cross-over designs when subject effects are random. *Journal of the American Statistical Association*, **101**, 1031–1038.

[552] Hellriegel, E.T., Bjornsson, T.D., Hauck, W.W. (1996) Interpatient variability in bioavailability is related to the extent of absorption: Implications for bioavailability and bioequivalence studies. *Clinical Pharmacology and Therapeutics*, **60**, 601–607.

[553] Helton, T., Bavry, A., Kumbahni, D., Duggal, S., Roukoz, H., Bhatt, D. (2007) Incremental effect of clopidogrel on important outcomes in patients with cardiovascular disease. *American Journal of Cardiovascular Drugs*, **7**, 289–297.

[554] Hennekens, C., DeMets, D. (2009) Doing more harm than good: Need for a cease fire. *The American Journal of Medicine*, **122**, 315–316.

[555] Herchuelz, A. (1996) Bioequivalence assessment and the conduct of bioequivalence trials: A European point of view. *European Journal of Drug Metabolism and Pharmacokinetics*, **21**, 149–152.

[556] Higgins, J., Spiegelhalter, D. (2002) Being sceptical about meta-analyses: A Bayesian perspective on magnesium trials in myocardial infarction. *International Journal of Epidemiology*, **31**, 96–104.

[557] Higgins, J.P.T., Thompson, S.G., Spiegelhalter, D.J. (2009) A re-evaluation of random effects meta-analysis. *Journal of the Royal Statistical Society, Series A*, **172**, 137–159.

[558] Hills, M., Armitage, P. (1979) The two period cross-over trial. *British Journal of Clinical Pharmacology*, **8**, 7–20.

[559] Hilton, J. (2006) Designs of superiority and non-inferiority trials for binary responses are non-interchangeable. *Biometrical Journal*, **48**, 934–947.

[560] Hilton, J. (2008) Noninferiority trial designs for odds ratios and risk differences. *Statistics in Medicine*, **29**, 982–993.

[561] Hinkelmann, K., Kempthorne, O. (1994) *Design and Analysis of Experiments, Volume I: Introduction to Experimental Design.* John Wiley and Sons, New York.

[562] Hirschfeld, S., Shapiro, A., Dagher, R., Pazdur, R. (2000) Pediatric oncology: Regulatory initiatives. *The Oncologist*, **5**, 441–444.

[563] Hirschfeld, S., Pazdur, R. (2002) Oncology drug development: United States Food and Drug Administration perspective. *Critical Reviews in Oncology and Hematology*, **42**, 137–143.

[564] Hochberg, Y. (1988) A sharper Bonferroni procedure for multiple tests of significance. *Biometrika*, **75**, 800–802.

[565] Hodges, J., Lehman, E. (1963) Estimates of location based on rank tests. *Annals of Mathematical Statistics*, **34**, 598–611.

[566] Hoenig, J., Heisey, D. (2001) The abuse of power: The pervasive fallacy of power calculations for data analysis. *The American Statistician*, **55**, 19–24.

[567] Holder, D., Hsuan, F. (1993a) Moment based criteria for determining bioequivalence. *Biometrika*, **80**, 835–846.

[568] Holder, D., Hsuan, F. (1993b) A moment based criteria for determining individual bioequivalence. *Drug Information Journal*, **29**, 965–979.

[569] Holford, N.H.G., Sheiner, L.B. (1981) Pharmacokinetic and pharmacodynamic modeling in vivo. *CRC critical reviews in bioengineering*, **July 1981**, 273–322.

[570] Holford, N.H.G., Hale, M., Ko, H.C., Steimer, J.-L., Sheiner, L.B., Peck, C.C. (1999) Simulation in drug development: Good practices. *Center for Drug Development Science*, www.dml.georgetown.edu/cdds

[571] Holford, N.H.G., Kimko, H. C., Monteleone, J.P.R., Peck, C.C. (2000) Simulation of clinical trials. *Annual Review Pharmacology*, **40**, 209–234.

[572] Holford, N., Karlsson, M. (2007) Time for quantitative clinical pharmacology: A proposal for a pharmacometrics curriculum. *Clinical Pharmacology and Therapeutics*, **82**, 103–105.

[573] Hollander, M., Wolfe, D. (1999) *Nonparametric Statistical Methods.* John Wiley and Sons, New York.

[574] Holm, S. (1979) A simple sequentially rejective multiple test procedure. *Scandinavian Journal of Statistics*, **6**, 65–70.

[575] Home, P.D., Pocock, S.J., Beck-Nielsen, H., Curtis, P.S., Gomis, R., Hanefeld, M., Jones, N., Komajda, M., McMurray, J.J., for the RECORD study team (2009) Rosiglitazone evaluated for cardiovascular outcomes in oral agent combination therapy for type 2 diabetes (RECORD): A multi-centre, randomised, open-label trial. *Lancet*, **373**, 2125–2135.

[576] Hommel, G. (1988) A stagewise rejective multiple test procedure based on a modified Bonferroni test. *Biometrika*, **75**, 383–386.

[577] Honig, P., Woosley, R., Zamani, K., Conner, D., Cantilena, L. (1992) Changes in the pharmacokinetics and electrocardiographic pharmacodynamics of terfenadine with concomitant administration of erythromycin. *Clinical Pharmacology and Therapeutics*, **52**, 231–238.

[578] Honig, P. (2007) The value and future of clinical pharmacology. *Clinical Pharmacology and Therapeutics*, **81**, 17–18.

[579] Honig, P. (2010) Systematic reviews and meta-analyses in the new age of transparency. *Clinical Pharmacology and Therapeutics*, **88**, 155–157.

[580] Horne, A., Lachenbruch, P., Getson, P., Hsu, H. (2001a) Analysis of studies to evaluate immune response to combination vaccines. *Clinical Infectious Diseases*, **33**, S306–S311.

[581] Horne, A., Lachenbruch, P., Goldenthal, K. (2001b) Intent-to-treat analysis and preventive vaccine efficacy. *Vaccine*, **19**, 319–326.

[582] Horne, A., Clifford, J., Goldenthal, K., Kleppinger, C., Lachenbruch, P. (2004) Preventive vaccines against bioterrorism: Evaluation of efficacy and safety. *Vaccine*, **23**, 84–90.

[583] Horton, J., Bushwick, B. (1999) Warfarin therapy: Evolving strategies in anticoagulation. *American Family Physician*, **59**, 635–648.

[584] Hosmane, B., Locke, C. (2005) A simulation study of power in thorough QT/QTc studies and a normal approximation for planning purposes. *Drug Information Journal*, **39**, 447–455.

[585] Hotta, K., Ueoka, H. (2005) New cytotoxic agents: A review of the literature. *Critical Reviews in Oncology and Hematology*, **55**, 45–65.

[586] Howard, G. (2007) Nonconventional study designs: Approaches to provide more precise estimates of treatment effects with a smaller sample size, but at a cost. *Stroke*, **38**, 804–808.

[587] Howe, W.G. (1974) Approximate confidence limits on the mean of X+Y where X and Y are two tabled independent random variables. *Journal of the American Statistical Association*, 69, 789–794.

[588] Hrobjartsson, A., Boutron, I. (2011) Blinding in randomised clinical trials: Imposed impartiality. *Clinical Pharmacology and Therapeutics*, **90**, 732–736.

[589] Hsiao, C.-F., Xu, J.-Z. (2005) A two-stage design for bridging studies. *Journal of Biopharmaceutical Statistics*, **15**, 75–83.

[590] Hsu, H.-C., Lu, H.-L. (1997) On confidence limits associated with Chow and Shao's joint confidence region approach for assessment of bioequivalence. *Journal of Biopharmaceutical Statistics*, **7, No. 1**, 125–134.

[591] Hsu, J.C., Hwang, J.-T.G., Liu, H.-K., Ruberg, S.J. (1994) Confidence limits associated with tests for bioequivalence. *Biometrika*, **81**, 103–114.

[592] Hsu, J. (1996) *Multiple Comparisons: Theory and Methods.* Chapman & Hall, CRC Press, London.

[593] Hsuan, F.C. (2000) Some statistical considerations on the FDA draft guidance for individual bioequivalence. *Statistics in Medicine*, **19**, 2879–2884.

[594] Hu, Z., Follmann, D. (2007) Statistical methods for active extension trials. *Statistics in Medicine*, **26**, 2433–2448.

[595] Huang, J., Liu, N., Pourahmadi, M., Liu, L. (2006) Covariance matrix selection and estimation via penalised normal likelihood. *Biometrika*, **93**, 85–98.

[596] Huang, S.-M., Temple, R. (2008) Is this drug or dose for you? Impact and consideration of ethnic factors in global drug development, regulatory review, and clinical practice. *Clinical Pharmacology and Therapeutics*, **84**, 287–294.

[597] Hudgens, M., Hoering, A., Self, S. (2003) On the analysis of viral load endpoints in HIV vaccine trials. *Statistics in Medicine*, **22**, 2281–2298.

[598] Hudgens, M., Gilbert, P., Self, S. (2004) Endpoints in vaccine trials. *Statistical Methods in Medical Research*, **13**, 89–114.

[599] Hughes, M.D., Daniels, M.J., Fischl, M.A., Kim, S., Schooley, R.T. (1998) CD4 cell count as a surrogate endpoint in HIV clinical trials: A meta-analysis of studies of the AIDS clinical trials group. *AIDS*, **12, No. 14**, 1823–1832.

[600] Huitson, A. (1955) A method for assigning confidence limits to linear combinations of variances. *Biometrika*, **42**, 471–479.

[601] Hulting, F.L., Harville, D.A. (1991) Some Bayesian and non-Bayesian procedures for the analysis of comparative experiments and for small-area estimation: Computational aspects, frequentist properties, and relationships. *Journal of the American Statistical Association*, **86**, 557–568.

[602] Hung, H.M., Wang, S.-J., O'Neill, R. (2005) A regulatory perspective on choice of margin and statistical inference issue in non-inferiority trials. *Biometrical Journal*, **47**, 28–36.

[603] Hung, H.M., Wang, S.-J., O'Neill, R. (2006a) Methodological issues with adaption of clinical trial design. *Pharmaceutical Statistics*, **5**, 99–107.

[604] Hung, H.M., O'Neill, R., Wang, S.-J., Lawrence, J. (2006b) A regulatory view on adaptive/flexible clinical trial design. *Biometrical Journal*, **48**, 565–573.

[605] Hung, H.M., Wang, S.-J. (2009a) Some controversial multiple testing problems in regulatory applications. *Journal of Biopharmaceutical Statistics*, **19**, 1–11.

[606] Hung, H.M., Wang, S.-J., O'Neill, R. (2009b) Challenges and regultory experiences with non-inferiority trial design without placebo arm. *Biometrical Journal*, **51**, 324–334.

[607] Hung, H.M., Wang, S.-J., O'Neill, R. (2011) Flexible design clinical trial methodology in regulatory applications. *Statistics in Medicine*, **30**, 1519–1527.

[608] Hunt, M.I. (2000) Prescription Drugs and Intellectual Property Protection. National Institute for Health Care Management: Foundation Issue Brief.

[609] Huque, M.F., Dubey, S., Fredd, S. (1989) Establishing therapeutic equivalence with clinical endpoints. *Proceedings of the American Statistical Association, Biopharmaceutics Chapter*, 46–52.

[610] Huson, L., Chung, J., Salgo, M. (2007) Missing data imputation in two Phase III trials treating HIV1 infection. *Journal of Biopharmaceutical Statistics*, **17**, 159–172.

[611] Husted, S., Emanuelsson, H., Heptinstall, S., Sandset, P., Wickens, M., Peters, G. (2006) Pharmacodynamics, pharmacokinetics, and safety of the oral reversible P2Y12 antagonist AZD6140 with aspirin in patients with atherosclerosis: A double blind comparison to clopidogrel with aspirin. *European Heart Journal*, **27**, 1038–1047.

[612] Huynh, H., Feldt, L.S. (1970) Conditions under which mean square ratios in repeated measures designs have exact F-distributions. *Journal of the American Statistical Association*, **65**, 1582–1589.

[613] Hwang, J.S. (1996) Numerical solutions for a sequential approach to bioequivalence. *Statistica Sinica*, **6**, 663–673.

[614] Hwang, J.T.G., Wang, W. (1997) The validity of the test of individual equivalence ratios. *Biometrika*, **84**, 893–900.

[615] Hwang, S., Huber, P.B., Hesney, M., Kwan, K.C. (1978) Bioequivalence and interchangeabiliy. *Journal of Pharmaceutical Sciences*, **67**, IV.

[616] Hyslop, T., Hsuan, F., Holder, D.J. (2000) A small sample confidence interval approach to assess individual bioequivalence. *Statistics in Medicine*, **19**, 2885–2897.

[617] Hyslop, T., Inglewicz, B. (2001) Alternative cross-over designs for individual bioequivalence. *Proceedings of the Annual Meeting of the American Statisticial Association.*

[618] Idanpaan-Heikkila, J.E. (2000) Current status of the international comparator (reference) product system. *European Journal of Drug Metabolism and Pharmacokinetics*, **25, No. 1**, 36–37.

[619] Ignarro, L., Balestrieri, M., Napoli, C. (2007) Nutrition, physical activity, and cardiovascular disease: An update. *Cardiovascular Research*, **73**, 326–340.

[620] Ihaka, R., Gentleman, R. (1996) R: A language for data analysis and graphics. *Computational and Graphical Statistics*, **5**, 299–314.

[621] International Conference on Harmonization (1994) E4: Dose response information to support drug registration. http://www.fda.gov/cder/guidance/

[622] International Conference on Harmonization (1995a) Q2a: Text on validation of analytical procedures. http://www.fda.gov/cder/guidance/

[623] International Conference on Harmonization (1995b) E1: The extent of population exposure to assess clinical safety for drugs intended for long-term treatment of non-life-threatening conditions. http://www.fda.gov/cder/guidance/

[624] International Conference on Harmonization (1998a) E5: Guidance on ethnic factors in the acceptability of foreign clinical data. http://www.fda.gov/cder/guidance/

[625] International Conference on Harmonization (1998b) E9: Statistical principles for clinical trials. http://www.fda.gov/cder/guidance/

[626] International Conference on Harmonization (2005) E14: The clinical evaluation of QT/QTc interval prolongation and proarrythmic potential for non-antiarrythmic drugs. http://www.fda.gov/cder/guidance/

[627] Imada, T., Douke, H. (2007) Step down procedure for comparing several treatments with a control based on multivariate normal response. *Biometrical Journal*, **49**, 18–29.

[628] Isaacsohn, J., Troendle, A., Orloff, D. (2004) Regulatory issues in the approval of new drugs for diabetes mellitus, dyslipidemia, and the metabolic syndrome. *The American Journal of Cardiology*, **93**, 49C–52C.

[629] Jackson, A. (2000) The role of metabolites in bioequivalency assessment. III. Highly variable drugs with linear kinetics and first-pass effect. *Pharmaceutical Research*, **17**, 1432–1436.

[630] Jackson, A.J. (2002) Determination of in vivo bioequivalence. *Pharmaceutical Research*, **19, No. 3**, 227–228.

[631] Jackson, A., Robbie, G., Marroum, P. (2004) Metabolites and bioequivalence — Past and present. *Clinical Pharmacokinetics*, **43**, 655–672.

[632] Jacobs, T., De Ridder, F., Rusch, S., Van Peer, A., Molenberghs, G., Bijnens, L. (2008) Including information on the therapeutic window in bioequivalence acceptance. *Pharmaceutical Research*, **25**, 2628–2638.

[633] James, S. (1991) Approximate multinormal probabilities applied to correlated multiple endpoints in clinical trials. *Statistics in Medicine*, **10**, 1123-1135.

[634] Japan MHLW (1997) Guideline for bioequivalence studies of generic products.

[635] Japan MHLW (2007) Basic principles on global clinical trials.

[636] Jennison, C., Turnbull, B.W. (2000) *Group Sequential Methods with Applications to Clinical Trials.* Chapman and Hall, New York.

[637] Jennison, C., Turnbull, B.W. (2005) Meta-analyses and adaptive group sequential designs in the clinical development process. *Journal of Biopharmaceutical Statistics*, **15**, 537–558.

[638] Jennison, C., Turnbull, B. (2006) Adaptive and nonadaptive group-sequential tests. *Biometrika*, **93**, 1–21.

[639] Jennrich, R.I., Schluchter, M.D. (1986) Unbalanced repeated-measures models with structured covariance matrices. *Biometrics*, **42**, 805–820.

[640] Jiang, W., Kim, S., Zhang, X., Lionberger, R., Davit, B., Conner, D., Yu, L. (2011) The role of predictive biopharmaceutical modeling and simulation in drug development and regulatory evaluation. *International Journal of Pharmaceutics*, **418**, 151–160.

[641] Jodar, L., Butler, J., Carlone, G., Dagan, R., Goldblatt, D., Kayhty, H., Klugman, K., Plikaytis, B., Siber, G., Kohberger, R., Chang, I., Cherian, T. (2003) Serological criteria for evaluation and licensure of new pneumococcal conjugate vaccine formulations for use in infants. *Vaccine*, **21**, 3265–3272.

[642] Johnson, N.L., Kotz, S., Balakrishnan, N. (1994) *Continuous Univariate Distributions, Vols. 1 and 2.* John Wiley and Sons, New York.

[643] Johanson, P., Armstrong, P., Barbagelata, N., Chaitman, B., Clemmenson, P., Delborg, M., French, J., Goodman, S., Green, C., Krucoff, M., Langer, A., Pahlm, O., Reilly, P., Wagner, G. (2005) An academic ECG core lab perspective of the FDA initiative for digital ECG capture and data management in large-scale clinical trials. *Drug Information Journal*, **39**, 345–351.

[644] Johnson, T.N. (2005) Modelling approaches to dose estimation in children. *British Journal of Clinical Pharmacology*, **59**, 663–669.

[645] Johnson, T., Taylor, J., Haken, R., Eisbruch, A. (2005) A Bayesian mixture model relating dose to critical organs and functional complication in 3D conformal radiation therapy. *Biostatistics*, **6**, 615–632.

[646] Johnston, A., Belitsky, P., Frei, U., Horvath, J., Hoyer, P., Helderman, J., Oellerich, M., Pollard, S., Riad, H., Rigotti, P., Keown, P., Nashan, B. (2004) Potential clinical implications of substitution of generic formulations for cyclosporine microemulsion (Neoral) in transplant recipients. *European Journal of Clinical Pharmacology*, **60**, 389–395.

[647] Jones, B., Jarvis, P., Lewis, J.A., Ebbutt, A.F. (1996) Trials to assess equivalence: The importance of rigourous methods. *British Medical Journal*, **313**, 36–39.

[648] Jones, B., Teather, D., Wang, J., Lewis, J. (1998) A comparison of various estimators of a treatment difference for a multi-centre clinical trial. *Statistics in Medicine*, **17**, 1767–1777.

[649] Jones, B., Wang, J. (1999a) Constructing optimal designs for fitting pharmacokinetic models. *Statistics and Computing*, **9**, 209–218.

[650] Jones, B., Wang, J., Jarvis, P., Byrom, W. (1999b) Design of cross-over trials for pharmacokinetic studies. *Journal of Statistical Planning and Inference*, **78**, 307–316.

[651] Jones, B., Deppe, C. (2000) Recent developments in the design of cross-over trials: A brief review and bibliography. *Proceedings of the Conference on Recent Developments in the Design of Experiments and Related Topics.*

[652] Jones, B., Kenward M.G. (2014) *Design and Analysis of Cross-over Trials, 3rd ed.* CRC Press, Boca Raton, FL.

[653] Jones, B., Lane, P.W. (2004). Procedure XOEFFICIENCY (Calculates efficiency of effects in cross-over designs). GenStat Release 7.1 Reference Manual, Part 3: Procedure Library PL15, VSN International, Oxford.

[654] Jones, B. (2005) Nonparmaetric methods for the analysis of data from cross-over trials with two or more treatments. *Presented at the Deming Annual Conference, Atlantic City, NJ.*

[655] Jones, B., Atkinson, G., Ward, J., Tan, E., Kerbusch, T. (2006) Planning for an adaptive design: A case study in COPD. *Pharmaceutical Statistics*, **5**, 135–144.

[656] Jones, B. (2009) Survival of the sickest: Tracking their progress. *Significance*, **6**, 184–186.

[657] Jones, B., Soaita, A., Weaver, J. (2010) Blinded sample size re-estimation in cross-over trials. *Proceedings of the Biopharmaceutical Section — Joint Statistics Meetings 2010*, 642–648.

[658] Joy, J., Coulter, C., Duffull, S., Isbister, G. (2011) Prediction of torsades de pointes from the QT interval: Analysis of a case series of Amisulpride overdoses. *Clinical Pharmacology and Therapeutics*, **90**, 243–245.

[659] Ju, H.L. (1997) On tier method for assessment of individual bioequivalence. *Journal of Biopharmaceutical Statistics*, 7, No. 1, 63–85.

[660] Julious, S., Debarnot, C.A.-M. (2000) Why are pharmacokinetic data summarized by arithmetic means? *Journal of Biopharmaceutical Statistics*, **10**, 55–71.

[661] Julious, S., Patterson, S. (2004a) Sample sizes for estimation in clinical research. *Pharmaceutical Statistics*, **3**, 213–215.

[662] Julious, S.A. (2004b) Designing clinical trials with uncertain estimates of variability. *Pharmaceutical Statistics*, **3**, 261–268.

[663] Julious, S.A., Swank, D.J. (2005a) Moving statistics beyond the individual clinical trial: Applying decision science to optimize a clinical development plan. *Pharmaceutical Statistics*, **4**, 37–46.

[664] Julious, S. (2005b) Sample size of 12 per group rule of thumb for a pilot study. *Pharmaceutical Statistics*, **4**, 287–291.

[665] Julious, S., Owen, R. (2006) Sample size calculations for clinical studies allowing for uncertainty about the variance. *Pharmaceutical Statistics*, **5**, 29–37.

[666] Julious, S. (2010) *Sample Sizes for Clinical Trials.* CRC Press, Boca Raton, FL.

[667] Julious, S., Whitehead, A. (2012) Investigating the assumption of homogeneity of treatment effects in clinical studies with application to meta-analysis. *Pharmaceutical Statistics*, **11**, 49–56.

[668] Kackar, R.N., Harville, D.A. (1980) Variance approximations for estimators of fixed and random effects in mixed linear models. *Proceedings of the American Statistical Association*, 52–58.

[669] Kackar, R.N., Harville, D.A. (1981) Unbiasedness of two-stage estimation and prediction procedures for mixed linear models. *Communications in Statistics*, **A10**, 1249–1261.

[670] Kadane, J.B., Wolfson, L.J. (1997) Experiences in elicitation. *The Statistician*, **46, No. 4**, 1–17.

[671] Kaitin, K., DiMasi, J. (2010) Pharmaceutical innovation in the 21st century: New drug approvals in the first decade, 2000-2009. *Clinical Pharmacology and Therapeutics*, **89**, 183–188.

[672] Kane, R.C., Bross, P.F., Farrell, A.T., Pazdur, R. (2003) Velcade: U.S. FDA approval for the treatment of multiple myeloma progressing on prior therapy. *The Oncologist*, **8**, 503–513.

[673] Kanfer, F.-H.J., Geertsema, J.C., Steyn, H.S. (1988) A two-stage procedure for testing bioequivalence. *Proceedings of the American Statistical Association*, 148–152.

[674] Kang, D., Schwartz, J.B., Verotta, D. (2004) A sample size computation method for non-linear mixed effects models with applications to pharmacokinetics models. *Statistics in Medicine*, **23**, 2551-2566.

[675] Karalis, V., Symillides, M., Macheras, P. (2009) Comparison of the reference scaled bioequivalence semi-replicate method with other approaches: Focus on human exposure to drugs. *European Journal of Pharmaceutical Sciences*, **38**, 55–63.

[676] Karalis, V., Symillides, M., Macheras, P. (2011) On the leveling-off properties of the new bioequivalence limits for highly variable drugs of the EMA guideline. *European Journal of Pharmaceutical Sciences*, **44**, 497–505.

[677] Kass, R.E., Wasserman, L. (1996) The selection of prior distributions by formal rules. *American Statistical Association*, **91, No. 435**, 1343–1370.

[678] Katsahian, S., Latouche, A., Mary, J.-Y., Chevret, S., Porcher, R. (2008) Practical methodology of meta-analysis of individual patient data using a survival outcome. *Contemporary Clinical Trials*, **29**, 220–230.

[679] Katz, D., D'Argenio, D.Z. (1983) Experimental design for estimating integrals by numerical quadrature, with applications to pharmacokinetic studies. *Biometrics*, **39**, 621–628.

[680] Kaul, S., Diamond, G. (2006) Good enough: A primer on the analysis and interpretation of noninferiority trials. *Annals of Internal Medicine*, **145**, 62–69.

[681] Kaul, S., Diamond, G. (2011) Is there clear and convincing evidence of cardiovascular risk with rosiglitazone? *Clinical Pharmacology and Therapeutics*, **89**, 773–776.

[682] Kawai, N., Andoh, M., Uwoi, T., Goto, M. (2000) Statistical approaches to accepting foreign clinical data. *Drug Information Journal*, **34**, 1265–1272.

[683] Kawai, N., Chuang-Stein, C., Komiyama, O., Li, Y. (2008) An approach to rationale partitioning sample size into individual regions in a multiregional trial. *Drug Information Journal*, **42**, 139–147.

[684] Keene, O. (2005) Design and analysis of trials with rare outcomes: Examples from trials in herpes transmission and influenza prophylaxis. *Contemporary Clinical Trials*, **26**, 311-322.

[685] Kehl, V., Ulm, K. (2006) Responder identification in clinical trials with censored data. *Computational Statistics and Data Analysis*, **50**, 1338–1355.

[686] Keitel, W., Couch, R., Quarles, J., Cate, T., Baxter, B., Maassab, H. (1993) Trivalent attenuated cold-adapted influenza virus vaccine: Reduced viral shedding and serum antibody responses in susceptible adults. *Journal of Infectious Diseases*, **167**, 305–311.

[687] Kelly, P.J. (2005a) Statistical design and analysis of pharmacogenetic trials. *Statistics in Medicine*, **24**, 1495–1508.

[688] Kelly, P.J., Sooriyarachchi, M.R., Stallard, N., Todd, S. (2005b) A practical comparison of goru-sequential and adaptive designs. *Journal of Biopharmaceutical Statistics*, **15**, 719–738.

[689] Kenward, M., Roger, J. (1997) Small sample inference for fixed effects from restricted maximum likelihood. *Biometrics*, **33**, 983–997.

[690] Kenward, M.G., Molenberghs, G. (1999) Parametric models for incomplete continuous and categorical longitudinal data. *Statistical Methods in Medical Research*, **8**, 51–83.

[691] Kenward, M., Roger, J. (2010) The use of baseline covariates in crossover studies. *Biostatistics*, **11**, 1–17.

[692] Kepner, J.L., Randles, R.H. (1982) Detecting unequal marginal scales in a bi-variate population. *Journal of the American Statistical Association*, **77**, 475–482.

[693] Kershner, R.P., Federer, W.T. (1981) Two treatment cross-over designs for estimating a variety of effects. *Journal of the American Statistical Association*, **76**, 612–619.

[694] Kershner, R.P. (1992) A note on the three-period two-treatment crossover designs. *Controlled Clinical Trials*, **13**, 248–249.

[695] Khuri, A.I. (2000) Designs for variance components estimation: Past and present. *International Statistical Review*, **68, No. 3**, 311–322.

[696] Kieding, N. (1991) Age-specific incidence and prevalence: A statistical perspective. *Journal of the Royal Statistical Society, Series A*, **154**, 371–412.

[697] Kieser, M., Hauschke, D. (2005) Assessment of clinical relevance by considering point estimates and associated confidence intervals. *Pharmaceutical Statistics*, **4**, 101–107.

[698] Kimanani, E.K., Potvin, D. (1997) A parametric confidence interval for a moment based scaled criterion for individual bioequivalence. *Journal of Pharmacokinetics and Biopharmaceutics*, **25**, 595–614.

[699] Kimanani, E.K., Lavigne, J., Potvin, D. (2000a) Numerical methods for the evaluation of individual bioequivalence. *Statistics in Medicine*, **19**, 2775–2795.

[700] Kimanani, E., Stypinski, D., Curtis, G., Stiles, M., Heessels, P., Logan, S., Melson, K., St. Germain, E., Boswell, G. (2000b) A contract research organization's response to the new FDA guidances for bioequivalence/bioavailability studies for orally administered drug products. *Journal of Clinical Pharmacology*, **40**, 1102–1108.

[701] Kimanani, E.K. (2000c) Definition of individual bioequivalence: Occasion-to-occasion versus mean switchability. *Statistics in Medicine*, **19**, 2797–2810.

[702] Kirkwood, T.-B.L., Westlake, T.J. (1981) Letter to the editor and response. *Biometrics*, **37**, 589–593.

[703] Knusel, L. (2004) On the accuracy of statistical distributions in Microsoft Excel 2003. *Computational Statistics and Data Analysis*, **48**, 445–449.

[704] Ko, F., Tsou, H., Liu, J., Hsiao, C. (2010) Sample size determination for a specific region in a multiregional trial. *Journal of Biopharmaceutical Statistics*, **24**, 870–885.

[705] Koch, G. (1972) The use of non-parametric methods in the statistical analysis of the two-period changeover design. *Biometrics*, **28**, 577–584.

[706] Koch, G.G., Gansky, S.A. (1996) Statistical considerations for multiplicity in confirmatory protocols. *Drug Information Journal*, **30**, 523–534.

[707] Kocherlakota, S. (1982) On the behaviour of some transforms of the sample correlation coefficient in samples from the bivariate t and bivariate x, density estimation procedures. *Commun Statist -Theor. Meth.*, **11, No. 18**, 2045–2060.

[708] Kocherlakota, K., Kocherlakota, S. (1981) On the distribution of r in samples from the mixtures of bivariate normal populations. *Commun. Statist.-Theor.Meth.*, **A10(19)**, 1943–1966.

[709] Koehne-Voss, S., Schmidli, H., Smtih, D., Pigeot, I. (2011) The impact of period effects on dose level contrasts in alternating cross-over designs for first-time-in-human studies. *Statistics in Medicine*, **10**, 45–49.

[710] Koenig, W., Khuseyinova, N. (2007) Biomarkers of atherosclerotic plaque instability and rupture. *Arteriosclerosis Thrombosis and Vascular Biology*, **27**, 15–26.

[711] Kong, F.H., Gonin, R. (2000) Optimal sampling times in bioequivalence tests. *Journal of Biopharmaceutical Statistics*, **10(1)**), 31–44.

[712] Kong, L., Koch, G., Liu, T., Wang, H. (2004a) Performance of some multiple testing procedures to compare three doses of a test drug and placebo. *Pharmaceutical Statistics*, **4**, 25–35.

[713] Kong, L., Kohberger, R., Koch, G.G. (2004b) Type 1 error and power in non-inferiority/equivalence trials with correlated multiple endpoints: An example from vaccine development trials. *Journal of Biopharmaceutical Statistics*, **14**, 893–907.

[714] Kong, M., Lee, J. (2006) A generalised response surface model with varying relative potency for assessing drug interaction. *Biometrics*, **62**, 986–995.

[715] Konkle, B., Schafer, A. (2005) Hemostasis, thrombosis, fibrinolysis, and cardiovascular disease. Chapter 80 in *Braunwald's Heart Disease, A Textbook of Cardiovascular Medicine*; Zipes et al., eds. Elsevier, Saunders.

[716] Kopec, J., Abrahamowicz, M., Esdaile, J. (1993) Randomized discontinuation trials: Utility and efficiency. *Journal of Clinical Epidemiology*, **46**, 959–971.

[717] Korn, E., Freidlin, B. (2007) A posterior tale. *Biometrical Journal*, **49**, 346–350.

[718] Koren, G. (2011) Pharmacokinetics in pregnancy: Clinical significance. *Journal of Population Therapeutics and Clinical Pharmacology*, **18**, e523–e527.

[719] Kortejarvi, H., Urtti, A., Yliperttula, M. (2007) Pharmacokinetic simulation of biowaiver criteria: The effects of gastric emptying, dissolution, absorption, and elimination rates. *European Journal of Pharmaceutical Sciences*, **30**, 155–166.

[720] Kraemer, H.C. (2009) Events per person time (incidence rate): A misleading statistic? *Statistics in Medicine*, **28**, 1028–1039.

[721] Krams, M., Lees, K., Hacke, W., Grieve, A., Orgogozo, J.-M., Ford, G., for the ASTIN Study Investigators (2003) Acute stroke therapy by inhibition of neutrophils: An adaptive dose-response study of UK-279276 in acute ischemic stroke. *Stroke*, **34**, 2543–2548.

[722] Krum, H., Tonkin, A. (2003) Why do phase III trials of promising heart failure drugs often fail? The contribution of 'regression to the truth'. *Journal of Cardiac Failure*, **9**, 364–367.

[723] Kroo, I. (2004) Innovation in aeronautics: 2004 AIAA Dryden Lecture. http://aero.stanford.edu/Reports/AIAA20040001b.pdf

[724] Krzyzanowska, M., Pintilie, M., Tannock, I. (2003) Factors associated with failure to publish large randomized trials presented at an oncology meeting. *Journal of the American Medical Association*, **290**, 495–501.

[725] Ku, M.S. (2008) Use of the biopharmaceutical classification system in early drug development. *The AAPS Journal*, **10**, 208–212.

[726] Kullback, S. (1968) *Information Theory and Statistics.* Dover Publications, New York.

[727] Kytariolos, J., Karalis, V., Macheras, P., Symillides, M. (2006) Novel scaled bioequivalence limits with leveling-off properties. *Pharmaceutical Research*, **23**, 2657–2664.

[728] Labes, D., Scheutz, H., Lang, B. (2015) R package PowerTOST. Power and Sample Size Based on Two One-Sided t-Tests (TOST) for (Bio)Equivalence Studies.

[729] Lacey, L.F., Keene, O.N., Bye, A. (1995) Glaxo's experience of different absorption rate metrics of immediate release and extended release dosage forms. *Drug Information Journal*, **29**, 821–840.

[730] Lacey, L.F., Keene, O.N., Pritchard, J.F., Bye, A. (1997) Common noncompartmental pharmacokinetic variables: Are they normally or log-normally distributed? *Journal of Biopharmaceutical Statistics*, **7**, 171–178.

[731] Lachenbruch, P. (1998) Sensitivity, specificity, and vaccine efficacy. *Controlled Clinical Trials*, **19**, 569–574.

[732] Lachenbruch, P. (2003) Proper metrics for clinical trials: Transformations and other procedures to remove non-normality effects. *Statistics in Medicine*, **22**, 3823–3842.

[733] Lachenbruch, P.A., Horne, A.D., Lynch, C.J., Tiwari, J., Ellenberg, S.S. (2003) Biologics. Chapter in *Encyclopedia of Biopharmaceutical Statistics*, 89–99. Marcel Dekker, New York.

[734] Lachenbruch, P., Rida, W., Kou, J. (2004) Lot consistency as an equivalence problem. *Journal of Biopharmaceutical Statistics*, **14**, 275–290.

[735] Lachenbruch, P. (2008) Some clinical trial design questions and answers, slide 15. http://www.amstat.org/chapters/northeasternillinois/pastevents/presentations/fall_08_lachenbruch_p.ppt

[736] Lachin, J., Foulkes, M. (1986) Evaluation of sample size and power for analyses of survival with allowance for nonuniform patient entry, losses to follow-up, noncompliance, and stratification. *Biometrics*, **42**, 507–519.

[737] Lachin, J. (1988a) Statistical properties of randomization in clinical trials. *Controlled Clinical Trials*, **9**, 289–311.

[738] Lachin, J., Matts, J., Wei, L. (1988b) Randomization in clinical trials: Conclusions and recommendations. *Controlled Clinical Trials*, **9**, 365–374.

[739] Lakatos, E. (1986) Sample size determination in clinical trials with time-dependent rates of losses and noncompliance. *Controlled Clinical Trials*, **7**, 189–199.

[740] Laird, N.M., Ware, J.H. (1982) Random effects models for longitudinal data. *Biometrics*, **38**, 963–974.

[741] Lalonde, R., Kowalski, K., Hutmacher, M., Ewy, W., Nicholds, D. et al. (2007) Model-based drug development. *Clinical Pharmacology and Therapeutics*, **82**, 21–32.

[742] Lambert, P., Thompson, J., Weston, C., Dickman, P. (2007) Estimating and modelling the cure fraction in population-based cancer survival analysis. *Biostatistics*, **8**, 576–594.

[743] Lange, S., Freitag, G. (2005) Special invited papers section: Therapeutic equivalence—clinical issues and statistical methodology in noninferiority trials. *Biometrical Journal*, **47**, 12–27.

[744] LaPlace, P.S. translated by Stigler, S.M. (1986) Memoir on the probability of the causes of events. *Statistical Science*, **1**, 364–378.

[745] Lathia, C.D., Amakye, D., Dai, W., Girman, C., Madani, S., Mayne, J., MacCarthy, P., Pertel, P., Seman, L., Stoch, A., Tarantino, P., Webster, C., Williams, S., Wagner, J.A. (2009) The value, qualification, and regulatory use of surrogate endpoints in drug development. *Clinical Pharmacology and Therapeutics*, **86**, 32–43.

[746] Latouche, A., Porcher, R. (2007) Sample size calculations in the presence of competing risks. *Statistics in Medicine*, **26**, 5370–5380.

[747] Lawless, J.F., Fredette, M. (2005) Frequentist prediction intervals and predictive distributions. *Biometrika*, **92**, 529–542.

[748] Lawrence, J. (2002) Designing group-sequential trials with survival endpoints. *Drug Information Journal*, **36**, 9–15.

[749] Lawrence, J. (2005) Some remarks about the analysis of active control studies. *Biometrical Journal*, **5**, 616–622.

[750] Lee, J., Feng, L. (2005) Randomized phase II designs in cancer clinical trials: Current status and future directions. *Journal of Clinical Oncology*, **23**, 4450–4457.

[751] Lee, Y., Shao, J., Chow, S.-C., Wang, H. (2002) Tests for inter-subject and total variabilities under cross-over designs. *Journal of Biopharmaceutical Statistics*, **12(4)**, 503–534.

[752] Lehmacher, W., Wassmer, G., Reitmeir, P. (1991) Procedures for two-sample comparisons with multiple endpoints controlling the experimentwise error rate. *Biometrics*, **47**, 511–521.

[753] Lehmacker, W., Wassmer, G. (1999) Adaptive sample size calculations in group-sequential designs. *Biometrics*, **55**, 1286–1290.

[754] Lehmann, E.L. (1975). *Nonparametrics: Statistical Methods Based on Ranks.* Holden-Day, San Francisco.

[755] Lekone, P.E. (2008) Bayesian analysis of severe acute respiratory syndrome: The 2003 Hong Kong epidemic. *Biometrical Journal*, **50**, 597–607.

[756] Lennernas, H., Abrahamsson, B., Persson, E., Knutson, L. (2007) Oral drug absorption and the Biopharmaceutical Classification System (BCS). *Journal of Drug Delivery, Science, and Technology*, **17**, 237–244.

[757] Lesko, L., Rowland, M., Peck, C., Blaschke, T. (2000) Optimizing the science of drug development: Opportunities for better candidate selection and accelerated evaluation in humans. *European Journal of Pharmaceutical Sciences*, **10**, iv–xiv.

[758] Lesko, L., Atkinson, A. (2001) Use of biomarkers and surrogate markers in drug development. *Annual Reviews in Pharmacology and Toxicology*, **41**, 347–66.

[759] Lesko, L. (2007a) Paving the critical path: How can clinical pharmacology help achieve the vision? *Clinical Pharmacology and Therapeutics*, **81**, 170–177.

[760] Lesko, L. (2007b) Personalised medicine: Elusive dream or imminent reality? *Clinical Pharmacology and Therapeutics*, **81**, 807–816.

[761] Leung, D., Wang, Y. (2001) A Bayesian decision approach for sample size determination in phase II trials. *Biometrics*, **57**, 309–312.

[762] Levy, G. (1995) The clay feet of bioequivalence testing. *Journal of Pharmacy and Pharmacology*, **47**, 975–977.

[763] Lewis, J., Facey, K. (1998) Statistical shortcomings in licensing applications. *Statistics in Medicine*, **17**, 1663–1673.

[764] Li, B., Davit, B., Lee, C., Pabba, S., Mahadevan, C., Caramenico, H., Haidar, S., Sanchez, A., Sigler, A., Stier, E., Conner, D. (2013) Common reasons for 'for-cause' inspections in bioequivalence studies submitted to the Food and Drug Administration. *The AAPS Journal*, **15**, 10–14.

[765] Li, B., Jin, F., Lee, S., Bai, T., Chowdhury, B., Caramenico, H., Conner, D. (2013) Bioequivalence for locally acting nasal spray and nasal aerosol products: Standard development and generic approval. *The AAPS Journal*, **15**, 875–883.

[766] Li, X., Mehrotra, D., Barnard, J. (2006) Analysis of incomplete longitudinal binary data using multiple imputation. *Statistics in Medicine*, **25**, 2107–2124.

[767] Li, X., Wang, W., Liu, G., Chan, I. (2011) Handling missing data in vaccine clinical trials for immunogenicity and safety evaluation. *Journal of Biopharmaceutical Statistics*, **21**, 294–310.

[768] Li, Z., Chuang-Stein, C. (2006) A note on comparing two binomial proportions in confirmatory noninferiority trials. *Drug Information Journal*, **40**, 203–208.

[769] Li, Z., Chuang-Stein, C., Hoseyni, C. (2007) The probability of observing negative sub-group results when the treatment effect is positive and homogeneous across all sub-groups. *Drug Information Journal*, **41**, 47–56.

[770] Liang, J., Patterson, S. (2014) Simulations on sample sizes and powers calculations for a registry vaccine study. *Proceedings of the American Statistical Association Joint Statistical Meetings, Biopharmaceutical Section*, 487–494.

[771] Liao, J.J.Z. (2005) Comparing the concentration curves directly in a pharmacokinetics, bioavailability/bioequivalence study. *Statistics in Medicine*, **24**, 883–891.

[772] Liao, J., Heyse, J. (2011) Biosimilarity for follow-on biologics. *Statistics in Biopharmaceutical Research*, **3**, 445–455.

[773] Lim, N., Park, S., Stanck, E. (2005) Bioequivalence trials with the incomplete 3×3 cross-over design. *Biometrical Journal*, **5**, 635–643.

[774] Lin, L. (1989) A concordance correlation coefficient to evaluate reproducibility. *Biometrics*, **45**, 255–268.

[775] Lin, L. (1992) Assay validation using the concordance correlation coefficient. *Biometrics*, **48**, 599–604.

[776] Lin, L. (2000) Total deviation index for measuring individual agreement with applications in laboratory performance and bioequivalence. *Statistics in Medicine*, **19**, 255–270.

[777] Lin, Y.-L., Kung, M.-F. (2009) Magnitude of QT prolongation associated with a higher risk of torsdaes de pointes. *Pharmacoepidemiology and Drug Safety*, **18**, 235–239.

[778] Lincoff, A., Wolski, K., Nicholls, S., Nissen, S. (2007) Pioglitazone and the risk of cardiovascular events in patients with type 2 diabetes mellitus. *Journal of the American Medical Association*, **298**, 1180–1188.

[779] Lindley, D.V. (1971) *Making Decisions, 2nd ed.* John Wiley and Sons, New York.

[780] Lindley, D.V., Singpurwalla, N.D. (1991) On the evidence needed to reach agreed action between adversaries, with application to acceptance sampling. *Journal of the American Statistical Association*, **86**, 933–937.

[781] Lindley, D.V. (1997) The choice of sample size (with discussion). *The Statistician*, **46**, 129–166.

[782] Lindley, D.V. (1998) Decision analysis and bioequivalence trials. *Statistical Science*, **13**, 136–141.

[783] Lindsey, J. K. (1974) Construction and comparison of statistical models. *Journal of the Royal Statistical Society*, **B36**, 418–425.

[784] Lindsey, J.K. (1996a) *Parametric Statistical Inference.* Clarendon Press, Oxford.

[785] Lindsey, J.K., Jones, B. (1996b) A model for cross-over trials evaluating therapeutic preferences. *Statistics in Medicine*, **15**, 443–447.

[786] Lindsey, J.K., Jones, B. (1997a) Treatment-patient interactions for diagnostics of cross-over trials. *Statistics in Medicine*, **16**, 1955–1964.

[787] Lindsey, J.K., Jones, B., Ebbutt, A.F. (1997b) Simple models for repeated ordinal responses with an application to a seasonal rhinitis clinical trial. *Statistics in Medicine*, **16**, 2873–2882.

[788] Lindsey, J.K., Wang, J., Byrom, W.D., Jones, B. (1999) Modeling the covariance structure in pharmacokinetic cross-over trials. *Journal of Biopharmaceutical Statistics*, **9**, 439–450.

[789] Lindsey, J.K., Syrom, W.D., Wang, J., Jarvis, P., Jones, B. (2000) Generalized nonlinear models for pharmacokinetic data. *Biometrics*, **56**, 81–88.

[790] Lindsey, J.K. (2001) *Nonlinear Models in Medical Statistics.* Oxford University Press, Oxford.

[791] Lindsey, J., Lindsey, P. (2006) Multivariate distributions with correlation matrices for nonlinear repeated measurements. *Computational Statistics and Data Analysis*, **50**, 720–732.

[792] Lindstrom, M.J., Bates, D.M. (1988) Newton-Raphson and EM algorithms for linear mixed-effects models and repeated-measures data. *Journal of the American Statisticial Association*, **83**, 1014–1022.

[793] Lionberger, R., Jiang, W., Huang, S.-M., Geba, G. (2013) Confidence in generic substitution. *Clinical Pharmacology and Therapeutics*, **94**, 438–440.

[794] Lipkovich, H., Duan, Y., Ahmed, S. (2005) Multiple imputation compared with restricted pseudo-likelihood and generalised estimating equations for analysis of binary repeated measures in clinical studies. *Pharmaceutical Statistics*, **4**, 267–285.

[795] Littell, R.C., Milliken, G.A., Stroup, W.W., Wolfinger, R.D. (1996) *SAS System for Mixed Models.* SAS Institute, Cary, NC.

[796] Little, R., Rubin, D. (2002) *Statistical Analysis with Missing Data.* John Wiley & Sons, Ltd., England, New York.

[797] Liu, G., Wang, J., Liu, K., Snavely, D. (2006) Confidence intervals for exposure adjusted incidence rate difference with applications to clinical trials. *Statistics in Medicine*, **25**, 1275–1286.

[798] Liu, J.-P. (1991) Bioequivalence and intrasubject variability. *Journal of Biopharmaceutical Statistics*, **1(2)**, 205–219.

[799] Liu, J.-P., Chow, S.-C. (1992) On the assessment of variability in bioavailability/bioequivalence studies. *Communications in Statistics, Theory and Methodology*, **21(9)**, 2591–2607.

[800] Liu, J.-P. (1995) Use of the repeated cross-over designs in assessing bioequivalence. *Statistics in Medicine*, **14**, 1067–1078.

[801] Liu, J.-P., Chow, S.-C. (1997a) A two one-sided tests procedure for assessment of individual bioequivalence. *Journal of Biopharmaceutical Statistics*, **7(1)**, 49–61.

[802] Liu, J.-P., Chow, S.-C. (1997b) Some thoughts on individual bioequivalence. *Journal of Biopharmaceutical Statistics*, **7(1)**, 41–48.

[803] Liu, J.-P., Chow, S-C. (2002a) Bridging studies in clinical development. *Journal of Biopharmaceutical Statistics*, **12**, 359–367.

[804] Liu, J.-P., Hsiao, C.-F., Hsueh, H. (2002b) Bayesian approach to evaluation of bridging studies. *Journal of Biopharmaceutical Statistics*, **12**, 401–408.

[805] Liu, J.-P., Hsueh, H., Hsiao, C.-F. (2004) A Bayesian non-inferiority approach to evaluation of bridging studies. *Journal of Biopharmaceutical Statistics*, **14**, 291–300.

[806] Liu, M., Wei, L., Zhang, J. (2006) Review of guidelines and literature for handling missing data in longitudinal clinical trials with a case study. *Pharmaceutical Statistics*, **5**, 7–18.

[807] Liu, R.Y., Sigh, K. (1987) On a partial correction by the bootstrap. *The Annals of Statistics*, **15, No. 4**, 1713–1718.

[808] Locke, C.S. (1984) An exact confidence interval for untransformed data for the ratio of two formulation means. *Journal of Pharmacokinetics and Biopharmaceutics*, **12**, 649–655.

[809] Logan, B., Tamhane, A. (2008) Superiority inferences on individual endpoints following noninferiority testing in clinical trials. *Biometrical Journal*, **50**, 693–703.

[810] Loke, Y., Tan, S., Cai, Y., Machin, D. (2006) A Bayesian dose finding design for dual endpoint phase I trials. *Statistics in Medicine*, **25**, 3–22.

[811] Longford, N.T. (1998) Count data and treatment heterogeneity in 2x2 crossover trials. *Applied Statistics*, **47**, 217–229.

[812] Longford, N.T. (1999) Selection bias and treatment heterogeneity in clinical trials. *Statistics in Medicine*, **18**, 1467–1474.

[813] Longford, N.T. (2000) An alternative definition of individual bioequivalence. *Statistica Neerlandica*, **14**, 14–36.

[814] Longford, N.T. (2001) Synthetic estimators with moderating influence: The carry-over in cross-over trials revisited. *Statistics in Medicine*, **20**, 3189–3203.

[815] Lori, W. (2010) In defense of human life. *Columbia*, **90**, 4–5.

[816] Lu, T.C., Graybill, F.A., Burdick, R.K. (1988) Confidence intervals on a difference of expected mean squares. *Journal of Statistical Planning and Inference*, **18**, 35–43.

[817] Lu, Y., Jin, H., Lamborn, K. (2005) A design of phase II cancer trials using total and complete response endpoints. *Statistics in Medicine*, **24**, 3155–3170.

[818] Ludbrook, J. (2002) Statistical techniques for comparing measurers and methods of measurement: A critical review. *Clinical and Experimental Pharmacology and Physiology*, **29**, 527–536.

[819] Lund, R.E. (1975) Tables for an approximate test for outliers in linear models. *Technometrics*, **17**, 473–476.

[820] Lui, K. (2005) A simple test of the homogeneity of risk difference in sparse data: An application to a multicentre study. *Biometrical Journal*, **47**, 654–661.

[821] Lunn, D.J., Aarons, L.J. (1997) Markov chain Monte Carlo techniques for studying interoccasion and intersubject variability: Application to pharmacokinetic data. *Applied Statistics*, **46, No. 1**, 73–91.

[822] Lunn, D.J., Best, N., Thomas, A., Wakefield, J., Spiegelhalter, D. (1997) Bayesian analysis of population PK/PD models: General concepts and software. *Pharmacokinetics and Pharmacodynamics*, **29, No. 3**, 271–307.

[823] Lunn, D.J., Wakefield, J., Thomas, A., Best, N., Spiegelhalter, D. *PKBUGS User Guide*. Imperial College of Science, Technology, and Medicine. Available at http://www.mrc-bsu.cam.ac.uk/bugs/winbugs/pkbugs.shtml

[824] Lupinacci, P., Raghavarao, D. (2000) Designs for testing lack of fit for a nonlinear dose-response curve model. *Journal of Biopharmaceutical Statistics*, **10**, 43–53.

[825] Lyles, R., Lin, H., Williamson, J. (2007) A practical approach to computing power for generalised linear models with nominal, count, or ordinal responses. *Statistics in Medicine*, **26**, 1632–1648.

[826] Ma, G., Chi, E., Ibrahim, J., Parker, R. (2012) Assessing similarity to existing drugs to decide whether to continue drug development. *Statistics in Biopharmaceutical Research*, **4**, 293–300.

[827] Ma, Y., Mazumdar, M. (2011) Multivariate meta-analysis: A robust approach based on the theory of U-statistic. *Statistics in Medicine*, **30**, 2911–2929.

[828] Machado, S., Miller, R., Hu, C. (1999) A regulatory perspective on pharmacokinetic and pharmacodynamic modelling. *Statistical Methods in Medical Research*, **8**, 217–245.

[829] Mahmood, I., Green, M.D. (2005) Pharmacokinetic and pharmacodynamic considerations in the development of therapeutic proteins. *Clinical Pharmacokinetics*, **4**, 331–347.

[830] Maki, E. (2006) Power and sample size considerations in clinical trials with competing risk endpoints. *Pharmaceutical Statistics*, **5**, 159–171.

[831] Malhotra, B., Glue, P., Sweeney, K., Anziano, R., Mancuso, J., Wicker, P. (2007) Thorough QTc study with recommended and supratherapeutic doses of tolterodine. *Clinical Pharmacology and Therapeutics*, **81**, 377–385.

[832] Mallet, A. (1986) A maximum likelihood estimation method for random coefficient regression models. *Biometrika*, **73**, 645–656.

[833] Mallinckrodt, C., Sanger, T., Dube, S., DeBrota, D., Molenberghs, G., Carroll, R., Potter, W., Tollefson, G. (2003) Assessing and interpreting treatment effects in longitudinal trials with missing data. *Biological Psychiatry*, **53**, 754–760.

[834] Mallinckrodt, C., Kaiser, C., Watkin, J., Molenberghs, G., Carroll, R. (2004) The effect of correlation structure on treatment contrasts estimated from incomplete clinical trial data with likelihood-based repeated measures compared with last observation carried forward ANOVA. *Clinical Trials*, **1**, 477–489.

[835] Malott Frey, C., Muller, K. (1992) Analysis methods for nonlinear models with compound-symmetric covariance. *Communications in Statistical Theory and Methods*, **21**, 1163–1182.

[836] Mancinelli, L., Frassetto, L., Floren, L., Dressler, D., Carrier, S., Bekersky, I., Benet, L., Christians, U. (2001) The pharmacokinetics and metabolic disposition of Tacrolimus: A comparison across ethnic groups. *Clinical Pharmacology and Therapeutics*, **69**, 24–31.

[837] Mandallaz, D., Mau, J. (1981) Comparison of different methods for decison making in bioequivalence assessment. *Biometrics*, **37**, 213–222.

[838] Mandema, J., Hermann, D., Wang, W., Sheiner, T., Milad, M., Bakker-Arkema, R., Hartman, D. (2005) Model-based development of gemcabene, a new lipid-altering agent. *The AAPS Journal*, **7**, E513–E522.

[839] Marcus, R., Peritz, E., Gabriel, K.R. (1976) On closed testing procedures with special reference to ordered analysis of variance. *Biometrika*, **63**, 655–660.

[840] Marston, S.A., Polli, J.E. (1997) Evaluation of direct curve comparison metrics applied to pharmacokinetic profiles and relative bioavailability and bioequivalence. *Pharmaceutical Research*, **14**, 1363–1369.

[841] Martin, M. (2007) Bootstrap hypothesis testing for some common statistical problems: A critical evaluation of size and power properties. *Computational Statistics and Data Analysis*, **51**, 6321–6342.

[842] Marzo, A., Balant, L. P. (1995) An updated reappraisal addressed to applications of interchangeable multi-source pharmaceutical products. *Arzneim-Forsch/Drug Res*, **45 (1)**, 109–115.

[843] Marzo, A. (1997) Clinical pharmacokinetic registration file for NDA and ANDA procedures. *Pharmacological Research*, **36, No.6**, 425–450.

[844] Marzo, A. (1999) Open questions on bioequivalence: Some problems and some solutions. *Pharmacological Research*, **40, No. 4**, 357–368.

[845] Marzo, A., Monti, N.C., Tettamanti, R.A., Crivelli, F., Bo, L.D., Mazzucchelli, P., Meoli, A., Pezzuto, D., Corsico, A. (2000) Bioequivalence of inhaled Formoterol Fumurate assessed from pharmacodynamic, safety, and urinary pharmacokinetic data. *Arzneim-Forsch./Drug Res.*, **50**, 559–563.

[846] Matthews, J.N.S. (1984) Robust methods in the assessment of multivariate normality. *Applied Statistics*, **33**, 272–277.

[847] Matthews, J.N.S. (1987) Optimal crossover designs for the comparison of two treatments in the presence of carryover effects and autocorrelated errors. *Biometrika*, **74, 2**, 311–320.

[848] Matthews, J.N.S. (1988) Recent developments in crossover designs. *International Statistical Review*, **56, 2**, 117–127.

[849] Matthews, J.N.S. (1989) Crossover designs for clinical trials. *Statistics in Medicine*, **8**, 633.

[850] Matthews, J.N.S. (1990a) The analysis of data from crossover designs: The efficiency of ordinary least squares. *Biometrics*, **46**, 689–696.

[851] Matthews, J.N.S. (1990b) Optimal dual-balanced two treatment crossover designs. *Sankhya: The Indian Journal of Statistics*, **52, Series B**, 332–337.

[852] Matthews, J.N.S. (1994a) Multi-period crossover trials. *Statistical Methods in Medical Research*, **3**, 383–405.

[853] Matthews, J. (1994b) Modelling and optimality in the design of cross-over studies for medical applications. *Journal of Statistical Planning and Inference*, **42**, 89–108.

[854] Matthews, J.N.S. (1995) Small clinical trials: Are they all bad? *Statistics in Medicine*, **14**, 115–126.

[855] Mauger, D.T., Chinchilli, V.M. (2000) An alternative index for assessing profile similarity in bioequivalence trials. *Statistics in Medicine*, **19**, 2855–2866.

[856] Maurer, W., Jones, B., Chen, Y. (To be Submitted) Controlling the type 1 error rate in two-stage sequential designs when testing for average bioequivalence. *Statistics in Medicine.*

[857] McCulloch, C.E. (1987) Tests for equality of variances with paired data. *Communications in Statistical Theory and Methods*, **16**, 1377–1391.

[858] McCullough, M., Lepor, N. (2007) The rosiglitazone meta-analysis. *Reviews in Cardiovascular Medicine*, **8**, 123–126.

[859] McGilveray, I.J. (2000) Differences in reference products: Dissolution and in vivo evidence. *European Journal of Drug Metabolism and Pharmacokinetics*, **25, No. 1**, 32–35.

[860] McLean, RA., Sanders, W.L. (1988) Approximating degrees of freedom for standard errors in mixed linear models. *American Statistical Association Proceedings*, **Volume**, 50–59.

[861] McLean, R.A., Sanders, W.L., Stroup, W.W. (1991) A unified approach to mixed linear models. *The American Statistician*, **45, No. 1**, 54–64.

[862] Mehring, G.H. (1993) On optimal tests for general interval-hypotheses. *Communications in Statistics, Theory and Methodology*, **22**, 1257–1297.

[863] Mehrotra, D., Adewale, A. (2012) Flagging clinical adverse experiences: Reducing false discoveries without materially compromising power for detecting true signals. *Statistics in Medicine*, **31**, 1918–1930.

[864] Mehta, C., Bauer, P., Posch, M., Brannath, W. (2007) Repeated confidence intervals for adaptive group sequential trials. *Statistics in Medicine*, **26**, 5422–5433.

[865] Mehvar, R. (2000) Development and application of an on-line module for teaching Bayesian forecasting principles in a clinical pharmacokinetics course. *American Journal of Pharmaceutical Education*, **64**, 121–125.

[866] Meibohm, B., Derendorf, H. (2002) Pharmacokinetic-pharmacodynamic studies in drug product development. *Journal of Pharmaceutical Sciences*, **91**, 18–31.

[867] Meier, Y., Cavallaro, M., Roos, M., Pauli-Magnus, C., Folkers, G., Meier, P.J., Fattinger, K. (2005) Incidence of drug-induced liver injury in medical patients. *European Journal of Clinical Pharmacology*, **61**, 135–143.

[868] Metzler, C.M. (1974) Bioavailability: A problem in equivalence. *Biometrics*, **30**, 309–317.

[869] Metzler, C.M., Huang, D.C. (1983) Statistical methods for bioavailability and bioequivalence. *Clinical Research Practices and Drug Regulatory Affairs*, **1**, 109–132.

[870] Meyer, M.C. (1995) Current scientific issues regarding bioavailability/bioequivalence studies: An academic view. *Drug Information Journal*, **29**, 805–812.

[871] Meyer, M.C., Straughn, A.B., Jarvi, E.J., Patrick, K.S., Pelsor, F.R., Williams, R.L., Patnaik, R., Chen, M.L., Shah, V.P. (2000) Bioequivalence of Methylphenidate immediate-release tablets using a replicated study design to characterize intra-subject variability. *Pharmaceutical Research*, **17**, 381–384.

[872] Meyer, M.C., Straughn, A.B., Mhatre, R.M., Shah, V.P., Chen, M.-L., Williams, R.L., Lesko, L.J. (2001) Variability in the bioavailability of Phenytoin capsules in males and females. *Pharmaceutical Research*, **18**, 394–397.

[873] Midha, K.K., Ormsby, E.D., Hubbard, J.W., McKay, G., Hawes, E.M., Gavalas, L., McGilveray, I.J. (1993) Logarithmic transformation in bioequivalence: Application with two formulations of Perphenazine. *Journal of Pharmaceutical Sciences*, **82**, 138–144.

[874] Midha, K.K., Rawson, M.J., Hubbard, J.W. (1997a) Individual and average bioequivalence of high variability drugs and drug products. *Journal of Pharmaceutical Sciences*, **86**, 1193–1197.

[875] Midha, K.K., Rawson, M.J., Hubbard, J.W. (1997b) Bioequivalence: Switchability and scaling. *European Journal of Pharmaceutical Sciences*, **6**, 87–91.

[876] Midha, K.K., Rawson, M.J., Hubbard, J.W. (2004) The role of metabolites in bioequivalence. *Pharmaceutical Research*, **21, No. 8**, 1331–1343.

[877] Midha, K., Rawson, M., Hubbard, J. (2005) The bioequivalence of highly variable drugs and drug products. *International Journal of Clinical Pharmacology and Therapeutics*, **43**, 485–498.

[878] Midha, K., McKay, G. (2009) Bioequivalence: Its history, practice, and future. *The AAPS Journal*, **11**, 664–670.

[879] Millard, S.P., Krause, A. (2001) *Applied Statistics in the Pharmaceutical Industry.* Springer, New York.

[880] Miller, M. (2001) Gender-based differences in the toxicity of pharmaceuticals — The Food and Drug Administration's perspective. *International Journal of Toxicology*, **20**, 149–152.

[881] Milliken, G.A., Johnson, D.E. (1992) *Analysis of Messy Data, Vol 1: Designed Experiments.* Chapman and Hall, New York.

[882] Mofsen, R., Balter, J. (2001) Case reports of the reemergence of psychotic symptoms after conversion from brand-name clozapine to a generic formulation. *Clinical Therapeutics*, **23, No. 10**, 1720–1731.

[883] Moher, D., Liberati, A., Tetzlaff, J., Altman, D. and the PRISMA Group (2009) (Reprint) Preferred reporting items for systematic reviews and meta-analyses: The PRISMA statement. *Physical Therapy*, **89**, 873–880.

[884] Moher, D., Hopewell, S., Schulz, K., Montori, V., Gotzsche, P., Devereaux, P., Elbourne, D., Egger, M., Altman, D. (2010) CONSORT 2010 explanation and elaboration: Updated guidelines for reporting parallel group randomised trials. *British Medical Journal*, **340**.

[885] Moldofsky, H., Lue, F., Mously, C., Roth-Schechter, B., Reynolds, W. (1996) The effect of zolpidem in patients with fibromyalgia: A dose ranging, double blind, placebo-controlled, modified cross-over study. *Journal of Rheumatology*, **23**, 529–533.

[886] Molenberghs, G., Kenward, M. (2007) *Missing Data in Clinical Studies.* John Wiley & Sons, Ltd., England, New York.

[887] Montalescot, G., White, H., Gallo, R., Cohen, M., Steg, P., Aylward, P., Bode, C., Chiariello, M., King, S., Harrington, R., Desmet, W., Macaya, C., Steinhubl, S. for the STEEPLE investigators (2006) Enoxaparin versus unfractionated heparin in elective percutaneous coronary intervention. *British Medical Journal*, **355**, 1006–1017.

[888] Montague, T., Potvin, D., DiLiberti, C., Hauck, W., Parr, A., Schuirmann, D. (2012) Additional results for 'sequential design approaches for bioequivalence studies with cross-over designs.' *Pharmaceutical Statistics*, **11**, 8–13.

[889] Morais, J.A.G. (2000) CPMP note for guidance on bioavailability and bioequivalence. *European Journal of Drug Metabolism and Pharacokinetics*, **No. 1**, 66–67.

[890] Morais, J., Lobato, M. (2010) The new European medicines agency guideline on the investigation of bioequivalence. *Basic and Clinical Pharmacology and Toxicology*, **106**, 221–225.

[891] Morgan, W.A. (1939) A test for the significance of the difference between two variances in a sample from a bi-variate normal population. *Biometrika*, **31**, 13–19.

[892] Morganroth, J. (2007) Cardiac repolarisation and the safety of new drugs defined by electrocardiography. *Clinical Pharmacology and Therapeutics*, **81**, 108–113.

[893] Morrison, D. (1990) *Multivariate Statistical Methods, 3rd ed.* McGraw Hill, New York.

[894] Moss, A. (1993) Measurement of the QT interval and the risk associated with QT interval prolongation. *American Journal of Cardiology*, **72**, 23B–25B.

[895] Moss, A. (2006) QTc prolongation and sudden cardiac death: The association is in the details. *Journal of the American College of Cardiology*, **47**, 368–369.

[896] Moyé, L. (2003) *Multiple Analyses in Clinical Trials.* Springer, New York.

[897] Moyé, L. with Commentary by Chaloner, K. and Rejoinder (2008) Bayesians in clinical trials: Asleep at the switch. *Statistics in Medicine*, **27**, 469–489.

[898] Muirhead, R.J. (1982) *Aspects of Multivariate Statistical Theory.* John Wiley and Sons, New York.

[899] Munk, A. (1993) An improvement on commonly used tests in bioequivalence assessment. *Biometrics*, **49**, 1225–1230.

[900] Munk, A. (1996) Equivalence and interval testing for Lehmann's alternative. *Journal of the American Statistical Association*, **91, No. 435**, 1187–1196.

[901] Munk, A., Czado, C. (1998) Nonparametric validation of similar distributions and assessment of goodness of fit. *Journal of the Royal Statistical Society, Series B*, **60**, 223–241.

[902] Munk, A., Pfluger, R. (1999) 1-α Equivalence confidence rules for convex alternatives are $\alpha/2$ tests with applications to the multivariate assessment of bioequivalence. *Journal of the American Statistical Association*, **94**, 1311–1319.

[903] Munk, A. (2000) Connections between average and individual bioequivalence. *Statistics in Medicine*, **19**, 2843–2854.

[904] Munk, A. (2001) On a problem in pharmaceutical statistics and the iteration of a peculiar nonlinear operator in the upper complex halfplane. *Nonlinear Analysis*, **47**, 1513–1523.

[905] Munoz, J., Alcaide, D., Ocana, J. (2015) Consumer's risk in the EMA and FDA regulatory approaches for bioequivalence in highly variable drugs. *Statistics in Medicine*, Published in Wiley Online Library on 28 DEC 2015.

[906] Munzel, U., Hauschke, D. (2003) A nonparametric test for proving noninferiority in clinical trials with ordered categorical data. *Pharmaceutical Statistics*, **2**, 31–37.

[907] Myers, R.H. (1990) *Classical and Modern Regression with Applications, 2nd ed.* PWS-Kent, Boston.

[908] N'Dri-Stempfer, B., Navidi, W.C., Guy, R.H., Bunge, A.L. (2009) Improved bioequivalence assessment of topical dermatological drug products using dermatopharmacokinetics. *Pharmaceutical Research*, **26**, 316–328.

[909] Nagata, R., Fukase, H., Rafizadeh-Kabe, J. (2000) East-West development: Understanding the usability and acceptance of foreign data in Japan. *International Journal of Clinical Pharmacology and Therapeutics*, **38**, 87–92.

[910] Nakai, K., Fujita, M., Ogata, H. (2000a) International harmonization of bioequivalence studies and issues shared in common. *Yakugaku Zasshi*, **120(11)**, 1193–1200.

[911] Nakai, K., Fujita, M., Ogata, H. (2000b) New bioequivalence studies: Individual bioequivalence and population bioequivalence. *Yakugaku Zasshi*, **120**, 1201–1208.

[912] Nakamura, T., Douke, H. (2007) Development of sequential multiple comparison procedure for dose response test. *Biometrical Journal*, **49**, 30–39.

[913] Nair, A., Margolis, M., Kuban, B., Vince, D. (2007) Automated coronary plaque characterisation with intravascular ultrasound backscatter: Ex vivo validation. *EuroIntervention*, **3**, 113–120.

[914] Naito, C. (1998a) Relevance of ethnic factors in global development: Historic overview. In *Proceedings of the Fourth International Conference on Harmonisation*, D'Arcy, P.F., Harron, D. eds., Greystone Books.

[915] Naito, C. (1998b) Ethnic factors in the acceptability of foreign clinical data. *Drug Information Journal*, **32**, 1283S–1292S.

[916] Narukawa, M., Yafune, A. (2005) A note on power and sampling schedule in population pharmacokinetic studies. *Drug Information Journal*, **39**, 353–359.

[917] National Academy of Sciences. (2010) *The Prevention and Treatment of Missing Data in Clinical Trials.* www.nap.edu/catalog/12955.html

[918] Nauta, J. (2010) *Statistics in Clinical Vaccine Trials.* Springer, London.

[919] Nayak, T.K., Kundu, S. (2001) Calculating and describing uncertainty in risk assessment: The Bayesian approach. *Human and Ecological Risk Assessment*, 7, No. 2, 307–328.

[920] Nedelman, J. (2005) On some "disadvantages" of the population approach. *The AAPS Journal*, **7**, E374–E382.

[921] Nelder, J.A. (1977) A reformulation of linear models. *Journal of the Royal Statistical Society, Series A*, **140, Part A**, 48–77.

[922] Newcombe, R.G. (1998) Interval estimation for the difference between independent proportions: Comparison of eleven methods. *Statistics in Medicine*, **17**, 873–890.

[923] Newell, D. (2005) How to develop a successful cancer drug — Molecules to medicines or targets to treatments? *European Journal of Cancer*, **41**, 676–682.

[924] Ng, H., Gu, K., Tang, M. (2007) A comparative study of tests for the difference of two Poisson means. *Computational Statistics and Data Analysis*, **51**, 3085–3099.

[925] Ng, T.-H. (2008) Noninferiority hypotheses and choice of noninferiority margin. *Statistics in Medicine*, **27**, 5392–5406.

[926] Nissen, S., Nicholls, S., Sipahi, I., Libby, P., Raichlen, J., Ballantyne, C., Davignon, J., Erbel, R., Fruchart, J., Tardif, J., Shoenhagen, P., Crowe, T., Cain, V., Wolski, K., Goormastic, M., Tuzcu, E., and the ASTEROID Investigators (2006) Effect of very high-intensity statin therapy on regression of coronary atherosclerosis. *Journal of the American Medical Association*, **295**, E1–E10.

[927] Nissen, S., Tardif, J.-C., Nicholls, S., Revkin, J., Shear, C. et al for the ILLUSTRATE investigators (2007) Effect of torcetrapib on the progression of coronary atherosclerosis. *New England Journal of Medicine*, **356**, 1304–1316.

[928] Nissen, S., Wolski, K. (2007) Effect of rosiglitazone on the risk of myocardial infarction and death from cardiovascular disease. *New England Journal of Medicine*, **356**, 2457–2471.

[929] Nissen, S. (2010) Setting the RECORD straight. *Journal of the American Medical Association*, **303**, 1194–1195.

[930] Noble, J. (2006) Meta-analysis: Methods, strengths, weaknesses, and political uses. *Journal of Laboratory Clinical Medicine*, **147**, 7–20.

[931] Nutescu, E., Wittkowsky, A. (2004) Direct thrombin inhibitors for anticoagulation. *The Annals of Pharmacotherapy*, **39**, 99–109.

[932] OBrien, P.C. (1988) Comparing two samples: Extensions of the t, rank-sum, and long-rank tests. *Journal of the American Statistical Association*, **83, No. 401**, 52–61.

[933] O'Donnell, M., Weitz, J. (2004) Novel antithrombotic therapies for the prevention of stroke in patients with atrial fibrillation. *The American Journal of Managed Care*, **10**, S72-S82.

[934] Offen, W., Chuang-Stein, C., Dmitrienko, A., Littman, G., Maca, J., Meyerson, L., Muirhead, R., Stryszak, P., Boddy, A., Chen, K., Copley-Merriman, K., Dere, W., Givens, S., Hall, D., Henry, D., Jackson, J., Krishen, A., Liu, T., Ryder, S., Sankoh, A., Wang, J., Yeh, C. (2007) Multiple co-primary endpoints: Medical and statistical solutions; A report for the multiple endpoints expert team of the Pharmaceutical Research and Manufacturers of America. *Drug Information Journal*, **41**, 31–46.

[935] Ogata, H. (2000) Equivalence in special populations. *European Journal of Drug Metabolism and Pharmacokinetics*, **1**, 72.

[936] Oldstone, M. (1998) *Viruses, Plagues, and History.* Oxford University Press, New York.

[937] Opara, J., Primozic, S., Cvelbar, P. (1999) Prediction of pharmacokinetic parameters and the assessment of their variability in bioequivalence studies by artificial neural networks. *Pharmaceutical Research*, **16, No. 6**, 944–948.

[938] O'Neill, R.T. (1995) Statistical concepts in the planning and evaluation of drug safety from clinical trials in drug development: Issues of international harmonization. *Statistics in Medicine*, **14**, 1117–1127.

[939] O'Neill, R.T. (1997) Secondary endpoints cannot be validly analysed if the primary endpoint does not demonstrate clear statistical significance. *Controlled Clinical Trials*, **18**, 550–556.

[940] O'Neill, R. (2006) FDA's critical path initiative: A perspective on contributions of biostatistics. *Biometrical Journal*, **48**, 559–564.

[941] O'Neill, R. (2008) A perspective on characterising benefits and risks derived from clinical trials: Can we do more? *Drug Information Journal*, **42**, 235–245.

[942] O'Neill, R., Temple, R. (2012) The prevention and treatment of missing data in clinical trials: An FDA perspective on the importance of dealing with it. *Clinical Pharmacology and Therapeutics*, **91**, 550–554.

[943] Ono, S., Yoshioka, C., Asaka, O., Tamura, K., Shibata, T., Saito, K. (2005) New drug approval times and clinical evidence in Japan. *Contemporary Clinical Trials*, **26**, 660–672.

[944] Ormsby, E.D. (1999) Invited Presentation: Individual Bioequivalence: A Canadian Perspective. *AAPS International Workshop on Individual Bioequivalence: Realities and Implementation.*

[945] O'Quigley, J., Baudoin, C. (1988) General approaches to the problem of bioequivalence. *The Statistician*, **37**, 51–58.

[946] O'Quigley, J., Pepe, M., Fisher, L. (1990) Continual reassessment method: A practical design for phase 1 studies in cancer. *Biometrics*, **46**, 33–48.

[947] O'Quigley, J. (2002) Continual reassessment designs with early termination. *Biostatistics*, **3**, **1**, 87–99.

[948] Ounpuu, S., Negassa, A., Yusuf, S. for the INTER-HEART Investigators (2001) INTER-HEART: A global study of risk factors for acute myocardial infarction. *American Heart Journal*, **141**, 711–721.

[949] Owen, D.B. (1965) A special case of a bi-variate non-central t-distribution. *Biometrika*, **52**, 437–446.

[950] Ozan, M., Stufken, J. (2010) Assessing the impact of carryover effects on the variances of estimators of treatment differences in crossover designs. *Statistics in Medicine*, **29**, 2480–2485.

[951] Pabst, G., Jaeger, H. (1990) Review of methods and criteria for the evaluation of bioequivalence studies. *European Journal of Clinical Pharmacology*, **38**, 5–10.

[952] Pan, Y., Liu, G., Dallas, M. (2011) Assessing non-inferiority to an aggregate response with an application to development of pneumococcal conjugate vaccines. *Pharmaceutical Statistics*, **10**, 332–340.

[953] Panhard, X., Mentre, F. (2005) Evaluation by simulation of tests based on non-linear mixed-effects models in pharmacokinetic interaction and bioequivalence cross-over trials. *Statistics in Medicine*, **24**, 1509–1524.

[954] Patel, H.I. (1994) Dose-response in pharmacokinetics. *Communications in Statistical Theory and Methodology*, **23(2)**, 451–465.

[955] Patel, H.I. (1996) Bioequivalence intervals: Conventional and bootstrap methods. *Journal of Applied Statistical Science*, **5, No. 1**, 93–104.

[956] Patnaik, P.B. (1949) The non-central χ^2 and F-distributions and their applications. *Biometrika*, **36**, 202–232.

[957] Patnaik, R., Lesko, L.J., Chan, K., Williams, R.L. (1996) Bioequivalence assessment of generic drugs: An American point of view. *European Journal of Drug Metabolism and Pharmacokinetics*, **21**, 159–164.

[958] Patnaik, R.N., Lesko, L.J., Chen, M.L., Williams, R.J., and the FDA Individual Bioequivalence Working Group (1997) Individual bioequivalence—New concepts in the statistical assessment of bioequivalence metrics. *Clinical Pharmacokinetics*, **33**, 1–6.

[959] Patterson, H.D. (1952) The construction of balanced designs for experiments involving sequences of treatments. *Biometrika*, **39**, 32.

[960] Patterson, H.D., Lucas, H. (1959) Extra-period change-over designs. *Biometrics*, **46**, 116–132.

[961] Patterson, H.D., Thompson, R. (1971) Recovery of inter-block information when block sizes are unequal. *Biometrika*, **58**, 545–554.

[962] Patterson, S., Francis, S., Ireson, M., Webber, D., Whitehead, J. (1999) A novel Bayesian decision procedure for early-phase dose-finding studies. *Journal of Biopharmaceutical Statistics*, **9**, 583–598.

[963] Patterson, S., Leonov, S., Mathur, A., Sparrow, P., Zhu, J. (2000) Dose-response technical policy document: Design and analysis of dose-response studies. *SmithKline Beecham Technical Policy Document* with Accompanying technical appendix by Leonov, S., Mathur, A., Zhu, J. (2001). Updated by Machin, A., Hamedani, A. (2004).

[964] Patterson, S. (2001a) A review of the development of biostatistical design and analysis techniques for assessing in vivo bioequivalence, Part 1. *Indian Journal of Pharmaceutical Sciences*, **63**, 81–100.

[965] Patterson, S. (2001b) A review of the development of biostatistical design and analysis techniques for assessing in vivo bioequivalence, Part 2. *Indian Journal of Pharmaceutical Sciences*, **63**, 169–186.

[966] Patterson, S., Zariffa, N., Howland, K., Montague, T. (2001c) Non-traditional study designs to demonstrate average bioequivalence for highly variable drug products. *European Journal of Clinical Pharmacology*, **57**, 663–670.

[967] Patterson, S., Jones, B. (2002a) Bioequivalence and the pharmaceutical industry. *Pharmaceutical Statistics*, **1**, 83–95.

[968] Patterson, S., Jones, B. (2002b) Statistical aspects of bioequivalence in the pharmaceutical industry. *Proceedings of the American Statistical Association Joint Statistical Meetings.*

[969] Patterson, S., Jones, B. (2002c) Clinical development planning and the use of pharmacokinetic data in ICH-E5 bridging assessments. *GSK BDS Technical Report 2002-04.*

[970] Patterson, S., Jones, B. (2004a) Simulation assessments of statistical aspects of bioequivalence in the pharmaceutical industry. *Pharmaceutical Statistics*, **3**, 13–23.

[971] Patterson, S., Agin, M., Anziano, R., Chuang-Stein, C., Dmitrienko, A., Ferber, G., Francom, S., Geraldes, M., Ghosh, K., Mills, T., Menton, R., Natarajan, J., Offen, W., Saoud, J., Smith, B., Suresh, R., Zariffa, N. (2005a) Investigating drug induced QT and QTc prolongation in the clinic: Statistical design and analysis considerations. *Drug Information Journal*, **39**, 243–266.

[972] Patterson, S., Jones, B., Zariffa, N. (2005b) Modelling and interpreting QTc prolongation in clinical pharmacology studies. *Drug Information Journal*, **39**, 437–455.

[973] Patterson, S., Jones, B. (2005c) *Bioequivalence and Statistics in Clinical Pharmacology.* Chapman and Hall, CRC Press, London.

[974] Patterson, S., Jones, B. (2007) A brief review of Phase 1 and clinical pharmacology statistics in clinical drug development. *Pharmaceutical Statistics*, **6**, 79–87.

[975] Patterson, S., Jones, B. (2010) Scaled average bioequivalence. *Proceedings of the American Statistical Association Joint Statistical Meetings, Biopharmaceutical Section*, 596–606.

[976] Patterson, S., Jones, B. (2012) Viewpoint: Observations on scaled average bioequivalence. *Pharmaceutical Statistics*, **11**, 1–7.

[977] Peace, K.E. (1986) Estimating the degree of equivalence and non-equivalence, an alternative to bioequivalence testing. *Proceedings of the American Statistical Association*, 63–69.

[978] Peace, K., ed. (1992) *Biopharmaceutical Sequential Statistical Applications.* Marcel Dekker, New York.

[979] Peace, K.E. (1993) Design and analysis considerations for safety data, particularly adverse events. *In Drug Safety Assessment in Clinical Trials*, Gibert, G.S. ed., 305–316. Marcel Dekker, New York.

[980] Peck, C., Desjardins, R. (1996) Simulation of clinical trials: Encouragements and cautions. *Applied Clinical Trials*, 30–32.

[981] Pereira, L. (2007) Bioequivalence testing by statistical shape analysis. *Journal of Pharmacokinetics and Pharmacodynamics*, **34**, 451–484.

[982] Peters, A., von Klot, S., Heier, M., Trentinaglia, I., Hormann, A., Wichmann, E., Lowel, H. for the Cooperative Health Research in the Region of Augsburg Study Group (2004) Exposure to traffic and the onset of myocardial infarction. *New England Journal of Medicine*, **351**, 1721–1730.

[983] Peterson, P., Carroll, K., Chuang-Stein, C., Ho, Y., Jiang, Q., Li, G., Sanchez, M., Sax, R., Wang, Y., Snapinn, S. (2010) PISC Expert Team White Paper: Toward a consistent standard of evidence when evaluating the efficacy of an experimental treatment from a randomized, active-controlled trial with Commentary and Rejoinder. *Statistics in Biopharmaceutical Research*, **2**, 522–539.

[984] Phillips, A. (1999) Guidelines for assessing the performance of statisticians involved in clinical research in the pharmaceutical industry. *Drug Information Journal*, **33**, 427–433.

[985] Phillips, K.F. (1990) Power of the two one-sided testing procedure in bioequivalence. *Journal of Pharmacokinetics and Biopharmaceutics*, **18**, 137–144.

[986] Phillips, K.F. (2009) Power for testing multiple instances of the two one-sided testing procedure. *The International Journal of Biostatistics*, **5**, 1–12.

[987] Pigeot, I. (2001a) The jackknife and bootstrap in biomedical research—Common principles and possible pitfalls. *Drug Information Journal*, **35**, 1431–1443.

[988] Pigeot, I. (2001b) The bootstrap percentile in Food and Drug Administration regulations of bioequivalence assessment. *Drug Information Journal*, **35**, 1445–1453.

[989] Pigeot, I., Schafer, J., Rohmel, J., Hauschke, D. (2003) Assessing non-inferiority of a new treatment in a three-arm clinical trial including a placebo. *Statistics in Medicine*, **22**, 883–899.

[990] Piotrovsky, V. (2005) Pharmacokinetic-pharmacodynamic modeling in the data analysis and interpretation of drug-induced QT/QTc prolongation. *The AAPS Journal*, **7**, E609–E624.

[991] Pitman, E.C.G. (1939) A note on normal correlation. *Biometrika*, **31**, 9–12.

[992] Plikaytis, B., Carlone, G. (2005a) Statistical considerations for vaccine immunogenicity trials. Part 1: Introduction and bioassay design and analysis. *Vaccine*, **23**, 1596–1605.

[993] Plikaytis, B., Carlone, G. (2005b) Statistical considerations for vaccine immunogenicity trials. Part 2: Noninferiority and other statistical approaches to vaccine evaluation. *Vaccine*, **23**, 1596–1605.

[994] Pocock, S.J. (1977) Group sequential methods in the design and analysis of clinical trials. *Biometrics*, **64**, 191–199.

[995] Pocock, S.J., Geller, N.L., Tsiatis, A.A. (1987) The analysis of multiple endpoints in clinical trials. *Biometrics*, **43**, 487–498.

[996] Pocock, S., Assmann, S., Enos, L., Kasten, L. (2002) Subgroup analysis, covariate adjustment and baseline comparisons in clinical trial reporting: Current practice and problems. *Statistics in Medicine*, **21**, 2917–2930.

[997] Pocock, S. (2006) The simplest statistical test: How to check for a difference between treatments. *British Medical Journal*, **332**, 1256–1258.

[998] Politi, M., Han, P., Col, N. (2007) Communicating the uncertainty of harms and benefits of medical interventions. *Medical Decision Making*, **27**, 681–695.

[999] Posch, M., Zehetmayer, S., Bauer, P. (2009) Hunting for significance with the false discovery rate. *Journal of the American Statistical Association*, **104**, 832–840.

[1000] Potvin, D., DiLiberti, C.E., Hauck, W.H., Parr, A.F., Schuirmann, D.J., Smith, R.A. (2008) Sequential design approaches for bioequivalence studies with cross-over designs. *Pharmaceutical Statistics*, **7**, 245–262.

[1001] Pound, N.J. (1999) Bioavailability and bioequivalence: Update on guidances from TPP. *AAPS International Workshop on Individual Bioequivalence: Realities and Implementation.*

[1002] Pradhan, R.S. (1997) Role of interoccasion variation in estimation of bioequivalence: A Bayesian approach. *Clinical Pharmacology and Therapeutics*, **61**, 186.

[1003] Prasad, P., Sun, J., Danner, R., Natanson, C. (2012) Excess deaths associated with tigecycline after approval based on noninferiority trials. *Clinical Infectious Diseases*, **54**, 1699–1709.

[1004] Pratt, J.W. (1961) Length of confidence intervals. *Journal of the American Statistical Association*, 549–648.

[1005] Pratt, C., Hertz, R., Elis, B., Crowell, S., Louv, W., Moye, L. (1994) Risk of developing life-threatening ventricular arrhythmia associated with terfenadine in comparison with other over the counter antihistamines. *American Journal of Cardiology*, **73**, 346–352.

[1006] Pratt, C., Ruberg, S., Morganroth, J., McNutt, B., Woodward, J., Harris, S., Ruskin, J., Moye, L. (1996) Dose-response relation between terfenadine (Seldane) and the QTc interval on the scalar electrocardiogram: Distinguishing drug effect from spontaneous variability. *American Heart Journal*, **131**, 472–480.

[1007] Prentice, R. (1989) Surrogate endpoints in clinical trials: Definition and operational criteria. *Statistics in Medicine*, **8**, 431–440.

[1008] Priori, S., Schwartz, P., Napolitano, C., Bloise, R., Ronchetti, E., Grillo, M., Vicentini, A., Spazzolini, C., Nastoli, J., Bottelli, G., Folli, R., Capelletti, D. (2003) Risk stratification in the long-QT syndrome. *New England Journal of Medicine*, **348**, 1866–1874.

[1009] Psaty, B., Weiss, N., Furberg, C., Koepsell, T., Siscovick, D., Rosendaal, F., Smith, N., Heckbert, S., Kaplan, R., Lin, D., Fleming, T., Wagner, E. (1999) Surrogate end points, health outcomes, and the drug-approval process for the treatment of risk factors for cardiovascular disease. *Journal of the American Medical Association*, **282**, 786–796.

[1010] Purkins, L., Love, E., Eve, M., Woolridge, C., Cowan, C., Smart, T., Johnson, P., Rapeport, W. (2004) The influence of diet upon liver function tests and serum lipids in healthy male volunteers resident in a Phase I unit. *British Journal of Clinical Pharmacology*, **57**, 199–208.

[1011] Putt, M. (2006) Power to detect clinically relevant carry-over in a series of cross-over studies. *Statistics in Medicine*, **25**, 2567–2586.

[1012] Putter, H., Fiocco, M., Geskus, R. (2007) Tutorials in biostatistics: Competing risk and multi-state models. *Statistics in Medicine*, **26**, 2389–2430.

[1013] Qazi, Y., Forrest, A., Tornatore, K., Venuto, R. (2006) The clinical impact of 1:1 conversion from Neoral to a generic cyclosporine (Gengraf) in renal transplant recipients with stable graft function. *Clinical Transplantation*, **20**, 313–317.

[1014] Qu, R., Zheng, H. (2001) Exact power and sample size calculations for bioequivalence studies with high order cross-over designs. *Proceedings of the American Statistical Association.*

[1015] Quan, H., Shih, J., Zhang, J., Bolongese, J., Capizzi, T., Oppenheimer, L., Simon, T. (2001) Evaluation of the impact of period and carry-over effects for a four-period cross-over study. *Proceedings of the American Statistical Association.*

[1016] Quan, H., Zhou, D., Mancini, P., He, Y., Koch, G. (2012) Adaptive patient population selection design in clinical trials. *Statistics in Biopharmaceutical Research*, **4**, 86–99.

[1017] Queckenberg, C., Fuhr, U. (2009) Influence of posture on pharmacokinetics. *European Journal of Clinical Pharmacology*, **65**, 109–119.

[1018] Quiroz, J., Ting, N., Wei, G., Burdick, R. (2002) Alternative confidence intervals for the assessment of bioequivalence in four-period cross-over designs. *Statistics in Medicine*, **21**, 1825–1847.

[1019] Quiroz, J. (2005) Assessment of equivalence using a concordance correlation coefficient in a repeated measures design. *Journal of Biopharmaceutical Statistics*, **15**, 913–928.

[1020] Racine-Poon, A., Grieve, A.P., Fluhler, H., Smith, A.F.-M. (1986) Bayesian methods in practice, experiences in the pharmaceutical industry (with discussion). *Applied Statistics*, **35**, 93–150.

[1021] Racine-Poon, A., Grieve, A.P., Fluhler, H., Smith, A.F.-M. (1987) A two-stage procedure for bioequivalence studies. *Biometrics*, **43**, 847–856.

[1022] Racoosin, J. (2003) The clinical evaluation of QT interval prolongation and proarrythmic potential for non-antiarrythmic drugs. *Presentation at Drug Information Agency/FDA Workshop*, www.diahome.org

[1023] Ramsay, T., Elkum, N. (2005) A comparison of four different methods for outlier detection in bioequivalence studies. *Journal of Biopharmaceutical Statistics*, **15**, 43–52.

[1024] Rao, C.R. (1973) *Linear Statistical Inference and Its Applications, 2nd ed.* John Wiley and Sons, New York.

[1025] Rao, S., Schoenfeld, D. (2007) Survival methods. *Circulation*, **115**, 109–113.

[1026] Reigner, B., Williams, P., Patel, I., Steimer, J., Peck, C., Brummelen, P. (1997) An evaluation of the integration of pharmacokinetic and pharmacodynamic principles in clinical drug development. *Clinical Pharmacokinetics*, **33**, 142–152.

[1027] Reigner, B., Blesch, K. (2001) Estimating the starting dose for entry into humans: Principles and practice. *European Journal of Clinical Pharmacology*, **57**, 835–845.

[1028] Reiser, B., Guttman, I. (1986) Statistical inference for $\Pr(Y < X)$. *Technometrics*, **28**, 253–257.

[1029] Ren, C., Sun, D., Speckman, P., He, C., Swan, S. (2005) Heirarchical models for the probabilities of conception. *Biometrical Journal*, **5**, 721–739.

[1030] Rescigno, A. (1992) Bioequivalence. *Pharmaceutical Research*, **9**, 925–928.

[1031] Rescigno, A., Powers, J.D. (1998) AUC and Cmax are not sufficient to prove bioequivalence. *Pharmacological Research*, **37**, 93–95.

[1032] Reynolds, S.M. (2004) ORI findings of scientific missconduct in clinical trials and publicly funded research, 1992-2002. *Clinical Trials*, **1**, 509–516.

[1033] Reynolds, M., Fahrbach, K., Hauch, O., Wygant, G., Estok, R., Cella, C., Nalysnyk, L. (2004) Warfarin anticoagulation and outcomes in patients with atrial fibrillation. *Chest*, **126**, 1938–1945.

[1034] Rheinstein, P.H. (1990) Therapeutic inequivalence. *Drug Safety 5*, **Suppl 1**, 114–119.

[1035] Rhodes, C.T. (1997) Acceptance limits for bioequivalence studies. *Clinical Research and Regulatory Affairs*, **14**, 127–137.

[1036] Ridker, P., Torres, J. (2006) Reported outcomes on major cardiovascular clinical trials funded by for-profit and not-for-profit organizations: 2000-2005. *Journal of the American Medical Association*, **295**, 2270–2274.

[1037] Riegelman, S., Collier, P. (1980) The application of statistical moment theory to the evaluation of in vivo dissolution time and absorption time. *Pharmacokinetics and Biopharmaceutics*, **8, No. 5**, 509–535.

[1038] Ring, A., Tothfalusi, L., Endrenyi, L., Weiss, M. (2000) Sensitivity of empirical metrics of rate of absorption in bioequivalence studies. *Pharmaceutical Research*, **17**, 583–588.

[1039] Robert, C., Casella, G. (1999) *Monte Carlo Statistical Methods.* Springer, New York.

[1040] Robinson, G.K. (1976) Properties of Student's t and of the Behrens-Fisher solution to the two means problem. *The Annals of Statistics*, **4, No. 5**, 963–971.

[1041] Robinson, G.K. (1991) The BLUP is a good thing: The estimation of random effects. *Statistical Sciences*, **6, No. 1**, 15–51.

[1042] Robinson, J.A. (1978) Sequential choice of an optimal dose: A prediction intervals approach. *Biometrika*, **65, 1**, 75–78.

[1043] Rosenkranz, G. (2011) The impact of randomization on the analysis of clinical trials. *Statistics in Medicine*, **30**, 3475–3487.

[1044] Rochester, G. (2009) Lifecycle planning for safety evaluation in support of risk-benefit activities. *Presented at the Biopharmaceutical Applied Statistics Symposium, XVI.*

[1045] Rocke, D.M. (1984) On testing for bioequivalence. *Biometrics*, **40**, 225–230.

[1046] Rodary, C., Com-Nougue, C., Tournade, M.-F. (1989) How to establish equivalence between treatments: A one-sided clinical trial in paediatric oncology. *Statistics in Medicine*, **8**, 593–598.

[1047] Rodda, B.E., Davis R.L. (1980) Determining the probability of an important difference in bioavailability. *Clinical Pharmacology and Therapeutics*, **28**, 247–252.

[1048] Roe, D., Vonesh, E., Wolfinger, R., Mensil, F., Mallet, A. (1997) Comparison of population pharmacokinetic modelling methods using simulated data: Results from the Population Modelling Workgroup. *Statistics in Medicine*, **16**, 1241–1262.

[1049] Rohmel, J., Gerlinger, C., Benda, N., Lauter, J. (2006) On testing simultaneously non-inferiority in two multiple primary endpoints and superiority in at least one of them. *Biometrical Journal*, **48**, 916–933.

[1050] Rolan, P., Danhof, M., Stanski, D., Peck, C. (2007) Current issues related to drug safety especially with regard to the use of biomarkers: A meeting report and progress update. *European Journal of Pharmaceutical Sciences*, **30**, 107–112.

[1051] Rom, D.M. (1990) A sequentially rejective test procedure based on a modified Bonferroni inequality. *Biometrika*, **77, 3**, 663–665.

[1052] Rosenbaum, D.H., Rowan, A.J., Tuchman, L., French, J.A. (1994) Comparative bioavailability of a generic phenytoin and dilantin. *Epilepsia*, **35(3)**, 656–660.

[1053] Rosenbaum, S.E. (1998) Effect of variability in hepatic clearance on the bioequivalence parameters of a drug and its metabolite: Simulations using a pharmacostatistical model. *Pharmaceutica Acta Helvetiae*, **73**, 135–144.

[1054] Rosenzweig, P., Miget, N., Brohler, S. (1999) Transaminase elevation on placebo during phase I trials: Prevalence and significance. *Clinical Pharmacology*, **48**, 19–23.

[1055] Rosner, G., Stadler, W., Ratain, M. (2002) Randomized discontinuation design: Application to cytostatic antineoplastic agents. *Journal of Clinical Oncology*, **20**, 4478–4484.

[1056] Rossell, D., Muller, P., Rosner, G. (2007) Screening designs for drug development. *Biostatistics*, **8**, 595–608.

[1057] Rothmann, M., Li, N., Chen, G., Chi, G., Temple, R., Tsou, H. (2003) Design and analysis of non-inferiority mortality trials in oncology. *Statistics in Medicine*, **22**, 239–264.

[1058] Rowland, M., Tozer, T.N. (1980) *Clinical Pharmacokinetics: Concepts and Applications.* Lea and Febiger, Philadelphia.

[1059] Roy, A., Ette, E. (2005) A pragmatic approach to the design of population pharmacokinetic studies. *The AAPS Journal*, **7**, E408–E420.

[1060] Royston, P., Matthews, J.N.S. (1991) Estimation of reference ranges from normal samples. *Statistics in Medicine*, **10**, 691–695.

[1061] Rubenstein, L., Korn, E., Freidlin, B., Hunsberger, S., Ivy, P., Smith, M. (2005) Design issues of randomised phase II trials and a proposal for phase II screening trials. *Journal of Clinical Oncology*, **23**, 7199–7206.

[1062] Rubins, J., Puri, A., Loch, J., Charboneau, D., MacDonald, R., Opstad, N., Janoff, E. (1998) Magnitude, duration, quality, and function of pneumococcal vaccine responses in elderly adults. *Journal of Infectious Diseases*, **178**, 431–440.

[1063] Russek-Cohen, E., Martinez, M., Nevius, A. (2005) A SAS/IML program for simulating pharmacokinetic data. *Computer Methods and Programs in Biomedicine*, **78**, 39–60.

[1064] Sabatine, M., Cannon, C., Gibson, C., Lopez-Sendon, J., Montalescot, G., Theroux, P., Claeys, M., Cools, F., Hill, K., Skene, A., McCabe, C., and Braunwald, E., for the CLARITY-TIMI 28 Investigators (2005) Addition of clopidogrel to aspirin and fibrinolytic therapy for myocardial infarction with ST-segment elevation. *New England Journal of Medicine*, **352**, 1179–1189.

[1065] Sager, P., Nebout, T., Darpo, B. (2005) ICH E14: A new regulatory guidance on the clinical evaluation of QT/QTc interval prolongation and proarrythmic potential for non-antiarrythmic drugs. *Drug Information Journal*, **39**, 387–394.

[1066] Sahin, S., Benet, L.Z. (2008) The operational multiple dosing half-life: A key to defining drug accumulation in patients and to designing extended release dosing forms. *Pharmaceutical Research*, **25**, 2869–2877.

[1067] Salsburg, D. (2010) Statistical aids for early management decisions in drug development. *Statistics in Biopharmaceutical Research*, **2**, 549–556.

[1068] Sampson, A.R., Sill, M.W. (2005) Drop-the-losers design: Normal case. *Biometrical Journal*, **47, 3**, 257–268.

[1069] Sankoh, A.J., Huque, M.F., Russell, H.K., D'Agostino, R.B. (1999) Global two-group multiple endpoint adjustment methods applied to clinical trials. *Drug Information Journal*, **33**, 119–140.

[1070] Sankoh, A.J., D'Agostino, R.B., Huque, M.F. (2003) Efficacy endpoint selection and multiplicity adjustment methods in clinical trials with inherent multiple endpoint issues. *Statistics in Medicine*, **22**, 3133–3150.

[1071] Santner, T., Pradhan, V., Senchaudhuri, P., Mehta, C., Tamhane, A. (2007) Small-sample comparisons of confidence intervals for the difference of two independent binomial proportions. *Computational Statistics and Data Analysis*, **51**, 5791–5799.

[1072] Sarkar, S., Watts, S., Ohashi, O., Carroll, R., Uesaka, H., Mason, T., Rivera, C. (2002) Bridging data between two ethnic populations. A new application of matched case-control methodology. *Drug Information Journal*, **36**, 349–356.

[1073] *Statistical Analysis Software, SAS/STAT User's Guide, Version 9.* (2004). SAS Institute, Cary, NC.

[1074] Satterthwaite, F. (1941) Synthesis of variance. *Psychometrika*, **6**, 309–316.

[1075] Satterthwaite, F. (1946) An approximate distribution of estimates of variance components. *Biometrics*, **2**, 110–114.

[1076] Sauter, R., Steinijans, V.W., Diletti, E., Bohm, A., Schulz, H.-U. (1992) Presentation of results from bioequivalence studies. *International Journal of Clinical Pharmacology*, **30, No. 7**, 233–256.

[1077] Schall, R. (1995) Assessment of individual and population bioequivalence using the probability that bioavailabilities are similar. *Biometrics*, **51**, 615–626.

[1078] Schall, R., Luus, H.G. (1993) On population and individual bioequivalence. *Statistics in Medicine*, **12**, 1109–1124.

[1079] Schall, R., Williams, R.L. (1996) Towards a practical strategy for assessing individual bioequivalence. *Journal of Pharmacokinetics and Biopharmaceutics*, **24**, 133–149.

[1080] Schall, R., Endrenyi, L., Ring, A. (2010) Residuals and outliers in replicate design crossover studies. *Journal of Biopharmaceutical Statistics*, **20**, 835–849.

[1081] Schall, R. (2012) The empirical coverage of confidence intervals: Point estimates and confidence intervals for confidence levels. *Biometrical Journal*, **54**, 537–551.

[1082] Scheffe, H. (1970) Practical solutions of the Behrens-Fisher problem. *Journal of the American Statistical Association*, **65**, 1501–1508.

[1083] Schellekens, H. (2008) The first biosimilar epoetin: But how similar is it? *Clinical Journal of the American Society of Nephrology*, **3**, 174–178.

[1084] Schildcrout, J., Jenkins, C., Ostroff, J., Gillen, D., Harrell, F., Trost, D. (2008) Analysis of longitudinal laboratory data in the presence of common selection mechanisms: A view towards greater emphasis on pre-marketing pharmaceutical safety. *Statistics in Medicine*, **27**, 2248–2266.

[1085] Schoenfeld, D., Borenstein, M. (2005) Calculating the power and sample size for the logistic and proportional hazards models. *Journal of Statistical Computation and Simulation*, **75**, 771–785.

[1086] Schlotzhauer, S., Littell, R. (1987) *SAS System for Elementary Statistical Analysis.* SAS Institute, Cary, NC.

[1087] Schuirmann, D.J. (1981) On hypothesis testing to determine if the mean of a normal distribution is contained in a known interval. *Biometrics*, **37**, 617.

[1088] Schuirmann, D.J. (1987) A comparison of the two one sided tests procedure and the power approach for assessing the equivalence of average bioavailability. *Journal of Pharmacokinetics and Biopharmaceutics*, **15**, 657–680.

[1089] Schuirmann, D.J. (1990) Design of bioavailability and bioequivalence studies. *Drug Information Journal*, **24**, 315–323.

[1090] Schulman, R.L. (1992) *Statistics in Plain English with Computer Applications.* Van Nostrand Reinhold, New York.

[1091] Schumaker, R.C., Metzler, C.M. (1998) The phenytoin trial is a case study of individual bioequivalence. *Drug Information Journal*, **32**, 1063–1072.

[1092] Schwartsmann, G., Ratain, M.J., Cragg, G.M., Wong, J.E., Saijo, N., Parkinson, D.R., Fujiwara, Y., Pazdur, R., Newman, D.J., Dagher, R., DiLeone, L. (2002) Anticancer drug discovery and development throughout the world. *Journal of Clinical Oncology*, **20, No. 18**, 47–59.

[1093] Schwartz, J. (2007) The current state of knowledge on age, sex, and their interactions on clinical pharmacology. *Clinical Pharmacology and Therapeutics*, **82**, 87–96.

[1094] Schwarz, G. (1978) Estimating the dimension of a model. *The Annals of Statistics*, **6(2)**, 461–464.

[1095] Scott, J., Hsu, H. (2011) Missing data issues at the FDA center for biologics evaluation and research. *Journal of Biopharmaceutical Statistics*, **21**, 196–201.

[1096] Searle, S.R. (1971) *Linear Models.* John Wiley and Sons, New York.

[1097] Searle, S. R. (1988) Mixed models and unbalanced data: Wherefrom, whereat and whereto? *Communications in Statistical Theory and Methodology*, **17(4)**, 935–968.

[1098] Seber, G.A. (1977) *Linear Regression Analysis.* John Wiley and Sons, New York.

[1099] Selwyn, M.R., Dempster, A.P., Hall, N.R. (1981) A Bayesian approach to bioequivalence for the 2×2 cross-over design. *Biometrics*, **37**, 11–21.

[1100] Selwyn, M.R., Hall, N.R. (1984) On Bayesian methods for bioequivalence. *Biometrics*, **40**, 1103–1108.

[1101] Selwyn, M., Fish, S. (2004) Choice of alpha spending function and time points in clinical trials with one or two interim analyses. *Pharmaceutical Statistics*, **3**, 193–203.

[1102] Senn, S. (1992) Is the 'simple carry-over' model useful? *Statistics in Medicine*, **11**, 715–726.

[1103] Senn, S. (1996) The AB/BA cross-over: How to perform the two-stage analysis if you can't be persuaded you shouldn't. In *Liber Amicorum Roel van Strik*, Hansen, B., and de Ridder, M., eds., 93–100. Erasmus University, Rotterdam.

[1104] Senn, S. (1997) *Statistical Issues in Drug Development.* John Wiley and Sons, New York.

[1105] Senn, S. (1998a) In the blood: Proposed new requirements for registering generic drugs. *The Lancet*, **352**, 85–86.

[1106] Senn, S., Lambrou, D. (1998b) Robust and realistic approaches to carry-over. *Statistics in Medicine*, **17**, 2849–2864.

[1107] Senn, S. (1998c) Some controversies in planning and analysing multi-centre trials. *Statistics in Medicine*, **17**, 1753–1765.

[1108] Senn, S., Grieve, A. P. (1999a) A comment on optimal allocations for bioequivalence studies. *Biometrics*, **55**, 1314–1315.

[1109] Senn, S. (1999b) Clinical cross-over trials in phase I. *Statistical Methods in Medical Research*, **8**, 263–278.

[1110] Senn, S. (2000a) Decisions and bioequivalence. *Conference Proceedings of Challenging Statistical Issues in Clinical Trials.*

[1111] Senn, S. (2000b) Consensus and controversy in pharmaceutical statistics. *The Statistician*, **49, Part 2**, 135–176.

[1112] Senn, S. (2001) Statistical issues in bioequivalence. *Statistics in Medicine*, **20**, 2785–2799.

[1113] Senn, S. (2002) *Cross-Over Trials in Clinical Research, 2nd ed.* John Wiley and Sons, New York.

[1114] Senn, S., Lee, S. (2004a) The analysis of the AB/BA cross-over trial in the medical literature. *Pharmaceutical Statistics*, **3**, 123–131.

[1115] Senn, S., D'Angelo, G., Potvin, D. (2004b) Carry-over in cross-over trials in bioequivalence: Theoretical concerns and empirical evidence. *Pharmaceutical Statistics*, **3**, 133–142.

[1116] Senn, S. (2005a) An unreasonable prejudice against modelling. *Pharmaceutical Statistics*, **4**, 87–89.

[1117] Senn, S. (2005b) Letter to the editor: Misunderstandings regarding clinical cross-over trials. *Statistics in Medicine*, **24**, 3675–3678.

[1118] Senn, S. (2006a) An early Atkins' diet: RA Fisher analyses a medical 'experiment'. *Biometrical Journal*, **48**, 193–204.

[1119] Senn, S. (2006b) Cross-over trials in *Statistics in Medicine*: The first '25' years. *Statistics in Medicine*, **25**, 3430–3442.

[1120] Senn, S. (2007a) Trying to be precise about vagueness. *Statistics in Medicine*, **26**, 1417–1430.

[1121] Senn, S., Amin, D., Bailey, R., Bird, S., Bogacka, B., Colman, P., Garrett, A., Grieve, A., Lachmann, P. (2007b) Statistical issues in first-in-man studies. *Journal of the Royal Statistical Society, Series A*, **170**, 517–579.

[1122] Senn, S., Bretz, F. (2007c) Power and sample size when multiple endpoints are considered. *Pharmaceutical Statistics*, **6**, 161–170.

[1123] Senn, S., Julious, S. (2011) Investigating variability in patient response to treatment — A case study from a replicate cross-over study. *Statistical Methods in Medical Research*, **20**, 657–666.

[1124] Senn, S. (2013) Seven myths of randomisation in clinical trials. *Statistics in Medicine*, **32**, 1439–1450.

[1125] Serfling, R. (1980) *Approximation Theorems of Mathematical Statistics.* John Wiley and Sons, New York.

[1126] Sethuraman, V., Leonov, S., Squassante, L., Mitchell, T., Hale, M. (2007) Sample size calculations for the power model for dose proportionality. *Pharmaceutical Statistics*, **6**, 35–41.

[1127] Shaffer, J. (1986) Modified sequentially rejective multiple test procedures. *Journal of the American Statistical Association*, **81**, 826–831.

[1128] Shah, B.K. (1979) On the method of internal least squares. *Biometrics*, **35**, 497–502.

[1129] Shah, R. (2005) Drugs, QTc interval prolongation, and final ICH E14 guideline. *Drug Safety*, **28**, 1009–1028.

[1130] Shah, V.P. (1987) Analytical methods used in bioavailability studies: A regulatory viewpoint. *Clinical Research Practices & Drug Regulatory Affairs*, **5(1)**, 51–60.

[1131] Shah, V.P., Yacobi, A., Barr, W., Benet, L.Z., Breimer, D., Dobrinska, M.R., Endrenyi, L., Fairweather, W., Gillespie, W., Gonzalez, M.A., Hooper, J., Jackson, A., Lesko, L.J., Midha, K.K., Noonan, P.K., Patnaik, R., Williams, R.L. (1996) Workshop report: Evaluation of orally administered highly variable drugs and drug formulations. *Pharmaceutical Research*, **13**, 1590–1594.

[1132] Shao, J., Tu, D. (1996) *The Jackknife and Bootstrap.* Springer, New York.

[1133] Shao, J., Chow, S.-C., Wang, B. (2000a) The bootstrap procedure in individual bioequivalence. *Statistics in Medicine*, **19**, 2741–2754.

[1134] Shao, J., Kubler, J., Pigeot, I. (2000b) Consistency of the bootstrap procedure in individual bioequivalence. *Biometrika*, **87**, 573–585.

[1135] Shapiro, S., Wilk, M. (1965). An analysis of variance test for normality (complete samples). *Biometrika*, **52**, 591–611.

[1136] Shapiro, E. (2012) Prevention of pneumococcal infection with vaccines. *Journal of the American Medical Association*, **307**, 847–849.

[1137] Sharma, A., Pilote, S., Belanger, P., Arsenault, M., Hamelin, B. (2004). A convenient five-drug cocktail for the assessment of major drug metabolizing enzymes: A pilot study. *British Journal of Clinical Pharmacology*, **58**, 288–297.

[1138] Sheiner, L.B. (1984) The population approach to pharmacokinetic data analysis: Rationale and standard data analysis methods. *Drug Metabolism Reviews*, **15**, 153–171.

[1139] Sheiner L.B., Beal, S.L., Sambol, N.C. (1989) Study designs for dose-ranging. *Clinical Pharmacology and Therapeutics*, **46**, 63–77.

[1140] Sheiner, L.B., Hashimoto, Y., Beal, S. (1991) A simulation study comparing designs for dose ranging. *Statistics in Medicine*, **10**, 303–321.

[1141] Sheiner, L.B. (1992) Bioequivalence revisited. *Statistics in Medicine*, **11**, 1777–1788.

[1142] Sheiner, L.B. (1997) Learning versus confirming in clinical drug development. *Clinical Pharmacology and Therapeutics*, **61**, 275–291.

[1143] Sheiner, L.B., Steimer, J.-L. (2000) Pharmacokinetic-pharmacodynamic modeling in drug development. *Annual Reviews of Pharmacology and Toxicology*, **40**, 67–95.

[1144] Sheiner, L.B. (2002) Letters to the editor. *Clinical Pharmacology & Therapeutics*, **April 2002**, 304–306.

[1145] Shen, M., Russek-Cohen, E., Slud, E. (2015a) Exact calculation of power and sample size in bioequivalence studies using two one-sided tests. *Pharmaceutical Statistics*, **14**, 95–101.

[1146] Shen, M., Russek-Cohen, E., Slud, E. (2015b) Letter to the editor by authors of 'Exact calculation of power and sample size in bioequivalence studies using two one-sided tests.' *Pharmaceutical Statistics*, **14**, 272.

[1147] Sheng, X., Carriere, K. (2005) Strategies for analysing missing item response data with an application to lung cancer. *Biometrical Journal*, **5**, 605–615.

[1148] Sheng, Y., He, Y., Huang, X., Yang, J., Wang, K., Zheng, Q. (2010) Systematic evaluation of dose proportionality studies in clinical pharmacokinetics. *Current Drug Metabolism*, **11**, 526–537.

[1149] Sherman, D. (2007) Stroke prevention in atrial fibrillation: Pharmacological rate versus rhythm control. *Stroke*, **38**, 615–617.

[1150] Sheshkin, D. (2000) *Handbook of Parametric and Nonparametric Statistical Procedures.* Chapman & Hall, CRC Press, London.

[1151] Shih, W. (2001) Clinical trials for drug registrations in Asian-Pacific countries: Proposal for a new paradigm from a statistical perspective. *Controlled Clinical Trials*, **22**, 357–366.

[1152] Shih, W. (2002) Problems in dealing with missing data and informative censoring in clinical trials. *Current Controlled Trials in Cardiovascular Medicine*, **3**, 3.

[1153] Shin, J., Kang, W., Shon, J., Arefayne, M., Yoon, Y., Kim, K., Kim, D., Kim, D., Cho, K., Woosley, R., Flockhart, D. (2006) Possible inter-ethnic differences in quindine-induced QT prolongation between healthy Caucasian and Korean subjects. *British Journal of Clinical Pharmacology*, **63**, 206–215.

[1154] Shumaker, R.C., Metzler, C.M. (1998) The phenytoin trial is a case study of "individual" bioequivalence. *Drug Information Journal*, **32**, 1063–1072.

[1155] Shun, Z., Chi, E., Durrleman, S., Fisher, L. (2005) Statistical consideration of the strategy for demonstrating clinical evidence of effectiveness—Open larger vs two smaller pivotal studies. *Statistics in Medicine*, **24**, 1619–1637.

[1156] Shuster, J., Jones, L., Salmon, D. (2007) Fixed versus random effects meta-analysis in rare event studies: The rosiglitazone link with myocardial infarction and cardiac death. *Statistics in Medicine*, **26**, 4375–4385.

[1157] Siber, G., Chang, I., Baker, S., Fernsten, P., O'Brien, K., Santosham, M., Klugman, K., Madhi, S., Paradiso, P., Kohberger, R. (2007) Estimating the protective concentration of anti-pneumococcal capsular polysaccharide antibodies. *Vaccine*, **25**, 3816–3826.

[1158] Siddiqui, O., Hung, H.M., O'Neill, R. (2009) MMRM vs. LOCF: A comprehensive comparison based on simulation study and 25 NDA datasets. *Journal of Biopharmaceutical Statistics*, **19**, 227–246.

[1159] Siewert, M., Roussel, H.M. (2000) International reference product-innovator industry's perspective. *European Journal of Drug Metabolism and Pharmacokinetics*, **25, No. 1**, 61–72.

[1160] Simon, C., Hegedus, S. (2005) Exploring websites on cancer clinical trials: An empirical review. *Contemporary Clinical Trials*, **26**, 530–533.

[1161] Simmonds, M., Higgins, J. (2007) Covariate heterogeneity in meta-analysis: Criteria for deciding between meta-regression and individual patient data. *Statistics in Medicine*, **26**, 2982–2999.

[1162] Singh, G.J.-P., Adams, W.P., Lesko, L.J., Shah, V.P., Molzon, J.A., Williams, R.L., Pershing, L.K. (1999) Development of in vivo bioequivalence methodology for dermatologic corticosteroids based on pharmacodynamic modeling. *Clinical Pharmacology and Therapeutics*, **66**, 346–357.

[1163] Singh, S.D., Williams, A.J. (1999) The prevalence and incidence of medical conditions in healthy pharmaceutical company employees who volunteer to participate in medical research. *British Journal of Clinical Pharmacology*, **48**, 25–31.

[1164] Siqueira, A., Whitehead, A., Todd, S., Lucini, M. (2005) Comparison of sample size formulae for 2×2 cross-over designs applied to bioequivalence studies. *Pharmaceutical Statistics*, **4**, 233–243.

[1165] Slob, W. (2002) Dose-response modeling of continuous endpoints. *Toxicological Sciences*, **66**, 298–312.

[1166] Smith, B., Vandenhende, F., DeSante, K., Farid, N., Welch, P., Callaghan, J., Forgue, S. (2000) Confidence interval criteria for assessment of dose proportionality. *Pharmaceutical Research*, **17**, 1278–1283.

[1167] Smith, B. (2004) Assessment of dose proportionality. In *Pharmacokinetics in Drug Development: Clinical Study Design and Analysis, Volume 1*, Bonate, P., Howard, D., eds., 363–382. AAPS Press, USA.

[1168] Smith, B. (2005) It's time. *The AAPS Journal*, **7**, E655–E658.

[1169] Smith, D.W., Murray, L.W. (1984) An alternative to Eisenhart's model II and mixed model in the case of negative variance estimates. *Journal of the American Statistical Association*, 79, No. 385, 145–151.

[1170] Smith, M. (2003) Software for non-linear mixed effects modelling: A review of several packages. *Pharmaceutical Statistics*, **2**, 69–75.

[1171] Smith, K., Wateska, A., Nowalk, M., Raymund, M., Nuorti, J., Zimmerman, R. (2012) Cost-effectiveness of adult vaccination strategies using pneumococcal conjugate vaccine compared with pneumococcal polysaccharide vaccine. *Journal of the American Medical Association*, **307**, 804–812.

[1172] Smith, M., Jones, I., Morris, M., Grieve, A., Tan, K. (2006) Implementation of a Bayesian adaptive design in a proof of concept study. *Pharmaceutical Statistics*, **5**, 39–50.

[1173] Snikeris, F., Tingey, H.B. (1994) A two step method for assessing bioequivalence. *Drug Information Journal*, **28**, 709–722.

[1174] Song, Y., Chi, G. (2007) A method for testing a pre-specified sub-group in clinical trials. *Statistics in Medicine*, **26**, 3535–3549.

[1175] Sooriyarachchi, M., Whitehead, J., Matsushita, T., Bolland, K., Whitehead, A. (2003) Incorporating data received after a sequential trial has stopped into the final analysis: Implementation and comparison of methods. *Biometrics*, **59**, 701–709.

[1176] Soy, D., Beal, S.L., Sheiner, L.B. (2004) Population one-compartment pharmacokinetic analysis with missing dosage data. *Clinical Pharmacology & Therapeutics*, **76(5)**, 441–451.

[1177] Stroke Prevention in Atrial Fibrillation Investigators (1991) Stroke prevention in atrial fibrillation study: Final results. *Circulation*, **84**, 527–539.

[1178] Spiegelhalter, D., Freedman, L. (1994) Bayesian approaches to randomised trials with discussion. *Journal of the Royal Statistical Society, Series A*, **157**, 357–416.

[1179] Spiegelhalter, D., Abrams, K., Myles, J. (2004) *Bayesian Approaches to Clinical Trials and Health-Care Evaluation.* John Wiley and Sons, West Sussex, England.

[1180] Spino, M., Tsang, Y.C., Pop, R. (2000) Dissolution and in vivo evidence of differences in reference products: Impact on development of generic drugs. *European Journal of Drug Metabolism and Pharmacokinetics*, **25**, 18–24.

[1181] Sprecher, D., Watkins, T., Behar, S., Brown, W., Rubins, H., Schaefer, E. (2003) Importance of high density lipoprotein cholesterol and triglyceride levels in coronary heart disease. *The American Journal of Cardiology*, **91**, 575–580.

[1182] Sprecher, D., Massien, C., Pearce, G., Billin, A., Perlstein, I., Willson, T., Hassall, D., Ancellin, N., Patterson, S., Lobe, D., Johnson, T. (2007) Triglyceride:high-density lipoprotein cholesterol effects in healthy subjects administered a peroxisome proliferator activated receptor δ agonist. *Arteriosclerosis, Thrombosis, and Vascular Biology*, **27**, 359–365.

[1183] Srinivasan, R., Langenberg, P. (1986) A two-stage procedure with controlled error probabilities for testing equivalence. *Biometrical Journal*, **7**, 825–833.

[1184] Stadler, W., Rosner, G., Small, E., Hollis, D., Rini, B., Zaentz, S., Mahoney, J., Ratain, M. (2005) Successful implementation of the randomized discontinuation trial design: An application to the study of the putative antiangiogenic agent carboxyaminoimidazole in renal cell carcinoma — CALGB69901. *Journal of Clinical Oncology*, **23**, 3726–3732.

[1185] Stallard, N., Whitehead, J., Cleall, S. (2005) Decision-making in a phase II clinical trial: A new approach combining Bayesian and frequentist concepts. *Pharmaceutical Statistics*, **4**, 119–128.

[1186] Stedman's Medical Dictionary, 25th ed. (1990) William and Wilkins, Baltimore.

[1187] Steg, P., Bhatt, D., Wilson, P., D'Agostino, R., Ohman, E., Rother, J., Liau, C.-S., Hirsch, A., Mas, J.-L., Ikeda, Y., Pensina, M., Goto, S., for the REACH Registry Investigators (2007) One-year cardiovascular event rates in outpatients with atherothrombosis. *Journal of the American Medical Association*, **297**, 1197–1206.

[1188] Steibuhl, S., Berger, P., Mann, J., Fry, E., DeLago, A., Wilmer, C., Topol, E. for the CREDO Investigators (2002) Early and sustained dual oral anti-platelet therapy following percutaneous coronary intervention: A randomized controlled trial. *Journal of the American Medical Association*, **288**, 2411–2420.

[1189] Steinijans, V.W., Diletti, E. (1983) Statistical analysis of bioavailability studies: Parametric and nonparametric confidence interval. *European Journal of Clinical Pharmacology*, **24**, 127–136.

[1190] Steinijans, V.W., Hauschke, V. (1990) Update on the statistical analysis of bioequivalence studies. *International Journal of Clinicial Pharmacology, Therapy, and Toxicology*, **28**, 105–110.

[1191] Steinijans, V.W., Hartmann, M., Huber, R., Radtke, H.W. (1991) Lack of pharmacokinetic interaction as an equivalence problem. *International Journal of Clinicial Pharmacology, Therapy, and Toxicology*, **29**, 323–328.

[1192] Steinijans, V.W., Sauter, R., Hauschke, D., Elze, M. (1995) Metrics to characterize concentration-time profiles in single and multiple-dose bioequivalence studies. *Drug Information Journal*, **29**, 981–987.

[1193] Steinijans, V.W., Hauschke, D., Schall, R. (1995) International harmonization of regulatory requirements for average bioequivalence and current issues in individual bioequivalence. *Drug Information Journal*, **29**, 1055–1062.

[1194] Steinjans, V.W., Diletti, E. (1997) Individual bioequivalence: A European perspective. *Journal of Biopharmaceutical Statistics*, **7**, 31–34.

[1195] Steinijans, V.W., Neuhauser, M., Bretz, F. (2000) Equivalence concepts in clinical trials. *European Journal of Drug Metabolism and Pharmacokinetics*, **25, No. 1**, 38–40.

[1196] Stephens, P. (2014) Vaccine R&D: Past performance is no guide to the future. *Vaccine*, **32**, 2139–2142.

[1197] Stevens, L., Greene, T., Levey, A. (2006) Surrogate endpoints for clinical trials of kidney disease progression. *Clinical Journal of the American Society of Nephrology*, **1**, 874–884.

[1198] Stokes, M., Davis, C., Koch, G. (2002) *Categorical Data Analysis Using the SAS System*. SAS Institute, Cary, NC.

[1199] Stram, D.O., Lee, J.W. (1994) Variance components testing in the longitudinal mixed effects model. *Biometrics*, **50**, 1171–1177.

[1200] Straus, S., Kors, J., De Bruin, M., van der Hooft, C., Hofman, A., Heeringa, J., Deckers, J., Kingma, J., Sturkenboom, M., Stricker, B., Witteman, J. (2006) Prolonged QTc interval and risk of sudden cardiac death in a population of older adults. *Journal of the American College of Cardiology*, **47**, 362–367.

[1201] Strnodova, C. (2005) The assessment of QT/QTc interval prolongation in clinical trials: A regulatory perspective. *Drug Information Journal*, **39**, 407–433.

[1202] Strom, B.L. (1987) Generic drug substitution revisited. *New England Journal of Medicine*, **316**, 1456–1462.

[1203] Suganami, H. (2004) Points to notice and proposal drug induced QT interval prolongation — Is your correction good enough? *Drug Information Association Meeting*, www.diahome.org

[1204] Suman, J., Laube, B., Dalby, R. (2006) Validity of in vitro tests on aqueous spray pumps as surrogates for nasal disposition, absorption, and biologic response. *Journal of Aerosol Medicine*, **19**, 510–521.

[1205] Swallow, W., Monahan, J. (1984) Monte Carlo comparison of ANOVA, MIVQUE, REML, and ML estimators of variance components. *Technometrics*, **26**, 47–57.

[1206] Sylvester, R., Bartelink, H., Rubens, R. (1994) A reversal of fortune: Practical problems in the monitoring and interpretation of an EORTC breast cancer trial. *Statistics in Medicine*, **13**, 1329–1335.

[1207] Symillides, M., Karalis, V., Macheras, P. (2013) Exploring the relationships between scaled bioequivalence limits and within-subject variability. *Journal of Pharmaceutical Sciences*, **102**, 297–301.

[1208] Taber, D., Baillie, M., Ashcraft, E., Rogers, J., Lin, A., Afzal, F., Baliga, P., Rajagopalan, R., Chavin, K. (2005) Does bioequivalence between modified cyclosporine formulations translate into equal outcomes? *Transplantation*, **80**, 1633–1635.

[1209] Tall, A., Yvan-Charvet, L., Wang, N. (2007) The failure of torcetrapib: Was it the molecule or the mechanism? *Arteriosclerosis Thrombosis and Vascular Biology*, **27**, 257–260.

[1210] Tallarida, R. (2000) *Drug Synergism and Dose-Effect Data Analysis.* Chapman and Hall, CRC Press, London.

[1211] Tamhane, A., Shi, K., Strassburger, K. (2006) Power and sample size determination for a step-wise test procedure for determining the maximum safe dose. *Journal of Statistical Planning and Inference*, **136**, 2163–2181.

[1212] Tan, C., Inglwicz, B. (1999) Measurement-methods comparisons and linear statistical relationship. *Technometrics*, **41**, 192–201.

[1213] Tanaka, A., Kawarabayashi, T., Fukuda, D., Nishibori, Y., Sakamoto, T., Nishida, Y., Shimada, K., Yoshikawa, J. (2004) Circadian variation in plaque rupture in acute myocardial infarction. *The American Journal of Cardiology*, **93**, 1–5.

[1214] Tang, D.-I., Gnecco, C., Geller, N.L. (1989) An approximate likelihood ratio test for a normal mean vector with nonnegative components with application to clinical trials. *Biometrika*, **76, 3**, 577–583.

[1215] Tanida, N. (2002) Ethical considerations for clinical trials in Asia. *Drug Information Journal*, **36**, 41–9.

[1216] Tate, R.F., Klett, G.W. (1952) Optimal confidence intervals for the variance of a normal distribution. *Journal of the American Statistical Association*, 674–682.

[1217] Temple, R. (1982) Government viewpoint of clinical trials. *Drug Information Journal*, **1**, 10–17.

[1218] Temple, R. (1994) Special study designs: Early escape, enrichment, studies in nonresponders. *Communications in Statistical Theory and Methods*, **23**, 499–531.

[1219] Temple, R. (1999a) Are surrogate markers adequate to assess cardiovascular disease drugs? *Journal of the American Medical Association*, **282**, 790–795.

[1220] Temple, R. (1999b) Meta-analysis and epidemiologic studies in drug development and postmarketing surveillance. *Journal of the American Medical Association*, **281**, 841–844.

[1221] Temple, R. (2002) Policy developments in regulatory approval. *Statistics in Medicine*, **21**, 2939–2948.

[1222] Temple, R. (2003) Overview of the concept paper, history of the QT/TdP concern; Regulatory implications of QT prolongation. *Presentations at Drug Information Agency/FDA Workshop*, www.diahome.org

[1223] Temple, R. (2005) Enrichment designs: Efficiency in development of cancer treatments. *Journal of Clinical Oncology*, **23**, 4838–4839.

[1224] Temple, R. (2006a) FDA perspective on trials with interim efficacy evaluations. *Statistics in Medicine*, **25**, 3245–3249.

[1225] Temple, R. (2006b) Hy's law: Predicting serious hepatotoxicity. *Pharmacoepidemiology and Drug Safety*, **15**, 241–243.

[1226] Temple, R. (2007) Quantitative decision analysis: A work in progress. *Clinical Pharmacology and Therapeutics*, **82**, 127–130.

[1227] Teo, K., Ounpuu, S., Hawken, S., Pandey, M., Valentin, V., Hunt, D., Diaz, R., Rashed, W., Freeman, R., Jiang, L., Zhang, X., Yusuf, S. on behalf of the INTERHEART Study Investigators (2006) Tobacco use and risk of myocardial infarction in 52 countries in the INTERHEART study: A case control study. *The Lancet*, **368**, 647–658.

[1228] Teveten NDA, Item 6. (1997) Human Pharmacokinetics and Bioavailability. *Private Files.*

[1229] Thall, P., Simon, R. (1994a) Practical Bayesian guidelines for phase IIb clinical trials. *Biometrics*, **50**, 337–349.

[1230] Thall, P., Simon, R. (1994b) A Bayesian approach to establishing sample size and monitoring criteria for phase II clinical trials. *Controlled Clinical Trials*, **15**, 463–481.

[1231] Thall, P., Wathen, J., Bekele, N., Champlin, R., Baker, L., Benjamin, R. (2003) Heirarchical Bayesian approaches to phase II trials in diseases with multiple subtypes. *Statistics in Medicine*, **22**, 763–780.

[1232] Thall, P., Cook, J. (2004) Dose-finding based on efficacy-toxicity trade-offs. *Biometrics*, **60**, 684–693.

[1233] Thompson, A., Gurtman, A., Patterson, S., Juergens, C., Laudat, F., Emini, E., Gruber, W., Scott, D. (2013) Safety of 13-valent pneumococcal conjugate vaccine in infants and children: Meta-analysis of 13 clinical trials in 9 countries. *Vaccine*, **31**, 5289–5295.

[1234] Thompson, R. (1980) Maximum likelihood estimation of variance components. *Math. Operations forsch. Statist., Ser. Statistics*, **11, No. 4**, 545–561.

[1235] Thompson, S., Pocock, S. (1990) The variability of serum cholesterol measurements: Implications for screening and monitoring. *Journal of Clinical Epidemiology*, **43**, 783–789.

[1236] Thompson, W. (1961) The problem of negative estimates of variance components. *The Annals of Mathematical Statistics*, **33**, 273–289.

[1237] Tilahun, A., Pryseley, A., Alonso, A., Molenberghs, G. (2007) Flexible surrogate marker evaluation from several randomised clinical trials with continuous endpoints, using R and SAS. *Computational Statistics and Data Analysis*, **51**, 4152–4163.

[1238] Ting, N., Burdick, R.K., Graybill, F.A., Jeyaratnam, S., Lu, T.-F.C. (1990) Confidence intervals on linear combinations of variance components that are unrestricted in sign. *Journal of Statistical Computing and Simulation*, **35**, 135–143.

[1239] Ting, N., ed. (2006) *Dose Finding in Drug Development.* Springer, New York.

[1240] Todd, S. (2007) A 25-year review of sequential methodology in clinical studies. *Statistics in Medicine*, **26**, 237–252.

[1241] Tonelli, M., Sacks, F., Pfeffer, M., Jhangri, G., Curhan, G. for the cholesterol and recurrent events (CARE) investigators (2005) Biomarkers of inflammation and progression of chronic kidney disease. *Kidney International*, **68**, 237–245.

[1242] Tong, T., Zhao, H. (2008) Practical guidelines for assessing power and false discovery rate for a fixed sample size in microarray experiments. *Statistics in Medicine*, **27**, 1960–1972.

[1243] Torling, J., Hedlund, J., Konradsen, H., Ortqvist, A. (2003) Revaccination with the 23-valent polysaccharide vaccine in middle-aged and elderly persons previously treated for pneumonia. *Vaccine*, **22**, 96–103.

[1244] Tothfalusi, L., Endrenyi, L. (2001a) Evaluation of some properties of individual bioequivalence (IBE) from replicate-design studies. *International Journal of Clinical Pharmacology and Therapeutics*, **39, No. 4**, 162–166.

[1245] Tothfalusi, L., Endrenyi, L., Midha, K., Rawson, M., Hubbard, J. (2001b) Evaluation of the bioequivalence of highly-variable drugs and drug products. *Pharmaceutical Research*, **18**, 728–733.

[1246] Tothfalusi, L., Endrenyi, L. (2003) Limits for the scaled average bioequivalence of highly variable drugs and drug products. *Pharmaceutical Research*, **20**, 382–389.

[1247] Tothfalusi, L, Speidl, S., Endrenyi, L. (2007) Exposure-response analysis reveals that clinically important toxicity difference can exist between bioequivalent carbamazepine tablets. *British Journal of Clinical Pharmacology*, **65**, 110–122.

[1248] Tothfalusi, L., Endenyi, L., Arieta, A. (2009) Evaluation of bioequivalence for highly variable drugs with scaled average bioequivalence. *Clinical Pharmacokinetics*, **48**, 725–743.

[1249] Tothfalusi, L., Endrenyi, L. (2012) Sample sizes for designing bioequivalence studies for highly variable drugs. *Journal of Pharmacy and Pharmaceutical Sciences*, **15**, 73–84.

[1250] Tozer, T.N., Bois, F.Y., Hauck, W.W., Chen, M.L., Williams, R.L. (1996) Absorption rate versus exposure: Which is more useful for bioequivalence testing? *Pharmaceutical Research*, **13**, 453–456.

[1251] Tozer, T.N., Hauck, W.W. (1997) Cmax/AUC, a commentary. *Pharmaceutical Research*, **14**, 967–968.

[1252] Trottet, L., Owen, H., Holme, P., Heylings, J., Collin, I., Breen, A., Siyad, M., Nandra, R., Davis, A. (2005) Are all aciclovir cream formulations bioequivalent? *International Journal of Pharmaceutics*, **304**, 63–71.

[1253] Trzaskoma, B., Sashegyi, A. (2007) Predictive probability of success and the assessment of futility in large outcome trials. *Journal of Biopharmaceutical Statistics*, **17**, 45–63.

[1254] Tsang, Y.C., Opo, R., Gordon, P., Hems, J., Spino, M. (1996) High variability in drug pharmacokinetics complicates determination of bioequivalence: Experience with Verapamil. *Pharmaceutical Research*, **13**, 846–850.

[1255] Tsiatis, A.A., Mehta, C. (2003) On the inefficiency of the adaptive design for monitoring clinical trials. *Biometrika*, **90, 2**, 367–378.

[1256] Tsong, Y., Zhang, J. (2005) Testing superiority and non-inferiority hypotheses in active controlled clinical trials. *Biometrical Journal*, 47, 1, 62–74.

[1257] Tsong, Y., Zhang, J., Zhong, J. (2009) Commentary on 'New confidence bounds for QT studies' by Boos et al. (2007) *Statistics in Medicine*. 26:3801-3817. *Statistics in Medicine*, **28**, 2936–2940.

[1258] Tsong, Y. (2013a) On the designs of thorough QT/QTc clinical trials. *Journal of Biopharmaceutical Statistics*, **21(3)**, 43–56.

[1259] Tsong, Y., Sun, A., Kang, S. (2013b) Sample size of thorough QTc clinical trial adjusted for multiple comparisons. *Journal of Biopharmaceutical Statistics*, **21(3)**, 57–72.

[1260] Tsou, H., Hung, H., Chen, Y., Huang, W., Chang, W., Hsiao, C. (2012) Establishing consistency across all regions in a multi-regional clinical trial. *Pharmaceutical Statistics*, **11**, 295–299.

[1261] Tsui, K.-W., Weerahandi, S. (1989) Generalized p-values in significance testing of hypotheses in the presence of nuisance parameters. *Journal of the American Statistical Association*, **84, No. 46**, 602–607.

[1262] Tu, X., Zhang, J., Kowalski, J., Shults, J., Feng, C., Sun, W., Tang, W. (2007) Power analyses for longitudinal study designs with missing data. *Statistics in Medicine*, **26**, 2958–2981.

[1263] Tudor, G., Koch, G. (1994) Review of nonparametric methods for the analysis of crossover studies. *Statistical Methods in Medical Research*, **3**, 345–381.

[1264] Tukey, J.W., Ciminera, J.L., Heyse, J.F. (1985) Testing the statistical certainty of a response to increasing doses of a drug. *Biometrics*, **41**, 295–301.

[1265] Uyama, Y., Shibata, T., Nagai, N., Hanaoka, H., Toyoshima, S., Mori, K. (2005) Successful bridging strategy based on ICH E5 guideline for drugs approved in Japan. *Clinical Pharmacology & Therapeutics*, **78(2)**, 102–113.

[1266] Vach, W., Christensen, R. (2006) Making efficient use of patients in designing Phase III trails investigating simultaneously a set of targeted therapies with different targets, with correspondence (Thompson, S.; Hasenclever, D.) and rejoinder. *Biometrical Journal*, **6**, 897–915.

[1267] Van Mieghem, C., Bruining, N., Schaar, J., McFadden, E., Mollet, N., Cademartiri, F., Mastik, F., Ligthart, J., Granillo, G., Valgimigli, M., Sianos, G., van der Giessen, W., Backx, B., Morel, M., Van Es, G., Sawyer, J., Kaplow, J., Zalewski, A., van der Steen, A., de Feyter, P., Serruys, P. (2005) Rationale and methods of the integrated biomaker and imaging (IBIS) study: Combining invasive and non-invasive imaging with biomarkers to detect subclinical atherosclerosis and assess coronary lesion biology. *The International Journal of Cardiovascular Imaging*, **21**, 425–441.

[1268] Van Peer, A. (2009) Variability and impact on design of bioequivalence studies. *Basic and Clinical Pharmacology and Therapeutics*, **106**, 146–153.

[1269] Van Velzen, E., Westerhuis, J., Van Duynhoven, J., Van Dorsten, F., Hoefsloot, H., Jacobs, D., Smit, S., Draijer, R., Kroner, C., Smilde, A. (2008) Multilevel data analysis of a cross-over designed human nutritional intervention study. *Journal of Proteome Research*, **7**, 4483–4491.

[1270] Verbon, F., Heuvel, E., Vermaat, C. (2005) The cluster design for the postmarketing stability surveillance program. *Drug Information Journal*, **39**, 361–371.

[1271] Vonesh, E.F., Chinchilli, V.M. (1997) *Linear and Nonlinear Models for the Analysis of Repeated Measurements.* Marcel Dekker, New York.

[1272] Vuorinen, J., Tuominen, J. (1994) Fieller's confidence intervals for the ratio of two means in the assessment of average bioequivalence from crossover data. *Statistics in Medicine*, **13**, 2531–2545.

[1273] Vuorinen, J., Turunen, J. (1996) A three step procedure for assessing bioequivalence in the general mixed linear framework. *Statistics in Medicine*, **15**, 2635–2655.

[1274] Vuorinen, J. (1997a) A practical approach for the assessment of bioequivalence under selected higher order cross-over designs. *Statistics in Medicine*, **16**, 2229–2243.

[1275] Vuorinen, J., Turunen, J. (1997b) A simple three-step procedure for parametric and nonparametric assessment of bioequivalence. *Drug Information Journal*, **31**, 167–180.

[1276] Wadhwa, M., Thorpe, R. (2007) Unwanted immunogenicity: Implications for follow-on biologicals. *Drug Information Journal*, **41**, 1–10.

[1277] Wagner, J.G. (1976) An overview of the analysis and interpretation of bioavailability studies in man. *Arzneim.-Forsch.(Drug Res.)*, **26**, 105–108.

[1278] Waite, D., Jaconson, E., Ennis, F., Edelman, R., White, B., Kammer, R., Anderson, C., Kensil, C. (2001) Three double-blind, randomized trials evaluating the safety and tolerance of different formulations of the saponin adjuvant QS-21. *Vaccine*, **19**, 3957–3967.

[1279] Wakana, A., Yoshimura, I., Hamada, C. (2007) A method for therapeutic dose selection in a Phase II clinical trial using contrast statistics. *Statistics in Medicine*, **26**, 498–511.

[1280] Wakefield, J.C., Smith, A.F.-M., Racine-Poon, A., Gelfand, A.E. (1994) Bayesian analysis of linear and non-linear population models by using the Gibbs sampler. *Applied Statistics*, **43**, 201–221.

[1281] Wakefield, J. (1996) The Bayesian analysis of population pharmacokinetic models. *Journal of the American Statistical Association*, **91, No. 433**, 62–75.

[1282] Wallentin, L., Wilcox, R., Weaver, W., Emanualsson, H., Goodvin, A., Nystrom, P., Bylock, A., for the ESTEEM Investigators (2003) Oral ximelagatran for secondary prophylaxis after myocardial infarction: The ESTEEM randomised controlled trial. *The Lancet*, **362**, 789–797.

[1283] Walpole, R.E., Myers, R.H., Myers, S.L. (1998) *Probability and Statistics for Engineers and Scientists, 6th ed.* Prentice Hall College Division.

[1284] Walsh, T.N., Noonan, N., Hollywood, D., Kelly, A., Keeling, N., Hennessy, T.P.J. (1996) A comparison of multimodal therapy and surgery for esophageal adenocarcinoma. *New England Journal of Medicine*, 335, No. 7, 462–467.

[1285] Wang, C.M. (1990a) On the lower bound of confidence coefficients for a confidence interval on variance components. *Biometrics*, **46**, 187–192.

[1286] Wang, C.M. (1990b) On ranges of confidence coefficients for confidence intervals on variance components. *Communications in Statistics, Simulation*, **19(4)**, 1165–1178.

[1287] Wang, H., Chow, S.-C. (2002a) On statistical power for average bioequivalence testing under replicated crossover designs. *Journal of Biopharmaceutical Statistics*, **12, No. 3**, 295–309.

[1288] Wang, H., Chow, S.-C. (2002b) A practical approach for comparing means of two groups without equal variance assumptions. *Statistics in Medicine*, **21**, 3137–3151.

[1289] Wang, M., Fitzmaurice, G. (2006) A simple imputation method for longitudinal studies with non-ignorable non-responders. *Biometrical Journal*, **2**, 302–318.

[1290] Wang, J. (2007) EM algorithms for non-linear mixed effects models. *Computational Statistics and Data Analysis*, **51**, 3244–3256.

[1291] Wang, S.-J., Hung, H.M. (1997) Use of two-stage test statistic in the two-period crossover trials. *Biometrics*, **53**, 1081–1091.

[1292] Wang, S.-J., Hung, H., O'Neill, R. (2006) Adapting the sample size planning of a phase III trial based on phase II data. *Pharmaceutical Statistics*, **5**, 85–97.

[1293] Wang, W. (1997a) Optimal unbiased tests for equivalence in intrasubject variability. *Journal of the American Statistical Association*, **88**, 939–946.

[1294] Wang, W., Hsuan, F., Chow, S.-C. (1997b) An adjusted two one-sided t-test for the assessment of bioequivalence with multiple doses. *Journal of Biopharmaceutical Statistics*, **7(1)**, 157–170.

[1295] Wang, W. (1999a) On testing for individual bioequivalence. *Journal of the American Statistical Association*, **94**, 880–887.

[1296] Wang, W. (1999b) On equivalence of two variances of a bivariate normal vector. *Journal of Statistical Planning and Inference*, **81**, 279–292.

[1297] Wang, W., Hwang, J.T.G. (2001) A nearly unbiased test for individual bioequivalence problems using probability criteria. *Journal of Statistical Planning and Inference*, **99**, 41–58.

[1298] Wang, Y. (1999) Use of jacknife influence profiles in bioequivalence evaluations. *Pharmaceutical Science and Technology Today*, **2**, 152–159.

[1299] Wassmer, G. (1994) Testing equivalence clinical trials using a new principle for constructing statistical tests. *Communications in Statistical Theory and Methodology*, **23(5)**, 1413–1427.

[1300] Watkins, P., Kaplowitz, N., Slattery, J., Colonese, C., Colucci, S., Stewart, P., Harris, S. (2006) Aminotransferase elevations in healthy adults receiving 4 grams of acetominophen daily: A randomized controlled trial. *Journal of the American Medical Association*, **296**, 87–93.

[1301] WAVE: Warfarin antiplatelet vascular evaluation investigators (2007) Oral anticoagulant and antiplatelet therapy and peripheral artery disease. *New England Journal of Medicine*, **357**, 217–227.

[1302] Waxman, H. (2009) Developing a legislative pathway for biosimilars in the United States. *Journal of Generic Medicines*, **6**, 295–302.

[1303] Weber, K.T. (2001) Aldosterone in congestive heart failure. *New England Journal of Medicine*, **345, No. 23**, 1689–1697.

[1304] Weerahandi, S. (1993) Generalized confidence intervals. *Journal of the American Statistical Association*, **88, No. 423**, 899–905.

[1305] Wei, L., Lachin, J. (1988) Properties of urn randomization in clinical trials. *Controlled Clinical Trials*, **9**, 345–364.

[1306] Weir, C., Walley, R. (2006) Statistical evaluation of biomarkers as surrogate endpoints: A literature review. *Statistics in Medicine*, **25**, 183–203.

[1307] Weise, K., Hubel, K., Rose, E., Schlager, M., Schrammel, D., Taschner, M., Michel, R. (2006) Bayesian decision threshold, detection limit and confidence limits in ionising radiation measurement. *Radiation Protection Dosimetry*, **121**, 52–63.

[1308] Weitz, J. (2006) Emerging anticoagulants for the treatment of venous thromboembolism. *Thrombosis and Haeomstasis*, **96**, 274–284.

[1309] Welch, B.L. (1956) On linear combinations of several variances. *Journal of the American Statistical Association*, 132–148.

[1310] Welham, S., Cullis, B., Gogel, B., Gilmour, A., Thompson, R. (2004) Prediction in linear mixed models. *Australian and New Zealand Journal of Statistics*, **46(3)**, 325–347.

[1311] Wellek, S. (1993) Basing the analysis of comparative bioavailability trials on an individualized statistical definition of equivalence. *Biometrical Journal*, **35**, 47–55.

[1312] Wellek, S. (1997) A comment on so called individual criteria of bioequivalence. *Journal of Biopharmaceutical Statistics*, **7**, 17–21.

[1313] Wellek, S. (2000) On a reasonable disaggregate criterion of population bioequivalence admitting of resampling-free testing procedures. *Statistics in Medicine*, 19, 2755–2767.

[1314] Wellek, S. (2003) *Testing Statistical Hypotheses of Equivalence*. Chapman and Hall, London.

[1315] Welty, T.E., Pickering, P.R., Hale, B.C., Arazi, R. (1992) Loss of seizure control associated with generic substitution of carbamazepine. *Annals of Pharmacotherapy*, 26, 775–777.

[1316] Westfall, P., Young, S. (1993) *Resampling-Based Multiple Testing*. John Wiley and Sons, New York.

[1317] Westfall, P. (1997) Multiple testing of general contrasts using logical constraints and correlations. *Journal of the American Statistical Association*, **92**, 299–306.

[1318] Westfall, P., Tobias, R., Rom, D., Wolfinger, R., Hochberg, Y. (1999) *Multiple Comparisons and Multiple Tests Using SAS*. SAS Institute, Cary, NC.

[1319] Westfall, P., Tsai, K., Ogenstad, S., Tomoiaga, A., Moseley, S., Lu, Y. (2008) Clinical trials simulation: A statistical approach. *Journal of Biopharmaceutical Statistics*, **18**, 611–630.

[1320] Westfall, P. (2011) On using the bootstrap for multiple comparisons. *Journal of Biopharmaceutical Statistics*, **21**, 1187–1205.

[1321] Westlake, W.J. (1972) Use of confidence intervals in analysis of comparative bioavailability trials. *Journal of Pharmaceutical Sciences*, **61**, 1340–1341.

[1322] Westlake, W.J. (1976) Symmetrical confidence intervals for bioequivalence trials. *Biometrics*, **32**, 741–744.

[1323] Westlake, W.J. (1979) Statistical aspects of comparative bioavilability trials. *Biometrics*, **35**, 273–280.

[1324] Westlake, W.J. (1986) Bioavailability and bioequivalence of pharmaceutical formulations. In *Biopharmaceutical Statistics for Drug Development*, Peace, K., ed., 329–352. Marcel Dekker, New York.

[1325] Wetherill, G., Glazebrook, K. (1986) *Sequential Methods in Statistics*. Chapman and Hall, New York.

[1326] Whitehead, A. (2002) *Meta-Analysis of Controlled Clinical Trials*. Wiley, England.

[1327] Whitehead, J. (1996) Sequential designs for equivalence studies. *Statistics in Medicine*, **15**, 2703–2715.

[1328] Whitehead, J. (1997) *The Design and Analysis of Sequential Clinical Trials*. Wiley, England.

[1329] Whitehead, J., Zhou, Y., Patterson, S., Webber, D., Francis, S. (2001a) Easy-to-implement Bayesian methods for dose-escalation studies in healthy volunteers. *Biostatistics*, **2**, **1**, 47–61.

[1330] Whitehead, J., Zhou, Y., Stallard, N., Todd, S., Whitehead, A. (2001b) Learning from previous responses in phase 1 dose escalation studies. *British Journal of Clinical Pharmacology*, **52**, 1–7.

[1331] Whitehead, J., Zhou, Y., Stevens, J., Blakey, G., Price, J., Leadbetter, J. (2006a) Bayesian decision procedures for dose-escalation based on evidence of undesirable events and therapeutic benefit. *Statistics in Medicine*, **25**, 37–53.

[1332] Whitehead, J., Zhou, Y., Mander, A., Ritchie, S., Sabin, A., Wright, A. (2006b) An evaluation of Bayesian designs for dose-escalation studies in healthy volunteers. *Statistics in Medicine*, **25**, 433–445.

[1333] M.R.Whitehead, M.R., A., Sooriyarachchi, Whitehead, J., Bolland, K. (2008) Incorporating intermediate binary responses into interim analysis of clinical trials: A comparison of four methods. *Statistics in Medicine*, **27**, 1646–1666.

[1334] Whitehead, J., Valdés-Márquez, E., Johnson, P., Graham, G. (2008) Bayesian sample size for exploratory clinical trials incorporating historical data. *Statistics in Medicine*, **27**, 2307–2327.

[1335] Wiens, B., Inglewicz, B. (1999) On testing equivalence of three populations. *Journal of Biopharmaceutical Statistics*, **9**, 465–483.

[1336] Wiens, B., Dmitrienko, A. (2005) The fallback procedure for evaluating a single family of hypotheses. *Journal of Biopharmaceutical Statistics*, **15**, 929–942.

[1337] Wiens, B. (2006) Randomisation as a basis for inference in non-inferiority trials. *Pharmaceutical Statistics*, **5**, 265–271.

[1338] Wierda, W.G., Kips, T.J., Keating, M.J. (2005) Novel immune-based treatment strategies for chronic lymphocytic leukemia. *Journal of Clinical Oncology*, **22, No. 26**, 6325–6332.

[1339] Willavize, S., Morgenthein, E. (2005) Comparison of models for average bioequivalence in replicate designs. *Proceedings of the American Statistical Association.*

[1340] Willavize, S., Morgenthein, E. (2006) Comparison of models for average bioequivalence in replicate designs. *Pharmaceutical Statistics*, **5**, 201–211.

[1341] Williams, R.L., Adams, W., Chen, M.-L., Hare, D., Hussain, A., Lesko, L., Patnaik, R., Shah, V., and FDA Biopharmaceutics Coordinating Committee (2000a) Where are we now and where do we go next in terms of the scientific basis for regulation on bioavailability and bioequivalence? *European Journal of Drug Metabolism and Pharmacokinetics*, **25**, 7–12.

[1342] Williams, R.L., Patnaik, R.N., Chen, M.-L. (2000b) The basis for individual bioequivalence. *European Journal of Drug Metabolism and Pharmacokinetics*, **25**, 13–17.

[1343] Williams, R.L., Chen, M.-L., Hauch, W.W. (2002a) Equivalence approaches. *Clinical Pharmacology & Therapeutics*, **72, No. 3**, 229–237.

[1344] Williams, R.L., Adams, P., Poochikian, G., Hauck, W.W. (2002b) Content uniformity and dose uniformity: Current approaches, statistical analyses, and presentation of an alternative approach with special reference to oral inhalation and nasal drug products. *Pharmaceutical Research*, **19, No. 4**, 359–366.

[1345] WINBUGS User Manual (2000) Available at www.mrc-bsu.cam.ac.uk/bugs.

[1346] Winterstein, A. (2011) Rosiglitazone and the risk of adverse cardiovascular outcomes. *Clinical Pharmacology and Therapeutics*, **89**, 776–778.

[1347] Wittes, J. (2002) On changing a long-term clinical trial midstream. *Statistics in Medicine*, **27**, 2789–2795.

[1348] Wittes, J., Lachenbruch, P. (2006) Opening the adaptive toolbox. *Biometrical Journal*, **48**, 598–603.

[1349] Wiviott, S., Antman, E., Winters, K., Weerakkody, G., Murphy, S., Behounek, B., Carney, R., Lazzam, C., McKay, R., McCabe, C., Braunwald, E., for the JUMBO-TIMI 26 Investigators (2005) Ramdomised comparison of prasugrel (CS-747, LY640315) a novel thienopyridine P2Y12 antagonist, with clopidogrel in percutaneous coronary intervention. *Circulation*, **111**, 3366–3373.

[1350] Wolfinger, R. (1993) Covariance structure selection in general mixed models. *Communications in Statistical Simulation*, **22(4)**, 1079–1106.

[1351] Wolfinger, R., Tobias, R., Sall, J. (1994) Computing Gaussian likelihoods and their derivatives for general linear mixed models. *Siam Journal on Scientific Computing*, **15**, 1294–1310.

[1352] Wolfinger, R.D. (1998) Heterogeneous variance-covariance structures for repeated measures. *Journal of Agricultural, Biological and Environmental Statistics*, **1, No. 2**, 205–230.

[1353] Wolfinger, R.D., Kass, R.E. (2000) Nonconjugate Bayesian analysis of variance component models. *Biometrics*, **56**, 768–774.

[1354] Wonnemann, M., Fromke, C., Koch, A. (2014) Inflation of the type 1 error: Investigations on regulatory recommendations for bioequivalence of highly variable drugs. *Pharmaceutical Research*, Published online: 18JUL2014.

[1355] Woodcock, J. (2012a) Evidence vs. access: Can twenty-first-century drug regulation refine the tradeoffs? *Clinical Pharmacology and Therapeutics*, **91**, 376–380.

[1356] Woodcock, J., Khan, M., Yu, L. (2012b) Withdrawal of generic budeprion for non-bioequivalence. *New England Journal of Medicine*, **367**, 2463–2465.

[1357] Woosley, R., Cossman, J. (2007) Drug development and the FDA's critical path initiative. *Clinical Pharmacology and Therapeutics*, **81**, 129–133.

[1358] World Health Organization, Expert Committee on Biological Standardization. (2009) Recommendations to assure the quality, safety, and efficacy of pneumococcal conjugate vaccines. *Adopted in Geneva, October 2009*, 1–57.

[1359] Wysowski, D., Corken, A., Gallo-Torres, H., Talarico, L., Rodriguez, E. (2001) Postmarketing reports of QT prolongation and ventricular arrhythmia in association with Cisapride and FDA regulatory actions. *American Journal of Gastroenterology*, **96**, 1698–1703.

[1360] Xiang, A., Sather, H., Azen, S. (1994) Power considerations for testing an interaction in a $2{\times}k$ factorial design with a failure time outcome. *Controlled Clinical Trials*, **15**, 489–502.

[1361] Xiao, W., Barron, A.M., Liu, J.-P. (1997) Robustness of bioequivalence procedures under box-cox alternatives. *Journal of Biopharmaceutical Statistics*, **7(1)**, 135–155.

[1362] Xu, H., Hsu, J. (2007) Applying the generalised partitioning principle to control the generalised familywise error rate. *Biometrical Journal*, **49**, 52–67.

[1363] Xu, J., Audet, C., DiLiberti, C., Hauck, W., Montague, T., Parr, A., Potvin, D., Schuirmann, D. (2016) Optimal adaptive sequential designs for cross-over bioequivalence studies. *Pharmaceutical Statistics*, **15**, 15–27.

[1364] Yacobi, A., Masson, E., Moros, D., Ganes, D., Lapointe, C., Abolfathi, Z., LeBel, M., Golander, Y., Doepner, D., Blumberg, T., Cohen, Y., Levitt, B. (2000a) Who needs individual bioequivalence studies for narrow therapeutic index drugs? A case for warfarin. *Journal of Clinical Pharmacology*, **40**, 826–835.

[1365] Yacobi, A. (2000b) Pharmacokinetic evaluation of controlled release dosage forms. *European Journal of Drug Metabolism and Pharmacokinetics*, **1**, 70.

[1366] Yahav, D., Paul, M., Fraser, A., Sarid, N., Leibovici, L. (2007) Efficacy and safety of cefepime: A systematic review and meta-analysis. *The Lancet Infectious Diseases*, **7**, 338–348.

[1367] Yamaoka, K., Nakagawa, T., Uno, T. (1978) Statistical moments in pharmacokinetics. *Journal of Pharmacokinetics and Biopharmaceutics*, **6**, 547–558.

[1368] Yan, Z., Hosmane, B., Locke, C. (2013) Cross-over versus parallel designs: Dose-escalation design comparisons for first-in-human studies. *Journal of Biopharmaceutical Statistics*, **23**, 804–817.

[1369] Yang, P., Fleming, T. (2006) Simultaneous use of weighted log-rank and standardized Kaplan-Meier statistics. *Journal of Biopharmaceutical Statistics*, **16**, 241–252.

[1370] Yao, Y.-C., Iyer, H. (1999) On an inequality for the normal distribution arising in bioequivalence studies. *Journal of Applied Probability*, **36**, 279–286.

[1371] Yan, L., Zhang, J., Ng, M., Dang, Q. (2010) Statistical characteristics of moxifloxacin-induced QTc effect. *Journal of Biopharmaceutical Statistics*, **20**, 497–507.

[1372] Yasuhara, H. (1994) Which is more important in pharmacokinetics: inter-ethnic variability or intra-ethnic variability? In *Proceedings of the Second International Conference on Harmonisation, 1993*, D'Arcy, P.F., Harron, D., eds.

[1373] Ye, H., Pan, J. (2006) Modelling of covariance structures in generalised estimating equations for longitudinal data. *Biometrika*, **93**, 927–941.

[1374] Ye, Y., Yao, B. (2012) Demonstrating biosimilarity via equivalence in clinical trials. *Statistics in Biopharmaceutical Research*, **4**, 264–272.

[1375] Yee, K.F. (1986) The calculation of probabilities in rejecting bioequivalence. *Biometrics*, **42**, 961–965.

[1376] Yeh, K.C., Kwan, K.C. (1978) A comparison of numerical integrating algorithms of trapezoidal, Legrange, and spline approximation. *Journal of Pharmacokinetics and Biopharmaceutics*, **6**, 79–81.

[1377] Yin, G., Li, Y., Ji, Y. (2006) Bayesian dose-finding in phase I/II clinical trials using toxicity and efficacy odds ratios. *Biometrics*, **62**, 777–787.

[1378] Yong, W., Lin-Xian, L., Zi-Can, W., Yue-He, W. (2001) Evaluate multiple adverse events in crossover design bioequivalence clinical trials. *Acta Pharmacologica Sinica*, **22(2)**, 187–192.

[1379] Yuh, L., Beal, S., Davidian, M., Harrison, F., Hester, A., Kowalski, K., Vonesh, E., Wolfinger, R. (1994) Population pharmacokinetic-pharmacodynamic methodology and applications: A bibliography. *Biometrics*, **50**, 566–575.

[1380] Yun, T., Dazhi, M., Hong, W. (2000) Mathematical model of extrinsic blood coagulation cascade dynamic system. *Tsinghua Science and Technology*, **15**, 360–364.

[1381] Yusuf, S., Hawken, S., Ounpuu, S., Dans, T., Avezum, A., Lanas, F., McQueen, M., Budaj, A., Pais, P., Varigos, J., Lisheng, L. on behalf of the INTERHEART Investigators (2004) Effect of potentially modifiable risk factors associated with myocardial infaction in 52 countries (the INTERHEART study): A case control study. *The Lancet*, **364**, 937–952.

[1382] Zabell, S. (2008) On Student's 1908 article "The probable error of a mean." *Journal of the American Statistical Association*, **103**, 1–20.

[1383] Zaccaro, D., Aertker, L. (2011) Use of zero-inflated mixture models to compare antibody titers in response to H1N1 vaccination. *Biopharmaceutical Report*, Fall, 17–26.

[1384] Zajicek, A., Giacoia, G. (2007) Obstetric clinical pharmacology: Coming of age. *Clinical Pharmacology and Therapeutics*, **81**, 481–482.

[1385] Zariffa, N., Patterson, S.D., Boyle, D., Hyneck, H. (1998) Case studies, comparison of the current and proposed bioequivalence criteria. *FDA/AAPS Workshop on Bioavailability and Bioequivalence.*

[1386] Zariffa, N., Patterson, S.D. (1999) A case review on the topic of subject by formulation interaction. *AAPS International Workshop on Individual Bioequivalence: Realities and Implementation.*

[1387] Zariffa, N., Patterson, S.D. (2000) Learnings and recommendations for population and individual bioequivalence based on the analysis of replicate study designs. *AAPS/FDA Workshop on Biopharmaceutics in the New Millennium: Regulatory Approaches to Bioavailability and Bioequivalence.*

[1388] Zariffa, N., Patterson, S.D., Boyle, D., Hyneck, H. (2000) Case studies, practical issues, and observations on population and individual bioequivalence. *Statistics in Medicine*, **19**, 2811–2820.

[1389] Zariffa, N., Patterson, S.D. (2001) Population and individual bioequivalence: Lessons from real data and simulation studies. *Journal of Clinical Pharmacology*, **41**, 811–822.

[1390] Zha, J., Endrenyi, L. (1997) Variation of the peak concentration following single and repeated drug administrations in investigations of bioavailability and bioequivalence. *Journal of Biopharmaceutical Statistics*, **7(1)**, 191–204.

[1391] Zhang, J. (2008) Testing for positive control activity in a thorough QTc study. *Journal of Biopharmaceutical Statistics*, **18(3)**, 517–528.

[1392] Zhang, L., Smith, B. (2007) Sex differences in QT interval variation and implications for sample size of thorough QT study. *Drug Information Journal*, **41**, 619–627.

[1393] Zhang, X., Zheng, N., Lionberger, R., Yu, L. (2013) Innovative approaches for demonstration of bioequivalence: The US FDA perspective. *Therapeutic Delivery*, **4**, 725–740.

[1394] Zhang, Z. (2006) Non-inferiority testing with a variable margin. *Biometrical Journal*, **48**, 948–965.

[1395] Zhao, P., Rowland, M., Huang, S. (2012) Best practice in the use of physiologically based pharmacokinetic modelling and simulation to address clinical pharmacology regulatory questions. *Clinical Pharmacology and Therapeutics*, **92**, 17–20.

[1396] Zhen, B. (2007) Consideration of operational α level with different approval strategies. *Drug Information Journal*, **41**, 23–29.

[1397] Zhou, Y., Whitehead, J., Bonvini, E., Stevens, J. (2006) Bayesian decision procedures for binary and continuous bivariate dose-escalation studies. *Pharmaceutical Statistics*, **5**, 125–133.

[1398] Zhou, Y., Whitehead, J., Korhonen, P., Mustonen, M. (2008) Implementation of a Bayesian design in a dose-escalation study of an experimental agent in healthy volunteers. *Biometrics*, **64**, 299–308.

[1399] Zia, M., Siu, L., Pond, G., Chen, E. (2005) Comparison of outcomes of phase II studies and subsequent randomised control studies using identical chemotherapeutic regimens. *Journal of Clinical Oncology*, **23**, 6982–6991.

[1400] Zimmerman, D.W. (1993) A note on the F test for equal variances under violation of random sampling. *The Journal of General Psychology*, **12(1)**, 77–83.

[1401] Zink, R. (2013) Detecting safety signals among adverse events in clinical trials. *American Statisical Association Webcast of October 2013.*

Index

2 × 2 Design, 17, 35, 36, 119, 129, 131, 192, 230, 236, 268, 286
p-value, 23, 210

Absolute bioavailability, 287
Absorption, 22, 25, 56, 230, 232, 286, 292, 293
Adaptive planning, 153
Adequacy of model fit, 137, 226, 266, 274, 275, 277, 280, 281, 283
Adjuvant, 311
ADME, 7, 130, 230, 232, 286, 296
Adverse events, 209
  Probability of, 210
  Serious, 209
Age, 10, 247, 284, 287–289, 298, 299
Allometric scaling, 211
Alpha-adjustment, 86
Antibody, 309
Area under the curve (AUC), 22
Area under the curve (AUC), 7, 19, 20, 23–25, 28, 29, 39, 41, 120, 128, 207, 211, 221, 279
Assumptions, 5, 26, 45, 53, 57, 58, 61, 71, 72, 118, 122, 131–133, 135–140, 206, 209, 215, 242, 253, 258, 259, 268, 291, 293

Baseline, 227, 247, 248, 252, 254, 264, 266–268
Bayesian statistics, 138, 242, 258, 270, 271, 283
  Prior distribution, 139, 242, 270
Binomial data, 24, 217, 218
Bioequivalence, 4, 11, 12, 14–17, 206
  75-75 Rule, 23
  80-20 Rule, 23
  Adverse events, 135
  Australia, 28
  Average, 25, 31
  Bayesian, 138
  Canada, 28, 30
  Carry-over, 124
  China, 28
  Distribution theory, 19
  Dose-exposure-response assessment, 119
  Endpoints, 19
  Europe, 28
  Failure to demonstrate, 117
  Generic substitution, 17
  Group-sequential design, 131
  Individual, 26, 190
  Issues with Cmax, 22
  Japan, 28
  Key assumption, 133
  More than two formulations, 79
  Multiple AUCs, 29
  No-effect claims, 298
  Nonparametrics, 56
  Outliers, 137
  Partial replicate design, 64
  Population, 26, 190
  power and sample size, 46
  Replicate design, 64, 129
  Restricted maximum likelihood, 115
  Scaled average, 190–192
  Special guidance, 26
  Standard design, 17, 129
  TOST, 28
  Two one-sided tests, 24
Bioinequivalence, 117
Biomarker, 9, 10, 206, 237, 260, 261, 263
Biopharmaceutical classification system, 28
Blinding, 12, 13, 18, 20, 209, 211, 217, 219, 248
Blocking, 12, 13, 18, 20, 209
Blood sampling limits, 130
Bonferroni, 87
Bootstrap, 88, 95, 96, 122, 124, 193, 214, 219, 222, 283

Carry-over, 18, 25, 34, 36, 38, 42, 44, 64–66, 73, 79, 83, 97–99, 127, 128, 254, 259, 337
Choice of weights, 164

Clearance, 221, 223, 224, 226, 281, 283, 284, 287, 288, 291, 293, 296, 299
    Creatinine, 299, 301, 302
    Renal, 234
Clinical outcomes, 260
Clinical pharmacology, 4, 6, 7, 10, 11, 13, 121, 122, 132, 133, 136, 207, 208, 256, 258, 260, 285, 286, 299
Coefficient of variation, 190
Conditional error, 151
Conditional power, 152
Confidence interval, 24–26, 35, 37, 39, 41, 57, 59, 72, 88, 118, 140, 219, 222, 237, 269, 280, 289
Confounding, 13, 22, 23, 119, 133, 137, 207, 212, 234, 238, 254, 258, 268, 289, 293
Convex hull plots, 38
Correlation, 27, 37, 39, 66, 99, 116, 227, 248, 250, 252, 253, 297
Critical values for maximum combination test, 148
Critical values for standard combination test, 144
Cross-over design, 4, 17, 18, 23–25, 28, 31, 33, 133, 207, 211, 220, 230, 258, 286, 287
Cytotoxic drugs, 207, 211, 215

Degrees of freedom (d.f.), 37, 47, 72, 73, 115, 134, 135, 192
Design
    Balaam, 332
    cross-over, 4
Distribution
    t, 47, 57, 72, 73, 192
    Chi-square, 91, 132, 135
    Log-normal, 19, 20, 25, 57, 58, 211, 224, 227, 265
    Normal, 19, 20, 22, 24, 27, 30, 39, 45, 46, 53, 57, 58, 61, 62, 65, 72, 224, 242
    Pharmacokinetic, 7, 230
Divergence, 193
Dose
    Escalation, 211
    Proportionality, 238, 239
    Supra-therapeutic, 248
    Therapeutic, 248
Dose-response, 4, 6, 7, 9, 16, 120, 121, 207, 215, 217, 218, 228, 229, 258, 260, 264, 267, 273, 277, 281, 292, 296
    Maximum-effective, 10
    Maximum-tolerated, 10, 210
    Minimum-effective, 10
    Pharmacokinetic-pharmacodynamic models, 271
Drop-outs, 31, 135
Drug development, 4

Efficacy, 6, 9, 13, 119–121, 206, 256, 258
Efficiency, 65, 83, 97
Electrocardiogram
    QT interval, 246
    QTc interval, 247
    RR interval, 247
Elimination, 7, 18, 29, 30, 64, 230, 293, 295, 296, 299
Error
    Type 1, 12, 13, 24, 25, 57, 117, 124, 131, 250, 251, 316
    Type 2, 12, 13, 25, 57, 250, 251, 316
Ethnicity, 229, 284, 291, 293, 295, 299
Example of maximum combination test, 149
Example of standard combination test, 145

Fixed effect model, 195
Formulation, 11, 12, 16, 17
Frequentist statistics, 138
Futility, 159, 160
Futility rule, 159

Gender, 10, 247, 284, 287, 289, 291, 293, 299
Generic, 17, 22, 26
Gibbs sampling, 139

Half-life, 8
Highly variable drugs, 26, 190
Histogram, 58, 60, 96
Hodges–Lehmann estimate, 59, 72, 73, 75, 78
Hypothesis test, 24, 47, 236, 270

Independence, 27, 36, 61, 65, 72, 132, 133, 224
Interaction
    Drug, 4, 230, 232, 233
    Drug-disease, 292
    Statistical, 42, 116, 117, 137, 138, 222, 227, 261, 263, 273
Intersection-union testing, 86, 251–253, 321

Kidney disease, 11, 298

Likelihood, 27, 114, 296, 299
Liver disease, 295, 298
Liver enzyme systems, 232
Liver function testing, 130, 220, 227
Logistic regression, 217
Lot consistency, 319

Mann–Whitney tests, 57
Maximum combination test, 142, 148
Maximum concentration (Cmax), 7, 18–20, 22, 28
Median, 60, 61, 72, 92, 95, 96, 136, 139, 140, 243, 270, 284
Metabolism, 64, 230, 232, 286, 292, 296, 299
  Inducing, 233, 236
  Inhibiting, 233, 234
Missing data, 49, 67, 68, 115, 135, 215
Model, 8, 10, 12, 14, 18, 20, 24, 34, 65, 120, 208, 209, 219, 258, 259, 264, 271, 279
  Assumptions, 45
  Emax, 276
  Fixed-effects, 35
  General linear, 25
  Interpretation, 277
  Logistic, 218
  Mixed, 29
  Nonlinear mixed effect, 223
  One-compartment, 223
  Power, 212, 222
  QTc, 248
  Random-effects, 36
  Repeated-measures, 248
  Restricted maximum likelihood, 114
  Validation, 124
Multiple comparisons, 86
Multivariate statistics, 263, 264

Narrow therapeutic index, 190
Narrow therapeutic index drugs, 26
No adverse effect level, 207, 211, 214, 215, 219, 221, 222, 226, 243, 283, 285, 286, 288, 289, 291, 296, 298
Non-compartmental Analysis, 7
Normal probability (Q-Q) plots, 45

Oncology, 10, 207, 211, 247
Operating characteristics, 157

Paired-agreement plots, 33
Parallel design, 28
Parallel group design, 133, 211, 238, 254, 259, 289
Period effects, 23, 25, 33–35, 43, 88, 98, 121, 212, 234, 238, 254, 336
Pharmacodynamics, 4, 9, 10, 20, 117, 125, 209, 211, 219, 258–260, 266, 271, 292, 299
Pharmacokinetics, 7, 10, 19, 28, 117, 124, 125, 128, 206, 208–212, 214, 219–221, 230, 233, 259, 279, 281, 284, 291, 293
  Population, 279, 280, 285, 292
Phase I, 4, 10, 16, 132, 209, 210, 219, 223, 258, 260, 261, 263, 266–268, 280–282, 289, 296, 311
Phase II, 10, 16, 254, 258, 267, 268, 277, 282
Phase III, 10, 17, 26, 267
Placebo, 10, 206, 207, 210, 211, 217, 219–221, 223, 248, 249, 251–255, 259, 261, 264, 266–270, 274–276
Pooling variability estimates, 132
Positive (active) control, 252
Positive control, 253, 255
Power, 47, 157, 159
PowerTOST, 47, 143
Precision, 13, 27, 50, 121, 130, 135, 236, 237, 251, 259, 286–288
Proof-of-concept, 258, 259, 268
Protein binding, 232, 292, 299
Protocol, 137, 208, 209, 211, 292, 298

R code, 48, 167
Radio-label bioavailability studies, 287
Randomization, 12, 14, 18, 20, 25, 61, 209
Regression, 242, 284, 291
Relative bioavailability, 287
Replication, 12, 13, 18, 20, 29, 79, 95, 97, 98, 116, 122, 130, 209
Residual, 36, 39, 45, 46, 53, 114, 135, 137, 224, 226, 261, 266, 274, 276, 277

Safety, 4–6, 9, 10, 13, 120, 130, 206, 247
Sample size, 47, 159, 163
Sample size re-estimation, 142, 146, 152
Simulation, 22, 23, 34, 120–122, 211, 223, 226, 282, 283
Smallpox, 308
Standard combination test, 142, 144, 147
Standard deviation, 19, 20, 26, 129, 136, 140

Standard error, 39, 46
Standard significance, 255
Steady state, 220, 233, 234, 268, 299
Surrogate marker, 6, 9, 10, 19, 28, 29, 230, 260, 264, 267, 268
Switchability, 26

Time of maximum concentration (Tmax), 8
Torsades de pointes, 247, 249, 255
Two-stage design, 142

Unbiased estimator, 65, 249
Union-intersection testing, 87, 253

Variance, 20, 25, 26, 36, 46, 64, 65, 68, 71, 72, 88, 97, 114, 116, 134, 190, 225, 249, 266, 289, 335

Weighted normal inverse combination of p-values, 142
Wilcoxon tests, 57, 61, 62, 88, 91, 92, 95
Williams design, 79, 83, 238

XOEFFICIENCY, 98